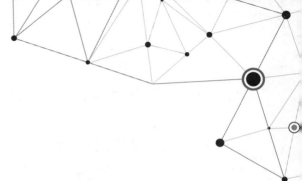

如何撰写
医学英文科研论文
How to Write
Medical Research Papers
in English

名誉主编　Jørgen Frøkiær
Honorary Editor-in-Chief　Jørgen Frøkiær
Aarhus University, Denmark

主　　审　王成增
Reviewer　Chengzeng Wang
The First Affiliated Hospital of Zhengzhou University, China

主　　编　文建国
Editor-in-Chief　Jianguo Wen
The First Affiliated Hospital of Zhengzhou University, China

副 主 编　王庆伟
Associate Editor-in-Chief　Qingwei Wang
The First Affiliated Hospital of Zhengzhou University, China

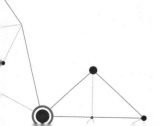

人民卫生出版社
·北 京·

版权所有，侵权必究！

图书在版编目（CIP）数据

如何撰写医学英文科研论文 / 文建国主编 . —北京：
人民卫生出版社，2024.6（2024.8重印）
ISBN 978-7-117-29154-5

Ⅰ. ①如… Ⅱ. ①文… Ⅲ. ①医学 – 英语 – 论文 – 写
作 Ⅳ. ①R

中国版本图书馆 CIP 数据核字（2019）第 237101 号

| 人卫智网 | www.ipmph.com | 医学教育、学术、考试、健康，购书智慧智能综合服务平台 |
| 人卫官网 | www.pmph.com | 人卫官方资讯发布平台 |

如何撰写医学英文科研论文
Ruhe Zhuanxie Yixue Yingwen Keyan Lunwen

主　　编：文建国
出版发行：人民卫生出版社（中继线 010-59780011）
地　　址：北京市朝阳区潘家园南里 19 号
邮　　编：100021
E - mail：pmph @ pmph.com
购书热线：010-59787592　010-59787584　010-65264830
印　　刷：天津市银博印刷集团有限公司
经　　销：新华书店
开　　本：787×1092　1/16　　印张：28
字　　数：699 千字
版　　次：2024 年 6 月第 1 版
印　　次：2024 年 8 月第 2 次印刷
标准书号：ISBN 978-7-117-29154-5
定　　价：139.00 元

打击盗版举报电话：010-59787491　E-mail：WQ @ pmph.com
质量问题联系电话：010-59787234　E-mail：zhiliang @ pmph.com
数字融合服务电话：4001118166　E-mail：zengzhi @ pmph.com

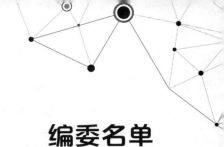

编委名单

编写秘书 何翔飞 崔林刚

编 委（按姓氏笔画排序）

马 源 王 焱 王亚仑 王庆伟 王志敏 王贵宪 王俊魁 毛淑萍 文一博 文建国
任川川 刘二鹏 芦 山 李天方 李云龙 李真珍 杨 静 杨 黎 何翔飞 冶 卓
宋 悦 张 艳 张国贤 张晓雪 陈 燕 胡金华 胡绘杰 贾 炜 贾亮花 黄书满
崔林刚 谢佳丰 薛 瑞

名誉编委（Honorary Editors）

按姓名首字母排序（Ordered by Name Initials）

Alan D. L. Sihoe, FRCSEd, FCCP. Chairman, Hong Kong Thoracic Surgery. Honorary Consultant in Cardio-Thoracic Surgery, Gleneagles Hong Kong Hospital, China.

Hans Stødkilde-Jørgensen, MD, PhD, Professor, Dr MedSc, The MR Research Centre, Aarhus University Hospital, Denmark.

Jens Chr. Djurhuus, MD, DMSc, Professor, Aarhus University/Aarhus University Hospital, Chairman of International Children's Continence Society, Chairman of the Institute of Experimental Clinical Research, Denmark.

Jørgen Frøkiær, MD, PhD, Professor, Aarhus University, Aarhus University Hospital, Denmark.

John Heesakkers, MD, PhD, Department of Urology, Maastricht University Medical Centre, Maastricht, Netherlands.

Jennifer D. Y. Sihoe, FRCSEd(Paed), FCSHK, FHKAM(Surg), Director, Hong Kong Paediatric Surgery and Paediatric Urology Centre; Honorary Clinical Assistant Professor, Department of Surgery, The Chinese University of Hong Kong, China.

Jianying Zhang, MD, PhD, Professor (Tenured), Director, Cancer Autoimmunity & Epidemiology Research Laboratory, Department of Biological Sciences & NIH-Sponsored Border Biomedical Research Center (BBRC), The University of Texas, El Paso, Texas, USA.

Jerzy B Gajewski, MD, FRCSC1, Professor of Urology, Dalhousie University, Halifax, Canada.

Jacques Corcos, MD, FRCS(S), Professor, Head of Department of Urology in Jewish Hospital of McGill University, Canada.

Stephen Shei-Dei Yang, MD, PhD, EMBA, Professor of Urology, School of Medicine, Buddhist Tzu Chi University, Hualien, Taiwan; Chief, Department of Surgery, Buddhist Tzu Chi General Hospital, New Taipei, Taiwan, China.

Tian-Fang Li, MD, PhD, Assistant Professor, Department of Biochemistry and Orthopaedics, Rush University Medical Center, Chicago, USA; Professor, First Affiliated Hospital of Zhengzhou University, China.

Wayne W. Zhang, MD, FACS, Division of Vascular and Endovascular Surgery, Louisiana State University Health Shreveport, Shreveport, Los Angeles, USA.

Wei Cheng, FRCS, FACS, MBBS, University of New South Wales, Australia; PhD, University of Toronto, Canada.

Yrjö T. Konttinen, MD, PhD, Professor of Medicine, Chief Physician, Institute of Clinical Medicine, Department of Medicine; Head of Research, ORTON Orthopaedic Hospital of the Invalid Foundation, Helsinki; Head of Research, COXA Hospital for Joint Replacement, Tampere, Finland.

Zhenhe Suo, MD, PhD, Professor, Department of Pathology, The Norwegian Radium Hospital, Oslo University Hospital, University of Oslo, Norway.

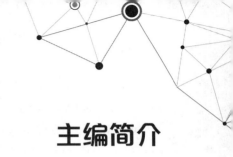

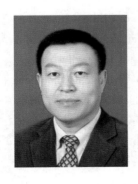

　　文建国,中国和丹麦双医学博士、郑州大学第一附属医院泌尿外科小儿尿动力中心教授/主任医师、硕士和博士研究生导师。现任河南省高等学校临床医学重点学科开放实验室和河南小儿尿动力国际联合实验室主任及丹麦奥胡斯(Aarhus)大学医学院荣誉教授(honor professor)。曾经获得"国务院政府特殊津贴专家"、"卫生部有突出贡献中青年专家"、"新世纪百千万人才工程"国家级人选、"河南省优秀留学回国人员成就奖"和"中原名医"等荣誉。

　　先后在荷兰林堡大学泌尿外科(Urology,University Hospital Maastricht of Limberg University)、鹿特丹大学儿童医院(Department of Pediatric Urology and Urological Oncology,Sophia Children's Hospital of Erasmus University Rotterdam)、丹麦奥胡斯大学(Department of Clinical Medicine,Aarhus University)、美国哈佛大学医学院小儿泌尿外科(Department of Pediatric Urology of Harvard University)、加拿大麦吉大学犹太人总医院(Jewish General Hospital of McGill University)和香港中文大学外科学系(Department of Surgery of Chinese University Hongkong)学习或工作。曾师从前国际尿控主席Corcos教授和国际小儿尿控主席Bauer教授进行神经泌尿外科和小儿尿动力学专业进修和学习。主要学术兼职有中国医师学会小儿外科分会副会长、中华医学会小儿外科专业委员会常务委员、小儿尿动力和盆底学组组长、《中华小儿外科杂志》副主编、《临床小儿外科杂志》副主编、国际尿控协会(ICS)儿童与青少年委员会委员、ICS尿动力委员会委员、ICS小儿泌尿学校校长、国际儿童尿控协会(ICS)理事、亚太小儿泌尿外科协会(APAPU)科学委员会副主席、ICS官方杂志 Continence 联合主编、美国泌尿外科杂志(J Urol)、欧洲泌尿外科杂志(Eur Urol)、美国儿科杂志(Pediatrics)、英国公共卫生杂志(BMC Public Health Journal)等10多种SCI杂志特约审稿人。承担完成了国家自然科学基金、卫生部和河南省等多项科研项目。获得省部级科技进步奖二等奖8项。拥有发明专利和实用新型专利12项。主编及参编教材和书籍30余部。先后在国内外学术期刊和国际学术会议发表论文800余篇,其中200余篇被SCI收录,单篇最高影响因子168。连续多年为郑州大学研究生开设英文科研论文写作课程,取得了良好的效果。

　　Qualified and awarded MD and PhD from Henan Medical University and Tongji Medical University China in 1984 and 1990, respectively, Second PhD awarded from Medical Faculty of Aarhus University Denmark in 2000. Professor Wen has been working for Urology/Pediatric Urology since 1984, and been the International Continence Society (ICS) member in 2007, ICS Children and Young Adult's Committee member in 2012 and ICS urodynamic committee member in 2013, ICCS Board Member in 2022, honor professor of Pediatric Urology of Aarhus University Hospital of Denmark since 2014. He is now the executive committee member of Chines Pediatric Surgery Association and Vice-Chairman of Chinese National Pediatric Urology Group, Vice Editor in Chief of Chinese Journal of Pediatric Surgery and Co-Editor of Continence (Official Journal of ICS) as well as invited reviewer of more than 10 international English Journals.

As a research fellow, he trained in Dept. of Pediatric Urology in Boston Children's Hospital of Harvard University in 2004. He got the first ICS Neurourology Fellowship and trained in Department of Urology, Jewish General Hospital of McGill University in 2009. From 1996–2000 as a postdoctoral research fellow, PhD candidate and surgical training in Institute of Clinical Research, Department of Urology of Skejby University Hospital and MR Research Center, Aarhus University, Denmark. From 1995–1996 as a postdoctoral training and research fellow in Dept. of Urology, University Hospital Maastricht and in Dept. of Pediatric Urology and Div. of Urological Oncology, Sophia Children's Hospital of Erasmus University Rotterdam, The Netherlands. More than 30 times as an invited speaker and organizer of international conferences and education courses, and more than 800 scientific research papers published either in Chinese and English (internationally). He became a professor of First Affiliated Hospital of Zhengzhou University, China, since 2001.

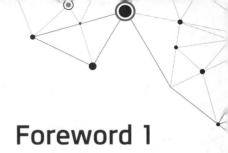

Foreword 1

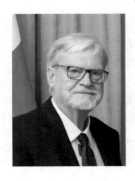

It is a great honor for me that professor Jianguo Wen has asked me to participate in prefacing in this book on how to write and publish medical research papers in English. Being a Dane, and thereby non-native as to an Anglo-Saxon heritage, I know most of the difficulties embedded in formulating and conveying medical research in a succinct mode so that the audience can get the full picture efficiently.

My own first articles were in Scandinavian Journals. Apart from a very rigid distinction between Material and Methods and Results and Discussion a formulation was allowed to reflect that our origin was non-Anglo-Saxon. However, when the first paper was sent to an American journal, the requirements became more strict, and the work in formulating more time and effort demanding.

Now with 351 articles listed in PubMed, a dissertation for the Doctor of Medical Science in 1980, having been chairman of Denmark's largest institute for 26 years, having had 26 DMSc and more than 75 PhD students as main supervisor, I still find it challenging to formulate medical science in English.

I have had the fortune of some so-called "lucky situations". One is that I was forced to use pigs as animal model, when everybody else used other animal models, for elucidating the activity of the upper urinary tract. The other "lucky situation" was when we by coincidence found nighttime polyuria in bedwetting, a finding which has revolutionized treatment of bedwetting all over the world, and also the foundation of the International Children's Continence Society which I founded together with two other colleagues.

The third "lucky situation" was when I received my first Chinese PhD student, Professor Jian Guo Wen, in 1996. I realized that he was something special, definitely with his own ideas, and during his stay, in which he acquired the PhD degree from Aarhus University, he developed some animal models which have been used in many studies, including PhD studies, in the time passed and at present.

The fruit of this cooperation has been an ongoing exchange of young researchers, scientific work and publications. As we are non-Anglo-Saxons, Danes as well as Chinese, albeit that we as Danes have some advantages in having a language which is closer to English than the Chinese have, we have been on equal terms facing the same challenges.

This book is trying comprehensively to give the researchers, especially the young ones, hints as to how a scientific paper should be formulated, how the rules are and where the pitfalls might be.

The first part of the chapters focuses on the basic knowledge of how to write research papers including the title, the authorship and address, the abstract and keywords, the introduction and aims, materials and methods, results, discussion and acknowledgements, the references, tables and illustrations, etc. In addition, this part also introduces how to write conference abstracts and exhibitions, book reviews, dissertations, and finally introduces how to do English paper submissions and reviews, and pay attention to some special English grammar notes, sentence patterns and various special English expressions etc.

The second part of chapters, written by invited well-known foreign and domestic experts, aimed to tell the readers how the postgraduates are cultivated to write English research papers in domestic and foreign famous university. In addition, some famous reviewers would also use some actual examples to introduce peer review experience, so that the readers will understand the review process clearly.

I firmly believe that this book is very useful to help medical students and medical workers to improve the ability of English scientific paper writing, and make their papers easier to be accepted and published, and to make the published papers understood and accepted by readers more easily.

Prof. JC Djurhuus, MD, DMSc
Aarhus University, Denmark

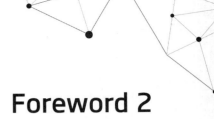

Foreword 2

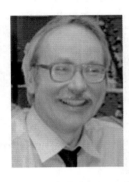

I was invited by Professor Wen to say a few words of this important book providing practical and theoretical guidance for young and senior scientists how to write scientific text. This is one of the main tasks of senior scientists, to help the new oncoming generation forward to successful careers in biomedical research.

I have been in scientific research field over 40 years. I love doing scientific research work and it is a bit like a hobby for me to work in lab, doing research work and instructing young researchers. I have 700-800 articles published at present, Hirsch Index 61 and 19 464 citations. I supervised 45 PhD thesis works and hosted post-doctors from 32 countries. In the year of 1994, I received my first Chinese PhD student, Tian-Fang Li, a hardworking young man, and he is now Associate Professor in Rush University, Chicago, USA. After that, I received two other young Chinese men as PhD students. And recently, Yan Chen, a young Chinese female PhD student, came to my lab for 2 years' joint PhD training. I also have a lot of Chinese researcher friends. Altogether I found that the Chinese researchers are really hard-working, but have naturally often somewhat poor English communication skills if they have not had any opportunity to work abroad; I understand this fully because English was for me first the fourth language. So I would like to uncover my experience in scientific research and English writing to guide young Chinese researches on the road, up and forward.

The aim of scientific research is to first generate good and important research questions and testable hypothesis and then to solve them and make the results available for the other members of the scientific community by publishing the research results. The medical scientific paper is still the most important form of report available for the transmission and dissemination of medical information, via which the scientific researchers and medical workers display their research achievements and clinical experience. A medical scientific paper should be an advanced, scientific and often also practical article, built on rules of logic, science theory and modern scientific knowledge. These also help to design the research plan, accomplish the experiments and make the clinical observations or field investigations to obtain the data files, which are analyzed by professional statistical methods to advance the knowledge and to produce new research questions and hypotheses. Scientific papers written in medical English are official and peer reviewed records of medical scientific research work, the prime results of the process and methods used by the mankind to struggle against disease and for progress. English is mainly used so that the development and medical literature could be followed by as wide audience as possible. Medical literature forms the most important worldwide platform and tool for communication in science and summarizes to advance of the medical knowledge and technology.

This book of "How to publish English Medical Scientific Papers" was produced in part as an international effort to help medical students and medical doctors and professionals to improve their ability of scientific writing in English, and make it easier to get the papers accepted and published, and to make the published papers easier understandable to and acceptable by their scientific and professional readers. This book will clearly and accurately clarify how to write and publish English medical research papers. The first part of the book focuses in separate chapters on how to write research papers, from the title, info on the authors and their addresses, the abstract and keywords, the introduction, hypothesis/research questions and aims, materials and methods, results, discussion and acknowledgements, to references, tables and illustrations. In addition, this part also introduces how to write conference abstracts and posters, book reviews, dissertations, and finally introduces submission process of international English papers and reviews, also paying attention to some special English grammar notes, sentence structures and various special expressions in English etc. The next chapters, written by invited well-known foreign and domestic experts, aimed to describe to the readers how the postgraduates are taught and guided to write English research papers in famous domestic and foreign universities. In addition, some experienced peer reviewers provide some actual examples and introduction to the peer review experience, so that the readers will understand the review process clearly.

This book has a strong group of editors. In addition to the many domestic experts, we have also invited well-known Professors from Denmark, Finland, United States, Australia, Norway, the Netherlands, Hong Kong, Taiwan and other countries and regions who are all actively engaged in research and clinical medicine. Readers will not only learn from the book technical and practical Medical English writing skills, but will also gain insight into medical science writing and an analysis of the process by internationally known experts. This book is a comprehensive, profound and solid source of universally applicable practical, theoretical and analytical information, guidance and advice for all medical personnel writing or reading and interpreting medical scientific papers. It will benefit students, scientific research beginners, junior and senior medical researcher, and even medical journal editors and peer reviewers.

I believe this book will play an important role in education of how research is translated to scientific medical papers published in international mostly English journals, and how to critically interpret papers published in such journals.

Yrjö T. Konttinen, MD, PhD, Professor of Medicine
University of Helsinki, Helsinki, FINLAND

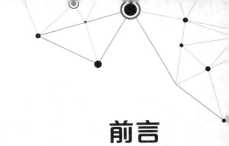

前言

　　医学科研论文是把医学科研成果公布于众的一种重要形式,也是取得科研成果的重要标志。医学英文科研论文写作是以英文记录医学科研工作,进行医学工作总结、交流和提高医疗技术水平的重要工具。文章只有发表出来,才能提高研究的价值和意义,尤其是发表在国际杂志的研究,具有更强的影响力和公信力,能更有力地促进相关专业发展。

　　除了学术方面的原因之外,国内的大环境也要求我们提高自己的英文论文写作能力,以应对不断提高的社会需求。国内外不少高校都将发表 SCI 文章作为研究生毕业的标准,使得发表英文论文成了研究生学业的一个奋斗目标。走上工作岗位之后,晋升职称、申报基金、申请成果等更加需要英文论文作为基础和支撑,这一现实极大地调动了大家学习英文论文写作的积极性。

　　要在国际杂志上发表文章,除了本身的研究内容之外,还需要很好的英文基础。目前,中国已经成为世界科研论文发表数量最多的国家。但是,由于庞大的人口基数,中国的人均科研能力还是比较落后,仍然有不少的好研究没能写成英文发表出来,没有得到国际的认可。在这种情况下,选择一本关于指导英文论文写作的好书便显得尤为重要了。

　　目前,关于指导写作医学英文论文的书籍,市场上有不少版本。但是综合评估之后发现,他们大多数集中在写作原则和规则的介绍方面,缺乏详细的实例指导。为了弥补这一缺憾,本书结合主编多年来的带教和写作经验,收集各方面的资料并邀请国内外的专家共同参与本书的编写工作。在初稿出来之后,又经过在郑州大学研究生"如何撰写英文科研论文"课程试用,充分凝聚了学生的要求之后,经过反复修改,历时 10 年,终于完成了本书的终稿。

　　本书旨在帮助医学生,尤其是研究生和广大医务工作者提高英文科研论文写作能力,使他们的论文更快被接收和发表。本书详细介绍了医学科研论文写作与发表所涉及的各方面内容。第一部分主要讲解如何撰写科研论文的基础知识,包括标题、作者和单位地址、摘要、关键词、前言和目的、材料和方法、结果、讨论和致谢、参考文献、表格和插图等,并详细介绍了综述写作、会议交流和壁展、书评、学位论文,最后介绍了英文论文如何投稿和审稿,以及英文语法注意事项、常用句型及各种数字英文表达方式等。第二部分是邀请国际知名专家介绍英文科研论文撰写的国际经验,包括国外著名大学如何培养研究生科研写作等。第三部分重点介绍了中英文计量单位及论文写作应注意的问题,供大家参考。

　　本书编委主要来自郑州大学第一附属医院和广州医科大学附属妇女儿童医疗中心有论文发表经验的硕士和博士,以及丹麦、芬兰、美国、澳大利亚、挪威、荷兰等国家和地区从事医学科研与临床研究的知名教授。读者不但能从书中学习到医学英文论文各部分的写作技巧,还能收获来自国际专家所贡献的写作经验及解析。以上特点使得本书的内容全面,深入浅出,普适性强,为读者提供全方位科研英文论文写作指导,无论是科研为零起点的在校学生,还是已经工作多年的医务工作者均能起到很好的借鉴和学习作用。

　　本书的缺点也在所难免,由于编者水平有限,在撰写过程中可能会出现许多不当之处,请广大读者给予批评指正。本书编撰历时十年,很多同事和研究生参与了不同阶段的内容修改和校稿,在此对他们的支持表示衷心感谢。由于篇幅有限,本书原计划的临床各专业医学英文撰写实例详解无法纳入,将来对这部分内容进一步修改完善后再另行出版。最后,对郑州大学第一附属医院和新乡医学院第一附属医院的支持表示诚挚的感谢!

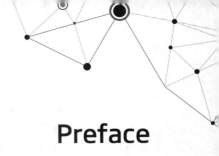

Preface

The aim of scientific research is to solve scientific problems and publish the research results. The medical scientific paper is an important form of reports for the transmission of medical information, by which the scientific researchers and medical workers exhibit their research achievements and clinical experience. The medical scientific paper should be a certainly advanced, scientific and practical article, based on pharmaceutical science theory and modern scientific knowledge to design the research protocol, accomplish the experiments and clinical observations or field investigations to obtain the first hand data, which are analyzed by professional statistic methods and a series of proceeding work. The medical English scientific papers is to record medical scientific research work, the process and methods of human struggling against disease, the development process of medical literature by English, which is also an important tool for the medical work communication and summary to improve the medical technology. Research needs to be written in the article and published in the international journal, so as to cause more concerns from people, and promote the progress of the related field.

In addition to the academic reasons, the domestic environment also requires us to improve our writing skills, in order to respond to the increasing needs of society. In recent years, with the continuous expansion of college enrollment, the number of undergraduate and graduate students is also increasing. Nowadays, more and more colleges regard SCI article as the graduate standards. Thus, publishing papers has become the ultimate goal for almost all the students. Moreover, publish an article is still important after you got a job, because it is closely related to title promotion, funds application, as well as awards application. The reality also makes us put a high value on article writing.

If you want to publish an article in international journals, in addition to the research itself, you also need to be good at English. In recent years, with the implementation of China's reform and opening-up policy, the English level among Chinese people has been greatly improved. At present, China has become one of the countries which have the largest number of scientific papers in the world. However, due to the huge population base, the status of China's scientific research is still not optimistic. There are still many good studies could not be written out and published in English. In this case, it is important to choose a good book for guiding English writing.

Currently, there are many versions of books that guiding on how to write medical papers in English, however, most of them only focused on the principles and rules of writing, lacking of detailed examples. To compensate for this shortcoming, we invited domestic and foreign experts to participate in planning and preparation of this book. After the first draft came out, it was used as a pilot edition for students in Zhengzhou University, in order to obtain relevant suggestions. After repeated modifications during the past ten years, we finally completed the final draft of this book.

This book is to help medical students and medical workers to improve the ability of English scientific paper writing, to make their papers easier to be accepted and published, and to make the published papers understood and accepted by readers more easily. This book will clearly and accurately clarify how to write and publish English medical research paper. The first part of the chapters focuses on each part of how to write research papers, from the title, the author and address, the abstract and keywords, the introduction and aims, materials and methods, results, discussion and acknowledgements, to references, tables and illustrations. In addition, this part also introduces how to write conference abstracts and exhibitions, book reviews, dissertations, and finally introduces how to do English paper submissions and reviews, and pay attention to some special English grammar notes, sentence patterns and various special English expressions etc.

The next chapters, written by invited famous foreign and domestic experts, intends to tell the readers how the postgraduates are cultivated to write English research papers in domestic and foreign famous university. In addition, some famous reviewers would also use some actual examples to introduce peer review experience, so that the readers will understand the review process clearly.

This book has a strong group of editors. In addition to many domestic experts, well-known professors from Denmark, Finland, the United States, Australia, Norway, the Netherlands and other countries and regions who engaged in research and clinical medicine are also included. Readers will not only learn from the book Medical English writing skills of each part, but also gain the writing and analytical experiences from international experts. In addition, we also have some graduate students as the editor for the book. They offered lots of suggestions on how to improve English writing based on their own experiences. All the above features make this book comprehensive as well as universal for the medical personnel. It will benefit students, scientific research beginners, junior and senior medical researcher, and even medical journal editors and workers.

Due to some limitation, errors and mistakes are unavoidable. Critiques from all readers are highly appreciated. In the course of writing this book, we got a lot of colleagues and friends to help us. We want to express our most sincere thanks to all of you!

目录
Contents

第二部分　国际知名专家介绍如何撰写医学英文科研论文

Part 2　Tips and Experiences of How to Write Medical Research Papers in English From Renowned Experts Internationally

第三部分　附录
Part 3　Appendix

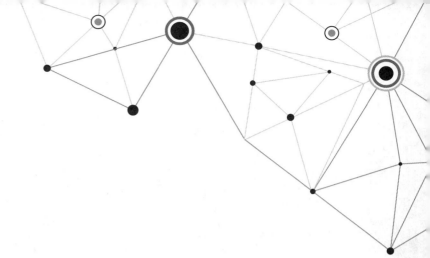

第一部分

医学英文科研论文写作基础知识

Part 1
Basic Knowledge of How to Write Medical Research Papers in English

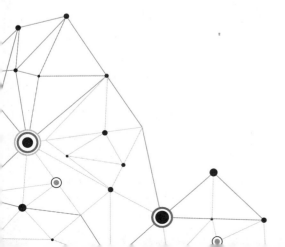

第1章
医学英文科研论文写作概述

Chapter 1
Overview of Medical Scientific Research Papers in English

前　言

科研论文（scientific paper）又称科技论文，是报道自然科学研究和技术开发创新工作成果的文章，是在科研调查、科学实验和科学研究的基础上，对一些自然科学理论或技术开发的研究成果进行分析。一般需要运用总结分析、统计学处理、推理、反驳、证明等科学手段和逻辑思维去完成。医学科研论文（medical scientific research paper）是其中最重要的一部分，是对现代医学科学知识或实验进行总结分析、统计学处理等，最终加工成具有一定科学性、先进性和实用性的文章。通常为医学科研工作者通过科研设计以及临床观察实验和调查来获得材料，再对这些材料分析并按照科研论文的要求撰写出来的文章。是其对所从事的医学基础和临床科研领域取得的经验和成果进行总结报道的一种重要形式，是人们传递医学信息的一个途径，也是作者取得科研成果的一种形式和重要标志。

英语是世界上使用最广泛的语言之一。由于上两个世纪英国和美国在文化、经济、军事、政治和科学上的领先地位，使其成为一种最重要的国际语言。因此，想要医学研究的成果得到世界各国相关领域人员的认可，必须采用英语作为媒介。作为医学科研论文写作范畴的一个重要组成部分，医学英文科研论文是以英文记录医学科研工作、人类同疾病作斗争和记录医学发展进步过程的文献，是医学科研和临床观察的书面总结，是进行医学交流和提高医疗技术水平的重要工具。正如 John Fowles（英国作家，1926—2005）指出的那样："For what good science tries to eliminate, good art seeks to provoke — mystery, which is lethal to the one, and vital to the other."。

医学科研论文承载着医学科学技术的成果，同时也对人类文明和现代科学技术的发展进步发挥着重要的作用。科学研究的最终目的是解决科学难题，把研究结果公布于众，这主要通过发表论文来实现。只有发表高质量医学研究论文的科研工作者才能逐渐成名。正如 RA Day 指出的那样："The goal of scientific research is publication. Scientists, starting as graduate students, are measured primarily not by their dexterity in laboratory manipulations, not by their innate knowledge of either broad or narrow scientific subjects, and certainly not by their wit or charm; they are measured and become known (or remain unknown) by their publications."。

科研结果只有发表才能得到认可，这已经是不争的事实。因此，科研人员不仅要会做科学研究，更要会写科研论文。否则，科研成果将难以发表或被推迟发表。正如 RA Day 在其书中指出的那样："The scientist must not only 'do' science but must 'write' science. Bad writing can and often does prevent or delay the publication of good science."。

医学英文科研论文的质量高低,直接影响医学科研成果的价值和水平,也是医学科研和临床工作者工作能力的具体反映。目前,医学英文科研论文是医学相关人员业务考核、职称评定、晋升晋级及医学院校学生毕业和取得学位的客观指标和主要依据,是医学临床和科研不可缺少的组成部分。因此,现代医学院校的研究生和其他医务工作者都应该知道如何进行医学英文科研论文写作。

许多医学科研人员未接受过医学英语科研论文写作方面的正规训练,硕士研究生攻读学位期间,常常只能完成简单的英文摘要,编写本书的目的就是帮助医学各学科的研究人员写好医学英文论文。为更好地理解和掌握医学英文科研论文的写作知识,广大医学工作者有必要了解医学英文科研论文的历史,明确医学英文科研论文的结构和写作要求,认识写作医学英文科研论文的重要意义。

第一节　医学英文科研论文历史

司马迁说过:"有国者,不可以不知《春秋》。"美国哥伦比亚大学戴安娜·诺维茨教授说过:"没有历史头脑的民族是健忘的民族,一觉醒来,他们就不知道自己是谁了。"的确,历史是人类过去的再现,重现以往可以"知今"。温故论文的发展历史有利于现代科研类论文的写作。

一、早期历史

人类文明持续了数千年,石洞壁画及石碑是人类遗留给后代的最早记录,也是传播医学知识的载体。在一定程度上,我们庆幸祖先选择这种材质来记录信息,才能留存至今,因为那些记录在容易变质腐烂材质上的信息很容易消失殆尽。

《洪水神话》(*A Chaldean Account of the Flood*)是我们所知道的最早的书籍,早于《圣经》(*Genesis*)约 2 000 年,这个故事记载在公元前 4 000 年的一块泥板上。河南安阳殷墟发现的记录 3 000 年以前中国历史的甲骨文(卜辞)是中国最古老的一种成熟文字。早在商朝,人们就用龟甲和兽骨占卜,然后在上面刻下占卜者的姓名以及占卜的内容和时间,内容包含了社会生活中的诸多方面,成为现代人研究商朝历史的重要参考资料。

显然,我们更需要一种轻型、便捷的材质作为交流载体。大约公元前 2 000 多年出现了第一种成功的交流载体——莎草纸(将纸莎草植物做成纸张,黏合在一起成长卷,系在木制的卷轴上,一般长 6~12 米)。公元前 190 年,羊皮纸(由动物皮制成)开始被使用。根据希腊历史学家的记载,帕加马图书馆在公元前 40 年的藏书就有 200 000 卷(Tuchman,1980)。

公元 105 年,中国的蔡伦发明了造纸术,纸张成为了一种现代交流载体。公元 1100 年,中国出现了活字印刷术(Tuchman,1980)。公元 1455 年,Gutenberg 利用印刷机印刷了 42 行《圣经》,西方世界给予其高度赞扬,Gutenberg 的发明迅速在欧洲传播起来,并有效投入使用。到了公元 1500 年,数百种书籍(古版本)的上千种拷贝本与世人见面。

科技期刊首次出现于 1665 年,当时同时出版了两种不同的期刊,分别是法国的《Scavans杂志》(*Journal des Scavans*)和英国的《伦敦皇家协会哲学会刊》(*Philosophical Transactions of the Royal Society of London*)。从此以后,期刊成为科学界最主要的交流方式。到 1981 年,全世界已经出版了 70 000 种科技期刊(Kingetal,1981)。

医学科研论文交流相对落后,第一本医学英文期刊出版在 300 年以前。随着医学英文论文写作的发展,在过去的 100 年间,逐渐形成了科研论文特殊的写作格式——IMRAD(Introduction, Method, Result And Discussion)格式,即引言、方法、结果和讨论。医学英文科研论文的出现,才使医学知识、科研成果等开始有效、广泛地交流。

二、IMRAD 写作形式的发展历史

早期期刊上发表的论文多为“描述性”论文。典型的写作形式是“首先,发现什么;接着,又发现什么”(First, I saw this, and then I saw that),或者是“首先,做了何种研究;接着,又做了何种研究”(First I did this, and then I did that)。观察结果通常是按照时间先后顺序进行简单的描述。这种描述性的写作形式适用于科研论文的报道。事实上,文学期刊目前仍在采用这种直接的写作形式。

到了 19 世纪后期,科学迅猛发展。尤其是 Louis Pasteur 证实了疾病的细菌学说,并发现了微生物培养方法,这两种发现极大地推动了科学的发展。同时,方法论显得至关重要。为了平息批评言论,Pasteur 发现有必要将实验描述得更细致些,以便有能力的同行能重复其实验。随后,实验重复原则成为基本准则。最终,方法部分从整体中被分离出来进行描述,这也促使了 IMRAD 写作形式的形成。

20 世纪初 Paul Ehrlich 和 20 世纪 30 年代 Gerhard Domagk 都开始效仿 Pasteur 的工作来研究磺胺类药物。第二次世界大战促使了青霉素的研发(1929 年 Alexander Fleming 首次描述)。1944 年链霉素被报道。通过接种疫苗可以使肺结核、败血病、白喉、瘟疫、伤寒、天花及小儿麻痹症(脊髓灰质炎)得到有效预防。

第二次世界大战之后,医学研究实验室大量涌现,科研资金投入增加。金钱成就了科学,同时,科学造就了科研论文的出现。如果无特殊原因,期刊编辑可以在文字修饰及语言组织上进行修改。期刊的空间有限,要求论文不能冗长或累赘。19 世纪后半叶,IMRAD 写作形式发展缓慢,但目前其几乎成为研究型期刊的通用模式。一些编辑支持 IMRAD 写作形式,因为他们认为这种写作形式简单且合乎逻辑,有利于交流。虽然有些编辑不认同这种写作格式,但由于 IMRAD 写作形式确实节省篇幅及费用,同时使论文几个主要部分醒目和更有条理;IMRAD 写作形式大大减轻了编辑和审稿人的工作量,使编辑及审稿人工作变得轻松。现在,几乎所有杂志都要求投稿符合 IMRAD 格式的要求。

按 IMRAD 形式写作的科研论文可以回答如下问题:文章研究的目的是什么? 怎样进行研究? 研究发现了什么? 研究的意义何在? 这些问题分别在引言、方法、结果和讨论中得到回答。正如 RA Day 在其著作中描述的那样:“What question (problem) was studied? The answer is the Introduction. How was the problem studied? The answer is the Methods. What were the findings? The answer is the Result. What do these findings mean? The answer is the Discussion.”。

三、英文科研论文杂志的历史

科学技术不断发展,学术团队也应运而生,团体的成员时常聚集在一起,互相讨论学术问题,展示取得的研究成果,其中的发言会被记录,印刷之后发给有需要的读者。部分科学家通过交谈和通信互相交流。在期刊问世之前,这些方式就是科学家互相交流的主要手段。

17 世纪中叶之后,科技活动的规模不断扩大,在学术通讯和学术会议的基础上产生了一种新的学术工具——期刊,标志着学术思想知识的收集、传播和交流更便捷的新时期到来。

1662 年建立的英国皇家学会是历史最悠久、享有盛誉的学术团队,世界上最早的杂志也是其 1665 年创刊(至今仍继续出版)的《哲学汇刊》和同年法国出版的《学者周刊》(1665—1938)。早期的这些学术团体和刊物大多是综合性的。伴随着现代科技的发展和新知识的不断涌现,科学门类也不断分支化,这些分支学科也产生了自己的学术团体和出版物。1679 年法国出版的《医学新进展》是世界公认的最早的医学期刊。之后各种医学杂志和科研论文相继出现,显著推动了医学科学的进展。正如 Gerard Piel 所说:"Without publication, science is dead."。

科技不断发展的同时也产生了更多的刊物和文献,学科之间互相渗透,想要从本专业的少量期刊中窥探某项研究课题的全貌也越来越难,为了方便研究就出现了提要、摘要、题录等形式的期刊来收集、浓缩和排序原始论文,被称为二次文献,即检索性文献。文摘杂志可以作为检索工具,同时也报道和交流了科学成果,不仅促进了科技情报活动的发展,也被看作科技情报诞生的标志。文摘言简意赅又能包含原文主要信息的特点,深受医务工作者的喜爱,其发展也相对较快。

在 300 多年的医学期刊发展史中,期刊种类越来越多,期刊的内容也从开始的综合性发展为专科以及之后的专题,如今已发展为一个完善的体系。在发展速度方面,医学期刊出现之后的近 200 年间,即 1679—1862 年,世界生物医学期刊仅有 20 种,到 1962 年增长到 6 000 种,而近 30 年迅速增长了 6 倍,几乎每 5 年增长 1 倍,已达到 35 000 种,是所有科技期刊中增长速度最快同时所占比重最大的一类。

说到医学英文期刊,不得不提及 SCI(Science Citation Index,简称 SCI)和 EI(Engineering Index)收录的杂志。SCI 和 EI 是什么? SCI 即《科学引文索引》,是一种世界闻名的综合性科技引文检索刊物,由美国科学情报研究所(Institute Scientific information,简称 ISI, http://www.isinet.com)出版。已经成为包括农业、生物学、物理学、化学、兽医学、生命科学、临床医学、工程学等各种领域的综合性检索刊物,在当今世界三大检索系统中占据首位,尤其能体现自然科学研究的学术水平,其中所占比例最大的是生命科学及医学、化学、物理,主要收录当年世界上的重要期刊,它的引文索引所具有的独特的科学参考价值,奠定了其学术界的重要地位。在很多国家和地区,被 SCI 收录和引证的论文情况已经成为评价学术水平的重要指标之一。SCI 具有严谨的选刊原则和完善的专家评审制度,所以它有一定的客观性,能够比较真实地反映出论文的水平和质量。所以被 SCI 收录和被引证的情况也就成为了衡量学术水平的发展情况的指标之一,每年一次的 SCI 论文排名是目前判断一个学校科研水平的非常重要的指标。

SCI 创刊于 1963 年,最初为年刊,1966 年改为季刊,1979 年改为双月刊。SCI 数据库随时间不断发展,如今已成为世界上最重要的大型数据库,位居国际著名检索系统之首。SCI 的数据来源于《期刊目次》(Current Content),其中自然科学数据库收录了 5 000 多种期刊,生命科学辑收录 1 350 种;工程与计算机技术辑收录 1 030 种;临床医学辑收录 990 种;农业、生物环境科学辑收录 950 种;物理、化学和地球科学辑收录 900 种期刊。

原始文献并不是 SCI 报道的核心内容,其核心内容是原始文献所附的参考文献。通过当前文献对先期文献的引用,来说明先期文献对当前文献的影响力,也能体现文献之间的相关性。其主要组成部分有"来源索引"(Source Index),"引文索引"(Citation Index),"轮排主题索引"(Permuterm Subject Index)等。SCI 通过自身严谨的评估程序和选刊标准,每年依次评价和调整入选的期刊,以此来保证其收录的文献能更充分的反映当今世界上最有影响力、最重要的研究成果。其收录的文献类型有:科技报告、图书、期刊、专利文献和会议录。

《期刊引用报告》(*Journal Citation Reports*,JCR)由 SCI 每年出版。SCI 收录的 4 700 种期刊(包括 3 500 种核心期刊)之间的引用和被引用数据被 JCR 统计、运算,按照每种期刊定义的评价指数如"影响因子"(Impact Factor)等加以报道。期刊的影响因子是指期刊前两年发表过的文献在当年被引用的次数的平均数。刊载文献被引用的次数越多,刊物的影响因子就越高,则该刊物的学术水平就越高,也说明文献报道的研究成果的学术影响力越大。作为论文的作者可以参考各期刊的影响因子排名来决定投稿的目标。

从上述影响因子的评估来看,许多杂志每年的影响因子都在变化之中。这里列一下大家比较关注的几个期刊的影响因子情况:

PloS ONE,JCR2014 是 3.234;2015 是 3.057;2016 是 2.806;2017(2018 年 6 月公布)是 2.766,2022—2023 影响因子 3.7。

Sci Rep,JCR2014 是 5.578;2015 是 5.228;2016 是 4.259;2017 是 4.122,2022—2023 影响因子 4.6。

NEJM、*The Lancet*、*JAMA*、*BMJ* 是公认的历史最为悠久和顶级的综合性临床期刊。2023 年影响因子分别为 158.5、168.9、120.7 和 105.7。《临床医师癌症杂志》(*CA: A Cancer Journal for Clinicians*)是由美国癌症学会主办的一份综述性、履行同行评议的学术期刊,论文内容涉及癌症诊断、治疗和预防。其影响因子 2023 年高达 254.7,冠绝所有期刊。汤姆森公司以原有的 SCI 文摘版源刊为基础加入精选的部分其他杂志产生的网络版就是 SCIE(SCI Expanded)。SCI 和 SCIE 的区别:SCI 是科学引文索引,SCIE 是科学引文索引扩展版(即网络版),收录的主要是自然科学、工程技术领域具有相当影响力的重要期刊,SCI 收录的期刊有 3 600 多种,SCIE 收录了多达 6 000 多种期刊,覆盖了 150 多个领域的学科。

1884 年创刊的 EI 即《工程索引》,由 Elesvier Engineering Information Inc. 编辑,美国工程信息公司出版。以收录工程技术领域的论文为主(多数为科技期刊和会议录论文),内容覆盖了生物工程、化学和工艺工程、农业工程和食品技术、应用物理、控制工程、机械工程、石油、汽车工程、核技术、交通运输、照明和光学技术、计算机和数据处理、电子和通信、土木工程、材料工程、宇航等学科领域。但是纯基础理论方面的论文 EI 是不收录的。

如果说 SCI 是 EI 的核心,那么 SCIE 就是 EI 的非核心。虽然在一些偶然的条件下会出现 SCIE 的影响因子高于 SCI 的情况,但是 SCIE 的影响价值还是低于 SCI 的。ISI 在挑选刊源时有严格的选刊标准和评估程序,每年的数量也略有变化,以此来保证全世界最有影响力最重要的研究成果被其收录的文献所覆盖。只有办的足够好的 SCIE 杂志才能成为 SCI 杂志,而且如果 SCI 杂志办的较差就会变成 SCIE 杂志,甚至被 SCIE 放弃。(SCI、EI 详细介绍见后面相关章节)。

Essential Science Indicators(ESI)是当今普遍用以评价大学和科研机构国际学术水平及影响的重要指标,也是全球公认的判断学科发展水平的重要参照之一,是汤森路透科技与医疗集团的产品;从 2002 年至今,该机构在统计的各学科篇均被引次数桂冠者中,预测到了 16 位诺贝尔奖获得者。

ESI 是一个基于 Web Of Science 核心合集数据库的深度分析型研究工具,通过对一万多种 Web Of Science(SCI/SSCI)收录期刊分析,能提供近十年各学科的科学家、机构、国家和期刊的排名数据。ESI 是基于 SCI 和 SSCI 权威数据建立的分析型数据库,能够为科技政策制定者、科研管理人员、信息分析专家和研究人员提供对 22 个学科研究领域中的国家、机构和期刊的科研绩效统计和科研实力排名。通过 ESI,您可以对科研绩效和发展趋势进行长期的定量分析。

ESI 数据库可以用于:分析机构、国家和期刊的论文产出和影响力,按研究领域对国家、期刊、论文和机构进行排名,发现自然科学和社会科学中的重大发展趋势,确定具体研究领域中的研究成果和影响力,评估潜在的合作机构,对比同行机构,确定某个学科领域中,哪些国家、研究机构的研究成果具有较高的影响力、本研究机构在全球各个学科领域中的排名、有哪些热点论文和高影响力的研究成果分布在全球各个学科领域中、本机构中科研人员发表的论文被引频次是否达到了全球平均水平、各学科领域中的研究前沿有哪些。ESI 数据每 2 个月更新一次。

通过 ESI,您可以对科研绩效和发展趋势进行长期的定量分析。基于期刊论文发表数量和引文数据,ESI 提供对 22 个学科研究领域中的国家、机构和期刊的科研绩效统计和科研实力排名。这些学科包括生物学与生物化学、化学、计算机科学、经济与商业、工程学、地球科学、材料科学、数学、综合交叉学科、物理学、社会科学总论、空间科学、农业科学、临床医学、分子生物学与遗传学、神经系统学与行为学、免疫学、精神病学与心理学、微生物学、环境科学与生态学、植物学与动物学、药理学和毒理学。

四、中国医学科研论文历史

我国医学科研历史源远流长,留下了许多医学科研工作者精心创作的科研论文——医学巨著。

闻名于世的汉代名医“医圣”张仲景,他的主要著作《伤寒杂病论》,记录的就是他的研究成果,对临床医学有着重大的贡献。晋代医学家王叔和所著的《脉经》整理探讨了晋代以前关于中医脉学的研究,内容包括了 24 种脉象并被应用至今。唐朝的王冰专注于研究《内经》,对其进行订正、整理,得出最流行的版本,这些都是了不起的科学研究和成就。唐代的药典《新修本草》,宋代的方典《和剂局方》和本草著作《证类本草》,都是古代学者们兢兢业业的研究成果。温病学说的理论来源于《温病条辨》,是明清时期的医家吴鞠通所著,在当今临床对于各种传染性、感染性疾病的治疗中仍发挥着作用,这一具有深远影响的成果也是由当时的科学研究实践得出的。

我们医学科研的先辈很早就知道进行实验研究。《本草纲目》中就有关于验证病因的动物实验的记载,《本草纲目》记载八世纪陈藏器认为脚气病的病因与食白米有关,说:“小猫、犬食之,亦脚屈不能行;马食之足重。”而且据文献记载对照研究在古代也已经出现,当时为了鉴别党参的真假,让嚼着党参的两个人一起跑步,坚持的更久的那个人嘴里的党参就是真的。这就是我们所说的对照实验。中国历史中还记载了最早的实验诊断方法,在晋唐时期,医生每天用黄疸患者的尿液浸染白布后晾干,通过比较颜色的变化来了解患者黄疸病情的变化。由此可知,古代中医在实验研究方面的很多创造是走在世界前列的。

我国医疗技术水平随时间不断进步发展,医学杂志和刊物也相应地不断涌现。唐大烈在 1792 年创刊的《吴医汇讲》是我国最早的医学杂志,同时也是具有史料和学术双重价值的医学刊物。唐大烈深思熟虑之后,在门口贴了一张亲笔写下的启事:“凡属医门佳话,发先人之未发可以益人学问者,不拘内、外、妇、幼各科,均可辑入;若是人云亦云者,因旧籍已多,则不复赘,凡高论赐光,不分门类,不限卷数,不以年龄先后,也不以先后受限制,以冀日增月益,可成大观……",就像现在的征稿启事一样。启事贴出没多久,稿件就从各地纷纷而来,唐大烈对这些稿件进行精心的编辑处理,不久后《吴医汇讲》第一卷就问世了。1792 年到 1803 年陆续出版了 11 卷《吴医汇讲》,每年出一大卷,当时江南一带由名医撰写的医疗学术文章大都记载其中,不仅涉及的内容广泛,产生的影响更是深刻而久远。

19 世纪中叶,广州、上海两大城市因为受西方资本主义影响较深,已经开始出现早期的西方医药期刊。《西医新报》是中国出现最早的西医药刊物,由美国传教医师主编,广州博医局在 1880 年(清光绪六年)发行出版。《博医学报》创刊于 1887 年,直到 1915 年 11 月改由中华医学会编辑出版并一直延续至今,是《中华医学杂志》中文版及其英文版的前身,也是中国历史最悠久、影响最深远的医学刊物。

1949 年国民政府败退,中华医学会的部分成员随之也迁至台湾,第一任理事长刘瑞恒邀集在台医界人士共同复会,1951 年台湾《中华医学会杂志》(*Journal of the Chinese Medical Association*)复刊,当时因经费等原因,台湾《中华医学会杂志》于 1954 年 3 月才开始发行复刊后第一卷第一期,并将台湾《中华医学会杂志》改为季刊。该杂志自 1997 年 1 月起被 SCIE 收录,是国内仅有的少数进入 SCIE 的期刊。2007 年该杂志正式进入 SCI 期刊门槛,2023 年影响因子 /JCR 分区 :3.0/Q2。

《中华医学杂志英文版》是中国大陆唯一被 SCI 收录的综合性医学期刊,是反映中国临床医学与基础医学发展动态的权威杂志。目前本刊被国内外 20 余个重要生物医学数据库、检索系统和文摘期刊收录,包括科学引文索引(SCI)、化学文摘(CA)、医学索引(IM)/Pubmed、生物医学文摘(BA)、荷兰医学文摘(EM)等国际著名检索系统,是我国唯一进入美国《科学引文索引》的综合性医学杂志。2022 年 CMJ 影响因子 6.1(Q1 区),跻身前 17%。

古人说得很好:"学史使人明智",确实如此,历史好比一艘船,装载着过去的记忆驶往未来。通过对医学英文科研论文历史的了解,我们更易理解和掌握医学科研论文写作,创作出更具影响力的科研作品。

五、电子时代

随着电子计算机技术的不断发展,出版过程较以前变得简单。文字处理器、图形绘制软件、数码影像等为发表论文的各个环节带来了极大的便利:期刊提供在线系统供作者投稿,编辑部和作者通过电子邮件进行沟通,编辑和作者都可以通过在线审阅和修改论文,电子期刊开始出现,作者可以通过网站获取参考文献或论文。但是,出版过程的变化对作者的网络和计算机技术有了更高的要求。虽然出版过程发生了很大变化,但是出版过程的许多要素仍然保持不变。科技论文的 IMRAD 的写作要求和科研论文从投稿到录用的程序等都没有发生变化。正如 RA Day 在其著作中强调的那样:"Whereas much regarding the mechanics of publication has changed, much else has stayed the same. Items that persist include the basic structure of a scientific paper, the basic process by which scientific papers are accepted for publication, the basic ethical norms in scientific publication, and the basic features of good scientific prose. In particular, in many fields of science, the IMRAD structure for scientific papers remains dominant."。

第二节 医学英文科研论文分类和结构

医学英文科研论文历经三个世纪发展,无论其定义还是论文的结构都发生了明显的改变,目前医学英文科研论文必须以一定的方式来撰写,并以特定的形式进行发表。了解医学英文科研论文的定义,方能知道其是什么;知道医学英文科研论文的特征和结构,方能对文章进行构思。对于刚刚接触医学英文科研论文写作的新手来说,很有必要理解医学英文科研论文的定义及其延伸,了解其特征和结构。

一、医学英文科研论文定义

医学英文科研论文是一种对原创性医学研究内容以英文写作和发表的方式进行报道,是医学科研成果的客观记录,是对医学科学研究最终阶段的总结,也是医学科研和临床工作者互相交流学习实践经验和学术观点、总结相关领域科学研究成果的一种手段。

想要对"医学科研论文"的定义有更深刻的理解,我们首先要明确何为医学英文科研论文的有效发表(valid publication)和初次发表(primary publication)。通常情况下,摘要、论文集、会议报道等其他论文形式并不被大家看作是有效地发表。此外,尽管科研论文经过重重审查,以整篇文章发表在杂志上,但是,如果其发表在不适当的期刊上,也不算是有效发表。如果论文被接受发表在合适的杂志(主要期刊或其他主要出版物),即使研究相对不完善,也算得上是有效发表。大多数政府出版物和会议论文,同公告和其他短篇报道一样,均不视为有效发表和作为主要文献。

生物学杂志编委会(Council of Biology Editors,CBE)是一个在生物学方面具有权威性的专业机构,1968 年其对初次发表进行了明确的定义:医学英文科研论文初次发表应是首次提供充分信息的公开发行,使同行专家能够对其实验研究进行观察评估、重复实验过程及结果,并能评估其学术价值;此外,文章可以被一个或多个主要机构定期进行检索。目前,检索机构主要有《生物学文摘》(*Biological Abstracts*)、《化学文摘》(*Chemical Abstracts*)、《医学索引》(*Index Medicus*)、《医学文摘》(*Excerpta Medica*)、《农业文献索引》(*Bibliography of Agriculture*)等。通过了解这个定义,可以帮助我们理解科研论文的真正含义。

一篇公认的医学英文科研论文必须是首次公布发表,呈现出大量的信息以使读者能够对其实验研究进行观察评估、重复实验过程及结果,并能评估其学术价值。读者可以通过论文数据判断结论是否与之相符。而且,科研论文一定要易于感官知觉的接受,公开发表的不只是可视资料(如:印刷期刊、缩微胶卷、单片缩影胶片等),还包括非印刷品及非可视资料,例如:以盒式录音磁带发行的"出版物"有其他不同的定义,但是其仍为有效出版物。当然,新型"电子期刊"符合有效发表的定义,如创办于 1992 年的《最新临床试验联机杂志》(*The Online Journal of Current Clinical Trials*)。

按照 CBE 的要求,可以将初次发表简单、笼统地概述为:①原创性研究结果的首次发表;②同行可以参考研究内容重复实验过程和结果;③在英文科学期刊或其他英文医学杂志上发表。这里所涉及"作者同行"意味着同行可以在正式出版之前对论文进行审核。因此,医学英文科研论文是一种被同行评审后才能够发表的文章。

科研论文是一种以 IMRAD 写作形式描述一定专业研究的特殊文献。如果研究生或科学家(即使他们中有些人已经发表过医学英文科研论文)完全理解其含义,撰写论文就会变得轻松自如。对撰写论文感到困惑源于对医学英文科研论文的定义界定不清。一旦明确医学英文科研论文应该写什么,怎样书写,撰写论文就会变得很容易。

二、医学英文科研论文的类型和体裁

(一)类型

根据科研论文的内容和涉及的学科领域、使用的研究方法等可以把论文分成以下几种类型:

1. 按论文的研究内容及学科分类

(1)应用型:即研究内容属于应用性学科范围,包括预防医学论文、调查报告等。

(2)实验型:即论文的研究内容属于实验性学科范围,包括基础科研论文和应用基础科研论文。

(3)理论型:即论文的研究内容属于理论学科范畴,涉及哲学、方法学、统计学、史学、伦理学、社会学、经济学、新闻学等。

2. 按研究方法分类

(1)理论型:主要是通过使用理论推理、证明和分析的研究方法,总结出新的观点、规律、理论等。

(2)实验型:是科研论文中最常见的类型,通过设计实验方案,收集实验数据,对数据进行分析,最后得出实验结果。

(3)调查型:是指通过调查的方法取得科学资料的一种研究方法,调查的方法包括前瞻性调查和回顾性调查两种。

(4)观察型:是依靠人的感觉器官和仪器对研究对象进行观察和研究的方法,然后做出科学地解释。

(5)综合型:是指论文中综合运用了两种或两种以上的上述的研究方法。

(二)体裁

国内学术期刊目前刊登的文稿可以大致分为论著类、综述、个案报道、专家共识、指南、学术讨论类、讲座类、会议文献类、评论类、简报类、消息类等几类。

投稿的第一步就是选择投稿的体裁。下面是杂志 *The New England Journal of Medicine* 可以发表的各种体裁的文章。

Step 1: Type, Title, & Abstract

Select the type of article you are submitting. The form will change according to the article type you select. For more information on which article type to choose, see "Instructions & Forms" at top. If you need to insert a special character or formatting, click the "Special Characters" button. Read More …

* =Required Fields

* Type:

CHOICE TYPE DESCRIPTION

Original Article

Brief Report

Special Article

Review Article

Image in Clinical Medicine

Perspective

Letter about NEJM Article

Letter NOT about NEJM Article

Other Article (all other article types, including Sounding Board, Medicine & Society, etc.)

下面介绍几种体裁的文章。

1. 评论类文稿　评论类常见类型有社评、专家论坛、编者语、编者的话、编者按、书刊评价、述评、专论、书评、文后评论等。书评类文稿是编者或作者对研究专题、科研项目、一个领域的研究工作、一个问题或一组科研论文进行深入、全面地阐述和精辟的评论,也可以深入地评论某一个方面,包括焦点论坛、专论、专家论坛、社论等。

2. 论著类文稿　论著类文稿是科研期刊发表类型最多的文稿。论著类文稿也称为原著类文稿,是总结科学研究成果的文章,主要报道相关领域的原始研究结果。论著类文章是期刊的核心部分。

列举一篇作者发表在美国《泌尿外科杂志》(*The Journal of Urology*)的论文,供参考,重点显示其写作格式。

Bilateral Renal Melamine Related Calculus in 50 Children:

A Single Centre Experiencein Clinical Diagnosis and Treatment

Author:

Author Affiliations:

* Corresponding author:

ABSTRACT

Purpose: To investigate the clinical diagnosis and treatment features of bilateral renal calculus in young children who were fed melamine-tainted infant milk formula.

Patients and Methods: The clinical data on 50 children (aged 23.4 ± 3.1 months) with a history of being fed melamine-tainted infant milk formula and suffering from bilateral renal calculus were analyzed retrospectively …

Results: Bilateral renal calculi peaked in 6-to 18-month-old infants (85% of cases). The male to female ratio was 3.1：1.0. …

Conclusions: Urinary melamine related calculi were seen most often in infants between the ages of 6 to 18 months after being fed melamine-tainted infant milk formula. …

Key words: urolithiasis, pediatrics, melamine, milk, kidney

INTRODUCTION

Urolithiasis is a common urological disease that affects approximately 10% of the population worldwide. The incidence of urolithiasis in children, approximately 2-3% in China, occurs most likely between the age of 2 and 6 years. Bilateral renal calculi are extremely rare in the absence of an underlying diagnosis. …

PATIENTS AND METHODS

Patients

More than 3 000 children with history of fed melamine-tainted infant formulas from local areas accepted free medical evaluation from September to October 2008. According to the diagnostic criteria established by WHO 165 children were diagnosed with melamine related urinary stones, 50 of them (23.4 ± 3.1 months, range 50 days to 7 years of age) …

Image evaluation

All patients were assessed by a color Doppler ultrasonic diagnostic apparatus (Aloka, SSD-α10, probe frequency 3.5MHz). …

Diagnosis

Urinary melamine related stone was diagnosed depend mainly on the guideline from WHO and regimen has been issued by the Ministry of Health, China. In brief, the diagnostic criteria is …

Treatment

All cases were treated according to diagnosis and treatment guidelines from the Chinese Ministry of Health. In short, all patients were immediately asked to stop the consumption of melamine-tainted infant milk formula. …

Discharged stone analysis

Discharged stone from 6 cases were analyzed by using combined liquid phase chromatography-mass spectrum methods (Esquire-LC MS analyzer, produced by Bruker Co).

Statistical analysis

Statistical analyses were performed with the Statistical Package for Social Sciences (SPSS), Version 1, for Windows. …

RESULTS

Incidence, age and sex distribution

Bilateral melamine-related calculi occurred most often in children less than 1.5 years old (32/50). The incidence peaked in patients 6 to 18 months of age, which accounted for 58% of cases …

Clinical features

The length of melamine-tainted infant milk formula feeding ranged from 47 days to 42 months (average 12.4 ± 1.5 months). …

Laboratory examination

Urinary pH ranged from 5.0 to 7.5, with 28 (56%) showing mildly acidic urine (pH ≤6). Eleven cases were diagnosed with renal failure. …

Ultrasound features

Single bilateral renal calculi were found in 72% (36/50). Bilateral renal calculi with unilateral ureteral calculi were observed in 16% (8/50) and …

Treatment response

After treatment in hospital (average 8.1 ± 0.7 days), the clinical symptoms in all patients disappeared and none died. Most of cases had a good treatment response to conservative treatment …

DISCUSSION

It has been reported that stones are rarely seen in children, especially bilateral renal calculi, in the absence of an underlying metabolic disorder The outbreak of urinary tract calculi after melamine-tainted infant milk formula consumption in China has caused an increase in the number of bilateral urinary calculi. …

…

CONCLUSIONS

Bilateral urinary melamine related calculi were more frequently observed after exposure to melamine-tainted milk than appears in otherwise normal children. …

ACKNOWLEDGMENTS

We thank Prof. S.B. Bauer, Department of Urology, Children's Hospital, HarvardMedicalSchool, Boston, MA, USA, Dr. J. Corcos, Department of Urology, McGillUniversity, Montreal, Quebec, Canada. …

References

…

从以上例子,可以初步了解论著的结构,包括标题(Title)、摘要(Abstract)、关键词(Key words)、前言(Introduction)、材料(Materials)和方法(Patients and Methods)、结果(Results)、讨论(Discussion)、结论(Conclusion)及参考文献(References),有时需要写上致谢(Acknowledgements)。

3. 简报类文稿　此类文稿是将原著中的重要内容高度概括后以简练的文字表达出来,内容包括方法、数据、结果等。简报类文稿常常刊登在简报、技术交流、经验交流、快讯等栏目中。

简报类文稿系已经报道过但在某一方面仍有一定的学术价值的初步研究或同类的内容,较论著的重要性相对较差。

技术交流类文稿介绍新方法、新技术或对某种方法、技术、器械的改进。

列举一篇摘自《新英格兰医学杂志》经验交流类文稿,如下。

Responses to 2009 H1N1 Vaccinein Children 3 to 17 Years of Age

Author:

Author Affiliations:

The current 2009 pandemic influenza A (H1N1) virus is associated with substantial morbidity in children, with 45% of hospitalizations occurring in patients under 18 years of age.1…

In a randomized, single-center study in Costa Rica, we tested various doses of egg-based 2009 H1N1 vaccine (Novartis) in subjects ranging in age from 3 to 64 years, including 194 subjects between the ages of 3 and 8 years and 196 subjects between the ages of 9 and 17 years (Clinical Trials. gov number, NCT00973700) …

Subjects in the two age groups, who were more than 99% Hispanic, were randomly assigned (in a 2:3:2 ratio) to receive one 7.5-μg hemagglutinin dose with adjuvant or either one or two 15-μg doses without adjuvant. After vaccination, local and systemic events were generally mild to moderate …

These preliminary data support the use of one 15-μg dose of 2009 H1N1 vaccine without adjuvant in children between the ages of 9 and 17 years. …

REFERENCES

…

　　从以上例子,可以初步了解经验交流类文稿的结构,可以无结构划分,通篇介绍某个领域的经验,也可以包括前言(Introduction)、材料和方法(Patients and Methods)、结果(Results)、讨论(Discussion)及参考文献(References)等结构。

　　快讯:是以快报的形式快速地报道科研工作中的新成果和新内容。

　　4. 学术讨论类文稿　学术讨论类文稿包括会议纪要、读者来信、学术讨论、专题笔谈等。杂志编辑部或编委会对于研究过程中出现的问题或是新的进展,组织相关的专家学者进行书面笔谈或者举办专题座谈会,然后总结整理得到的就是会议纪要和专题笔谈类文稿。此类文稿能及时地体现最新的科研成果和进展,对于具体的科研工作也有着普遍的指导意义。

　　5. 综述、讲座文稿　研究进展、继续教育、名词解释、综述、讲座、基础知识等是刊登该类稿件的常见栏目。

　　综述类文稿:这种文稿是体现一个领域或专题的科研进展和动态的文稿。包括叙述性综述和系统性综述两种。叙述性综述是归纳、分析一个专题在一段时间内的所有文献之后进行带有评价性和倾向性的综合阐述。系统性综述是依据特殊人群,系统地检索一个具体问题的文献,根据一定的科学标准,选出达到要求的研究,然后进行全面分析和统计学处理得到准确的结论。综述可以涉及任何层面,尽管其大部分或全部内容先前已经被发表,但是正常情况下重复发表并不会出现。因为综述的性质很明确,多数情况下,题目会惯用如:《微生物评论》(*Critical Reviews in Microbiology*)、《生物化学年度回顾》(*Annual Review of Biochemistry*)等方式。若非如此,综述则没有任何新意。从一篇好的综述中,我们可以提炼出整合后新的信息、思路、理论及范式。

　　列举一篇《新英格兰医学杂志》的综述如下。

Melamine and the Global Implications of Food Contamination

Author:

Author Affiliations:

* Corresponding author:

Food contamination, whether accidental or intentional, has been a sad, recurrent theme throughout recorded history, going back some 8 000 years and described in the Old Testament.

However, a new dimension has been added in this new millennium: …

In addition to its catastrophic health effects, the contamination has had major economic effects, with the United States and other countries banning the importation of milk and other food products from China …

Now melamine is being discovered in other foods, which are turning up worldwide. Melamine (1, 3, 5-triazine-2, 4, 6-triamine, or $C_3H_6N_6$) (see diagram), a chemical developed in the 1830s, has had varied and widespread legitimate uses …

But why would one intentionally add a non-nutritious substance such as melamine to food? Nitrogen content has long been used as a surrogate for assessing the protein content of foods, and melamine contains a substantial amount of nitrogen-66% by mass …

How much melamine must food contain to pose a risk to humans? Given the lack of data, regulatory bodies such as the FDA and international agencies such as the World Health Organization (WHO) are trying hard to develop useful recommendations …

The present epidemic illness resulted from melamine's tendency to form stones and gravel in the urinary system. Young children exposed to the median level of the brand with the highest melamine content, according to the executive summary from the WHO meeting …

A further problem is that melamine food contamination is more pervasive than was originally thought. Since melamine is in animal feed in China, it has now been detected in eggs; it has also been found in wheat gluten and other foods …

Yet it is not certain what should be done going forward. In the United States, commonsense suggestions have been posted on the Web sites of both the FDA …

In today's world, it is crucial to understand and deal with the global implications of foodborne diseases if problems like the melamine epidemic are to be prevented …

REFERENCES

…

从以上例子,可以初步了解综述类文稿的结构,可以无结构地划分,层次分明,通篇介绍某个领域的进展,也可以包括前言、研究领域不同方面最新的进展、展望及参考文献。

讲座及继续教育类文稿:此类文稿是向读者系统地介绍某一专业或专题研究知识的文稿。其特点是比教科书的内容新颖,且有作者的经验或评价。

6. 专家共识和指南类文稿　专家共识指医学领域专家针对某一个疾病的诊断和治疗或某一个新的诊疗技术等达成的共同认识,取得一致的意见。专家共识可以作为诊疗护理常规的参考依据。但是,在临床工作中,若遇医疗纠纷,专家共识并不具有法律效应,不能成为法律依据。医学专家共识的英文定义为:"Medical consensus is a public statement on a particular aspect of medical knowledge at the time the statement is made that a representative group of experts agree to be evidence-based and state-of-the-art (state-of-the-science) knowledge. Its main objective is to counsel physicians on the best possible and acceptable way to diagnose and treat certain diseases or how to address a particular decision-making area. It is usually, therefore, considered an authoritative, community-based expression of a consensus decision-making and publication process."。

临床指南的定义为:"A medical guideline (also called a clinical guideline or clinical practice line) is a document with the aim of guiding decisions and criteria regarding diagnosis, management, and treatment in specific areas of healthcare."。

指南提供指导性资料,是辨别方向的依据。临床实践指南指根据特定的临床情况系统制定出的帮助临床医生和患者做出恰当处理的指导意见,集中了当前最佳医学证据。最佳证据即指有循证医学的证据,避免了对权威和经典的迷信,是严格检验之后得出的事实。这些证据有五个等级:一级证据是最可靠的,是对若干个具有优良设计的 RCT(即随机对照双盲临床试验)进行总结分析得出的。五级证据包括专家意见、临床总结和病理报告。循证医学是由具有一定学术水平的不同专业的临床专家、社会医学家、临床流行病专家、临床和卫生统计学家、医学科学信息工作者等共同合作,收集、分析、评价文献中最好的科研成果,最后得出指南。这些指南展现了各个领域的最新进展,是临床医生工作的依据。

临床指南的目的:"Clinical guidelines are to standardize medical care, to raise quality of care, to reduce several kinds of risk (to the patient, to the healthcare provider, to medical insurers and health plans) and to achieve the best balance between cost and medical parameters such as effectiveness, specificity, sensitivity, resolutiveness, etc. It has been demonstrated repeatedly that the use of guidelines by healthcare providers such as hospitals is an effective way of achieving the objectives listed above, although they are not the only ones."。

NIH 给专家共识定义为："Consensus statements synthesize new information, largely from recent or ongoing medical research, that has implications for reevaluation of routine medical practices. They do not give specific algorithms or guidelines for practice."。这是专家共识和指南的区别。

制定共识和指南的方式很多。最常见的方式是由行业协会或政府指定一个专家委员会或独立专家小组就医学问题或疾病等参考该领域最新发表的成果或新知识达成一致,供临床或医学实践参考。共识需要根据该领域的新进展进行不断更新。

下面的三大主要原因迫使现代医学去寻找临床决策更科学更可靠的证据即制定临床指南。医疗费用的与日俱增已超过社会的负担能力,这就迫使我们必须更加高效的使用而不是滥用有限的卫生资源。传统经验医学根据自身的专业训练和临床经验来决定病人的诊疗方案,是通过理论推导或从过去案例中得到的个人经验。这些经验不一定都是可靠的。例如,对急性缺血性脑卒中处理方案中英两个曾有对比研究发现 69% 的中国医生使用甘油 / 甘露醇,英国仅 1%;19% 的中国医生用激素、53% 的中国医生用钙拮抗剂,英国小于 1%。中外医生间的差异也呼唤国际指南的出台。

7. 消息类文稿　时讯、信息及会议消息、科研简讯、国际学术动态、国内学术动态等栏目常常刊登这类文稿。消息类文稿具有时效性强,内容覆盖范围广的特点。

列举一则国际尿控协会(ICS)年会会议消息,如下。

Abstract Submission for ICS 2009, San Francisco

Submit your abstracts for the opportunity to present your work at the ICS 2009 Annual Meeting in San Francisco. Visit the ICS Abstract Centre now to access the abstract submission guidelines, instructions and application form. THE DEADLINE FOR SUBMISSION OF ABSTRACTS IS WEDNESDAY, 1 APRIL, 2009.

Deadline for Expressions of Interest and Nominations for ICS Committees 1 April 2009; The following committees are specifically calling for interest in membership: Ethics Committee · Publications and Communications Committee; Please send your nominations for the following ICS posts by 1 April 2009 · Continence Promotion Chair · Neurourology Chair; In order to stand for a position as Chair you need to be nominated and seconded by two ICS members. Deadline for applications to host 2013 ICS ANNUAL MEETING are to be received at the ICS office by 1 April 2009.

For more information on any of these items please contact the ICS office click here International Continence Society Educational Course in cooperation with the Thai Urological Association, 3-4 April 2009 Venue: Zign Hotel, Pattaya, Thailand; The ICS is pleased to announce an Educational Course to be held in Thailand in collaboration with the Thai Urological Association (TUA). The ICS course will take place on the first days of the TUA's annual meeting. The TUA meeting will then continue from the end of the ICS course until 5 April. As well as using local Thai experts, the ICS will bring internationally renowned speakers to speak on topics that include: Neurourology, Good Urodynamic Practice, Overactive Bladder, LUTS, Dysfunction and Prolapse Surgery.

All ICS members and non-members are welcome. For further information, visit www.icsoffice. org If you are interested in participating in any of the mentioned activities or have any questions, please do not hesitate to contact the ICS office on info@icsoffice.org.

ICS e-News, is a regular information service designed to keep you informed about all relevant events in a timely fashion. Contributions and feedback are most welcome. If you wish to see this e-News as a PDF, please go to the News Section on the ICS website www.icsoffice.org International Continence Society 19 Portland Square, Bristol BS2 8SJ, UK

Web: www.icsoffice.org

E-mail: info@icsoffice.org

Tel:+44 (0) 117 9444881

Fax:+44 (0) 117 9444882

从以上例子,可以初步了解会议消息文稿的结构。

8. 会议文献类文稿　国家性学术会议的重要讲话、开幕词、闭幕词、会议通过的决议及章程等都属于此类文稿。

9. 会议论文　会议报道是一种发表在书籍或期刊上的论文形式,为专题报告会、全国或国际会议、研讨会、圆桌会议或其他会议的一部分。正常情况下,报道不包括原始数据及结果部分,不认为是初次发表。会议论文通常是评论论文,是对近来特殊科学家或实验室的研究进行的报道。一些会议(尤其是一些有意义的会议)首次报道了某些研究,数据新且原创,观察意义较大。但是,这些初次报道通常不符合科研论文的要求。之后,这些研究被接受发表在主要期刊上;与此同时,一些细节被完善,所有必要的实验数据被详细地描述在论文中(以至于有能力的科研工作者能够重复实验),先前的推断变成了结论。

印刷出版的大量会议资料通常并不是主要期刊。如果原稿发表在会议资料中,那么其可以而且应该发表(或再次发表)在主要期刊上。否则,研究内容可能会不为人知。如果会议报道发表后又继续在主要期刊上发表,那么就存在版权和许可问题。

会议摘要与会议论文集一样,存在多种类型,通常包含一些原创资料。会议摘要并不是初次发表,也不应该将其视为之后全文发表的一种阻碍。论文出现在会议上随后通常可以发表在主要期刊上。近来,对摘要(或概要)进行扩展成为一种趋势。因为,如果要在国际大型会议上发表全文是非常昂贵的,而且不能取代在主要期刊上进行发表。所以,扩充摘要意义重大,可以提供给大家更多的信息。

三、医学英文科研论文的结构

科研论文应按照投稿杂志格式要求准备文章的结构,在医学英文科研论文中,最常见的论文结构为引言、方法、结果和讨论(IMRAD)四部分。事实上,"材料和方法"这个标题中,"材料"比"方法"更常用,但是,我们选用两者的首字母 M 作为简写中的字母。

推荐采用 IMRAD 的写作形式已经很多年。直到目前为止,这种写作形式仍受到许多期刊和编辑的青睐。从 1972 年 IMRAD 写作形式首次被美国国家标准协会(American National Standards Institute)推荐为科研论文的标准写作形式以来,这种形式就一直没有改变。但最近,《细胞》(*Cell*)及一些其他杂志对 IMRAD 写作形式进行了改动。在新的变动中,方法部分被安排在最后而非第二部分,也许我们应该称之为 IRDAM。

IMRAD 写作形式的基本顺序完全符合逻辑性,以至于其渐渐成为其他一些说明性文章的写作形式。不管是创作一篇化学、考古学、经济学论文,还是描述一个街头犯罪事件,

IMRAD 写作形式通常都是最好的选择。

报道实验室研究的论文通常采用此写作形式。当然,也有例外。例如:对地质学的现场研究报道及对临床医学病例进行的报道并非采用此组织形式。但是,尽管如此,从提出问题到解决问题这样相同的逻辑方式仍然适用。

对实验室研究论文的组织有时不尽相同。如果在方法部分中直接列出相关结果,那么将材料和方法部分与结果部分融合成"实验"部分则是可行的。结果部分很少出现复杂情况或进行对比分析,以至于讨论部分显得尤为重要,将结果和讨论部分融合在一起亦是可行的。另外,许多主要期刊发表的"短篇报道"或"短篇交流"已经取消了 IMRAD 的写作形式。

摘要是对文章主要内容的浓缩,是医学英文科研论文必不可少的部分。多数医学英文科研论文采用 IMRAD 结构,但文章摘要的结构变化较大,即使文章结构相同,其摘要要求也可能不尽一样。如:"① *The New England Journal of Medicine*: Provide an abstract of not more than 250 words. It should consist of four paragraphs: labeled Background, Methods, Results, and Conclusions. They should briefly describe, respectively, the problem being addressed in the study, how the study was performed, the salient results, and what the authors conclude from the results; ② *JAMA, the Journal of the American Medical Association*: Reports of original data should include an abstract of no more than 300 words using the following headings: Context, Objective, Design, Setting, Patients (or Participants), Interventions (include only if there are any), Main Outcome Measure(s), Results, and Conclusions. For brevity, parts of the abstract may be written as phrases rather than complete sentences; ③ *The Lancet*: Include an abstract, with five paragraphs (Background, Methods, Findings, Interpretation, and Funding), not exceeding 300 words. Our electronic submission system will ask you to copy and paste this section at the submit abstract stage."。

各种不同类型的组织形式被用于描述性科研论文的写作当中。决定以什么样的写作形式组织一篇论文,及选用什么样的题目,需要参考投稿期刊简介。如果对此期刊持怀疑态度,或其涉及面广,不同类型的论文均可发表,那么就需要从恰当的书籍资料当中获取信息。例如:1990 年 Huth 详细记录了医学论文的许多写作类型,同年,Michaelson 总结了工程学论文及报道的许多写作类型。

总之,医学英文科研论文的准备与文学技巧的关系不大,而与写作组织形式关系密切。医学英文科研论文并不是文学作品,创作者并非文学意义上的作者。有人认为医学英文科研论文就是文学作品,作者的写作风格及天赋是最重要的,写作形式的多样性会吸引读者,这种观点是不正确的。医学科研交流不需要浮夸之词,要求提交的论文数据统一、简洁和易懂。

第三节　医学英文科研论文写作要求

科研论文是以文字的方式体现科研成果,严谨的科研设计、客观的实验观察、全面分析推理的观点以及能准确表达客观事实的写作造诣,这是论文质量的保证也是撰写科研论文的基本要求。有的论文有很好的素材,科学的研究方法,可成立的结论,但是从论文写作的角度来看,不能充分反映科学内容,没有好的逻辑性、可读性,结论就变得难以让人信服,甚至经过多次修改也未能达到在刊物上发表的标准,这是论文评审中常常出现的情况。这说明，客观地、真实地表现事物的本质是写好一篇论文的必要条件；不仅要有严谨科学的方法，令人信服的正确观点，还要有足够的写作水平。

论文的写作绝不是把所有的科研工作、实验过程、观测数据、结果都记录到论文中，而应该是整理分析所得到的数据和资料，用统计学方法加工处理，取其精华，得其本质，有所发现、发明、创新地进行分析总结，这样才能把握事物内部的客观规律，得出的结论才能令人信服。要做到这些，"三严"精神——严谨的学风、严肃的态度、严密的方法——是最基本的要求，精益求精，慎重立论。

科研论文不允许丝毫的夸大和渲染，更不能捏造，甚至做假，切忌为了塑造典型而偷梁换柱。脍炙人口，千古传诵的诗句"白发三千丈"，就绝不能模仿运用于学术论文中，而应该本着实事求是的精神。早在 1930 年在美国 Ohio 州立大学任教的 Ward G. Recoler，曾就此问题提出 5 个词，在 70 多年后的今天，这 5 个词仍具有重要意义，即：正确性（accuracy）、客观性（objectivity）、公正性（impartiality）、确证性（verifiability）、可读性（readability）。作者只有遵循一定的写作方法和形式才能撰写出达到这些标准的科研论文。"Accuracy"用我们的话来说，即实验数据精确可靠，内容论点正确无误。现在姑且用"正确性"一词概括。"Objectivity"即不含任何主观臆测，实事求是、客观实际。对结果有所预测是可以且应该出现的，但在收集整理实验数据资料撰写学术论文时，应当遵从客观事实，摒弃主观愿望。这一条叫"客观性"。"Impartiality"是处理实验数据和研究结果要公正，不偏不倚，不能任意取舍。不能舍弃自己觉得不该出现的某些现象、数据和结果，不能忽视偶然性，偶然之中存在着必然，一些重要的突破就孕育在偶然性中。我们称为"公正性"。"Verifiability"即论文中的数据和实验结果是经过反复验证的，具有重复性、再现性，而且经得起别人的验证。以相同实验条件任何人、任何地点、任何时间，都可以得到相同的实验结果．可以名曰"确证性"。"Readability"指论文必须通顺易懂，可以成诵，切忌言语晦涩。要尽量地丰富词汇，润饰文字，文章内容吸引人，读物具有阅读和欣赏价值。

符合下面几点基本要求才能成为一篇好的论文。

（一）思想性

论文的主题和内容要以国家的方针政策为依据，体现科研工作者向经济建设看齐、为国民经济发展服务的方针；要贯彻"理论和实践相结合，普及和提高相结合"的方针；遵守国家法令法规，遵守保密和技术专利等相关法律规定，杜绝政治错误和泄密；重视科学道德。

（二）科学性

科研论文与其他文学的、美学的、神学的文章区别就在于其在方法论上的特征，即科学性。科研论文不仅要体现科学和技术领域的进展，而且必须具有客观真实性、再现性、精确性、逻辑性和公正性，要把"三严"精神贯彻于论文的选题、科研设计、观察整理、分析推理到得出结论的整个过程。

1. **真实性**　选题要以充足的科学依据为基础，科研设计严谨、合理、可操作，取材精确可靠、客观真实，实验方法准确无误，可比性和随机性也必不可少，实验结果完全来源于原始资料，不随意取舍、不弄虚作假、不夸大，实事求是，客观的记录观察数据。

2. **再现性**　在任何时间和地点的任何人在相同的实验条件下进行整个实验过程或是重复论证实验数据，得出的实验结果相同。即证明具有再现性。

3. 准确性　有明确的目标,言之有物,客观真实的实验数据,确保内容论点正确无误,用词合理引文准确可靠。

4. 逻辑性　表现在论文的结构上。论文概念明确,有条有理,结构清晰严谨,数据真实准确,判断精准,符合标准,图表简洁准确,行文通顺易懂,整个论文前后呼应,自成系统。

5. 公正性　对待实验数据和结果要公正客观,不偏不倚,排除个人主观观念的影响,评价自己和别人的工作也应该实事求是,保持公正客观。

（三）独创性

这是科研论文的灵魂,也被称为首创性、先进性和创造性。它指论文的科研内容、实践方法、理论观点都优于或有别于已发表的科研论文。要求揭示前人尚未发表或做过的事物现象、本质、特征、属性及所遵循的规律,即所记录的研究是首创或部分首创,应当做到有所发现、发明、创造、进展,而不是简单的重复、复述、模仿和解释前人的工作。如果是对前人的研究进行重复或效仿,则必须是仿中有创,即从新的角度观察,阐述新的问题,提出自己的论点,有独创性的论文才值得被刊登。

（四）实用性

科研论文还应该有实用价值。科研论文通过各种形式刊登交流之后,能否吸引读者,看后能否运用,用后能否解决实践中的问题,能否在社会上推广应用,是否具有一定的社会效益和经济效益,这些问题决定了一篇论文的价值。

（五）双向性

科学交流是双向的。正如任何形式的信号只有被接收才会有意义一样,一篇发表的科研论文只有被预期的读者接受才有意义。因此,科学的原则是:只有结果被发表并被理解,科学实验才是成功的。

（六）可读性

论文结构合理严谨,层次清晰分明;文字表达言简意赅,用词和标点符号准确规范,句子通顺易懂,可以成诵,没有词不达意,不晦涩;使读者可以轻松的了解文章的内容,获得知识和信息,不用浪费不必要的时间和精力。

（七）清晰性

科研论文写作的重要特征是清晰。成功的科学实验包括:清晰的思路下解决了存在的难题,得出清晰的结论。清晰是任何形式交流的特征。当第一次说某事时,清晰是基本要求。科研论文写作要求绝对清晰。

（八）理解性

科研论文写作是把一个清晰的信号传导给读者。这个信号的语言应该尽可能清晰、简洁而有序。科研论文中几乎不需要装饰,那些词藻华丽的文学修饰（暗喻、明喻等）很可能引起混淆,因此应尽可能少地用于研究性论文的写作。

总之,对科研论文写作的要求是数据精准可靠,论点明确清晰,同时突出核心,遵循实际,言简意赅,逻辑清晰合理,要做到具有创造性的科研成果被生动,明确,鲜明的传达给读者。R. B. McKerrow 提倡:"State your facts as simply as possible, even boldly. No one wants flowers of eloquence or literary ornaments in a research article."。

一篇科研论文除了结构外,第二重要因素是适当的语言。

许多写作的目的是为了娱乐,但科研论文的写作却有不同的目的,即交流科学新发现。所以,词语表达必须准确、清晰。科研工作者需要有很强的驾驭文字的能力。大卫·杜鲁门在他任职哥伦比亚学院院长时说:"在当代复杂社会中生存的专家如果只是受过训练而非系统教育,只有专门技能而修养不全,这将是很危险的。"

在科研论文写作中,英文最好以最简单的语句表达出其含义。文学设计、暗喻等形式在科研论文写作中应少用。研究者花费数月或数年辛苦统计分析数据,如果因为表达不清楚而使研究重要性降低,得不偿失。

写作英文科研论文前了解上述要求很有必要。掌握了这些基本知识,就会感觉写作并不难。但要记住,任何科研写作都需要付出艰辛劳动。正如 Gene Fowler 指出的那样:"Writing is easy. All you do is stare at a blank sheet of paper until drops of blood form on your forehead."。

第四节 医学英文科研论文的重要性

医学英文科研论文已成为科技文献中不可或缺的一部分,记载着医学进步足迹,是医学研究和发展的源动力,是医务工作者、科学研究人员、教学人员在临床、科研、教学实践中通过调查研究所取得成果的记录,是医学科学研究成果的纸质或电子文稿并且具有标准的结构和格式,是医学研究工作重要的组成部分。新的研究成果和发明创造只有以标准、科学的文体格式记录下来,然后刊登于合法的医学科研刊物载体上,在社会上广泛传播和推广之后,最终达到生产和转化研究成果的目的。具体来说,医学科研论文的重要性包括如下几方面。

(一)记录和储存医学科研信息

在完成临床观察或科学研究之后,立即总结得出的结果,将发现或发明以论文或报告的形式记录下来。否则,其发明与发现可能随时间流逝而逐渐消失,致使后人需要浪费不必要的人力物力再次重复这些工作。因此,把这些医学科研发现或观察结果以论文的方式记录下来,才能以此为基础催生出新的发明、发现,使人类的医学科技宝库不断壮大丰富。正是因为这种连续性,在不断地记录、创造、再记录、再创造的过程中人类的文明才能得以延续和不断向上发展。因此,医学论文承载着医学科研信息,而撰写医学科研论文则是总结医学科研发现的重要方法。

(二)传播医学科研结果,促进学术交流

英国科学家法拉第在 19 世纪就曾指出,对于科研工作,必须"开始它,完成它,发表它"(to begin, to end, to publish)。因为,任何一项科研成果与发明创造都是由社会成员的个体劳动或组织团体进行科研活动得出的结晶。从全人类角度思考,将少数人的科研成果变成全人类共享的共同财富是很有必要的,这就需要相互学习、借鉴、交流,才能不断发现更先进科学技术。而通过发表科技论文就是相互交流的重要方式之一。如英国《自然》杂志在 1997

年 2 月 27 日,第一次刊登了培育绵羊的无性繁殖技术,这项技术无疑是生物基因工程研究领域的一个历史性突破,轰动了整个世界。因此,科研信息的传播需要以医学论文为载体,而且按照国际惯例,科学研究成果的首创权想要得到承认,必须以科研论文的形式刊登在合法的学术期刊上。

(三)促进医学研究成果转化为生产力

医学论文的写作、发表是使医学研究成果转化为社会生产力的重要手段之一。在撰写论文的过程中,科研人员对涉猎的信息、自己所做的工作进行由表及里的分析、探讨,从而使工作不断地深入、完善。医学研究成果一经发表,为世人所知后,就会促使人们将其投入生产和实践中,产生社会效益和经济效益,这些效益可能会以无法估量的力量推动人类医学事业的发展。

(四)交流临床实践经验和科研信息

工作在临床一线的医护人员,在日常的实践工作中,日积月累得到很多成功经验和失败教训。而将这些经验教训进行科学地分析和总结,写成论文之后发表交流,就可以起到更大的指导与借鉴作用,不仅能造福于患者,同时也促进科学的进步和发展。科研论文在期刊上公开发表是最好的交流形式。这种交流形式不会被地域、时间、历史更迭、社会发展条件和国家所限制。随着互联网的诞生和发展,如今已进入信息时代,科学情报也随着迅猛发展,将论文储存在情报中心检索系统中,全世界的读者都可以查阅。

(五)启迪学术思想

各种学术思想以大量的科研成果和实践经验为依据逐渐发展起来,这些学术思想被写作成论文发表,然后又被其他人学习与交流,并相互印证启迪,产生新的学术思想,科学事业就这样得到了发展。

(六)提高医学科研能力和学术水平

医学论文写作是一种含有巨大艰辛的创造性的脑力劳动。在写作论文的同时,随着思维不断扩展深化,医疗科研工作中发现问题、分析问题与解决问题的能力也进一步提高,同时医学科研能力和学术水平也跟着提高。

(七)考核业务水平

评价医务工作者业务能力和科研能力的重要标准,一是发表医学论文的数量,二是其发表论文的质量也就是论文产生的社会效益和经济效益的大小。也是如今进行职称评定、业务考核、晋升晋级及医学院学生毕业与取得学位的客观指标和主要依据。授予学位和考核业务能力的重要依据就包括研究生期间的学位论文、大学期间的毕业论文、科研工作者的学术论文等。如我国多数医学院校的硕士研究生必须在核心期刊上发表 1 篇与本专业相关的论著,才能被授予硕士学位;博士研究生在核心期刊上发表 3 篇与本专业相关的论著,方能参与毕业答辩,发表 1 篇 SCI 文章才能授予博士学位;某些重点医学院校要求博士研究生发表 1 篇影响因子为 3.0 以上的文章才能授予博士学位。

（八）有助于人才培养和选拔

科研论文真实地记录了科研的成果,可以体现出论文作者及其所在单位、地区、国家的科学技术研究水平。一个单位的面貌、成就、人才资源及科研能力、教学水平的高低,通过发表科研论文的数量、质量都可以体现出来。好的论文是发现培育科研人才的重要渠道之一,也可以体现人员本身及技术、科研的水平。

（九）促进学科建设

科学研究是学科建设与发展的基础。在学科建设过程中,通过对科研研究工作成果的逐步积累和对各学科理论体系的总结和完善,在原有学科的基础上,不断地进行学科的分割、划分和构建,完善学科建设的环境和条件,形成新的学科框架,使学科建设得以不断完善、发展和壮大。发表医学英文科研论文的数量和质量具体反映了一个单位科学研究的水平和能力,也是学科建设评估和水平提高的重要依据。

（十）提高国家学术地位,增强国际医学界影响力

近年来,我国许多研究成果被国际颇具影响力的杂志发表,国家学术地位得到很大的提高。同时,国内医学期刊也在蓬勃发展,我国医药卫生事业也在其带动下迅速发展。

第2章
如何准备标题

Chapter 2
How to Prepare a Title

标题（title）是论文的眼睛，是科研论文最重要的组成部分。论文的标题不仅应简洁明了可概述全文，还应具有准确性、鲜明性、生动性、更要富有吸引力，要对整篇文章起到画龙点睛、引人注目的效果，要启发读者兴趣，便于读者快速确定全文中心内容，给人以深刻的印象。因此，文章的标题应当以最确切、简洁的词语来反映文章中最重要的核心内容，使读者看到标题的瞬间就诱发出阅读该论文的兴趣，进而选择阅读全文。正如 T. Clifford Alibutt 指出的那样："First impressions are strong impressions; a title ought therefore to be well studied, and to give, so far as its limit permit, a definite and concise indication of what is to come."。因此，一定要重视标题的写作。

一、标题的重要性

阅读一篇论文时，首先接触到的就是标题。标题犹如商标。俗话说先入为主。标题的作用之一是吸引阅读者。标题能否引起读者的兴趣决定着读者的选择，即是否会进一步浏览摘要及全文，甚至下载并给予保存。

通常读者会根据标题来决定是否继续阅读摘要及全文。如果标题表达不准确，会失去应用价值，让读者错误理解论文中心内容进而失去阅读兴趣。科技论文中的标题概括了论文的中心内容，是反映研究方向及深度最适当、简洁的逻辑组合。

标题也有检索及追踪文献的作用。查阅文献时常选择标题中的关键词进行检索，那么这些关键词必须准确地表达出论文的核心内容，不然会增加漏检率。图书馆以及研究机构大都选择自动检索系统，其中一部分就是选择标题中的关键题词或主题词来查寻资料的。因此，导致论文"丢失"的原因很可能就是标题不恰当，不能被读者正确检索出来。

在文章拟题的过程中，作者必须牢记的是，对大多数人来说，可能只会阅读文章的标题，只有少数对标题感兴趣的人会阅读全文。读者从文摘、索引或题录等检索中最先查找到文章的标题。美国《医学索引》(*Index Medicus*)、我国的中文科技目录等，都只标引论文标题。标题的单词必须精挑细选。一个好的标题能很好地展示你的研究方向、研究对象、研究条件和设计方案，从标题中应能窥见全篇论文的实质和精华所在，标题应以最少的单词来最充分地描述全文的内容。

二、如何确定一个好的标题

（一）好的标题离不开正确的选题

如何确定一个好的标题,是写科研论文首先要考虑的问题。医学论文写作时常需要考虑两个问题,即写什么和如何写。选好研究方向,课题有意义,写出的论文才会有价值,才能获得比较好的效果。因此,提出一个研究问题,有时要比解决一个问题还重要。好的选题往往要求与作者进行的科研工作、临床诊疗紧密配合,并且结合学科前沿的发展方向。同时,也应考虑能使研究成果或医疗经验在成文后更易交流。下面就以笔者选择的题目"Voiding pattern in newborns"为例来说明确定好的标题应从哪几个方面考虑。

（二）注重创新和有可行性

尽量选取在本专业和交叉学科前沿而且他人没有做过的科研课题。对于"Voiding pattern in newborns"课题的选择,我们查阅大量的文献,包括中文、外文,证实相关领域这方面的研究资料确实不多,保证了课题的创新性。换句话说,提前应进行充分的文献检索,了解相关的领域情况,避免重复劳动,也保持在该领域的领先地位。作者开展的另一个课题"Melamine related bilateral renal calculi in 50 children: single center experience in clinical diagnosis and treatment",从题目就可以看出该研究在该领域的重要性。

医学科研离不开客观条件的支持,尽管许多课题非常需要,而且十分的先进和科学,但倘若现有的支持条件不够,比如缺少人才、信息、经费、实验手段及现代管理不完备,就很难完成课题,不能达到所期望的研究结果。因此,要注重科研人员、基金和实验条件等准备,增加课题的可行性。

（三）选题难易适中,量力而行,围绕课题研究方向和目的开展研究

选择课题要符合自己的实际情况,不要好高骛远,或开展不切实际的课题,或完成全面论述性过大的问题。结合笔者选择的题目"Voiding pattern in one-week-old newborns"。我们限定了年龄并局限在新生儿进行,避免课题过大,有利于实际操作。一周的新生儿可以是正常新生儿,也可以包括排尿异常新生儿。当然也不要选择的题目太小,轻而易举。如果笔者选题为"Voiding pattern in one-week-old normal newborns",题目过小,只包括一周龄正常新生儿,进行课题的意义就减少了许多。

一般来说,不管课题的大小和难易程度如何,研究内容越具体越好,研究方向越清晰越好。否则,研究结果将会受到不同外在因素的干扰,达不到实验目的。回视笔者的选题《出生后一周正常和脑缺氧新生儿排尿方式的观察》具有内容具体、方向清晰的特点,并且具有延续性,可以在前面研究的基础上衍生出这个课题。

在此,总结一下选题的基本步骤:①要进行实际问题的考察和文献资料的检索,全面掌握本专业、本学科研究的现状;②通过已掌握的实际问题和文献资料,进行深入细致地分析以发现问题。比如要进行的科研价值如何,能否在当前的学科技术发展中产生重大的现实意义,能否达到预期的实验结果;③进行自我评议、初步论证和课题筛选。比如,分析课题能否完成的主客观条件和优势,组织和举行开题会,也可请专家帮助进行评议和论证等;④为

了减少人力和财力资源的浪费,进行实验研究之前一定要进行多次反复论证,采用"先定题后研究"的原则,从社会和临床实践中寻得课题加以研究,只有保持严谨的科学态度,才能获得较满意的研究结果;⑤如果不能拿到国家相应科研机构的课题,也可以采用"先研究后定题",这是研究者进行自由选择的一种方式,先查阅相关的文献资料,了解本专业的现状和历史、现存的研究成果、争论的要点等。

三、标题的基本要求

（一）标题撰写

准确（Accuracy）、简洁（Brevity）和清楚（Clarity）是标题撰写的基本要求。"准确"指标题要准确地反映论文的内容。"简洁"指标题选词应简明扼要,用简单词语去概述更多的内容。"清楚"指标题清晰、明白、有条理地表达出文章的特色和具体内容,明确研究目的,要求简捷有效、突出重点。下面分别详述。

1. **准确**　标题要提供准确的信息或关键词,这是文献检索的重要部分。目前,大部分摘要服务系统和索引都已采取查询"关键词"系统,因此,标题中的专业术语应起到启示文章重点内容的作用,并且容易被读者理解和检索。作为论文的"标签",标题既不能空泛和一般化,也不宜太过繁琐,使读者没有鲜明的印象。如果标题不能引起读者的注意,或关键词不堪理解,就会错失读者。为了确保标题的定义准确,要尽可能避免使用一些非定量的、含义不明确的词语。

2. **简洁**　标题通常不是一个完整的句子,不需要主谓宾等结构,说明题目比句子短小。只有少数杂志允许标题采用完整的句子。有时保留单词如"is"等的完整句子做标题能引起误解。比如 *Science* 308:1291,2005 的题目是:"Amalthea's Density Is Less Than That of Water",显然,"Is"在标题中是多余的字眼,去掉它也可以理解含义。通常读者不愿意看到作者用这种武断的方式陈述结果。Rosner（1990）把这种题目称为 assertive sentence title（断言式整句题目）。为了使题目简洁,标题一般不超过 10~12 个单词,若能用一行文字表达,则尽量不用两行。为了使标题简练,标题的选词应尽量简短,用最简练的词语概括最核心的内容。但是,在撰写标题时,也不能因为要追求形式上的简短,而忽视对论文内容的概述。过于简短的标题,常不能帮助读者正确理解论文含义。标题过长,则读者在浏览时不能迅速了解信息,如有作者建议将 "Preliminary observations on the effect of Zn element on anticorrosion of zinc plating layer" 改为 "Effect of Zn on anticorrosion of zinc plating layer"。为了使标题简短,标题中常可删去不必要的冠词（a,an 和 the）和多余的说明性词。这些词有 Development of, Evaluation of, Experimental, Investigation of (on), Observations on, On the, Regarding, Report of (on), Research on, Review of, Studies of (on), The preparation of, The synthesis of, The nature of, Treatment of, Use of, 等。在内容层次较多的情况下,如果难以简短化,最好采用主标题和副标题相结合的方法,如 "Importance of replication in microarray gene expression studies: statistical methods and evidence from repetitive CDNA hybridizations (Proc Nat Acad Sci USA,2000,97(18): 9834-9839)"。其中的副标题起补充、阐明作用,效果很好。

为使标题表达明确、清楚,应尽量将反映中心内容的关键词放在标题开头。如 "The effectiveness of vaccination against in healthy, working adults (N Engl J Med,1995,333:889-893)"

中;如果作者的标题开头的关键词是 vaccination,读者可能产生这是一篇方法性文章的误解:"How to vaccinate this population?"相反,第一个主题词用 effectiveness 的话,就更加直接的指明了研究问题"Is vaccination in this population effective?"

标题中应慎用缩略词,特别是对于有多个解释的缩略词,更应严加限制,必要时需在括号中注明全称。对于全称较长,缩写后已得到科技界公认的,可使用缩略词,且使用时仍需相应期刊读者群的认可,如 DNA(deoxyribonucleic acid,脱氧核糖核酸)、AIDS(acquired immune deficiency syndrome,获得性免疫缺陷综合征,艾滋病)等已为整个科技界公认和熟悉,可以在各类科技期刊的标题中使用;CT(computerized tomography)、MRI(magnetic resonance imaging,磁共振)等已为整个医学界公认和熟悉,可以在医学期刊的标题中使用。在设计标题时,作者应先思考一个问题"我如何检索到这个标题?"有些术语是以地名或人名命名的,并不常用。因此应用于标题中似不妥(如"坐骨神经痛"应使用 sciatica,而不是 Cotunnius' disease)。标题中应避免使用化学式、上下角标、特殊符号(数字符号、希腊字母等)、公式、不常用的专业术语和非英语词汇(包括拉丁语)等。

(二)标题内容

1. 展示写作目的 首先需要明确写该论文的目的,是要介绍并推广一项新的技术研究成果,还是要反映最新进展的综述或者讲座? 是一篇经验性的总结,还是一则病案报道。标题就是论文中心内容的提示,读者阅完标题,即知论文论述的宗旨,可大致了解论文的核心内容,吸引读者注意,符合读者兴趣,正是读者所需的。如标题"Normal voiding pattern and bladder dysfunction in infants and children"让读者一看就知道这是一篇综述,而标题"Family and segregation studies: 411 Chinese children with primary nocturnal enuresis"就是一篇典型的论著。读者可以根据标题提示的内容决定是否阅读全文。

如何撰写论文才能切题呢? 有的学者选择先定标题,再写论文,即预设几个不同的标题,再根据计划撰写的论文内容相互比较,选择其中贴切、醒目者。有的作者在已有的科技成果的基础上,先写出论文,然后再根据论文的主要意思再确定标题。一般说来,前者常用于撰写前瞻性研究、调查报告、综述讲座等论文,如标题"Partial unilateral ureteral obstruction in rats"就是作者在一系列研究基础上撰写的综述标题。后者常用于撰写回顾性分析、临床总结、病例报告等类型论文,如标题"Bilateral Renal Melamine Calculus in 50 Children: A Single Centre Experience in Clinical Diagnosis and Treatment"就是作者对 50 例服用三聚氰胺污染奶粉儿童出现双肾结石的研究,先总结临床诊断和治疗经验后再决定论文标题,是"文先于题"。

2. 题目新颖和准确得体 题目首先要突出论文的创新性,确切反应全文的特定内容,既不抽象,也不笼统,画龙点睛,能够吸引读者,在读者阅读后即可初步了解该研究的目的和价值,不要影响于整篇论文内容的表达。例如标题"Inositol trisphosphate and calcium signaling"是 Nature 杂志发表的一篇引用率很高的高质量文章,标题简明醒目;而如:"First report of three cases of abnormal chromosome karyotype"即《世界首报染色体异常核型 3 例》,能明确地告诉读者,这篇论文是报道 3 例染色体异常核型的,而且又是世界范围的首先报道;再如"手术治疗高反射性神经源性膀胱",其正文中仅述及膀胱自扩大术,因其题目过大、不够具体,欠醒目,有词不达意之嫌,如改为"膀胱自扩大术治疗高反射性神经源性膀胱"则使该文的题目更加鲜明和具体,读者能一目了然。

过于标新立异,有时也易失真实,应尽量去掉题目中的所谓"研究"、"观察"、"分析"或

"探讨"此类的惯加词和俗语。去掉这些字后,有时能使标题变得更加清晰。例如:标题"Bed-wetting in Chinese children: Epidemiology and predictive factors"没有提及任何多余的"study"、"evaluation"等词;而如"儿童和青少年原发性夜遗尿症患病率调查分析","调查分析"过于笼统,去掉这样的单词并改成"儿童和青少年原发性夜遗尿症患病率回顾性调查",加上"回顾性"便能突出这项研究的特点;又如"阴茎癌切除后阴茎再造术研究"就可省去"研究"而改为"阴茎癌切除后一期阴茎再造术"以突出笔者实施这项手术的治疗特色。

所谓"文要切题、题要得体"就是强调论文的标题应该紧扣主题,能够准确的表达论文的核心内容,实事求是地去反映该研究方向和深度,防止小题大做或容量小而冠以大标题。换句话说,就是要求撰稿时不要跑题。例如:标题"Family and segregation studies: 411 Chinese children with primary nocturnal enuresis",把文章研究的内容限定得很准确;又如把"硅橡胶套管人工腱的临床应用"修改成"硅橡胶套管人工腱移植修复手屈肌腱损伤 26 例",使得这篇论标题目更为主次分明、具体得当。

3. 简明扼要　标题,是用少量单词去尽可能概述论文的核心内容。从形式上来说,标题简短而且没有累赘。标题切忌使用模棱两可、含糊不清的词语,不用过于笼统的泛指性词语,更要切忌华而不实。

大多数烦琐超长标题里都有些多余的字,且常出现在标题的开始部分,如"observations"、"studies on"、"investigation"等。此外,放在标题开头部分的"A"、"An"、"The"等也是多余的。如有文章标题过大,使用上面的单词,翻译成中文一般就是如"……规律的探讨"、"……药物作用机制研究"。也有的题目虽短,内容过多(大)不符合实际情况也不合适,如标题"Genetic variants at 10p11 confer risk of tetralogy of fallot in Chinese of Nanjing"就不宜写成"Genetic variants at 10p11 confer risk of tetralogy of fallot in China",后者题目过大。该研究实际上写中国南京的研究,如果写成中国的研究则不切合实际。

但是,如果标题因为过短以至于过于笼统而没有表达出特异性内容也不合适。Robert A Day 在其知名论著《如何撰写和发表科技论文》中的举例"The role of antibiotics on bacteria",即"抗生素对细菌的作用",题目虽短,但过于笼统而没有表达出特异性内容。标题"Preliminary observation of a certain type of antibiotics on the role of a variety of bacteria"即"某一类抗生素对各种细菌的作用的初步观察",表达出了特异性内容,但又略显长了一些。

显然这个标题并不是说测定所有的抗生素对全部细菌的作用。那么,这个标题的意义是什么? 如果只研究一种或者几种抗生素,应该在标题中单独列出;如果只测试了抗生素对一种或者几种生物的作用,也应该在标题中单独列出;如果抗生素的种类或者生物体(这里指细菌)的种类过多,列在标题里过于冗长,则可以用一组名称来代替。例如,下面的标题就更恰当:

Action of Streptomycin on *Mycobacterium tuberculosis*
(链霉素对结核分枝杆菌的作用)

Action of Streptomycin, Neomycin, and Tetracycline on *Gram-Positive Bacteria*
(链霉素,新霉素和四环素对革兰氏阳性菌的作用)

Action of Polyene Antibiotics on *Plant-Pathogenic Bacteria*
(多烯类抗生素对植物病原菌的作用)

Action of Various Antifungal Antibiotics on *Candida albicans* and *Aspergillus fumigatus*
(各类抗真菌药物对白色念珠菌和烟曲霉的作用)

虽然这几个标题较之前过于简单的标题更能让人接受,但是这几个标题仍然不够完美,因为依然过于笼统。如果能够简单明确的定义这种"作用",那么标题的意思就明确了,例如:上面的第一个标题可以改为"链霉素对结核分枝杆菌的生长抑制作用"(Inhibition role of Streptomycin on *Mycobacterium tuberculosis*)。

(三)标题格式

1. 标题的位置 阅读一篇论文时,首先接触到的就是标题。标题理所当然应该位于全文之首,并用特殊的字体和字号表示,而不同的杂志有不同的要求,在此不用详列。为了帮助读者阅读,杂志的每一页的最上部都会印有"页头书名"或者是"页头标题",英文是 running title,即印在文章每一页(或每隔一页)上部的书名(或其缩写)。通常不同期刊杂志也有不同要求,多数杂志或者书名都印刷在每一页头的左侧,而文章或者章节的题目都印刷在页头的右侧。因为页头的空间有限,文章标题就需要缩写。因此在论文中确定一个页头标题是非常明智的。

2. 标题的长度 标题应该在紧扣主体思想的前提下,经过反复推敲提炼,删减掉"废"字,一般中文标题以 20 个字以内为宜,英文标题则以 10 个单词以内为宜。例如:美国 *Journal of the National Cancer Institute* 明文规定不得超过 14 个词,美国医学协会杂志 *Archives of Internal Medicine* 规定不能超过两行,包括副标题。下面是 *Blood* 杂志中读者须知对标题页的说明,其中明确规定了标题的长度 "article title; short title for the running head (not to exceed 50 characters, including spaces between words)",即题目,副标题以及单词之间的空格合计不超过 50 个字符。

题目要很具体的表达文章研究的内容和结果,使读者一目了然。标题一般不用缩写词,也不能用所从事研究的学科或分支学科的"类"、"目"作为标题,标题中尽量不使用标点符号。例如,我们被 *Scandinavian Journal of Urology and Nephrology* 杂志录用的一篇文章,题为 "Expression of renal aquaporins is down-regulated in children with congenital hydronephrosis"(先天性肾积水患儿肾脏水通道蛋白表达下调),题目具体表达了文章研究的内容和结果,使读者一目了然。一般来说标题不能过短,有一篇投稿细菌学杂志的文章标题则为 "Brucella research"(布鲁氏菌的研究)。很明显,这个标题对潜在的读者来讲没有多少的帮助。至少我们想知道这个研究是否是关于细菌分类学、基因学、生物化学抑或是临床研究。而标题过长更常见,例如,"对显微镜研究法补充一种物体和它底色之间或物体本身各部分间产生色差的新方法"若作为一篇论文的标题,实在过于烦琐、冗长,简直像一个摘要。

毫无疑问,过分冗长的标题都含有"垃圾"单词。标题中常可删掉非必要的冠词(a,an 和 the)及说明性"废词"。如 "the usage of disposable diaper usage increase the prevalence of nocturnal enuresis in mainland of China" 可以精简为 "Disposable diaper usage increase the nocturnal enuresis prevalence in mainland China"。另外还需注意避免标题中的词意重叠。当然,这些单词对于检索来讲也是毫无用处的。如果内容层次很多,难以选择简短化,最好使用主标题和副标题相互配合的方法。如 "Importance of replication in microarray gene expression studies: statistical methods and evidence from repetitive CDNA hybridizations (Proc Nat Acad Sci USA 2000 97 (18): 9834-9839)",其中副标题起到补充和阐明的作用。

3. 标题中的数字 除了作为"名词"或"形容词"的数字使用汉字或英文外,论文标题出现数据均要统一采用阿拉伯数字。例如:"创伤性十二指肠破裂 33 例的外科治疗"这个题目中"十二指肠"不用"12",而"33 例"不能写成"三十三例"。

4. **英文标题的书写方式**   标题的书写有两种方式:①标题中第一个单词的首字母大写,末尾不用句号。例如 "Diet and nutrition" 就只有第一个单词的首字母大写;②标题中每个词的第一个字母都大写,只有某些虚词才小写,例如 "Surgical Treatment of Hyperparathyroidism"除了虚词 of 之外,每一个词的首字母都需大写。冠词、三个字母以内的连词、介词都属于虚词都需要小写,但是四个字母以上的,如 with、from、after、before、during、against、between 等仍要用大写,例如 "Left Ventricular Function Before and Following Surgical Treatment of Mitral Valve Disease"。

5. **标题中的缩写与术语**   标题中几乎不能有缩写、化学式、专有(非一般)名称、术语等。在拟题的过程中,作者需要问自己:检索时我怎么才能得到这篇文章的信息? 如果文章的内容是关于盐酸(hydrochloric acid)的作用,那么标题中是用 hydrochloric acid 这个单词还是用它的缩写 HCL? 多数情况下我们都会用 hydrochloric acid 而不是 HCL 这个词来检索,而且,如果一些作者使用了 HCL(杂志编辑允许)而另外一些作者使用的却是 hydrochloric acid,书目服务的读者可能就只得到了部分这方面的著作,并没有注意到另外一些参考文献列在缩写的目录下。通过 Medline 网上检索我们需要的有关水通道蛋白 AQPs 的文章时,我们输入关键词 AQPs 能查到 392 篇文献报道,而输入 aquaporins 却能查到 3 955 篇文献。事实上我们在书写论文标题的时候,使用的都是 aquaporins,而不是缩写 AQPs,这也符合国际上大多数期刊杂志的要求。实际上,大的二级检索服务的计算机程序能够将诸如此类 hydrochloric acid 和 HCL 的文献总结到一起。但是目前作者和编辑最好避免在标题中使用缩写。当然这个规则包括专有名称、术语、不常见或者过时的术语。

(四)标题形式

1. **正标题**   正标题(main title)是指论文的总题目,亦称"总标题",与"副标题"和"层次标题"相互对称,表现形式则为单行标题,这种标题形式是大部分论文所采用的。例如:"Urine flow acceleration is superior to Qmax in diagnosing BOO in patients with BPH"(尿流加速度优于最大尿流率诊断前列腺增生患者膀胱出口梗阻),"The effect of unilateral ureteral obstruction on renal function in pigs measured by diffusion-weighed MRI"(磁共振弥散成像评估猪单侧输尿管梗阻对肾功能的影响)。需要明确:如果论文没有副标题及层次标题,则可将论文的正标题定为标题或者题目。而英语科研论文中并不主张用副标题,一般有正标题即可。例如 Berridge M J 的 "Inositol trisphosphate and calcium signaling"(三磷酸肌醇和钙信号表达)[*Nature*,1993,361(6410):315-325],该文被引用了 4 377 次。作者用 5 个单词简练、清晰地表达出论文的主题:inositol trisphosphate 与 calcium signaling。需要注意的是,作者使用 signal 的分词形式 signaling 较为准确地表述出论文内容 "Inositol trisphosphate is a second messenger that controls many cellular processes by generating internal calcium signals"(该文摘要的首句)。

2. **副标题**   副标题(sub-title)是指对正标题进行说明、补充或者加以限制性的标题。如遇到以下情况时可应用副标题:①正标题语意不明了,需补充说明其核心内容;②系列性报道文章、研究的课题需分阶段才能得到成果,需对其中心内容进行区别;③其他有必要进行说明和引申的。副标题被用来突出论文的特定内容,例如研究方法、病例数等。其格式为用冒号隔开正副标题。例如 "Long-term effects of partial unilateral ureter obstruction on renal

hemodynamic and morphology in newborn rats: a magnetic resonance imaging study"（新生鼠单侧输尿管梗阻对肾脏形态和局部血流的长期影响:磁共振成像研究）则用副标题突出研究方法。而副标题还具有很多功能,下面从杂志上摘抄一些例句显示副标题有以下几个方面的应用:

（1）突出病例数:Surgical treatment of pancreatic pseudocysts: Analysis of 119 cases（假性胰腺囊肿手术治疗——199 例分析）。此例中突出了研究的病例数——199 例,而且又补充说明正标题中必要的特定内容。

（2）突出研究方法:Diffuse pulmonary in filtrates in immunosuppressed patients: prospective study of 80 cases（免疫功能抑制患者弥漫性肺损害——前瞻性研究 80 例）。

（3）突出重点内容:Bed-Wetting in Chinese Children: Epidemiology and Predictive Factors（中国儿童的尿床率——流行病学与危险因素）。

（4）表示同位关系:Prazodine — A new vasodilator used for treatment of hypertension（哌唑嗪:一种新型血管扩张剂治疗高血压）。

（5）提出疑问:Unresolved issues: Do drinkers have less coronary heart disease?
（尚未解决的问题——饮酒者冠心病发生率少吗?）。

（6）表示长篇连载论文的各分篇主题:长篇形式论文分篇章发表时,一般以副标题表示分篇的内容,可在副标题前加罗马数字Ⅰ、Ⅱ、Ⅲ、Ⅳ、Ⅴ等,示为连续性。

Physical and chemical studies of human blood serum: Ⅰ. A study of normal subjects
（人类血清的理化研究:Ⅰ. 正常人研究）

Physical and chemical studies of human blood serum: Ⅱ. A study of 29 cases of nephritis
（人类血清的理化研究:Ⅱ. 29 例肾炎患者的研究）

Physical and chemical studies of human blood serum: Ⅲ. A study of miscellaneous disease conditions
（人类血清的理化研究:Ⅲ. 多种病例的研究）

四、标题的语法

（一）标题语法的重要性

应用简明扼要的标题不能缺少正确的语法,或者是标题中每个单词的具体形式。例如"生物学的新比色标准"主要是叙述动植物标本的颜色规格的发展。但是,标题"生物学家的新颜色标准"（*Bioscience* 27:762,1977）是说这种新的标准对生物学家的分类学有用,使得我们能将他们分为绿色生物学家和蓝色生物学家。

标题中引起歧义的常见错误是语法（单词顺序）错误。标题中应该尤其注意语法,标题中最常见的语法错误是由单词错误引起的。

一篇投稿到《细菌学》杂志文章的标题为 "Mechanism of Suppression of Nontransmissible Pneumonia in Mice Induced by Newcastle Disease Virus"（鼠非传染性新城疫病毒肺炎的抑制机制）,除非作者某些时候指出了物种的起源,否则无法表明肺炎是由鼠新城疫病毒引起而不是导致鼠发病的原因。这个标题应该改为 "Mechanism of Suppression of Nontransmissible Pneumonia Induced in Mice by Newcastle Disease Virus"（新城疫病毒导致鼠非传染性肺炎

的抑制机制）。这里再列举一个论文标题"Wistar rat and evaluation of immune response after moderate and overtraining exercise"显然应该写成"Evaluation of immune response after moderate and overtraining exercise in wistar rat"。

写作时用到"use"这个词时要认真斟酌。有一篇文章让人很迷惑，题目为"Using a fiberoptic bronchoscope, dogs were immunized with sheep red blood cells"（狗应用纤维支气管镜，对绵羊红细胞免疫），显然"use"这个词没有用对。

（二）标题的语法

文章的标题就是一个标签，而不是一个句子。正因为标题不是一个句子，因此不会出现主语、谓语、宾语这些严格的排列，通常标题都较句子简单（或者至少较句子短）。正因为如此，标题中单词的顺序更为重要。

有少数杂志允许标题是一个完整的句子，例如标题"Oct-3 is a maternal factor required for the first mouse embryonic division"（Cell 64：1103，1991）。有两个理由反对这个标题。首先，系动词 is 是一个"垃圾单词"。在这里完全可以删去而不会影响题目的意思；其次，含有 is 使这个标题看起来像一个结论。有一个规律是我们不习惯作者将他的结论以现在时态写出来。Rosner（1990 年）将这种标题定义为"陈述句（肯定句）标题"（assertive sentence title），列举了众多原因来说明这种标题不可取。不合适的、轻率的"陈述句标题"更不可取，这是因为在某些情况下，"陈述句标题"已经有了结论，但是同时又在摘要或者其他地方得出了其他不确定的结论。

标题中单词的含义和顺序对浏览杂志目录的读者来讲尤为重要。因此，标题要适合如化学索引，医学索引或者其他检索的格式。多数的检索或者文摘服务都依赖于"关键词"系统，分为上下文内关键词，上下文外关键词。因此，提供正确的关键词极其重要，也就是说，标题中的词必须是能够反映文章亮点而且要能够为读者所理解，并且容易检索。例如"Bed-Wetting in Chinese Children: Epidemiology and Predictive Factors"（中国儿童的尿床率：流行病学与危险因素），就很好地反映出文章的要点：bed-wetting（尿床）；epidemiology（流行病学）；predictive factors（危险因素）。

标题是由名词性质的短语构成。如果出现了动词，大多是分词或者动名词形式。由于陈述性标题常常具有判断式的语意，一般语句会显得不够简洁，因此，大部分的编辑和学者会认为标题不应该由陈述句构成。因为标题比句子简练，无须注意主、谓、宾，所以词序的重要性就凸显出来了，尤其要注意的是词语之间的修饰关系，如果使用不当，会影响读者对标题的正确理解。例如"Isolation of antigens from monkeys using complement-fixation techniques"，会使读者误解为"猴子使用了补体结合技术"。应改为"Using complement-fixation techniques in isolation of antigens from monkeys"（用补体结合技术从猴体中分离抗原）。此外，读者一般不习惯作者使用现在时来表达研究成果，而陈述形式的标题又显得武断，因此其作为标题可大胆地提出结论，但是在总结时或者在正文中却常常以探讨性质的论证出现。有时候可以使用疑问句型作为标题，如探讨性质的疑问句型标题应用于评论性论文的标题中会显得比较生动，易吸引读者兴趣。如"When is a bird not a bird?"（*Nature* 1998 393：729-730）；"Should the K-Ar isotopic ages of olivine basalt be reconsidered?"［*Chinese Science Bulletin* 1998 43（19）：1670-1671］等，生动且切题。

多数英文标题使用单部句，一般有如下特点。

1. 标题一般选择单部句　即由一个名词或者多个并列名词,加上必要性的修饰语构成,一般不含谓语成分,如:

Haemorrhagic cholecystitis

(出血性的胆囊炎)

Myocardial infarction, Alcohol use, sudden cardiac death, and hypertension

(心肌梗死、饮酒、心源性猝死及高血压病)

以上例句均为单部句,省略了谓语。部分医学杂志,如美国的 *Journal of the National Cancer Institute* 甚至规定了标题不可以写完整的句子。

2. 偶尔可见标题为双部句　双部句即"主谓句",但句尾没句号。例如:

Dietary cholesterol is co-carcinogenic for human colon cancer

(胆固醇饮食对人类结肠癌具有协同致癌作用)

Cytochrome b is present in neutrophils from patients with chronic granulomatous disease

(慢性肉芽肿患者中中性粒细胞中存在细胞色素 b)

上述两例均为双部句,但没有标点符号。

3. 标题也可用疑问句句式　疑问句可是单部句或双部句。句尾一般是疑问号,如果使用了疑问代词或者疑问副词,可省略疑问号。

单部句示例:

Home or hospital births?

(家庭还是医院分娩?)

What to look for in rib fracture and how

(肋骨骨折时应注意的问题及治疗方案)

双部句示例:

Is treatment of borderline hypertension good or bad?

(治疗临界型高血压的利与弊)

What does exercise mean for menstrual cycle?

(锻炼对月经周期有什么影响)

五、英语标题的特点

首先,让我们比较以下两组英文标题:

第一组

(1) Oral immunization of mice with at tenuated Salmonnella typhimurium expressing Helicobacterpylori urease B subunit

(2) Multivariate analysis by Cox Proportional Hazards Model on prognoses of patients with bile duct carcinoma after resection

第二组

(1) Establishment, safety and efficiency of attenuated Salmonella typhimurium expressing Helicobacterpylori urease B subunit as an oral vaccine in mice

(2) Influence of various clinicopathologic factors on the survival of patients with bile duct carcinoma after curative resection: a multivariate analysis

　　这两例都是描述性标题。通过比较,我们发现,于同一篇论文来讲,第二组标题更加清楚明了。比如对题目(1)在第一组中表达,我们只了解在该研究中,对小鼠进行的免疫方法是口服,但是为什么要实验,是针对小鼠还是针对疫苗的进一步研究就不甚明了。而在第二组标题中,我们一眼便可清楚,该研究是以小鼠作为研究对象观察研究某口服疫苗使用中的安全性及有效性。对这项研究有兴趣的读者可选择继续阅读论文,不感兴趣的读者则会弃读。例题(2)也存在同样的问题。

　　在上述英标题目的写作中,还体现出以下几条相同的原则:

　　(1)重要内容前置原则:像 detection、effect、establishment 等所引导的短语大多是研究的核心内容。

　　(2)研究对象明确原则:需注意的是,细胞或实验动物等都应在研究对象里,应该在此交代清楚,不能省略或简化。如果是来自于人体,研究对象则可省略不提。但出自某特殊人群,如某地理环境,或者某患病群体等,则需注明 human 或 patient 等词。

　　(3)研究方法随意原则:事实上,可以反映研究内容的一个重要方面就是研究方法,但因标题字数常常是有限制的,研究方法与其他重要指标相比略弱些,在书写标题时,研究方法是否忽略,应视情况而定。假如需列出,则不放在开头,置于标题的中间或者末尾[英文标题(2)]。

　　在 18 世纪,科技论文(英语版)标题喜欢采用"Some thought of …","A few observations on …"的格式,而现在已经很少用了。如今的科技论文越来越趋向简短扼要,而上述句式并无实质性内容,即所谓的"垃圾单词",甚至"Investigation of …","Study of …","A report of …"这样的句式也并不多见。例如:"Cystometry in infants and children with no apparent voiding symptoms"(无排尿异常婴幼儿的膀胱测压)。在上例中就省略了"观察"、"研究"、"分析"、"报告"等垃圾单词,同样在汉语标题中也要省略这些。另外,值得注意的是,在标题中冠词一般是省略的,这在中文和英文标题中都是一样的。比如上例,就在 Cystometry 前省略了冠词 the。

　　不同民族语言具有不同形式的表达方法,科技论文方面,汉语和英语的描述方式有许多相同之处,也有许多不同的地方。而英语科技论文的标题又有着它自身的特点。例如带"as"的句式怎样翻译,病例数的表达又怎样处理,这些都将在下面详细介绍。

　　(1)带 as 的句式:科技论文(英语)的标题中不用有主系表的句型,需要表示"是"这个概念时,常常用带 as 的句型。例如 "Gastrocolic fistula as a complication of benign gastric ulcer"(胃结肠瘘是为良性溃疡的并发症)。

　　(2)病例数的处理:在我国医学论文中,为达到吸引读者的目的,有很多将病例数放于正标题中,而很少用副标题,而在英语论文的标题中应该怎样表达,在下面列举实例以说明。例如 "Analysis of 80 cases of SLE"(系统性红斑狼疮 80 例分析)用"of … cases"这样的句式可以表达。另外还有用更巧妙的方法突出病例数的例子,例如 "Family and segregation studies on 411 Chinese children with nocturnal enuresis"(411 例遗尿症儿童和青少年的家族史和家系分析)。而在国外,病例数大多放在副标题中。所以在翻译为英文时,最好用副标题。

　　(3)"原因"的表达方式:标题中如果需要表示原因,一般用 due to,而不用 owing to 或 because of,有时也可用 caused by 代替。例如:"Bacteremia due to gram-negative bacilli"(革兰氏阴性菌菌血症)。

（4）汉语标题中常用词的译法

1）"探讨"的译法：表达"探讨"的词有 evaluation，discussion，study，approach，investigation 等。

Discussion on experimental pulmonary insufficiency（实验性肺动脉瓣闭锁不全的探讨）

An evaluation of treatment for fracture of patella by combined Chinese traditional and Western medicine（中西医结合治疗髌骨骨折的探讨）

"探讨"用介词 on 来表达这个概念。如：On clinical diagnosis of primary carcinoma of liver（原发性肝癌临床诊断的探讨）

一般情况下，"探讨"一词可以省略不译。如：A simplified scheme of diagnosing and treating rickets in children（佝偻病简易诊治标准的探讨）

2）"体会"的译法："体会"译为 experience

Experience in treating 818 patients with diabetes mellitus（818 例糖尿病患者治疗体会）

在美、英杂志中，experience 常与介词 with 配合，可直接和疾病名称一起用，不需要加"治疗"一词，如：

Recent experiences with bacillemia due to gram negative organisms（治疗革兰氏阴性杆菌菌血症的新体会）

"体会"一词也可忽略不译，如：

Tumor and tumor-like hyperplasia complications of chronic hepatitis and their Chinese traditional treatment（迁延型肝炎合并瘤或瘤样增生及中医治疗的体会）

3）"总结"的译法：

"总结"一词常用 experience 表达

Renal embryonal carcinosarcoma（Wilms' tumor）：A twenty years' clinical experience（肾胚胎瘤 20 年临床资料总结）

"总结"一词也可删去不译。如：

Operative treatment of congenital heart diseases in childhood: Analysis of 464 cases（464 例小儿先天性心血管手术总结）

4）"问题"的译法："问题"一词可译成 problem 或者 aspect。

Certain problems of total parenteral nutrition in clinical practice（完全肠道外营养实践中的几个问题）

Some aspects on surgical treatment of portal hypertension（关于门脉高压症外科手术的几个问题）

5）"初步"的译法：我国医学论文中的标题带有表示谦虚意思的词语，如"初步研究""初步分析""初步应用""初步观察""初步报告""初步小结""初步体会"等字眼。这种句式在国外标题中较为少见。按照欧美人的观点讲，科技论文实质便是事实材料，不必要谦虚客套。译法如下。

A preliminary report on anesthesia for liver transplantation（肝移植术麻醉的初步报告）

表示谦虚的字眼往往可略去不译，如：

Electron microscopic observation on the transformed lymphocytes（转化淋巴细胞的电子显微镜观察初步报告）

The etiological investigation of myocarditis among children in Shanghai（上海地区小儿心肌炎病因学的初步研究）

（5）常用词（组）和表达方式

1）用……（手段 / 方法）对……进行研究 / 观察 / 评价 / 分析

study (analysis/evaluation/observation/assessment) of (on) ... (by) using（by 方法 /with 工具）...

e.g. In vivo study of pituitary enlargement in normal pregnancy using magnetic resonance imaging。

2）A 对 B 的作用：effect of A on B

e.g. Immunomodulatory effect of alkaloid sinomenine on the mouse acute graft versus host disease (aGVHD) model

3）A 与 B 的相关性（关系）：correlation (relation/relationship) between A and B，there be correlation of A with B and C, there be A (be) correlated with B

常用修饰词：positively（正）/negatively（负）/significantly（明显）/insignificantly（不明显）/ strongly（很大）/little（很小）

e.g. Positive correlation of CD44v6 expression with invasion and metastasis of human gastric cancer

4）用……治疗……：use of ... in the treatment of ...（病）in ...（生物）

e.g. Use of sulphamethizole in the treatment of urinary tract infection in the elderly

5）A 是 B：A as B

e.g. Thyroid cancer as a late consequence of head-neck irradiation

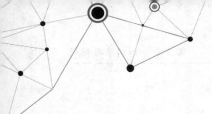

第3章
作者和作者单位地址

Chapter 3
Authors and Their Addresses

第一节　作　者　署　名

作者署名（authorship）是科技论文本身必要的组成部分，署名的意义在于明确论文由谁负责。它是作者对科学事业所付出辛勤劳动应得的荣誉，也是对作者的贡献和权力的尊重，对作者著作权的尊重，同时也满足文献检索的需要。一旦科技论文上签署作者姓名，即为该论文著作权人，著作权受法律保护。

一、署名的意义

署名的意义可归纳总结为以下 5 项。

（一）署名作为拥有著作权的声明

《中华人民共和国著作权法》规定：著作权属于作者。作者的著作权包括发表权、修改权、署名权和保护作品的完整权等。署名除了表明该论文的著作权只属于作者外，也是作者劳动成果被社会尊重和认可的前提条件。

（二）署名表示文责自负的承诺

所谓的文责自负，就是该论文已经发表，作者便对论文负有学术上、道义上、政治上和法律上的责任，如果该论文存在剽窃或抄袭现象，或者是在政治上、技术上和学术理论上存在错误，署名者就要完全负起责任。因此，署名则表明作者是愿意承担上述责任的。

（三）署名便于读者与作者进行联系

若读者针对于该论文中有学术上的问题想和作者商榷、咨询甚至是质疑，则通过署名便可以直接联系到作者。因此，署名则表明作者是愿意与读者联系的。

（四）署名为文献资料的重要检索信息

在数据库中作者的姓名是重要信息源和检索信息。因此，查阅署名便为查阅文献资料、提供了重要的依据和检索信息。

（五）署名人地址

论文中的署名地址、所在单位是对署名人成果、荣誉等评定的依据，也是对署名人个人学术水平认定的依据。

二、署名的原则

国际上公认的对"作者"的定义是："Only those who actively contributed to the overall design and execution of the experiments are included. The authors should be listed in order of importance to the experiments."。具体内容包括以下几个方面。

（一）根据对论文科研贡献大小决定是否署名——坚持实事求是的原则

科技论文中可集体署名，也可署名个人。个人署名时要突显出创造性，需尊重客观事实，根据论文写作给予的贡献大小来决定作者署名的顺序。国际标准 GB7713-87《科学技术报告，学位论文和学术论文的编写格式》对科技论文的作者署名条件的规定：学术论文的正文前署名的个人作者，只限于那些设计研究课题和制定研究方案，直接参加全部或主要部分研究工作并做出贡献，以及参加撰写论文并能对内容负责的人，按其贡献大小排列名次。至于参加部分工作的合作者、按研究计划分工负责具体小项的工作者、某一项测试的承担者，以及接受委托进行分析检验和观察的辅助人员等不得列入。这些人可以作为参加工作的人员列入致谢部分。上述规章制度建立于以下原则上。

1. 署名必须是做出了较大贡献者。

2. 循名责实的原则：署名应循名责实，不可以只图其名，而不符合其实，一定得是名副其实。

3. 文责自负的原则：只要是作者在论文上署名了就要能对论文内容负责，即为"文责自负"的原则。如不能负责、不能解释该论文的人是不可以在论文上署名的。

因此，论文的署名者应具备以下 3 个条件：

1. 参与课题研究的部分或全部工作，且做出了主要贡献者；

2. 论文的主要撰写者；

3. 能对论文修回时提出的问题做出满意回答，而且是论文的主要责任者。

美国《内科学记事》编辑部规定作者署名的 5 个条件，这些条件有：

1. 必须要参加与该项研究的设计及开创工作，如是后期才参与该工作，必须认可前期的所有研究和设计；

2. 必须要参加该论文中的某项获取数据和观察者的工作；

3. 必须要参加实验工作、观察实验对象或者对获取的数据能作出合理解释，并可得出论文的最后结论；

4. 必须要参与论文的撰写工作或讨论工作；

5. 必须阅读过该论文的全文，并同意将其发表。

而"Uniform Requirements for Manuscripts Submitted to Biomedical Journals: Ethical Considerations in the Conduct and Reporting of Research: Authorship and Contributorship"一文中也指出："Authorship credit should be based on ① substantial contributions to conception and design, acquisition of data, or analysis and interpretation of data; ② drafting the article or revising it critically for important intellectual content; and ③ final approval of the version to be published. Authors should meet conditions ① , ② and ③ ."。

实事求是是署名的重要原则,它是署名原则中其他原则的前提和基础。而对于该研究有贡献但不满足作者条件的贡献者,可以放在文章后的致谢部分。

(二)杜绝弄虚作假的原则

如今的社会崇尚知识、重视科技性人才,科技论文不仅可以展现出作者的科研能力,也是专业职称晋升的重要砝码。但是,科技论文的署名也存在很多弄虚作假的现象。

针对各种不当署名,要大力宣扬科学道德规范,牢记严谨务实的科学态度,按贡献大小合理署名,为了避免署名争议,可提前商定署名问题,编辑也要本着对作者负责、对期刊负责、对社会负责的态度认真履行编辑的责任,而各单位科技主管部门也要认真负责,严格把关。

关于科技论文的署名有一种错误观点需要纠正,即第一作者享有论文的绝对的著作权,可以完全凭自己意愿处置署名权。实际上著作权并不完全属于第一作者,所有的署名者都拥有著作权。因此,第一作者没有对署名权进行处置的权利,必须要按照《著作权法》的署名条件来决定是否署名,按照对论文的实际贡献大小确定署名的次序。

(三)将致谢对象和作者严格区别的原则

需确定论文的署名者时,必须将致谢对象和作者加以区别。那些对全面工作并不了解,且仅仅只参加了部分工作的人,或者只是课题研究组的成员,参加了部分研究或者实际工作,但此工作只是辅助性的,均不可列为作者。他们虽达不到署名的条件,但也对该研究成果做出了贡献。因此,要列为致谢对象。

(四)署名应署真名的原则

根据《著作权法》规定,署名可署真名,也可署化名。但因科技论文的发表牵扯到实际的科研成果归属和收益权的问题,科技论文如果没有特殊原因,均应该签署真实姓名。共同完成科技论文的作者在进行作者署名时,除了应署真实姓名外,还应该按对论文付出的贡献大小来进行排序。第一作者必须是论文的直接创作者和主要贡献者,同时也应该对论文负直接责任,如无特别声明,第一作者应享有第一权利,同时承担首要责任,履行第一义务。

三、作者署名的格式

(一)欧美人名署名

欧美人的 name 既指名,也指姓。first name 指名字,last name 指姓,还有 family name 和 surname,都和 last name 一样指姓。如诺贝尔的姓名全称 Alfred Bernhard Nobel,Alfred 为 first name,Bernhard 是 middle name,等同于我国的名,Nobel 是 last name,等同于我国的姓。也有只有 first name 无 second name 的情况,如爱因斯坦的姓名全称是 Albert Einstein。由此可知,欧美人的姓名书写次序与我国刚好相反,先名后姓。在论文上署名时,一般将 first name 与 last name 书写全文,而 middle name 缩写,例如:Alfred B. Nobel。

如今科学上有一种错误的发展趋势,作者仅仅使用名字的大写字母,如果这样继续下去那么科学文献可能会变得混乱。例如这里有两个称为 Jonathan B. Jones 的作者,那么文献查询系统很可能按照不同地址将他们区分开来,但是如果有些 Jonathan B. Jones 以 J. B. Jones 的名字来发表论文,而另外一些 Jonathan B. Jones 使用 Jonathan B. Jones 发表文章,或者同一个 Jonathan B. Jones 有时用 Jonathan B. Jones,有时用 J. B. Jones 发表文章,那么检索系统必定会变得混乱。

另外很多国外科学家由于结婚、宗教或法律要求等原因要改变他们的姓,如女科学家在结婚后要用丈夫的姓,这在作者署名上也造成很多的麻烦,所以很多科学家很排斥改变他们的姓名,以确保让他人和自己容易区分出版的论文。因而,很多科学家都沿用在变更以前的姓名来署名,这在大多数杂志的投稿须知中没有明确的规定。

目前许多数字化图书馆的目录和文献检索系统依据截词原则进行检索。因此,不必键入一个长的题目或一个完整的名字,而是通过缩写登记来节约时间。但是,如果某个人名为 Day, RA,搜索后将出现所有 Rachel Days、Ralph Days 和 Raymond Days 等表示的名称,但不是要查的作者 Robert A. Day。因此,不用全名而使用缩写可能引起一些筛选的麻烦。

（二）中国人名在中文文章的英语摘要中署名

中文期刊的英文摘要中,中国人的姓名要按照汉语拼音对应的字母翻译为英文,例如"吕布"即翻译为 Lv Bu;"文建国"则翻译为 Wen Jianguo 或 Wen Jian-guo,而双名和双姓在其中间是否加入连字符即"-",在不同的杂志有不同的习惯,却没有固定的格式。例如:《中华泌尿外科杂志》和《中华实用儿科临床杂志》中"文建国"多翻译为 Wen Jian-guo。而有些杂志中也用名在前姓在后的格式,例如"文建国"则翻译为 Jianguo Wen 或 Jian-guo Wen 甚至应用缩写,这就和下面讨论的中国人名在英语文章中的署名相同。然而,在中文论文中英文摘要中的姓名一般不参与检索的功能,所以并不重要。

（三）中国人名在英语文章中的署名

以现如今科技文献出版的情况而言,中国作者署名的形式有以下三类:

第一类为中国式姓名的传统表述形式,即汉语拼音全部拼写完整,姓于名前,姓与名中间有空格,双字之间不用加连字符,只有首字母大写。比如:"李四光"写为 Li Siguang。由于西方英文媒体报道中国越来越多,该表述的使用频率也呈上升趋势。比如:习近平、胡锦涛等中国领导人在英文报道中普遍以 Xi Jinping、Hu Jintao 的形式出现,这与我国出版的英文报纸、杂志保持一致,也可以减少中国姓名误报的概率。但该表述也有突出的缺陷,毕竟普通科技工作者是不能与领袖人物相比知名度的。如果作者粗心在校样阶段时并未注意署名,可能出现名变成姓,姓变成名的现象,导致一系列错误和麻烦,尤其在检索和查询时。因此,上述署名在英文科技论文中并不常见。

第二类表述采用了西方姓名的表述习惯,即名在姓前。这一类表述形式又分成四种:一是采用全名,即单或双字名将汉语拼音全拼出,双字之间不用加连字符,比如:"李四光"表述为 Siguang Li;二是用全名,但双字名之间加连字符连接,每个字的首字母大写,比如:Si-Guang Li;三也是用全名,双字名中间也用连字符相连,但第二个字的首字母小写,如 Si-guang Li。严格地讲第三种用法并不规范,因为连字符连接的部分应对称。但一般英文期刊编辑及出版社对此并不予计较。总体而言,这种表述保留了中国作者署名的完整性,便于通讯联系。尤其双字名加短线的用法,强调出这部分是名,而不是姓。在排版过程中可减少错误率,在姓名索引时比较容易排列正确。但也有缺点,主要是单字姓名出错率比较高,在排版时名和姓容易混淆。第四种,就是将双名的两个名分开写,不加短线连接,首字母均大写,如 Si Guang Li,目前这种应用在英文杂志中越来越普遍。因为在投稿时候写成 Si Guang Li,在杂志刊登后检索时,很多杂志将在检索工具中自动将姓名简写成 Li SG,这就更符合中国人姓名书写的习惯。如果姓名写成 Siguang Li,最后刊登后查询就会发现简写成 Li S。

第三类是按西方的姓名顺序,名在姓前,但名不用全拼,只用缩写。这一类表述也有三种缩写形式:一是不论单或双字字名,都只要拼音的首字母,即"李四光"表述为 SG. Li;二是双字名均需取首字母,之间用连字符连接,两个首字母均要大写,外加缩写点,如 S.-G. Li;三是双字名的第一个字首字母大写,第二个字的首字母小写,中间用连字符连接,如 S.-g. Li。该表述笔者认为并不完全正确,理由如上所述,应该避免。字母缩写的表述形式,在英文期刊中比较普遍出现,也是发表英文期刊的风格之一。该表述的优点是不论是编辑还是排版的工作者均可一目了然地判断出姓与名,解决了外国人最头痛的难题,判断中国人姓名。

现在,中国人名在英文文章中的署名并没有太大的问题,因为大多数杂志都有网上投稿系统,在网上投稿系统中"作者"这一项有专门的对话框,分别列出 first name、second name 和 last name 项。只要分别填写,杂志编辑就会按要求署名。但有些没有 second name 项的,则只能将姓名写在一起。

欧美人姓名的格式在前面已经讨论,而中国人名在投稿时一般采用姓在前,全大写;名在后,首字母大写,姓与名应分开写,而双姓与双名不必分开,中间也不必加连字符,但笔者建议双名分开写,并且名的首字母均大写,下面举例说明。例如:"文建国"在投稿时按照汉语拼音翻译为 WEN Jian-guo 或 WEN Jianguo。而按照欧美期刊在发表论文时常要保持与欧美人的习惯相同,即把 WEN 后置,作为 last name,而 Jianguo 或者 Jian-guo 作为 first name。然而这样就会出现问题,即在检索时,参考文献中的缩写就会为 J Wen,如果还有一位叫作"文君"的科学家发表文章也会出现 J Wen 的缩写就会搞混,检索系统就会出现类似于前面讨论过的欧美人姓名简写时的情况。要想尽量避免这种情况,笔者建议用含 second name 形式的姓名署名即用 Jian Guo WEN 的名字投稿,这样发表文章后在检索系统中简写就为 Wen JG。从而尽量减少名字的重复,也方便读者的查阅。这种写法就是我们上面说到的第二类第 4 种姓名的写法。

(四)作者署名的各种称谓(M.D 或者 MD)

一般来说,科学期刊不在作者名字之后添加学位或头衔(BS、MS、PhD、MD)。但是部分医学期刊在作者名字后注明学位。有医学期刊也列出头衔,或者位于名字和学位后,或者在题目页的脚注中。投稿人可以参考期刊的作者投稿说明,或者参照最近一份期刊中有关作者投稿的说明。

英、美医学杂志中,论文作者的姓名之后附有学位的格式为姓名之后用逗号隔开再加上学位缩写。如:

S. Francis, MD(S. Francis 医学博士)

Joseph L. Gerry, MD(Joseph L. Gerry 医学博士)

有时还可同时附有几个学位。如:

Roger R. Dozois, MD, PhD(Roger R. Dozois 医学博士,哲学博士)

常见的学位名称有：

Bachelor of Medicine［医学学士，M. B.（MB）］

Magister Chirurgiae［外科硕士，M. C.（MC）］

Master of Surgery［外科硕士，M. S.（MS）］

Doctor of Medicine［医学博士，M. D.（MD）］

Bachelor of Arts［文学学士，B. A.（BA）］

Master of science［理学硕士，M. Sc.（MSc）］

Doctor of philosophy［哲学博士，Ph. D.（PhD）］

除学位外，作者姓名之后还可附有"某学会会员"的缩写词，这是因为这些学会在国际上享有较高声誉。如：

John F. Goodwin，MD，FRCP［Fellow of the Royal College of Physicians 皇家内科医师学会（特别）会员］。

四、作者顺序的确定

（一）作者顺序确定的基本原则

根据上述作者署名原则来确定作者的排列顺序。作者应该只包括那些积极参与整体设计和具体实验操作的人员。排序通常将按照其在实验中的重要性来排列。第一作者为论文的主要撰写者，对论文负主要责任。第二作者是主要的协作人员，第三作者可能等同于第二作者，但是很可能参与论文研究相对较少。如果没有参与相关研究就不能询问在原稿中是否有他们的名字，也不应该允许他们名字出现在自己没有密切参与的论文研究中。下面介绍一下当前存在的一些作者排序模式。

"如果你有合作者，那么有关作者顺序问题需要按照对文章的贡献排列"（O'Connor，1991）。有时候，准备科学论文最容易的部分就是作者署名和单位，而且很少听到因为作者排列顺序而争论的，但是也可能因为不同意谁的名字被列出或不同意以什么顺序来排列作者，而使通力协作的团队之间出现矛盾。那么什么是正确合理的作者次序呢？不幸的是目前没有一致的规定或普遍接受的协议，一些期刊（主要是英国）需要作者按照字母顺序列出，像这样一个简单无意义的排序系统值得推荐。但是，按字母排序作者还不是很普及，尤其在美国。

过去，一般习惯于把实验室主任作为合作者，不论他或她是否积极参与研究。通常，主任在最后列出（两名作者中第二位，三名作者中第三位，等等）。结果看上去就是以获取一定的声望为主要目的。然而，如果只有两位作者，而他们既不是实验室主任也不是资深教授，那么两人势必会争夺后面的位置。如果这里存在三名或更多的作者，那么"重要"作者将喜欢在第一或最后的位置，而不是中间位置。以发表在《新英格兰医学杂志》的一篇有关三聚氰胺有毒奶粉的文章"Melamine-contaminated powdered formula and urolithiasis in young children"为例，能被影响因子全球排名前三的杂志接受发表，我们可以想象这篇文章的作者序列的确定可能会异常艰难，特别是第一、第二作者的顺序问题。可是我们发现作者在文章的旁边是这样注明的："Dr. Guan and Fan contributed equally to this article."。即第一作者和第二作者对本文的贡献是一样的。于是有效地解决了第一作者和第二作者的潜在矛盾，此方案值得大家借鉴。

现在倾向于使用"详细列出名单"的方法,实事求是地标注实验室中每个人,包括在试验结束后清洁试管的技术人员。因此,每篇论文作者的平均数量呈现出增加的趋势。

不可否认的是,这一问题的解决并不容易。通常计算一篇论文智力方面的投入是很困难的。一起工作数月或数年来解决同一研究问题的人员很难记得谁是参与研究的原创人员或者是谁的观点对实验成功起到关键作用,而且这些同事做什么。出版文献中列出的每名作者应在所发表的论文中做出重要贡献,"重要"一词指的是在原创科学论著中有创造性的贡献。

高水平科研人员不会允许增加一些贡献微小的人员而削弱了自己的工作价值,也不会允许增加很多无足轻重的人来损害自己的名声。

简而言之,科学论文应该仅仅列出那些对工作有实质性帮助的作者。下面举例说明如何有效地确定一篇科研论文的作者序列。

(二)如何确定作者次序

下面的例子将有助于从概念水平或应该涉及原作者的专业水平上来进行阐明。假设科学家 A 设计了一系列可能导致重要新发现的试验,然后科学家 A 详细告诉技术人员 B 如何进行这些试验。如果试验得出结果,并给予出版,那么科学家 A 将是唯一作者,即使技术人员 B 做了全部工作(当然,技术人员 B 的贡献将在致谢中得到认可)。

现在,让我们假设上述试验没有得出结论,那么技术人员 B 给科学家 A 得出一个无效结果,而且可能类似于"我认为如果改变孵化温度从 24℃到 37℃,同时增加人血白蛋白到介质中,那么可能促进菌株生长",科学家 A 同意这一改变,而且试验期间产生令人兴奋的结果,在这一情况下,发表文章时应该同时列出科学家 A 和技术人员 B。

让我们把这一例子往前再推进一步。假如这一试验在 37℃ 和增加人血白蛋白的情况下出现一个结果,但是科学家 A 认为目前这一结果的改变是不彻底的;换句话说,该条件下的生长显示该测试物是一个病原体,但是先前出版文献显示这一有机物是非病原体,那么科学家 A 现在将请求病原微生物学专家的同事科学家 C 来测试这一有机物的病原性,科学家 C 按照任何医学生物学家使用的标准程序给实验室小鼠注射检查物来进行快速检测并证实病原性,然后把一条简短但很重要的句子添加到原稿中,之后这一稿件被发表,那么科学家 A 和技术人员 B 将以作者列出,而科学家 C 的帮助将在致谢中注明。但是,假如科学家 C 对这一特殊菌株感兴趣的话,而且从一系列设计较好的试验中获益,并且得出这一特殊菌株不仅仅存在致病鼠中,而且是长久以来在某些人类罕见疾病中寻找的罪魁祸首。因此,有两项新的数据表增加到原稿中,同时结果和讨论给予重写。然后,这一论文出版时将列出科学家 A、技术人员 B 和科学家 C 作为作者(一些情况下将把科学家 C 作为第二作者)。

五、通讯作者

通讯作者(corresponding author)是研究论文的指导者,负责选题、实验设计和选择研究的先进性及使用首创性方法的合理性、结论的可信性、负责科研经费的申请和回答读者的提问。读者有质疑或咨询时,首先应该和通讯作者联系反映意见。和第一作者不同是,通讯作者不用直接在第一线操作,但是都对原始数据的真伪负有一定责任,但不是负首要责任。而论文的第一作者必须是第一线操作的实施者和原始数据的收集和处理人,又是初稿的执笔人。因此,第一作者要对研究结果和数据的真实性负首要责任。研究生导师一般是通讯作者,研究生论文的第一作者必须是研究生本人,而不是导师或领导。作为通讯作者有责任指导第一作者严格把好文章署名的关。在本人未参加实验又未曾看过本论文稿件下,其姓名不得写到作者的行列中。

另一单位合作从事了文章中的某一部分检测并提供了数据的人应该而且必须成为作者之一,并注明该作者的工作单位,以示同意负相应责任。每一位作者都要对本文的结果、结论负有责任。

杂志特邀有权威性的专家亲笔撰写专评(Editorial)或综述,第一作者和通讯作者当然是同一人。这一点和一般的研究论文不同。这样的特邀专家作为第一作者自己是高级或副高级职称,又亲自选题,在第一线做实验研究,亲自撰写论文,这样由一人兼任第一作者和通讯作者是符合实际的。这些观点可以在中国实验血液学杂志编辑部的文章《维护第一作者和通讯作者的责任和尊严》(中国实验血液学杂志 J Exp Hema tol 2010;18(4):862)查到。

按照国际惯例,有关稿件的一切事宜均联系通讯作者(corresponding author),国内多数期刊也启用该惯例。通讯作者并非只是起到通讯联系作用,而是论文的责任作者,对论文负全责,一般应是论文的指导者,研究生导师或课题负责人。通讯作者一般为一位,特殊情况下可以有两位。一般在论文标题页(title page)标明通讯作者的联系电话、E-mail 及地址等。就对论文的责任而言,通讯作者高于第一作者。

下面这段话是《欧洲泌尿外科》杂志对通讯作者的标注(图 3-1),这些要求可以在作者须知部分查阅。通讯作者列出了姓名、工作单位、联系方式和 E-mail。

☆ This study was supported by "The Innovation and Talent Research Foundation of Henan Province China (0221002000)", "Henan Innovation Project For University Prominent Research Talents (HAIPURT) (2001KYCX004)"and "National Natural Science Foundation of China (NSFC) (30571931)"
* Corresponding author. Pediatric Urodynamic Centre, The First Affiliated Hospital of Zhengzhou University, Zhengzhou, 450052, China. Tel. +86 371 65107278.
E-mail address: jgwen@zzu.edu.cn (J.G. Wen).

图 3-1 《欧洲泌尿外科》杂志对通讯作者的标注

六、作者署名应该注意的问题

(一)正确区分个人署名和多作者署名关系

凡是研究成果由个人完成并撰写的论文或是由个人搜集的资料和累积的经验撰写成的论文,理应单独署名。当然也应该避免以个人的名义去发表集体研究的成果,更不可以发表别人研究的成果。

由多人(多单位)合作完成的研究成果,是否需要撰文发表应共同商量决定,不可以单方擅自决定撰文发表。这类论文的发表需要参与作者共同署名。需注意,凡在论文上署名的作者,必须是参与研究课题选定、研究方案的制定者,直接参加全部或参加了主要部分研究工作,并有着主要贡献,以及参加了撰写论文并对该论文内容可以负责的人。

多作者排列次序,一般主要撰写论文者为第一作者,需对论文的内容负主要责任,其余按照所做工作多少以及贡献大小排列,绝不能以职位和资历排序。例如:研究生在读研期间独立完成科研成果并撰写的毕业论文,在科技期刊或者学报上发表时,研究生本人应为第一作者,导师可放在第二位并作为通讯作者。

（二）正确区别团体和单位署名与执笔人的界限

对于科研团体(如课题组)或者单位集体研究出的成果撰写出的论文,尤其该团体或单位的成员(实际参加研究的人员)较多时,署名应该是该团体或集体。若论文是由一个或两个人执笔写的,则可以注明执笔人署名。执笔人需对该论文负主要责任。

（三）区别作者和其他合作者的关系

仅参与部分工作并对整个研究缺乏基本了解的合作者,按研究分工中负责小项目的工作者、某一项测试的承担者,以及因接受委托而进行分析检验者和观察辅助人员,均不应列为作者。如需列出这些人姓名,可用脚注或者致谢的方式列出。

（四）正确署名学位、职称

论文署名前一般不加学位和职称,但研究生写的论文需要加上指导老师的姓名、职称及职务,以表明该项研究是在具有硕士、博士学位的专家教授指导下完成的。但也有一些杂志例外,他们有的要求在第一作者和(或)通讯作者署名后加学位、职称等,有的甚至要求所有罗列的作者后面加上学位、职称等。

第二节　作者单位地址和联系方式

一、单位地址的一般要求

一个作者对应一个地址(所在实验室的名称和地址)。论文出版前,如果作者已经搬迁到不同的地址,那么新地址将在"当前住址"的脚注中显示。当两个或更多的作者被列出,每个人有不同的研究机构时,地址将按照作者的相同排序来列出。

当一篇论文发表时,如果三名作者隶属于两个实验机构,那么每名作者的名称和地址应该有适当的标注,例如在作者名字之后和适当地址之前(或之后)标注指导者 a,b 或 c。这一惯例通常对读者是有用的,可能他们想知道是否 R. Jones 在耶鲁或哈佛。明确标明作者和地址对一些二级系统也是最重要的。对于那些功能强大的机构来说,他们需要知道是否一篇 J. Jones 的论文是来自于爱荷华州的 J. Jones,康奈尔的 J. Jones 或者英国牛津大学的 J. Jones。只有当作者适当被区分时,他们的论文在索引引用时才可能被分在一组。

作者的工作机构和地址可用来区分作者,同时它也提供(或应该提供)作者的联系地址。虽然不是必须提供研究机构的街道门牌号,但是近年来很多杂志期刊对邮政编码也是要求提供的。

一些期刊使用星号、脚注或致谢方式来标明"与文章相关的人"的单位地址。在这一点上作者应该认识到期刊的规定,而且他们将优先决定谁将购买和出版论文(由于正常情况下是科研机构购买出版物,而不是个人)。除非科学家希望匿名出版,否则作者的全名和详细地址是必要的。

二、单位地址的标注原则

（一）准确性原则

标注作者的单位时必须用全称，不能用简称。不能为了简便，或是"想当然"，把口头中的单位简称标注在科技论文上。例如：不可以将"中国科学院植物研究所"简单写成"中科院植物所"；也不能将"郑州大学第一附属医院尿动力学中心"简称为"郑大一附院尿动力"。

（二）简明性原则

论文标注的作者单位和通讯地址有利于交流和联系，所以，既要精确，又要简明。工作单位邮政编码已清楚表明所属市区，因此，不必写出详细通讯地址，但是须在邮政编码前加注单位所在省自治区、直辖市名称以及具体城市名称。例如："郑州大学第一附属医院小儿外科，河南郑州 450052"，直辖市只标注直辖市的城市名即可，而不写"河南省郑州市二七区建设东路 1 号"。再例如"北京大学第一临床医学院，北京 100034"，而不写"北京市西城区西什库大街 8 号"。

三、单位地址的一般译法

（一）"教研室"与"科"的译法

在以英语为母语的国家，医学院校所属"教研室"和医院所属"科室"，通常用 department 一词。如 Department of Surgery, Louisiana State University Medical School, New Orleans, Louisiana（路易西安那州立大学医疗系外科教研室，路易西安那州新奥尔良）。

（二）"组"的翻译方法

"组"通常是指科以下组织，在国内外常用 division、section 或 unit 等词表示。例如：Division of Gastroenterology, Department of Medicine（内科胃肠道小组）。这种"科"跟"组"的从属关系往往不是绝对的，在墨西哥，"科"用 division，而"组"却用 department，如：Department of Thoracic Surgery, Division of Surgery（外科胸组）。Division 与 section 两词，除后接 of 介词短语外，还可接名词或形容词定语。如：Gastroenterology Division, Department of Medicine, University of Texas Medical School, Houston, Texas（德克萨斯大学医疗系内科教研室胃肠组）。Unit 一词通常搭配名词前置定语使用。如：Oncology Unit of the Department of Medicine（内科肿瘤组）。通常在一些研究机构中，"组"也用 branch 表示。如：Pulmonary Branch, National Heart, Lung, and Blood Institute（国家心、肺及血液研究所肺组）。

（三）Laboratory 的搭配用法

Laboratory 一词不仅有"实验室"的意义，还可有"研究室"的意义。该词可后接 of 介词短语,也可前接名词或形容词定语,如:Laboratory of Radiobiology and Department of Anatomy,University of California(加利福尼亚大学放射生物学研究室和解剖教研室)。

（四）工作单位名称的单、复数问题

"科""室""组"等名称在应用时要注意单、复数的问题。如:Department of History and Embryology(组织胚胎教研室)(department 用单数,因为是一个单位)。disease 一词的单复数问题比较复杂,一般来说,disease 处在 of 介词短语中时,一般用复数,如:Department of Infectious Diseases(传染病教研室)。但也有用单数的,如:Department of Biostatistics and Neoplastic Disease,Mount Sinai School of Medicine,New York(纽约州纽约市蒙西拿医疗系生物统计及肿瘤科)。disease 一词用作前置定语时,一般应用单数,如:Renal and Infectious Disease Sections(肾病及传染组),但也有用复数的,如:Rheumatic Diseases Unit(风湿病组)。我们在写作时,应按一般的习惯来处理 disease 的单复数问题。

（五）工作单位排序

通常工作单位排序是小的单位放在前,大的单位放在后,如:Division of Digestive Diseases,University of Mississippi Medical Center. Jackson,Mississippi(密西西比州杰克逊市密西西比大学医学中心内科消化组)。

四、工作单位的排版位置

（一）英美杂志中,作者所属工作单位通常置于标题下方,用注脚形式备注。此时,介词 from 一般要放在工作单位名称前,如:From the Department of Medicine,University of California Los Angels School of Medicine(加利福尼亚洛杉矶大学医疗系内科教研室)。

如作者来自不同单位,在英、美杂志中则有不同的处理方法,如:

Paul R. Beining[1,3], Geraldine M. Flannery[2], Benjamin Prescott[3], and Philip J. Baker[3]

University of Scranton, Pennsylvania 18510[1]; Biomedical Research Institute, Rockville, Maryland 20852[2]; and laboratory of Microbial Immunity, National Institute of Allergy and Infectious Diseases, Bethesda, Maryland 20205[3](宾夕法尼亚州 Scranton 大学 18510[1];马里兰州 Rockville 生物医学研究所 20852[2];马里兰州 Bethesda 国家变态反应及传染病研究所微生物免疫研究室 20205[3])。

（二）以脚注的形式将工作单位标注在标题页的下方,介词 from 置于单位名称前:用相同印刷符号分别标记在作者姓名和单位名称之后,如:Peter C. Burger,MD,M. Stephen Mahaley,Jr.,MD,PhD,from the Department of pathology。

（三）工作单位以脚注形式置于标题的下方,工作单位名称前要用介词 from。在每一个工作单位名称之后,将该工作单位的作者用括号形式列出,如:Charles P. Darby,MD;From the Departments of Pediatrics(Dr Darby and Chatellier)。

在我国中华医学杂志英文版中,对来自不同工作单位的作者,处理办法如下:

1. 工作单位置于作者姓名之下。

Wang Yan

Urodynamic Center of Fist Affiliated Hospital of Zhengzhou University

2. 以脚注的形式将工作单位置于标题页之下,用相同印刷符号分别标记在作者姓名和单位名称之后,但介词 from 一般不置于单位名称前。

Wang Xi, *Liu Pengli, **Liu Yuehan ……

*Department of Surgery, Fist Affiliated Hospital of Zhengzhou University

**Institute of Clinical Medicine, Fist Affiliated Hospital of Zhengzhou University, China

五、常用医疗、医学教学和科研单位名称

College of traditional Chinese medicine 中医学院

College of pharmacy 药学院

Military medical college 军医大学

Medical college of the Ministry of Railways 铁道医学院

Affiliated hospital 附属医院

Teaching hospital 教学医院

Provincial people's hospital 省人民医院

County people's hospital 县医院

Hospital of traditional Chinese medicine 中医医院

Army hospital 陆军医院

General hospital 综合医院

Chest hospital 胸科医院

Tumor hospital 肿瘤医院

Workers' hospital 职工医院

Hospital for infectious diseases 传染病医院

Hospital for mental diseases 精神病医院

Hospital for obstetrics and gynecology 妇产科医院

Hospital for tuberculosis 结核病医院

Institute of antibiotics 抗生素研究所

Institute of acupuncture and moxibustion 针灸研究所

Institute of cardiovascular diseases 心血管疾病研究所

Institute of dermatology 皮肤病研究所

Coordinating/cooperative group 协作组

Research unit 研究室

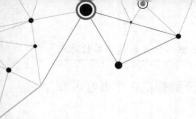

第4章
如何准备摘要和关键词

Chapter 4
How to Prepare the Abstract and Key Words

第一节 摘 要

一、摘要的定义

摘要(abstract)又称文摘、内容简介或提要,是对正文的精练概括,是论文的重要组成部分,通常位于文献的署名和前言之间。一篇摘要可以看作是微缩的正文,不插入任何解释或评论,要求文字精练、论点明确、内容概括、结论具体、篇幅简短。摘要将对论文的每一主要章节进行简短概述,包括目的、材料和方法、结果和结论。

好摘要能吸引读者,使其产生兴趣,快速并准确地了解文章的基本内容并产生想进一步阅读论文全文的冲动。相反,如果一个摘要写得不好,不仅影响文章的发表,也影响该研究的交流。正如 Sheila M. McNab 指出的那样:"I have the strong impression that scientific communication is being seriously hindered by poor quality abstracts written in jargon-ridden mumbo-jumbo."。国际检索系统使摘要(尤其是英文摘要)成为一种信息高度密集的相对独立文体,为科研人员在浩如烟海的文献中找寻自己所需提供了便利。因此,摘要的写作要引起我们的重视。

一般摘要不能超过 250 个单词,而且需要条理清楚地表述论文的主要内容。摘要通常以单一段落列出(许多医学期刊现在使用"结构式"摘要,它包括几个简短的段落)。许多人阅读的摘要来源于原始学报期刊、生物学摘要索引、化学摘要索引或者其他出版物(印刷版本或者在线网络搜索)。

《中华泌尿外科杂志》对摘要的要求为:论著必须附中、英文摘要,摘要须包括目的、方法、结果(包括主要数据)、结论四部分,各部分需有相应的标题。通常采用第三人称撰写,不用"本文""作者"等主语。考虑到国内读者可参考中文原著资料,为节省篇幅,中文摘要可适当简略(200 字左右),英文摘要则需要相对具体(400 个实词左右)。英文摘要需要包括题目、作者姓名(汉语拼音)、所属单位名称、所在城市及邮政编码。作者应全部列出,如不属同一单位,可以在第一作者姓名的右上角加"*",同时也要在单位名称首字母左上角加"*"。例如:WEN Jianguo *,LI Zhenzhen,WANG Yan,* Department of Urodynamic, The First Affiliated Hospital of Zhengzhou University, Zhengzhou 450052,China。

JAMA 详细规定了摘要的所用内容,并指出 "Abstracts should be prepared in JAMA style",即"摘要必须按照 JAMA 的要求编写"。这也说明不同的杂志有不同的格式要求。

　　总之,摘要应该陈述主要目的、研究范围、描述采用的方法、概述结果和主要结论。因为摘要指的是过去所做的东西,所以大多数摘要以过去时态来写。摘要不应给出任何文章中没有说明的信息或结论,参考文献所提及的内容不能在摘要中引用(除了在极少数情况下,如对先前发表的方法进行修正)。

二、摘要的类型

　　论文摘要一般置于论文正文之前,置于论文之尾的称为小结(summary)。但也有英美医学杂志(如 *Clinical Science*)将置于论文正文之前的摘要称为 summary。摘要为二次文献提供材料,便于引用和检索。

　　目前有部分期刊要求的摘要形式采用结构式摘要(structured abstract),其内容包括四大要素,即目的、方法、结果和结论(本章第四部分)。它可以说是整篇论文的高度概括,包括简短陈述问题、研究方法、原始数据和结论。大多数期刊会采用这种类型摘要。通常情况下,阅读摘要可替代阅读全文,可以说如果没有论文摘要,科学家要及时跟上研究的进展将会需要更多时间。

　　另外一种常见的摘要是指示性摘要或被称为说明性摘要(informative-indicative abstract)。作者首先应该对论文的写作背景简单介绍,然后应该对文章的主要内容进行简要说明,最后对文章的研究意义进行介绍。但是,由于它的描述不是实体,所以它不能代替全文。因此,在研究性论文中指示性摘要将不作为“主要”的摘要形式,但是它们能用于其他类型出版物(如述评论文、会议报告、政府报告文献等),这些指示性摘要对于图书馆查阅通常有很高价值。不同用途和类型的摘要虽然不包含目录、图或参考表格,但它是完整的,可以单独出版。因此,摘要的用语一定是读者所熟悉的,而且应省略意义含糊的首字母缩写词。如果可能的话,写摘要之前最好先把文章写好。除非在摘要中多次使用较长的术语,否则不要将这些词语缩写。在文章中首次使用的较长术语要引入适当的缩写(可以出现在引言中)。

　　一般而言,向学术性期刊投稿,多采用结构式摘要(报道性摘要),即包括文章的目的、方法、结果和结论四部分内容。毕业论文的摘要多采用指示性摘要的写法,即概括文章的主题和主要内容。下面详细介绍各种摘要的写作要点。

(一)结构式摘要

　　结构式摘要的优点是内容完整,层次清楚,一目了然,便于阅读时选择性查阅,也利于计算机系统的贮存和检索;既可提供固定的格式,便于作者撰写,避免费时构思,易成文,又不会遗漏重要内容。

(二)评论性摘要

　　评论性摘要(critical abstract)不常用,见于部分综述。内容包括研究背景和对研究的评价。下面的例子就是评论性摘要,介绍了研究背景。

Ureterorenoscopy: avoiding and managing the complications.

Abstract: Retrograde exploration of the ureter and kidneys is currently a widely used and well-established procedure to deal with problems of a diagnostic and therapeutic nature with reduced invasiveness. The process of miniaturizing the instruments combined with the steady improvement in video quality has continuously amplified its potential applications, maintaining the procedure safe and rapid. During an operation, however, unexpected events may condition a change to the program or determine the onset of even more serious complications. Our aim is to analyze such events and complications and recommend potential solutions to prevent and/or deal with such happenings. Urol Int. 2011; 87 (3): 251-259.

（三）说明性摘要

说明性摘要（descriptive abstract），又称通报性摘要或指示性摘要（indicative abstract）。它只说明论文的内容范围，简单地描述研究主题，不涉及具体内容，泛泛而谈。这种文体常常使用一般现在时。例如："We describe two patients who developed pleural fibrosis after treatment with practolol."。（我们报道两例患者应用普拉洛尔后继发胸膜纤维化。）下面请看另一个例子。

Late development of colorectal cancer subsequent to pelvic irradiation

Two cases of irradiation-associated carcinoma of the colon are reported and literature reviewed. The clinical courses and operative difficulties in treating these patients are emphasized, the necessity for life-long follow-up examinations with proctoscopic and barium-enema evaluations in high risk patients is stressed. Irradiation-associated carcinoma of the colon occurs almost exclusively in women, but should be investigated in patients of either sex who live for long periods after pelvic irradiation.

标题：继发于盆腔放疗的迟发性结直肠癌

此摘要报道两例与放疗有关的结肠癌，并介绍了有关文献。文章着重叙述临床诊治过程与手术难度，并强调对发病可能性较大的患者，必须终身进行直肠镜及钡灌肠的随访检查。放疗诱发的结肠癌几乎仅见于女性，但盆腔放疗后长期存活的患者，不论男女，均应作长期观察。这篇摘要原文共四句。第一句是通报本文的主题；第二、三句是通报本文侧重谈什么问题；第四句是作者的结论。四句全用现在时态表达。

（四）资料性摘要

资料性摘要（informative abstract），与说明性摘要正好相反，内容比较具体、丰富，可以按IMMRD（Introduction，Materials and methods，Results，Discussion）格式撰写，要求一定要写出关键性数据。这样可以使读者在没有阅读全文的情况下也能得到明确概念，有时甚至可直接引用其中某些研究成果。这种摘要可以说是文章的微型化。

资料性摘要一般包括下述内容：①研究背景：介绍论文的研究背景、研究目的或解题性说明；②研究方法与结果；③结论；④对未来的展望。

一篇摘要并不一定非要包括上述全部内容。在上述内容中，研究过程与结果以及作者结论是关键。所以，有的资料性摘要只写研究过程与结果，或只写结论。但大多数资料性摘要会同时写出这两方面的内容，至于研究背景与研究目的以及展望，相对次要，可根据作者的需要决定取舍。总之，这里没有一成不变的格式。下面我们对常见的几种情况进行举例说明。

1. 只叙述研究过程与结果　有些摘要内容比较单一，只涉及研究过程与结果。这是一种较为客观的写法，不加作者评论，用事实说明问题，研究过程与结果的描述用一般过去时表达。

以作者发表的文章摘要为例:

A study of staccato urine flowcurve in healthy chinese children

【Abstract】Objective　To investigate the incidence of staccato urine flow curve and analyze the parameters of urine flow rate in healthy children. Methods　One hundred sixty nine Chinese healthy children (81 boys, 88 girls) aged from 8 to 13 years was included in this uroflowmetry study. Residual urine was evaluated using ultrasonography after voiding. Voided volume (VV) in all cases was more than 50ml. The cases with staccato urine flow curve were analyzed to evaluate the incidence and its relationship to age, gen der and VV. Results　Fifty four cases (24 boys, 30 girls) had the characteristics of staccato urine flow curve. The incidence of that curve was 29.6% in boys and 34.1% in girls, respectively. In boys, the incidence of staccato urine flow curve was decreased with age increased while it had nothing to do with age in girls. With VV increased, the incidence of that curve was also increased in both boys and girls. In boys with staccato urine flow curve, maximum flow rate, mean flow rate, VV and post void residual (PVR) incidence were (26.9 ± 10.5)ml/s, (13.2 ± 4.1)ml/s, (198.2 ± 118.7)ml, and 12.5%, respectively. Meanwhile, these indices were (25.9 ± 9.3)ml/s, (13.1 ± 4.9)ml/s, (243.7 ± 164.0)ml, and 6.7% in girls with staccato urine flow curve, respectively. Moreover, VV, flow time and time to maximum flow rate in children with staccato urine flow curve were higher than those with normal curve. No significant difference was noted in maximum flow rate, mean flow rate and PVR incidence between children with staccato flow curve and those with normal curve. Conclusions　Staccato urine flow curve may serve as a parameter for screening the bladder dysfunction in children.

标题:正常儿童 Staccato 尿流曲线分析

【摘要】目的　探讨正常儿童 staccato 尿流曲线的发生率和尿流率表现。方法　对 169 例无下尿路症状儿童[男 81 例,女 88 例,年龄 8~13 岁,平均(10.3 ± 1.6)岁]进行自由尿流率检测,并用 B 超测量残余尿量。全部儿童尿量均大于 50ml。对其中表现为 Staccato 尿流曲线的儿童的检查结果进行回顾性分析。结果　8~13 岁正常儿童 Staccato 尿流曲线的总体发生率为 31.9%,其中男 29.6%,女 34.1%,二者之间无显著性差异。随着年龄增长男性发生率逐渐下降;女性发生率与年龄无相关性。Staccato 尿流曲线的发生率受尿量影响,随尿量增加而增加。男性最大尿流率(26.9 ± 10.5)ml/s,平均尿流率(13.2 ± 4.1)ml/s,尿量(198.2 ± 118.7)ml,残余尿发生率 12.5%(残余尿量均小于 5ml);女性最大尿流率(25.9 ± 9.3)ml/s,平均尿流率(13.1 ± 4.9)ml/s,尿量(243.7 ± 164.0)ml,残余尿发生率 6.7%(残余尿量均小于 5ml)。Staccato 尿流曲线儿童尿量、尿流时间和达最大尿流时间均显著大于正常尿流曲线儿童;最大尿流率、平均尿流率和残余尿发生率与正常尿流曲线儿童无显著性差异。结论　正常小儿的 Staccato 尿流曲线常见,其发生率受年龄大小和尿量多少影响。如果发现小儿 Staccato 尿流曲线应结合残余尿是否增多来考虑其临床意义。Staccato 尿流曲线可用做初步筛查小儿排尿异常参考指标之一。

解析:这篇摘要叙述研究过程中所发生的情况,故均用过去时态表达。

再举其他文献发表的摘要为例:

Oral mucosal ulceration in systemic lupus erythematosus

【Abstract】Objective: In 182 patients with systemic lupus erythematosus (SLE), oral mucosal ulceration occurred in 47 patients (26%), was usually painless (82%), and most often involved the hard palate (89%). Oral ulceration was associated with an increase in overall clinical activity, although this was not accompanied by significant changes in the levels or titers of C3, anti-DNA antibodies, and anti-nuclear antibodies. Necrotizing vasculitis was not observed. Microscopic changes were similar to the skin lesions of SLE and immunoglobulin and complement were found in both the basement membrane and blood vessel walls.

标题：系统性红斑狼疮与口腔黏膜溃疡

【摘要】目的　我们观察了 182 例系统性红斑狼疮（SLE）患者，其中有口腔黏膜溃疡者 47 例（26%），这种溃疡一般不伴有疼痛（82%），往往累及硬腭（89%），虽然患者口腔溃疡与总的临床表现加剧有关，但患者补体 3，抗 DNA 抗体及抗核抗体的滴度无明显变化，未发现有坏死性脉管炎。口腔黏膜溃疡变化在显微镜下所见与 SLE 皮肤病变相似。在基底膜与血管壁均见有免疫球蛋白与补体沉积。

解析：这篇摘要共四句，叙述了研究过程中所发生的情况，用过去时态表达。

2. 只叙述作者的结论　与上述摘要写作完全不同，有的摘要不涉及研究过程与结果，只有作者的结论与看法，这种写法的优点为直截了当，引人注目。结论一般用现在时态表达。例如：

Alcohol use, myocardial infarction, sudden cardiac death and hypertension

Abstract: Studying coronary risk factors, this article concludes that: regular use of alcohol may protect against major coronary events; regular use of three or more drinks daily is a probable risk factors for hypertension; the relations of alcohol used to coronary disease, hypertension and cardiomyopathy are disparate.

饮酒 - 心肌梗死 - 心源性猝死与高血压

摘要　我们对冠心病的有害因素进行了研究，结论是：经常饮酒可防止冠心病严重发作；每天饮酒三次以上，可能是产生高血压的危险因素；饮酒对冠心病、高血压及心肌病三者的影响并不相同。

解析：这篇摘要只有一个复合句，由一个主句和三个分句组成。整句话是叙述作者的研究结论，用现在时态表达。

3. 研究过程、结果和作者结论　在摘要中先写研究过程与结果，最后写结论是一种最常见的摘要形式。研究过程与结果一般用过去时表达，作者结论用现在时表达。举其他文献发表的摘要为例：

Malignant hypertension and cigarette smoking

Abstract: The smoking habits of 48 patients with malignant hypertension were compared with those of 92 consecutive patients with non-malignant hypertension. Thirty-three of the patients with malignant and 34 of the patients with non-malignant hypertension were smokers when first diagnosed. This difference was significant and remained so when only men or black and white patients were considered separately. Results suggest that malignant hypertension is yet another disease related to cigarette smoking.

恶性高血压与吸烟

摘要　作者将 48 例恶性高血压与 92 例非恶性高血压患者做了吸烟习惯的对比研究。在初诊时就已吸烟的恶性高血压患者有 33 例，非恶性患者 34 例。两者之间有显著差异。

如仅对男性患者进行比较,或将白人与黑人分别进行比较,这种差异也仍然显著。本研究表明:恶性高血压也是一种与吸烟有关的疾病。

解析:这篇摘要共四句。第一句首先叙述作者在研究过程中做了哪些工作,第二、三句接着叙述研究过程中所得到的结果,这三句都用过去时表达;第四句是作者的结论,应用现在时表达。

举其他文献发表的摘要为例:

Diabetes after infection of hepatitis

Eleven patients (nine men, one woman, and one girl) aged 11 to 62 years old who developed diabetes mellitus after an attack of infectious hepatitis during the eastern Nigerian epidemic of 1970 to 1972 were followed up for two to nine years. One patient aged 60 years old remained diabetic after the original illness. In the remaining ten patients the diabetes remitted after three to nine months (mean 6.7 months) but in four it recurred after a remission lasting one and a half to hour years (mean 2.6 years). Results of this study seem to confirm that the pancreas is sometimes permanently damaged during infectious hepatitis.

继发于传染性肝炎的糖尿病

1970—1972 年,在东尼日利亚传染性肝炎流行期间,有 11 例 11~62 岁的患者(男性 9 例、妇女 1 例、女孩 1 例)患了传染性肝炎后继发了糖尿病,随访时间为 2~9 年。一例 60 岁的患者在原发病后糖尿病一直未愈,其余 10 例在 3~9 个月后(平均 6.7 个月)糖尿病症状缓解,但其中 4 例缓解 1.5~4 年后(平均 2.6 年)又复发。这一研究结果证实,在传染性肝炎病期间胰腺有时会受到永久性损害。

解析:原文共四句,第一句叙述研究当时的情况和研究的对象,第二、三句是研究的结果,第四句是结论。

4. 开场白与对未来的展望　如上所述,有很多摘要不用开场白,开门见山地叙述研究过程、结果或结论,但必要时也要有一两句开场白。开场白需包括研究背景、研究目的,或仅仅是解题性说明。

(1)交代研究背景:在摘要开头就叙述所研究课题的已知情况即研究的背景。研究背景一般用现在时或现在完成时态。举例如下:

Impaired pancreatic polypeptide release in chronic pancreatitis with steatorrhoea

Abstract: Pancreatic polypeptide (PP) is a newly discovered hormonal peptide localized in a distinct endocrine cell type in the pancreas. PP circulates in plasma and in normal subjects levels rise substantially on the ingestion of food (mean rise 138 pmol/L). in 10 patients with chronic pancreatitis with exocrine deficiency, the PP response to a test breakfast was greatly reduced (mean rise 20pmol/L, $P<.001$) PP response to the meal was normal in 10 patients with active coeliac disease and 12 patients with acute tropical sprue with steatorrhoea.

慢性胰腺炎合并脂肪痢患者的胰多肽释放受损

摘要　胰多肽(PP)是最近发现的一种激素肽,仅由胰腺特殊的内分泌细胞分泌。PP 随血浆循环,正常人进食后其浓度会大大升高(平均升高 138pmol/L)。10 例慢性胰腺炎合并外分泌不足的患者,其 PP 对早餐试验反应能力下降(平均升高 20pmol/L,$P<0.001$),而 10 例急腹症患者及 12 例急性热带口炎性腹泻并伴有脂肪痢患者,PP 对进餐试验反应正常。

解析:这篇摘要原文共四句。前两句是叙述着手研究时的已知情况,即研究背景,用现在时表达;后两句是叙述研究中发生的情况,用过去时表达。

（2）交代研究目的:在摘要一开始就叙述研究的目的。研究目的一般用过去时态。摘要举例如下。

Relation between mammary cancer growth kinetics and the intervals of screening

Abstract: The purpose of this study was to consider the time interval for periodic mammographic screening for breast cancer. One hundred fifteen breast cancers occurring in 10,128 women receiving over 30,000 mammograms over a four year period were reviewed. Tumors were diagnosed at three time intervals: first screening (39/115); annual examination (27/115); and at an examination that occurred less than twelve months from a previous annual examination (10/115). Also, there were tumors that grew to palpable dimensions and were self-detected between annual examinations (39/115). Our opinion is that screening intervals should be individualized to each patient according to risk factors and suspicious mammographic. Furtherly, there is a significant number of breast cancers that grow too fast to be detected effectively by annual mammography. Suspicious mammographic findings did not exist before these cancers reached palpable dimensions, other risk factors characterizing the hosts who develop these fast growing cancers are yet to be determined.

乳腺癌生长动力学与普查间隔时间的关系

摘要　本研究旨在探讨定期乳腺 X 线摄影检查乳腺癌的间隔时间。四年来,作者对 10 128 名妇女做了 30 000 次以上的 X 线摄片检查,并复查了其中的 115 例乳房癌患者的 X 线检查资料。诊断出癌症的时间有如下三种:第一次检查(39/115);每年一次的检查(27/115);离上次年度检查不到 12 个月的检查(10/115)。还有 39 例是在两次年度检查之间肿瘤已长到可触及的程度患者自己发觉的。我们的观点是:定期检查的间隔时间应因人而异,要根据患者是否有引起乳腺癌的有害因素及乳腺 X 线摄片是否可疑来决定。此外,有不少患者肿瘤生长太快,以致一年一次的乳腺 X 线摄片也不能及时发现,或者在肿瘤尚未达到可触及的程度之前,乳腺 X 线摄影未能发现可疑的病变。其他一些使癌肿迅速生长的有害因素尚待查明。

解析:这篇摘要原文共八句。第一句是开场白,交代研究目的,用过去时表达;第 2~4 句是叙述研究及获得数据的分析,用过去时表达;第 5、6 句是作者的结论,用现在时表达;第 7 句又回头陈述研究过程中所遇到的情况,用过去时态表达;最后一句是讲述对今后工作的展望,用含有将来意味的"be+ 不定式"的结构来表达。

（3）解题性说明:有的医学论文摘要在开头用一句开场白来解题,说明本文的要旨(不是叙述研究背景与目的)。这类解题性的开场白往往用一般现在时,常见的动词有:describe (描述),report(报告)、present(介绍)等。举例如下。

Angiosarcoma of the heart

Two cases of angiosarcoma of the heart are described. In one the tumor, which arose from the right atrium, was demonstrated during life by angiography. In the other, diagnosed only at necropsy, the tumor arose from the right ventricle, both cases illustrate many of the typical features of this rare tumor and difficulties of antemortem diagnosis.

心血管肉瘤

本文报道两例心脏血管肉瘤,一例发生于右心房,是生前通过血管造影确诊的。另一例起源于右心室,是死后尸检时确诊的。此两例罕见肿瘤有多种典型表现,并且在生前难以确诊。

解析:这篇摘要原文共四句。第一句是解题性说明,阐明本文的主题,用现在时表达;第二、三句是叙述研究过程中所发现的情况,用过去时表达;最后一句是作者的结论,用现在时表达。

(4) 作者对未来的展望:在摘要收尾处有时可以写上作者对未来的展望。这类内容常用一般将来时。举例如下。

The efficacy of calcifediol in renal osteodystrophy

The results are in agreement with previous reports on small numbers of patients, although no direct comparison studies are available, it would seem that calcifediol offers some advantages over other forms of vitamin D therapy in these patients. Ultimately, comparison studies will be required to determine the relative efficacy and convenience of the various forms of vitamin D that are now being developed for use in patients.

骨化二醇治疗肾性骨营养不良的疗效

本研究结果与过去所报道的少数病例相同,虽未进行直接的比较研究,但骨化二醇对肾性骨营养不良的疗效比其他类型的维生素 D 制剂要好。最后,目前正在研制中的各种维生素 D 制剂的疗效高低及使用方便与否,尚需进行比较研究。

解析:这篇摘要原文共三句,前两句是叙述作者的结论,用现在时表达;最后一句叙述作者对未来的展望,用将来时表达。

(5) 资料性结合通报性写法:资料性摘要有时也可掺杂通报性摘要的写法,即对部分内容不详细叙述,而是按通报性摘要的手法提示一下。举例如下。

Malignant lymphoma associated with marked Eosinophilia

A 60-year-old black man with poorly differentiated lymphocytic lymphoma presented with generalized lymphadenopathy and marked eosinophilia. Extensive evaluation of the eosinophils revealed them to be normal morphologically and functionally. The patient responded to corticosteroid therapy with resolution of the lymphadenopathy and reversion of the peripheral blood counts to normal limits, recurrence of the original clinical picture within months prompted institution of systemic chemotherapy. Response was transient, and the patient expired after an unremitting downhill course. Recent advances in our knowledge of mechanisms of eosinophilia and eosinophil function are reviewed. The relationship of lymphoma to eosinophilia is discussed.

恶性淋巴瘤合并明显的嗜伊红细胞增多症

一名 60 岁的黑人患分化程度低的淋巴细胞型淋巴瘤,呈现全身性淋巴结肿大及嗜伊红细胞明显增多。对嗜伊红细胞进行了广泛研究后,发现其形态与功能均属正常。患者经过可的松治疗后,肿大的淋巴结消失,周围血细胞计数恢复到正常范围。可是仅维持了几个月,原来的临床症状复发,随即开始全身性化疗。疗效是暂时的,之后患者病情急转直下,最后死亡。本文综述了嗜伊红细胞增多症的发病机制和嗜伊红细胞功能研究的最新进展,并探讨了淋巴瘤与嗜伊红细胞增多症的关系。

解析:这篇摘要原文共七句。第一、二句说明患者的病名、主要症状和检查结果;第三、四、五句叙述治疗的经过和疗效;第六句是患者的转归,即结局;第七句指出了这篇论文探讨的重点内容。

三、摘要的特点

如果你的论文摘要不能吸引审稿人的眼球,那么论文将丧失发表机会。通常审稿人在单独阅读摘要后所做出的判断与对你论文最后的判定结果很接近。

摘要尽可能简明扼要。有一位科学家发现了与物质能量相关的伟大理论。接着他写了一篇伟大的论文。但是,这位科学家知道编辑的局限性,认识到如果这篇论文能被接受的话,其论文摘要必须是简短的,所以他花费很多时间琢磨摘要,逐字进行删减,直到最后移去所有的冗词。最后,他留下最短的摘要"$E=mc^2$"。

写摘要时,仔细推敲每一句话。如果你能在 100 个单词内叙述你的报道,就不要使用 200 个单词。从经济学和科学的角度来说,浪费单词没有任何意义。整体的交流沟通系统只能负担一定数量的文字。因为大多数期刊需要标题式摘要,会议式摘要则出现在大多数国内和国际会议中,科学家需要掌握摘要编写的基本原则。对你来说更为重要的是,使用准确、简洁的单词将给编辑和审稿人留下较好的印象(更不用说读者),然而使用难以理解且冗长的结构很可能在审稿过程中就被拒绝。

一篇好的摘要通常具有以下特点:

1. 准确性　一篇摘要能准确反映文章的目的和内容,在摘要中不包括未在文章正文列出的信息。如果研究者扩展或重复先前的研究,那么它必须在摘要中显示,并简要说明作者等信息。

2. 独立性　一篇完整的摘要是一篇文章主要内容的浓缩,可以完整独立地表达全文的观点,应是一个完整独立的部分。

3. 简洁特异性　每个句子要尽可能提供更多的信息,尤其是首句,尽可能使其简短。如果可能,摘要尽量为一段。摘要的起始部分是最重要的信息,但是不能与标题重复。

4. 紧凑易读性　遵循如下建议可使表达更为清楚:①使用动词而不是名词;②使用主动语态而不是被动语态;③使用现在时描述结果;④使用过去时描述特定操作;⑤使用第三人称而不是第一人称。

下面我们通过文献中这方面摘要例子进行详细说明。

题目:食管癌组织中水通道蛋白 3 的表达变化及意义

摘要:采用免疫组化 SP 法对 56 例食管癌组织及 45 例正常食管组织中水通道蛋白 3(AQP3)进行检测,结果显示食管癌组织中 AQP3 高表达者 41 例、低表达者 15 例,正常食管组织分别为 23、22 例,两种组织相比,$P<0.05$;32 例有淋巴结转移食管癌组织中 AQP3 高表达 27 例、低表达 5 例,24 无淋巴结转移者中分别为 14、10 例,两种组织相比,$P<0.05$;21 例 Ⅰ 级食管癌组织中,AQP3 高表达 11 例、低表达 10 例,20 例 Ⅱ 级者分别为 16、4 例,15 例 Ⅲ 级者分别为 14、1 例,三种组织相比,$P<0.05$。认为食管癌组织中 AQP3 的表达可能在食管癌分化和转移过程中发挥作用。

解析:本摘要符合写作要求:①能正确反映文章的目的和内容,在摘要中不包括未在文章正文列出的信息;②本篇中没有唯一性术语、缩写和首字母缩略词;③每个句子都信息量充足,尤其是首句,它简短且明确地告诉读者——当前研究采用免疫组化 SP 法对 56 例食管癌组织及 45 例正常食管组织中水通道蛋白 3(AQP3)进行检测。

总之,一篇好的摘要应该注意以下方面:简要描述主要发现和结论;包括所有文中包含的主要信息;在不同地方适当强调文章主体;对于简短文章,摘要将以单一句型写作;对于长篇文章,如果为了使摘要更清晰,可以把摘要分为两段或更多;对于发现的东西使用过去式;摘要中包括文中尽可能多的关键词;避免不熟悉的术语,首字母缩略词,缩写词或标志,或者如果没有选择就定义它们;对于化学物和药品来说,使用通用名称,不是商品名;摘要中不包括表格,图表和方程式,或者结构性公式;避免引用参考文献,除非参考文献促使作者对进一步研究产生灵感;摘要中第一次出现英文缩写词应该给出英文全称。

四、英文摘要的撰写

（一）论著类文章的结构式摘要

大部分医学期刊中,较为常见的论著类结构式摘要在向简化的趋向发展,通常采用的结构式摘要有 4 个层次:目的、方法、结果、结论。部分期刊又在此基础上有了创新,就是将结论（conclusion）改成解释（interpretation）。应该指出,四段式中用"背景"和"解释"做标题,是对摘要内容的拓展、信息的增加,相比单纯用"目的"和"结论"更为丰富。下面结合作者的写作经验进行描述。

四段式趋简的结构式英文摘要举例如下。

Objective　To investigate the relationship between aquaporin-1,-2,-3,-4 mRNA (AQP1-4) and renal parenchyma thickness in congenital hydronephrotic kidney in children.

Methods　The expression of aquaporin 1,-2,-3, and-4 mRNA in hydronephrotic kidney of 37 children (aged 60.3 ± 48.8 months) were evaluated with congenital hydronephrosis and normal kidney of 6 children (aged 62.7 ± 17.1 months) using semi-quantitative reverse transcriptase polymerase chain reaction technique. Hydronephrotic kidney parenchyma thicknesses measured by B-Ultrasound preoperatively and were verified at operation. The relation of aquaporin 1,-2,-3, and-4 mRNA to the hydronephrotic kidney parenchyma thickness were analyzed by linear regression.

Results　The aquaporin 1,-2,-3, and-4/beta-actin ratio in the hydronephrotic kidney and normal kidney were AQP1: 0.39 ± 0.22 VS 0.90 ± 0.10; AQP2: 0.42 ± 0.20 VS 0.92 ± 0.09; AQP3: 0.52 ± 0.22 VS 0.98 ± 0.12; AQP4: 0.30 ± 0.18 VS 0.74 ± 0.21 respectively, and the differences were significant ($P<0.01$). Hydronephrotic kidney parenchyma thickness measured by B-Ultrasound is averaged 5.01 ± 2.38 mm, which is identical with those measured at operation. Significant correlation was found between the levels of aquaporin 1,-2,-3, and-4 mRNA and hydronephrotic kidney parenchyma thickness (r=0.773, 0.772, 0.557, 0.625, respectively; $P<0.01$)

Conclusions　Significant correlation exists between decrease expressions of aquaporin 1,-2,-3, and-4 mRNA and atrophic change of renal parenchyma providing evidence to explain the mechanism why the thinner renal parenchyma thickness, the weaker renal concentration and dilution function.

中文结构式摘要相应为:

目的　观察先天性肾积水肾组织水通道蛋白 14（aquaporins，AQP1-4）mRNA 表达及其与肾实质厚度变化之间的关系。

方法　采用逆转录 - 聚合酶链反应（RT-PCR）法检测先天性肾盂输尿管连接部狭窄患儿 37 例［年龄（60.3 ± 48.8）月］和正常对照组 6 例［年龄（62.7 ± 17.1）月］肾组织中 AQP1-

4 mRNA 的相对表达量。术前 B 超检测积水肾脏的实质厚度,并与术中测定结果比较。AQP1-4 mRNA 相对表达量与肾实质厚度之间进行回归相关分析。

结果　积水肾组织中 AQP1-4 mRNA 表达分别为 AQP1:0.90 ± 0.10,AQP2:0.92 ± 0.09,AQP3:0.98 ± 0.12,AQP4:0.74 ± 0.21,正常对照组中 AQP1-4 mRNA 表达分别为 AQP1:0.39 ± 0.22,AQP2:0.42 ± 0.20,AQP3:0.52 ± 0.22,AQP4:0.30 ± 0.18,两者差异均有统计学意义。B 超测得积水肾实质厚度平均为(5.01 ± 2.38)mm,术中肾盂放水后测量梗阻肾脏实质厚度平均为(5.12 ± 1.81)mm,两者之间无显著性差异。梗阻肾脏实质厚度与 AQP1-4 mRNA 相对表达量呈正相关(r 分别为 0.773,0.772,0.557,0.625;$P<0.01$)。积水肾实质厚度越薄,AQP1-4 表达越低。

结论　梗阻肾实质厚度变化与 AQP1-4 mRNA 表达下降有一定相关性,为了解肾实质厚度越薄肾脏尿液浓缩稀释功能越差现象的机制研究提供了客观依据。

(二)结构式摘要的利弊

作者在进行课题研究设计时需要考虑摘要层次,不仅可使课题设计严密、科学、合理,也可使作者按层次写作,力求内容准确、具体、完整、不易遗漏;另外还能让审稿人审稿、修稿便捷、省时、省力;它能体现出类似中文简洁的优点,如无主语句的应用。同样在英文中,部分层次的文字可直接以短语形式出现。如:

Objective: Our purpose was to investigate the expressions of aquaporin 2, 3 and 4 in mild hydronephrotic kidney (HnK) in children. 可写成:

Objective: To investigate the expressions of aquaporin 2, 3 and 4 in mild hydronephrotic kidney (HnK) in children.

在字数上,结构式摘要比传统摘要略多,英文一般会超过 400 字。如果按四个层次写,则可压缩到 350 字以内。

(三)常用时态

科技论文中的时态应用,听起来似乎比较容易,然而目前在国内医学刊物中,时态应用的错误非常常见。这主要是因为部分作者与编者不清楚论文摘要中时态不仅要看所叙述的具体内容,而且与摘要这一特定体裁有关。作者需要通过动词时态的应用,让读者明白有些工作是研究过程中做的,有些是着手研究前就已做过的,有些只是当时的结果,而有些是客观真理。这一切都与论文摘要的内容相关联。此外,论文摘要的体裁也为研究提供了特定的背景。现结合文献中查找到的例句将论文摘要中常用的时态分述如下。

1. 过去时态

(1)在研究过程中所进行过的活动:一般用过去时态。因为作者在撰写论文时,研究工作已结束,研究过程中所做的已成为过去。如:Thirty-seven consecutive renal transplant recipients were studied prospectively for joint disease(连续对 37 例肾移植患者是否有关节病变做了前瞻性观察)。

(2)研究目的一般采用过去时态:The purpose of this study was to investigate factors that may participate in the production of innocent ejection murmurs(本研究目的为调查产生非病理性喷射性杂音的可能因素)。

2. 过去完成时态

（1）着手研究之前已进行过的工作或已存在的状态，一般用过去完成时表示。

In a 22-year-old male, who had been irradiated 16 years previously for Hodgkin's disease, a radiation-induced thyroid carcinoma developed.

一例16年前因患霍奇金氏病接受过放射治疗的22岁男患者发生放疗诱发的甲状腺癌。

（2）研究过程中如果有两个前后相连的动作，先发生的动作往往用过去完成时态。

Two patients with primary spontaneous pneumothorax died despite intensive treatment. In the first the pneumothorax had been present for 10 days, …

两例原发性自发性气胸患者，虽得到积极治疗，仍死亡。第一例患者气胸已持续达 10 天之久……

3. 现在时态

（1）论文发表时的当时情况要用一般现在时态表达：如：

About 50 cases of leptospirosis are diagnosed each year in the United Kingdom, with an overall mortality of 5%, renal failure, in association with jaundice, is commonly held responsible for this figure. Over a period of 18 years, 6 cases of leptospirosis complicated by renal failure were treated at the Royal Air Force Renal Unit; there were 4 survivors …

美国每年确诊螺旋体病约 50 例，总死亡率达 5%。造成这些死亡的原因一般认为是肾衰竭合并黄疸。18 年来，有 6 例合并肾衰竭的患者在皇家空军肾病科进行治疗。有 4 例存活……

（2）介绍本研究的内容一般用现在时态：这类动词常见的有：report（报告）、describe（描述）、present（提出，介绍）、discuss（讨论）、review（评述）、emphasize（强调）、stress（强调）等。

In this paper, we report the effect of plasma exchange in a patient with this syndrome.

本文报道一例这种综合征患者换血浆疗法的效果。

A case of a 27 year old man who developed anemia after fracture of sella turcica is reported.

本文报道一例 27 岁患者在蝶鞍骨折后发生贫血。

介绍本研究的内容，除上述动词外，还可用系动词 be。如"本文是一篇……报道"，"本文是一篇……分析"等句式中的"是"均要用现在时。

This study is a description of a patient who exhibited diabetic ketosis associated with an alkalosis rather than acidosis and a review of eight previously reported cases.

本文报道一例有碱中毒而不伴有酸中毒的糖尿病酮症患者，并对既往报道的 8 例做了综述。

介绍"本文"的内容，包括"本文"的目的，同样要应用现在时态。这与前面说过的"表示研究的目的"不同。"研究的目的"是指在开始研究前要确定所研究的目的。既然研究过程中的全部行为都应用过去时态，在开始研究之前确定一下研究的目标更应当用过去时态。"本文"的目的却不同。"本文"的目的是指介绍本文的中心思想，其所用的不定式动词一般都含有"叙述""说"的意思。如：

The purpose of this report is to emphasize the value of radiation therapy.

本文旨在强调放射治疗的价值。

（3）表示作者的结论：作者进行各种研究工作最终要得出一个结论，不管结论是肯定还是否定。在叙述结论时要用一般现在时态，因为科学结论往往具有普遍真理的性质。

We conclude that the principles of the test system allow increased safety and accuracy in hospital drug handling.

我们的结论是：这种试验制度的一些原则可以提高医院药物管理的安全性与精确性。

The authors conclude that labetalol when combined with a thiazide diuretic is an important therapeutic advance in the treatment of the difficult hypertensive subject.

我们的结论是：拉贝洛尔与噻嗪类利尿剂合用治疗难治性高血压症更具有优势。

由上述例句可以看出，作者应该用一般现在时态表示得出的研究结论。当然，有时也会出现用一般过去时态的情况。用现在时态或过去时态虽然都合于语法，但却隐含作者对该结论两种截然不同的态度。用现在时态表明作者认为该结论具有普遍真理的性质；用过去时态则表明作者并不认为这是一个普遍性的结论，而仅仅是当时的研究结果。如：

This trial showed both drugs to be effective and there was no statistically significant difference between them in their effect.

这一试验表明，两种药物都有效，其效果在统计学上无明显差异。

4. 现在完成时态

（1）代表持续到撰写论文时的行为或状态。

Three patients have been now free from recurrences for 5 years, 13 patients for 4 years, 11 patients for 3 years, and 9 patients for 2 years.

迄今为止，5 年未复发者 3 例，4 年 13 例，3 年 11 例，2 年 9 例。

（2）代表在另一现在时态动作之前就已完成的动作，而那个现在时动词往往表示不受时间限制的永恒现象。

Radionuclide examinations provide considerable information in evaluating patients who have received renal transplants.

用放射性同位素检查能为评价肾移植的患者提供重要资料。

（3）用来提供一个过去时间的背景：在报道性文献中，往往一开始用一个现在完成时态作为先导，紧接着用一连串的一般过去时。这种现在完成时起到提供过去时间背景的作用。

The authors have examined the lungs from five patients who died with the adult respiratory distress syndrome. Pressure volume curves were obtained and bronchoalveolar lavage fluid was studied on a surface balance. The pressure volume curves revealed reduced compared to normal or near normal lungs. A significant loss of volume was also found …

我们检查了 5 例死于呼吸窘迫综合征成人患者的肺脏，取得了加压容量曲线资料，对支气管肺泡灌洗液的表面平衡做了研究。与正常或接近正常的肺脏相比，加压容量曲线提示顺应性降低，肺活量也显著减少。

5. 将来时态表示以后要做的工作或预期的结果

As greater clinical correlation is obtained, usefulness of thyroglobulin determinations will increase.

随着甲状腺球蛋白测定与临床的相关性增强，其使用价值也将提高。

（四）论文摘要中几个常用动词不同时态的意义

1. report 与 describe

（1）一般现在时态：表示"本文报道"。

Three patients with rheumatoid arthritis who appeared to have allergy to prednisolone are reported.

本文报道了 3 例对泼尼松龙过敏的类风湿性关节炎患者。

（2）一般过去时态：表示在撰写论文时也已报道过。因此不是"本文报道"，而是其他文章已经报道过。

In 1968, studies of infectious hepatitis in volunteers were reported.

对志愿人员进行传染性肝炎的研究，在 1968 年就已有报道。（本句中的 report 根据内容可以看出不是"本文"报道，而是"别的文章"已有报道。

（3）现在完成时态：用现在完成时态即可表示"另外的报道"，也可表示"本文报道"。

A patient with plasma cell leukemia and Ig G (K) M-component, who developed a hyperviscosity syndrome is reported. To our knowledge, this complication has not yet been reported in plasma cell leukemia.

本文报道一例合并有 IgG（K）M 血症的浆细胞白血病患者出现高黏稠综合征。就我们所知，浆细胞白血病的这一并发症迄今未见报道。（本句中第一次出现的 report 是"本文"报道；第二次出现的现在完成时态的 report 则不是"本文"，而是"别的文章"没有报道过。）

2. present

present 一词用一般现在时态与 report 相同，表示"本文报道"或"本文介绍"。

Two cases of hemobilia due to haemorrhagic cholecystitis are presented.

本文报道 2 例出血性胆囊炎引起的胆道出血。

在英美医学杂志中出现的一般过去时态的 present，用"本文报道"或"另外报道"之类含义来解释，往往讲不通。在目前国内出版的英汉辞典中也找不到恰当的解释。

在"Webster's Third New International Dictionary"中对 present 有一段释文可以用得上：to come forward as a patient。如：

Three elderly patients presented at one hospital in a 2-week period with acute urinary retention precipitated by the hyperosmolar non-ketotic diabetic state.

在两周内有三名老年患者因高渗性非酮症糖尿病继发急性尿潴留而来同一医院就诊。

present 的过去时态与 with 连用时，含有"呈现""表现"之意。如：

A successful pancreatogram was obtained at endoscopic retrograde holangiopancreatography in 53 patients with calculous biliary disease. Twenty-eight patients presented with jaundice and 25 with pain.

我们对 53 例胆道结石患者经内窥镜做逆行胰胆管造影，成功地获得了胰造影图。表现为黄疸的患者 28 例，表现为腹痛的患者 25 例。

3. review

review 一词在论文摘要中往往因时态应用的不同，而具有不同的意义，而其时态的应用又与该动词的宾语有关。

（1）一般现在时：review 用于一般现在时态，含有"本文综述"或"本文评述"的意义。与 review 搭配连用的各词一般要有一定的内容可以加以叙述。如：

The (pertinent) literature is reviewed.

本文综述了相关文献。

Chemotherapy experience is briefly reviewed.

本文扼要地评述了化学治疗的经验。

（2）一般过去时：review 用于一般过去时态时，就不能表示"本文综述"或"本文评述"。因"综述"与"评述"是作者在撰写论文时的行为，所以用现在时。过去时态是表示作者在撰写论文之前的研究行为，即是作者在研究过程之中所进行的工作，这时，它含有"复述""回顾"的意义。

Eighty-seven cases of male breast cancer seen over 30-year period were reviewed.

我们对 30 年来所遇到的 87 例男性乳腺癌做了回顾性研究。

我们不少医务工作者已习惯将 review 一词译成"复习"，如"复习文献"等。我们认为"复习功课"是汉语的固定搭配用法，而"复习文献"似嫌搭配不当。

（五）英文摘要撰写常见问题

1. 夸张、失实　科学报道与事实不符的情况屡见不鲜。比如某些作者喜欢说自己的工作"never reported in the literature""a new methods""the first report"，在学术论文摘要中最好不要出现这类"拔高"词语，应由研究内容去说明。

论文中有许多常见的不必要的程度副词，如 most、always、never、markedly 等。这类词与别的词结合，不能说明程度，却给人一种夸张、失实的印象，最好能写出客观具体的数字、年龄和作用等资料。

2. 冗词赘语　医学论文英语摘要中普遍存在很多冗词赘语。如果从论文中删去这些冗词，可以大大节省篇幅。举例如下。

【原句】The Aquaporin-1/beta-actin ratio in the mild hydronephrotic kidney, severe hydronephrotic kidney and normal kidney were 0.624 ± 0.084, 0.237 ± 0.154 and 0.858 ± 0.122 respectively, and the differences were significant（$P<0.00$）. The Aquaporin-2/beta-actin ratio in the mild hydronephrotic kidney, severe hydronephrotic kidney and normal kidney were 0.583 ± 0.112, 0.283 ± 0.124 and 0.976 ± 0.134 respectively, and the differences were significant（$P<0.00$）. The Aquaporin-3/beta-actin ratio in the mild hydronephrotic kidney, severe hydronephrotic kidney and normal kidney were 0.76 ± 0.066, 0.46 ± 0.146 and 1.001 ± 0.084 respectively, and the differences were significant（$P<0.00$）. The Aquaporin-4/beta-actin ratio in the mild hydronephrotic kidney, severe hydronephrotic kidney and normal kidney were 0.439 ± 0.076, 0.196 ± 0.124 and 0.739 ± 0.201 respectively, and the differences were significant（$P<0.00$）.

【改正】RT-PCR showed that the expressions of AQP1-4 was significantly decreased in the severe HnK group compared with those of mild HnK group and normal kidney（AQP1：0.237 ± 0.154 Vs. 0.624 ± 0.084 Vs. 0.858 ± 0.122；AQP2：0.283 ± 0.124 Vs. 0.583 ± 0.112 Vs. 0.976 ± 0.134；AQP3：0.46 ± 0.146 Vs. 0.76 ± 0.066 Vs. 1.001 ± 0.084；AQP4：0.196 ± 0.124 Vs. 0.439 ± 0.076 Vs. 0.739 ± 0.201, $P<0.01$ respectively）.

3. 矛盾、重复　作者撰写文章顾前不顾后，粗心大意，使论文摘要中出现不合逻辑、自相矛盾的语句。

【原句】The diagnosis and treatment of internal medicine

【改正】Diagnosis and medication

4. 被动语态泛滥　被动语态在描述实验过程、实验操作时，可以适当使用。但是前提是在实际环境中可以理解，关键是要使用得体。主动语态的句子可以替代一些被动语态，这样比较简洁。

【原句】It was not felt advisable that any further therapy should be given at this time.

【改正】We considered further treatment inadvisable.

5. **中式英文及其他**　我们在写论文时经常会遇到受汉语思维影响的情况。此外,英文论文摘要标题便是一个明显的例子。中文论文中经常出现"研究""探讨""调查""评价"等一类词语,翻译成英文标题时不能照译成"study of""investigate of""observation of""evaluation of",这样会让摘要显得冗长多余。查阅一下国外文献,这类词语很少使用。中文标题直译成英文,常会出错或表达不恰当。

第二节　关　键　词

为了引起读者对论文主题的注意,绝大部分杂志会要求作者在摘要后面提供 3~10 个关键词(key words)或短语。这些词应能反映论文的主题内容,也可以帮助标引员对论文进行标引,并且随摘要一起刊出。关键词包括主题词以及自由词两部分。一般而言,正规的关键词标引要使用美国国立医学图书馆的《医学索引》(Index Medicus)主题词表(MeSH)中的词汇。但如果是近期才提出的专用名词,尚没有被 MeSH 主题词表收录,那么使用现有的名词或词组以自由词的形式列出也是可以的,以补充关键词个数不足,并更好的表达论文的主题内容。如有关水通道蛋白的系列文章刚发表时,其中关键词水通道蛋白 AQPs(aquaporins)就不是 MeSH 中的词汇,但被作为自由词加入文章关键词部分。

确定关键词的时候,可通过上网检索 Medline 中相关课题的关键词。同时可以查阅主题词总表(由美国国立医学图书馆出版)。值得注意的是,一篇论文的关键词多数应该集中出现在文题中,这也是评价论文题目好坏的标准之一。我们在确定文章关键词的时候需要注意以下几点:①关键词最好采用已经定型的名词原形,多是单词或词组;②关键词必须具备检索价值;③化学分子式等符号类不能作为关键词;④未被本专业普遍接受或采用的缩写词不能作为关键词;⑤论文中提到的常规技术,应用过于普遍且不具有区分价值的词语不能作为关键词。

例如:笔者发表过的文章《原发性遗尿症尿动力学检查评估》中关键词为"遗尿;尿动力学";《终末型逼尿肌过度活动患者的尿动力学表现》关键词为"尿动力学;膀胱过度活动症;逼尿肌过度活跃";"Uroflowmetry combined with ultrasonic residual urine: good approach to evaluate detrusor function for benign prostate hyperplasia patients"(尿流率联合超声残余尿评估良性前列腺增生症逼尿肌收缩功能)其中关键词为"urodynamics; benign prostate hyperplasia; detrusor function; ultrasound; reflow"(尿动力学;良性前列腺增生症;逼尿肌;超声;残余尿)。

目前,不少 SCI 杂志对文章的关键词都有自己的要求,包括关键词个数、写作方式等。一般可以在杂志主页上的"author guidelines"下级菜单中找到。下面我们就一些不同领域 SCI 杂志对关键词的要求进行举例:

例 1　在泌尿外科杂志 *The Prostate* 中,其对关键词的要求只有言简意赅的一句话:"Supply a list of 3 to 6 key words or phrases (not in title) that will adequately index the subject matter of the article."。提供可以对文章主题进行确切索引的 3~6 个单词或短语(排除文章题目中已经出现的内容)。

在很多情况下,文章的题目和位于文章摘要之后的关键词一样,被认为是可以用来对文章进行索引的主要内容,单词重复的出现在标题以及关键词中其实是一种资源的浪费。因此,一些杂志在关键词书写中对这方面进行了限制。

例2 在生物化学与生物物理学杂志 *Biochemical and Biophysical Research Communication* 中,有关关键词的要求相对而言比较细致:"Immediately after the abstract, provide a maximum of 6 keywords, using American spelling and avoiding general and plural terms and multiple concepts (avoid, for example, 'and', 'of'). Be sparing with abbreviations: only abbreviations firmly established in the field may be eligible. These keywords will be used for indexing purposes."。在摘要部分之后,请紧接着提供最多6个关键词,采用美式拼写,避免一般性用语或词语的复数形式,避免多概念情况(如避免"and""of"的出现)。尽量不采用缩写形式,除非该缩写被该领域广泛认可和接受。这些关键词将用于对文章进行索引。

我们看出该杂志对关键词的要求非常细致,从书写规范、关键词个数,到选取关键词需要遵守的条件,无不一一列举。从这里也反映出杂志的特点和偏好,从而可以使我们对文章整体构架的布局起到了一个提示作用。比如该杂志对关键词的要求中提到了美式拼写这一规定,提示我们该杂志更倾向于美语的表达方式,因此对整篇文章进行写作的时候要更倾向于采用美式英语来进行表达。

例3 在消化系统杂志 *Clinical Gastroenterology and Hepatology* 中,则对关键词的要求精确到了标点符号方面,并对其应用方面进行了详细的举例说明:"Include three-to-four keywords associated with your manuscript, separated by semicolons (e.g., active vitamin D; parathyroid hormone-related peptide; hypercalcemia; bone resorption)."。包括3~4个与本文相关的关键词,词与词之间用分号进行分隔(如:活性维生素D;甲状旁腺激素相关肽;高血钙;骨重吸收)。

关键词是需要采用符号进行分隔的,一般不会出现词与词之间没有符号而只有空格的情况。但在有些已经发表的文章中,由于篇幅和排版的关系,关键词的位置有可能不在abstract部分之后,而是处于页面角落的位置并且以竖排的形式从上而下的进行排列。在这种情况下,关键词之间不需要分隔,当然在写作的具体要求中会进行细致的要求。

通常情况下,关键词之间多用逗号","或者分号";"进行分隔。对于大多数没有在关键词说明中给出详细要求的杂志,我们可以自由选择采用逗号或分号。但是对部分在这方面进行细致要求的杂志而言,我们在写作时必须完全按照要求进行。

例4 同样属于消化系统的顶级杂志 *Gastroenterology* 中,我们可以看出其对我们上述举例提到的内容进行了一个总结:"Include 3-4 keywords associated with your manuscript, separated by semicolons (e.g., active vitamin D; parathyroid hormone-related peptide; hypercalcemia; bone resorption). The keywords should be different than the words in the title of your manuscript. Should your manuscript be accepted, the keywords will appear with the published manuscript, making it easier to find in literature search engines such as PubMed."。包括3~4个与本文相关的关键词,词与词之间用分号进行分隔(如:活性维生素D;甲状旁腺激素相关肽;高血钙;骨重吸收)。关键词不能与标题所用词汇重复。如果您的稿件被接收,关键词会出现在出版的手稿中,使其在文献搜索引擎如PubMed中更容易被检索到。

由于 *Clinical Gastroenterology and Hepatology* 与 *Gastroenterology* 同属消化系统文章,使得它们在关键词的要求方面也有高度的重合性。不同的是,*Gastroenterology* 杂志对关键词的要求更加细致,除了对标点符号的限制外,还要求标题中出现过的词汇不可出现在关键词中,以避免造成重复检索的浪费。这一点与例 1 中所提出的观点相同。

例 5　在生物医学学杂志 *Antibodies* 中,将摘要部分与关键词部分的要求放在了一起进行规范,且对关键词的要求多了来自内容方面的规定:"Three to ten pertinent keywords need to be added after the abstract. We recommend that the abstract and the keyword list use words that are specific to the article yet reasonably common within the subject discipline."。在 abstract 部分后加入 3~10 个相关的关键词,我们建议摘要与关键词必须是特有的且能反映文章内容,并且在本领域内较为常见。

对于很多杂志而言,对关键词内容方面的约束要远远重要于格式方面的规定。这也反映出关键词本身所包含的价值,即文章索引的能力。我们需要能反映文章内容且常用的词汇作为关键词,这样在搜索引擎上进行检索时,能够很容易的让自己的文章出现在需要它们的学者面前,以提高文章的影响力和增加引用次数。能够达到这个效果的,便是我们所能提供的准确关键词了。

除此之外,其实相当多的杂志对于关键词的要求并不高,也不细致。如 Springer 出版社旗下的大部分杂志,在关键词一栏的要求中仅仅出现了 "Please provide 4 to 6 keywords which can be used for indexing purposes"(提供 4~6 个关键词用于索引目的)"这样简单的一句话,不涉及任何针对内容或格式方面的规定。但在这种情况下,我们也不要因为杂志的规定过于简单而对关键词部分的写作过于疏忽。因为,无论杂志有没有对关键词部分进行严格要求,关键词的书写都需要遵守一些约定俗成的规则,即我们前面提到的几个要点。要知道,杂志的要求是相对的,对自己时时刻刻的高要求才是写好一篇文章的重中之重。

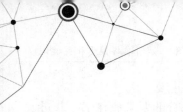

第 5 章
如何写作前言和研究目的

Chapter 5
How to Write Introduction and Objectives

前言(Introduction)即引言、序言或导语,是论文的开端,告诉读者为什么进行本研究并对正文主要内容进行解释。前言引导读者大概了解论文的背景和内容,突出论文的核心论点,让读者对论文的主旨或结论有所了解,使读者理解本文的核心和纲领。前言需要阐述研究问题的起因,此次研究的领域、设想和理论来源,可选择性追溯本研究问题的历史依据,以及此次研究内容方向前人的研究成果和知识空缺;言简意赅阐述当下国内外该研究的进程;也可以简单描述一下本研究的重要发现。A bad beginning makes a bad ending(Euripides),只有重视前言的写作,才能为写好整个论文打好基础。

一、前言的基本内容

前言是开场白,要将读者由浅入深地引入你研究的领域。正如英文描述的那样:"The purpose of an introduction is to bring the reader into the general area of your study and then state the specific area of study (move from the general to the specific. The introduction shows the scope of your investigation efforts).”。前言首先将带领读者了解文章所做研究的相关背景,即作者文章中所涉及范围的研究状况、现存的问题,以及当前新发展等。前言中还应包括对本研究重要性和研究意义的分析,并要使读者对于研究的总体范围和目的有较为直观的了解。总之,前言的内容通常包括以下 4 个方面:①研究背景:说明所研究问题的目前总体情况或历史(statement of general area or history of problem);②研究意义:说明本研究的意义或必要性(statement of significance or need);③研究目的:说明本研究的目的(statement of purpose of current study);④研究内容:简明扼要地介绍要研究的具体问题(statement of specific area of problem to be studied)。有的文献喜欢简要介绍自己的研究结果以便进一步吸引读者。

(一) 研究背景

研究背景主要介绍文中所研究问题的历史及现状。总的来说,理论性、学术性科技论文在前言中要将作者自己最新研究的结论与该方向的国内外同行已获取的学术理论成就相结合,并且纳入其中。与作者论文最新研究成果同范围的国内外同行的研究报道,包括已经取得的进展,以及对现存问题的评述,就形成了此类论文的研究背景。通常,研究背景的介绍要精练且有针对性,无需过多,其主要作用是使读者对文章所涉及的领域有一个初步的认知。医学科研论文作为学术性科技论文的一种,其有关研究背景的写作也要遵循上述原则。

但是,因医学研究涉及的疾病多,范围广,且各种疾病之间具有很强的交叉性,因此常常需要涉及较多内容。这就引出了大背景和小背景两方面的内容,这也是医学论文研究背景写作过程中独特的一面。

大背景即作者文章中研究所涉及的医学及社会学背景,如涉及疾病的研究要首先对该疾病的相关背景做一简单介绍,包括疾病的流行情况、诊疗情况、目前遇到的问题等。待读者了解研究的基本知识后,便可引入针对所做研究的相关介绍了,为读者介绍小背景即专业背景的内容,这将精确到某个方法、某种现象或某种机制的水平。下面以文献中的例子说明如何介绍研究背景。

例 1　Association between left ventricular hypertrophy with retinopathy and renal dysfunction in patients with essential hypertension

Shirafkan A, Motahari M, Mojerlou M, Rezghi Z, Behnampour N, Gholamrezanezhad A.

Hypertension (HTN) is the most common cardiovasculardisease. (1) The disease which was considered to be rareoutside of Europe and America in the early 1900s, is now diagnosed in more than 25% of the population throughout the world. (1, 2) Although HTN is often asymptomatic, the disease is related to different types of target organ damage (TOD) and associated clinical conditions. (2) SubtleTOD, such as left ventricular (LV) hypertrophy (LVH), retinopathy, microalbuminuria and cognitive dysfunction, occurs early in the course of hypertensive disease, while catastrophic events, such as stroke, heart attack, renalfailure and dementia, are usually a result of a long period of uncontrolled HTN complications. (3, 4) On the other hand, echocardiographically-determined LV mass (LVM) indices, corrected for either body surface area or patients' height, are independent risk predictors of cardiovascular disease and chronic heart failure. (5-9) Hence, these indices as well as other factors, such as the severity of retinopathy and renal dysfunction (all evidences of TOD), were confirmed to be major predictors of cardiovascular mortality and morbidity among hypertensive patients. (10-12) …

例 2　Expression of renal aquaporins is down-regulated in children with congenital hydronephrosis

* Jian Guo Wen, Zhen Zhen Li, Hong Zhang, Yan Wang, Guixian Wang, Qingwei Wang, Søren Nielsen, Jens Christian Djurhuus, Jørgen Frøkiaer

Congenital hydronephrosis due to pelviureteric junction obstruction (PUJO) is a frequent cause of renal failure in infants and children[1]. Developmental renal and urinary tract abnormalities have been reported responsible up to 54% of chronic renal insufficiency cases with a predominance of congenital obstructive nephro-uropathies[2]. Antenatal screening detects fetal hydronephrosis in about 1 of 100 births, with at least 20% being clinically significant[3]. Despite the impact of this devastating disease, the pathophysiologic mechanisms in most congenital obstructive cases in humans are not yet known …

以上两个例子均是前言部分有关背景介绍的内容。第一个例子对高血压发展的大背景做了概括性的介绍,包括高血压在欧洲的发展史,高血压的发病特点等,小背景则主要集中在高血压所产生的各种并发症,以及预测高血压严重程度的参数等。在第二个例子中,作者则介绍了先天性肾盂积水的发病原因、发病特点、诊断方法,以及目前对该疾病的研究现状等背景知识。通过对上述举例的研读,我们应当明白在进行某一疾病的背景介绍时,要按照上述写作格式,遵循该写作特点可以使读者对该疾病的重要性、复杂性以及研究该疾病的迫切性有一个直观的了解,同时点明了文章研究的意义所在,激发读者继续研读此文的浓厚兴趣。

(二)研究意义

研究需要说明其理由及必要性,这也是研究的意义所在。前言需要列举理论依据或实验数据来证明本研究的重要性,需要引用大量的文献,用来介绍自己或他人的工作,并对已有的理论或观点进行阐述和分析。在这个过程中,可以指出前人研究的缺陷,也可以对针对有争议的研究结果进行介绍,并指出亟待解决的问题,从而引出自己所做研究的重要性和创新点,凸显文章的意义所在。另外,这部分写作中如需引出新概念,则需要附上具体的说明和解释,不必留待正文中再去阐述。下面用文献中的例子加以说明。

Aquaporin 1 Is Over expressed in Lung Cancer and Stimulates NIH-3T3 Cell Proliferation and Anchorage-Independent Growth

Mohammad Obaidul Hoque, * Jean-Charles Soria, Janghee Woo* et al

… Most recently, we reported that the expression of AQP1and AQP5 is induced in the early stages of colorectal carcinogenesis. 10 other reports have alluded to the role of other AQPs in the development of human cancer … As a firststep in examining the role of AQPs in human lung carcinogenesis, we studied AQP1 expression during the development of non-small cell lung cancer (NSCLC). We initially used reverse transcriptase-polymerase chain reaction (RTPCR) to screen the expression profiles of human AQP1 in 10 NSCLC cell lines, and confirmed our results by Western blotanalysis …

这个例子告诉我们,在叙述自己研究理由的时候,一定要详细罗列证据,并对所举的例子进行较为详细的分析,从而引出自己所涉及的研究目前存在的问题,顺理成章地对自己所做的研究进行介绍。

(三)研究目的

前言需要对写作目的进行简单介绍,包括针对何种问题进行研究,主要解决了哪方面的难题等。研究目的是前言中必不可少的部分,但并不需要对其进行冗长的叙述。下面用文献中的例子加以说明。

Association between left ventricular hypertrophy with retinopathy and renal dysfunction in patients with essential hypertension

Shirafkan A, Motahari M, Mojerlou M, Rezghi Z, Behnampour N, Gholamrezanezhad A.

… In selected populations such as those with HTN, renal dysfunction was found to be related to LVH. (11) Some authors also claimed that LVH is an independent predictor for extracardiac TODs in essential HTN. (13) Infact, some of the previous reports revealed that there is a significant association between different types of TOD in hypertensive populations. (14-16) Unfortunately, discordant conclusions on this matter emphasis the need for further investigation on such relationships. (17, 18). Therefore, the aim of this study was to examine the relationship between LVH and other signs of TODs (retinopathy and renalfailure) secondary to systemic HTN.

通过上述例子我们不难看出,在引出自己所做研究的目的之前,首先要对该研究方向现有的研究结果进行总结,指出其不足之处或者尚未解决的问题,同时强调该遗留问题的重要性、复杂性以及紧迫性,随后再对文章目的作一介绍。一般而言,对文章目的的叙述不宜过长,一两句话即可。但该目的一定要承接上文,即对解决了一个遗留问题或者对解决该问题具有潜在的贡献。

(四)研究内容

在前言写作的最后,可以对本研究的基本内容进行一个笼统的总结,其目的是使读者对文章大概的框架有所了解。该总结除了简介研究得出的结论之外,还需要对研究中所涉及的理论创新、方法创新等内容加以说明。因为是否具有创新性是一篇文章的核心价值所在,也是审稿人和读者重点关注的问题。此外,作者还可以根据研究所得结论的内容,对文章的意义和研究前景进行介绍,以再次强调文章的重要性。下面用文献中的例子加以说明。

Expression and Immunohistochemical Localization of Aquaporin-1 in Male Reproductive Organs of the Mouse

D. Y. Lu, Y. Li, Z. W. Bi, et al

… This study investigated the expression of AQP-1 mRNA and protein in the testis, epididymis, vasdeferens, ventral prostate and seminal vesicle from maturemice by using reverse transcription polymerase chain reaction (RT-PCR) and Western blotting and the cellular localization of AQP-1 by immuno histochemistry.

由上述例子我们可以看出,研究方法和结果的写作在前言部分只需要略有提及,因为其具体的介绍会放在正文的"材料与方法"以及"结果"部分。前言中提及这部分内容的主要作用是引起读者对文章的兴趣,有继续读下去的动力。

二、前言的写作要求

(一)言简意赅、意精词明,点明主题即可

引言的语言要求简洁明了,对读者阅读正文具有明确的指导作用。因此,无需做过多的铺垫,而是一语中的,不绕圈子。篇幅不宜过长,一般约占全文的 1/10~1/8,例如一篇四五千字的论文,前言应控制在 300~500 字。前言应突出重点,一般教材上已有的内容或为人熟识、显而易见的机制或意义,在前言中不必过多论述,应言简意赅地介绍研究工作的来龙去脉及课题的概况、价值和意义。介绍背景时可选择性借鉴以往重要的文献,并加以对比分析,切记不要长篇大论的回顾历史,列举文献不作系统综述,无需过多回顾和评价。

(二)叙述清楚

引言与结论相呼应很重要。引言中涉及的问题,通常在结论中作出相应的回应。所以,引言的写作要层次分明且具有缜密的逻辑性,首先写什么,其次写什么,以及如何去论述。这些都是撰写引言必须思考的问题。但无论怎么写,引言的作用在于使读者思路清晰,更好地为阅读论文正文做铺垫,即引言的引导作用始终不变。因此,引言必须依据逻辑顺序来布局。只有如此,才能层次分明,文理贯通。

（三）用词恰当，客观评价

一方面要避免对自己研究工作的吹捧，要把握好分寸，避免使用夸大其辞的语句，如"前人不曾探索过""文献也未发表过""本文在国内外首次发表""本文达到世界最高水平或在国内外遥遥领先""填补了一项空白"等自夸性的语言。一方面要防止过度自夸，同时也要避免过分谦虚，言之无物，如"才薄智浅，能力不足""疏漏谬误之处，恳乞指教""不足之处，期望多提出宝贵意见""不足之处在所难免"等的客套话。因为一篇论文的水平如何，具有何种意义，内容是否准确，不是由作者所决定，而是由广大读者做出的客观评价所决定的。另一方面，也要避免过度贬抑他人、文人相轻的趋势，在指出他人研究工作中存在的问题时，一定要实事求是、有凭有据，用语要恰如其分。要客观地评价前人在相关研究方向已做出的成绩，绝不能有意贬低，以免造成不良影响。

（四）缩略词说明

如果在论文中使用专业化语言，或缩略词、符号等，应在前言中给予解释说明，即在对应词后用括号标注。

Functionality of aquaporin-2 missense mutantsin recessive nephrogenic diabetes insipidus

N. Marr, E.J. Kamsteeg, M. van Raak

The vasopressin-regulated water channel aquaporin-2 (AQP2) plays an important role in the reabsorption of water in the kidney collecting duct and consequently in concentrating urine[2]. Binding of arginine vasopressin (AVP) to the V2 receptor at the basolateral side of principal cells of collecting ducts leads to an increase in the intracellular concentration of cAMP, resulting in the phosphorylationof AQP2 by protein kinase A (PKA) and the subsequent re-distribution of AQP2 from subapical storagevesicles to the apical plasma membrane … The congenital form of nephrogenic diabetes insipidus (NDI), a disease in which the kidney is unable to concentrate urine in response to AVP, can be caused by mutations either in the gene coding for the V2 receptor, the X-linked form, or in the AQP2 gene, the autosomal form of NDI[7, 14] … Expression in oocytes of missense mutants in recessiveNDI revealed that all were impaired in their export fromthe endoplasmic reticulum (ER), presumably through misfolding of the mutants, providing the molecular basisfor NDI caused by these mutants[1, 7]. High expression levels in oocytes and later in Chinese hamster ovary (CHO) cells revealed that three AQP2 mutants in recessive AQP2-A147T, AQP2-L22 V)[7, 12] …

一个好的前言建议按如下规则进行书写：①前言要尽量简明扼要，包括调查问题的类型和范围；②应该回顾相关文献；③应该说明研究方法，如果觉得有必要，应说明选择特殊方法的原因；④应该陈述研究的主要结果；⑤应该陈述由结果得出的主要结论。

第一个规则（提出问题）是最重要的，因为如果没有合理而且容易理解的方法来介绍问题，读者将对你的文章后面部分没有兴趣。在前言中，你应该有一个"诱饵"来吸引读者的注意力。为什么你选择那个课题？它为什么重要？第二个规则和第三个规则与第一个规则联系密切。文献回顾和选择的方法应该使读者能够理解问题是什么以及你试图用怎样的方式解决它。这三个规则自然而然引出了第四和第五个规则，即主要结果和结论的陈述。

三、前言写作注意事项

（一）把握好全面和精练的问题，既要介绍当前领域概况，又要突出重点，论文的背景来源要避免过于空洞。

（二）避免与论文摘要、结论相似，或防止对摘要进行解释说明。要明确不同部分的侧重点和界限。

（三）避免文不对题，写作思路不清晰，在前言中提出的问题在结论中没有回答。

（四）注意文献的引用。前言是大量信息量的汇总，需要相当多的文献对你的观点提供支持，因此详细而恰当地选择引用文献对前言的写作非常重要。

（五）避免出现图画、列表，不要阐述基本理论，不要推导数学公式，不要叙述基本方法，在前言中不要重复出现教科书已有内容。

（六）如果前言过于简短，不应分段。

（七）在阐明自己的最新研究成果时，别人的成果和自己的成就要有所区别，否则容易造成所述的创新内容含糊其辞，引发不必要争议。

四、举例说明如何写好前言

例 1 作者利用国内三聚氰胺的公共事件，对患者进行随访，探讨三聚氰胺对儿童生长发育的影响。该论文的前言如下。

It has been a year since the melamine-tainted milk powder scandal occurred in China in the fall of 2008. Chinese authorities provided free screening and treatment to all infants with melamine-related urinary stones (MUS). Many research results regarding MUS epidemiology, diagnosis, clinical symptoms and treatment have been published since that time（介绍文章的研究背景）。

Although more than half of MUS cases recovered after a short-time stay in the hospital, there were still many infants and young children with residual stones at the time of discharge from hospital. Prognosis and post hospital treatment effects of these cases need to be further investigated. The clinical features of infants and young children with residual MUS, the effects of toxic milk powder on kidney, bladder and body growth are still unclear in the past one year.（介绍本研究领域存在的问题和为什么要进行本研究目的的研究背景）。

The compound melamine is a synthetic product used primarily as a plastics stabilizer and fire retardant. In animal models, urogenital lesions, urolithiasis and bladder carcinoma have been found with long-term in take of melamine.（目前的研究现状）。

Based on these observations, we hypothesized: ① Most of residual MUS may disappear with conservative treatment during the past one year; ② Melamine milk powder consumed by infants in last year may have no effects on growth of kidney, bladder and body after one year due to the fact that the contents of melamine in milk powder was lower than those used in animal studies.（提出亟待解决的问题和假设）。

The aim of this study was to summarize clinical features and effects of toxic milk powder on the kidney, bladder and body growth in infants and young children with diagnosed MUS in the past one year after discharging from hospitals.（最后提出本文的研究目的）。

该前言的书写言简意赅，重点突出，值得大家借鉴。

例 2 是发表在 *J Urol*（美国《泌尿外科杂志》）的一篇文章。

Melamine Related Bilateral Renal Calculi in 50 Children: Single Center Experience in Clinical Diagnosis and Treatment

Jian Guo Wen, * Zhen Z. Li, Hong Zhang, Yan Wang, Rui F. Zhang, Li Yang, Yan Chen, Jia X. Wang and Sheng J. Zhang

Urolithiasis is a common urological disease that affects approximately 10% of the population worldwide. The incidence of urolithiasis in children, approximately 2%~3% in China, occurs most likely between the age of 2 and 6 years. Bilateral renal calculi are extremely rare in the absence of an underlying diagnosis. Since the first media reports linking an outbreak of renal diseases among children on mainland China to the consumption of milk products contaminated with melamine on September 11, 2008, more than 50 000 children have been exposed to melamine-tainted milk products. All infants and children fed with melamine-tainted milk formula received free screening and treatment in a hospital. At the same time, the incidence of bilateral renal calculi in Chinese children has increased, but cases were rarely reported.（介绍文章的研究背景）。

Melamine is a chemical compound. Little is known about the adverse effects of melamine consumption in humans, especially in young children. Melamine was added illegally in milk-collecting stations to increase apparent protein concentration readings to meet the national standard on the protein content of milk before Oct. 2008 in China. It has been reported that outbreak of urinary stone in young children is related to consumption of melamine-tainted formula. After Oct. 2008, the test of new batch of formula from Chinese government didn't show any melamine. Thereafter no new melamine-related urinary stone cases have been diagnosed. Accordingly, a close tie may exist between the consumption melamine-tainted milk powder and the outbreak of pediatric urinary stone.（目前的研究现状，提出仍然存在的问题）。

Our clinical practice showed that bilateral renal calculi have been found in one-third of all patients diagnosed with stones from September to October 2008. However, their clinical manifestation and treatment response have not been reported. Therefore, the purpose of this report was to investigate clinical features and treatment response in children with bilateral renal melamine-related calculi.（最后提出本文的研究目的）。

下面再看一个反例，供读者借鉴。

Introduction　Septum pellucid tumor is seldom and accounts for about 0.5% of intracranial tumors. Previous studies focused mostly on central neurocytoma but the number of cases is inadequate。In our study, we reviewed 41 patients with septum pellucidum tumor treated at our hospital from January 1998 to September 2004. The diagnosis of these patients was confirmed by imaging and operation. Clinical manifestations and pathological findings were analyzed to determine which of transcortical, transulcal or transcallosal approaches is applicable for the resection of septum pellucidum tumor in consideration of factors of extent of the resection and postoperative complications.

Chinese Medical Journal, 2005, 118 (1): 812-816.

例 3 中的前言过于简单，背景知识交代内容较少。

五、前言常用英语句型

（一）研究背景

1. 国内外相关课题的研究成果和现状 在对研究背景进行介绍时,熟练掌握一些常用词和常用句型对于文章的写作将大有裨益。在此笔者收集英文撰写相关书籍中的例子对其进行简要的介绍。

常用词:demonstrate（演示）,carry out（完成）,conduct（进行）,perform（做）,present（提出）,test（测试）,develop（开发、研制）,investigate（研究）,examine（考察）

常用句型:

（1）描述特定人物进行的研究（以下例句中人名以 A 和 B 代替）:A. et al. tested（developed,reported,conducted,used）… ,they found that … Something were（was）conducted（performed,made）by A.

A 和 B 在 1931 年提出关于……的最早报道之一。

One of the earliest reports of … was made in 1931 by A and B.

A 在 1932 年做了关于……的早期研究。

Early studies in … were reported in 1932 by A.

A 和 B 所著的文章是最早研究关于……之一。

The paper by A and B is one of the earliest which considered the …

A 与其他人采用了另一种方法（见 1993 年发表的文章）。

Another method of … has been used by A et al. (1993).

A 采用了一个略微不同的方法来……。

A (1987) adopted a slightly different approach to …

A 与其他人描述了一项技术……。

A et al. (1984) described a technique for …

（2）对已有研究进行分类:研究者们所用方法包括两种:一种是……,另一种是……。

The ways that researchers have put forward may be concluded in two sorts: One is … The other is …

这些理论大致分为两类:一类是……,另一类是……。

Generally speaking, these theories fall into two categories: One is … ; and the other is …

基于……的模式可分为两组。

The models based on … can be divided into two groups.

（3）对研究结果进行总结:

已有几位研究者从理论上研究了……

Several researchers have theoretically investigated …

基于……的结果,A 提出……

Based on … results of A et al. confirmed that …

过去对……的研究工作说明……

The previous work on … has indicated that …

……所做的近期试验已表明……

Recent experiments by … have suggested …

近期的研究工作在下列文章中都有报道,如 A(见 1984 年文章),以及……

Some work has also been presented recently by authors such as A (1984), and …

A 与其他人报道过关于……的最新研究(见 1998 年文章)。

The most recent work on … has been reported by A et al. (1998).

对……的使用可追溯到 20 世纪末。

The history of the use of … dates back to the end of the last century.

2. 相关课题未得到充分研究及研究的不足之处　对某研究的国内外现状进行回顾后,接着要提及目前关于该研究存在的问题,以便为自己所做研究的创新性和重要性进行铺垫。其常用句型包括:

……未得到充分研究。

… has not yet been thoroughly investigated.

尽管关于……的一般领域有不少论著,但对于…少有研究。

Although a number of papers have been published in the general area of … little work has been carried out for …

然而,对于……的问题以前还没有研究过。

However, no prior work exists on the problem of …

未曾报道过对于……的进一步研究。

No further study on the … has been reported.

尽管最近有些进展,但关于……仍然没有一致认同的理论。

Despite the recent progress, there is no theory concerning …

迄今为止,没有足够令人信服的证据表明……

So far there is not enough convincing evidence showing …

在……方面没有相关的发现。

No such finding could be available in …

文献资料未能证明……

The data available in literature failed to prove that …

对……的性质还不是了解得很清楚。

The character of the … is not yet very well known.

尽管在……方面做了大量研究,但在……方面却少有研究。

While much research has been undertaken on … , less work has addressed the …

回顾文献资料,似乎没有关于……的相关研究。

From a literature survey, it appears that none of the previous investigators is concerned with …

然而,这种方法不能用来分析更加实际的情况,比如……

However, this method cannot be used to analyze more practical cases in which …

人们早就意识到……的局限性,一个经常遇到的问题是……

The limitations of … have long been recognized. One problem frequently encountered is that …

然而,这些算法要求……实际上有时很难满足。

However, these algorithms require … , which can be problematic in practice.

在运用……时,存在一些缺点。

There are some shortcomings in the use of …

该方法的另外一个缺点是……

Another disadvantage of this approach is that …

该理论不能应用于关于……的其他情况。

The theory cannot apply to other cases of …

以上所有模型都忽视了……

All of the above models ignored …

对…的研究存在着两个主要问题:一个是……;另一个是……

The study of … gives rise to two main difficulties: One is … ; and the other is …

……的理论无法解释……

The theory of … did not explain …

此类方法的主要缺点是……

The main drawback of this type of methods is that …

尽管它们……,但缺点是:更加复杂,成本高,无法大量供应。

Although they … , they have the disadvantage of greater complexity and higher cost, and are not commercially available.

3. 相关课题引起关注情况　在介绍了针对某研究的不足之处后,继续为自己所做研究进行铺垫的内容还包括目前与本研究相关的课题进展情况,所引起的关注与影响等,从侧面凸显自己所选取研究方向的重要程度。具体例句包括:

句型:Sth. has received (significant, considerable …) attention.

近年来对……的研究已引起足够关注。

Research on … has received significant attention in recent years.

与……相关的问题长期以来都为研究者们所关注。

The problem associated with … has for a long time been of interest to investigators.

与……相关的问题已经受到长期的关注和研究。

During the past several years, there has been considerable interest in …

因此,近几年人们对……的使用越来越关注。

For this reason, increased attention has been paid in recent years to the use of …

最近以来对……的研究较为活跃。

… has been an active area of research recently.

近年来人们对……的兴趣日增。

… has undergone a remarkable increase in interest and attention in recent years.

鉴于……,人们正在对……进行大量研究。

In view of the … , considerable effort is being expanded into …

（二）研究内容

在详细介绍研究背景后,我们需要对自己所做研究的内容也进行简要介绍,以提高人们对阅读该文章的兴趣。其相关句型简要介绍如下:

常用词和词组:examine,purpose,describe,analyze,introduce,explain,discuss,deal with, present, focus on, concentrate on.

句型:This paper examines (is concerned with, deal with, presents, describes and evaluates, concentrates on) …

本研究考察 IT 对……的作用。

This research examines the effect of IT use on …

本文提出两种新技术。

This paper proposes two new techniques.

本文分析了……

The article presents an analysis of …

本文说明……的各种设计方法。

The paper describes various designs for …

本文讨论了……的三种基本方法。

The paper discussed the three basic methods that …

本文论述了……的问题。

The paper addressed the problems of …

本文旨在描述……

The paper intended to describe …

本研究特别针对……

It is the particular intention of this work to remark upon the …

本文着重于……

In this paper, attention is focused on …

本文重点是调查……

The emphasis of this paper is to survey …

因此,本研究着重于……

The present study will therefore focus on …

在本文中我们设计出对于……的一些方法。

In this paper, we develop some methods for …

在本工作中,我们研究……

In the present work we study …

课题主要是关于……的研究。

The subject is concerned chiefly with the study of …

作者的研究侧重于……的几个相关方面。

The author has limited his studies to the related aspects of …

本文探讨的问题是在……的范围内。

The problem under discussion is within the scope of …

下面是一些实例。

The following are some examples.

(三)研究目的

前言的最后,我们往往需要用一句或几句话将本文所研究的目的进行简要概括,包括研究得到的结果以及其意义等。具体例句如下。

常用词：purpose，objective，aim，goal

句型：The（primary，overall，major）objective（purpose，goal，aim）of this study（research，paper，project，investigation，experiment）is …

本文旨在描述和分析……

The purpose of this study is to describe and analyze …

本研究的目的在于……

The objective of the study consists in …

本研究的目的旨在为……找到一个解决方法。

The aim of the research presented in this paper is to find a way for …

进行此项研究工作可以加深我们对……的理解。

This research work has been undertaken to enhance our understanding of the …

本研究的目的是调查……

The goal of this work is to investigate the …

本研究的一个重要目的是研究……

It was, therefore, our objectives to study …

参考目前的文献资料，我们为……而进行此项研究。

On the basis of existing literature data, we carried out studies in an effort to …

在本文中，我们的目的是……

In this paper, we aim at …

本研究目的有三个：1）……2）……3）……

The study has three objectives: 1) … 2) … 3) …

This study was undertaken to assess the effect of glucagon on biliary tract opacification during intravenous cholangiography.

本研究旨在评定静脉胆管造影时高血糖素对胆道显影的作用。

A study was undertaken to find out the mechanism of cholestasis in amoebic liver abscess.

本研究旨在查明阿米巴肝脓肿时胆汁郁滞的机制。

In this study, an attempt was made to determine if the electrocardiogram or vectorcardiogram might show previously unrecognized evidence of myocardial infarction.

本研究旨在测定心电图及心向量图是否能发现潜在的心肌梗死。

Attempt were made to find prognostic factors in myeloma.

我们试图找到骨髓瘤的预后因素。

In an attempt to determine which type of antihypertensive drug is more effective in reducing left ventricular hypertrophy, thiazide a-methyldopa. hydralazine and propranolol were administered singly or in combination to patients with essential hypertension, and to spontaneously hypertensive rats.

作者单一或联合使用噻嗪类，甲基多巴、肼本哒嗪及普萘洛尔治疗原发性高血压患者患者及自发性高血压小鼠，以期确定哪种类型降压药物对消减左心室肥厚更为有效。

The preoperative clinical and hemodynamic findings of 139 consecutive patients with aortic stenosis were analyzed in an attempt to determine the incidence and influence of coronary heart disease on the mode of presentation of patients with aortic stenosis.

作者分析了连续 139 例主动脉狭窄患者的术前及血流动力学资料,以期测定其发病率及冠心病对主动脉狭窄患者临床类型的影响。

In an effort to determine the usefulness of prodromata for predicting a myocardial infarction, a prospective analysis was made of 211consecutive patients with chest pain who were admitted to the Stanford University Medical Center Coronary Care Unit

作者对 Stanford 大学医疗中心冠心病监护室连续收治的 211 例胸痛患者做了前瞻性分析,试图确定前驱症状对预测心肌梗死的效用。

In order to investigate the mechanisms of severe growth failure in children with Crohn's disease, 7affected patients were studied before, during, and after parenteral nutrition as a supplement to oral intake.

为了研究克罗恩病患儿严重发育障碍的发病机制,我们给 7 例患儿肠道外补充营养,并对补充营养前、补充过程中,以及补充营养后三个阶段分别进行了研究。

A total of 70 cases of cholestatic jaundice have been studied by gray scale ultrasonography in order to evaluate how this technique may be used to differentiate between intra-and extrahepatic cholestasis.

我们采用灰级超声显像对 70 例胆汁淤积性黄疸患者进行了研究,以期确定如何使用这一方法来鉴别肝内及肝外胆汁淤积。

六、前言常用语态和时态

(一)叙述有关现象或普遍事实时,常用现在时。

(二)描述特定研究领域中最近的某种趋势,或者强调表示某些“最近”发生的事件对现在的影响时,常采用现在完成时。如:

Few studies have been done on bone marrow stem cells.

Little attention has been devoted to bone marrow stem Cells.

(三)在阐述作者本人研究的方法及结果的句子时,多使用过去时。

(四)在阐述作者本人研究目的的句子中应有类似“In this study, …”“The experiment reported, …”等词,以表示所涉及的内容是作者现在的工作,而不是指其他学者或者作者过去的研究。

(五)适当地使用第一人称如 we 或 our,以明确地指明是作者本人的工作。

【推荐】We conducted this study to determine whether …

【不推荐】The study was conducted to determine whether …

总之,在前言的写作过程中,最好能做到层层递进,环环相扣,由大背景介绍至小背景,并提出问题,从而引出自己的研究,为文章后续部分的写作埋下伏笔。前言就像舞台上华丽的序幕,用五光十色的丰富内容牢牢吸引住读者的眼球,从而对后续即将发生的整个故事产生出浓厚的兴趣。

第 6 章
如何写作材料和方法

Chapter 6
How to Write Materials and Methods

　　材料和方法（Materials and Methods）是论文的基础，如果材料方法描述不当，所得的实验结果将会受到质疑。可见科研方法非常重要。Whitehead 曾经指出 19 世纪最大的发明就是发现了能够创造发明的科研方法（The greatest invention of the nineteenth century was the invention of the method of invention）。材料方法描述主要包括：实验对象（实验材料）及其性质特征，研究的方法（处理方法）和实验设计，实验的目的，使用的仪器、设备、器材、化学制剂及成分，生物制剂和型号来源，实验研究的方法与过程，统计学分析采用的方法和标准。

　　国际期刊发表的文章，在材料和方法部分，描述比较详细完整，读者可根据实验资料来判断实验设计和实验过程是否可信，而且按照描述的过程，完全可以重复该实验。材料和方法部分应该用过去时态来表述，因为所叙述的这些实验设计、实验材料和实验过程均已完成。下面结合作者在 SCI 期刊美国生理杂志《肾脏生理》（Wang G. Am J Physiol Renal Physiol. 2008 Aug；295（2）：F497-506.）上发表的一篇动物实验的基础研究论文来说明材料和方法部分如何撰写。

Materials and methods

Experimental protocols

All procedures conformed with the Danish national guidelines for the care and handling of animals and to the published guidelines from the National Institutes of Health. The animal protocols were approved by the board of the Institute of Clinical Medicine, University of Aarhus, according to the licenses for use of experimental animals issued by the Danish Ministry of Justice. Studies were performed on male Munich-Wistarrats initially weighing 250 g (Møllegard Breeding Centre, Eiby, Denmark). Rats were maintained on a standard rodent diet (Altromin, Lage, Germany) with free access to water. Rats were assigned randomly to either the sham-operated control or the experimental groups and kept in individual metabolic cages, with a 12: 12-h artificial light-dark cycle, a temperatureof (21 ± 2)℃, and a humidity of (55 ± 2)%. Rats were allowed to acclimatize to the cages for 3 days before surgery. Water intake, urine output, and body weight of the rats were monitored every 24 h during study.

Rats were anesthetized with isofluran (Abbott Scandinavia), and during surgery the rats were placed on a heated table to maintain constant temperature (rectal temperature at 37~38℃). In protocol 1, through a midline abdominal incision, both ureters were occluded by silk ligature for 24 h, and then rats were sacrificed. In protocols 2, the ureters were exposed and a 4-mm-long piece of bisected polyethylene tubing (PE-50) wasplaced around the midportion of each ureter (12; 25; 26). The ureter wasthen occluded by tightening the tubing with a 4-0 silkligature. After surgery rats were allowed to regain consciousness. Twenty-four hours later, rats were anesthetized again and the obstructed ureters were decompressed by removal of the ligature and the PE tubing. With this technique, the ureters could be completely occluded for 24 h without evidence of impaired ureter function. Rats were randomly allocated to the protocols indicated below. Age-and time-matched, sham-operated controls were prepared and wereobserved in parallel with each experimental group in the following protocols.

上面段落主要描述了研究所使用动物的一般情况，包括动物的名称、产地、体重、喂养条件、动物模型制作方法等。

Protocol 1. BUO was induced for 24h (BUO, n=12), and the two kidneys were removed and separately prepared for semiquantitative immunoblotting (n=7) or immunocytochemistry (n=5). For time-and age-matched sham-operated controlrats (Sham, n=12), the two kidneys were also removed and separately prepared for semiquantitative immunoblotting (n=7) or immunocytochemistry (n=5).

Protocol 2. BUO was induced for 24h, followed by release, and rats were observed for the following 4 days (n=19). To examine whether release of BUO (BUO-R) was associated with an acidification defect, BUO-R rats were subjected to either vehicle (BUO-R, 3ml of water, n=11) or acid loading (BUO-A, 0.033mmol NH_4Cl/g body wt in 3ml of water (11; 14), n=8) by gavage once a day during the last 2 days before termination. In parallel sham-operated animals were also subjected to acid loading (Sham-A, n=7) or vehicle (Sham, n=7). Semiquantitative immunoblotting was performed in BUO-R and Sham groups.

上面两段介绍了该动物研究的两种方案，包括各组的例数、标本采集、观察指标等。

Clearance studies

Body weight, water intake, food intake and urine output were observed during the time rats were maintained in the metabolic cages. Urine was collected during 24 hours periods throughout the study. The pH of urine was measured with a 744 pH meter (Metrohm, Switzerland).

Clearance studies were performed during the last 24 hours in each protocol. During anesthesia, at the end of each protocol, 3~4ml of arterial blood was drawn in gas-tight syringes from the abdominal aorta before removal of the kidneys. One aliquot of the blood sample was used immediately for blood-gas analysis with an ABL system 615 (Radiometer). The remaining blood was centrifuged for the determination of plasma electrolytes and osmolality. The plasma concentrations of creatinine, urea, sodium, and potassium were determined (Kodak Ektachem 700XRC). The osmolality of plasma was measured with a vapor pressure osmometer (Osmomat 030, Gonotec, Berlin, Germany).

上面的内容重点介绍了本研究中一个重要的观察指标"clearance studies"。

Membrane fractionation for immunoblotting

After rapid removal of kidneys, the left kidney was frozen in liquid nitrogen and the right kidney was split into inner medulla (IM), inner stripe of outer medulla (ISOM), and cortex and outer stripe of outer medulla (C+OSOM), using a microscope. Tissue (IM, ISOM or C+OSOM) was minced finely and homogenized in 1ml (IM), 1.5ml (ISOM) or 2ml (C+OSOM) of ice cold dissecting buffer (0.3 M sucrose, 25mM imidazole, 1mM EDTA, pH 7.2, and containing the following protease inhibitors: 8.5μM leupeptin, 1mM phenylmethylsulfonyl fluoride), with five strokes of a motor-driven Potter-Elvehjem homogenizer at 1,250 rpm. This homogenate was centrifuged in a Universal 30RF centrifuge (Hettich, Tuttlingen, Germany) at 4 000g for 15 min at 4℃. The supernatants were assayed for protein concentration using the method of BCA protein assay. Gel samples (in Laemmli sample buffer containing2% SDS) were made from this membrane preparation, and then stored at −20℃.

Electrophoresis and immunoblotting

Samples of membrane fractions from IM, ISOM, and C+OSOM were run on 12% or 9% SDS-polyacrylamide minigels (Bio-Rad Mini Protean III). For each gel, an identical gel was run in parallel and subjected to Coomassie blue staining. The Coomassie-stained gel was used to verify identical loading or to allow for potential correction for minor differences in loading after scanning and densitometry of major bands. The other gel was subjected to Western blotting analysis. After transfer by electroelution to nitrocellulose membranes, blots were blocked with 5% milk in PBS-T (80mM Na_2HPO_4, 20mM NaH_2PO_4, 100 mMNaCl, 0.1% Tween 20, pH 7.5) for 1 h and incubated with primary antibodies overnight at 4℃. After being washed with PBS-T, the blots were incubated with horse radish peroxidase-conjugated secondary antibody (P447 or P448, DAKO A/S, Glostrup Denmark, diluted 1 ∶ 3 000) for 1 h. After a final washing as above, antibody binding was visualized using the (ECL) enhanced chemiluminescence system (Amersham International). ECL films with bands within the linear range were scanned (Arcus II, Agfa, and Corel Photo paint software). The labeling density was corrected by densitometry of the Coomassie blue-stained gels.

Immunocytochemistry

The kidneys from BUO rats and sham-operated rats were fixed by retrograde perfusion via the abdominal aorta with 3% paraformaldehyde, in 0.1 M cacodylate buffer pH 7.4. For immunoperoxidase microscopy, kidney blocks containing all kidney zones were dehydrated and embedded in paraffin. The paraffin embedded tissues were cut at 2 micrometer on a rotary microtome (Leica, Germany). The sections were deparaffinated and rehydrated. For immunoperoxidase labeling, endogenous peroxidase were blocked by 0.5% H_2O_2 in absolute methanol for 10 min at room temperature. To reveal antigens, sections were put in 1mmol/L TRIS solution (pH 9.0) supplemented with 0.5mM EGTA (3.6-di-oxa-octa-methylen-di-nitrilo-tetra-acetic-acid) and heated using a microwave oven for 10 min. Nonspecific binding of immunoglobulin was prevented by incubating the sections in 50mM NH_4Cl in 30 min followed by blocking in PBS supplemented with 1% BSA, 0.05% saponin and 0.2% gelatin. Sections were incubated overnight at 4℃ with primary antibodies diluted in PBS supplemented with 0.1% BSA and 0.3% Triton X-100. After rinsing with PBS supplemented with 0.1% BSA, 0.05% saponin and 0.2% gelatin for 3 x 10 min, the sections were washed, then incubated with horseradish peroxidase-conjugated immunoglobulin (DAKO A/S, Glostrup, Denmark, P448, 1 ∶ 200) diluted in PBS supplemented with 0.1% BSA and 0.3% Triton-X-100. The sections were washed for 3 x 10 min and followed by incubation with diaminobenzidine for 10 minutes. The microscopy was carried out using a Leica DMRE light microscope (Leica, Heidelberg, Germany).

上述段落重点介绍了 membrane fractionation for immunoblotting, electrophoresis, immuno-blotting, immunocytochemistry 4 种基础实验方法和相关化学试剂, 这是材料和方法部分的重点内容。

Primary antibodies

For semiquantitative immunoblotting and immunocytochemistry, we used previously characterized polyclonal antibodies to several key acid-base transporters, as follows:

1) NHE3: type 3 Na^+/H^+ exchanger (26)

2) NBC1: rat kidney electrogenic Na^+/HCO_3^- cotransporter (23)

3) NBCn1: electroneutral Na^+/HCO_3^- cotransporter (23)

4) NKCC2 (BSC-1): bumetanide-sensitive Na^+-K^+-$2Cl^-$ cotransporter (10)

5) Pendrin: anion exchanger pendrin (11)

6) H^+-ATPase: B_1 subunit of vacuolar type H^+-ATPase (20)

上面内容主要介绍了本研究使用的抗体等具体生物制剂的情况, 这是基础研究必须阐明的内容。

Statistical analysis

For the densitometry of immunoblots, samples from experimental kidneys were run on each gel with corresponding sham kidneys. Renal acid-base transporter expression in the samples from the experimental animals was calculated as a fraction of the mean sham control value for that gel. Parallel Commassie-stained gels were subjected to densitometry and used for correction of potential minor differences in loading. Values are presented in the text as means ± SE. Comparisons between two groups were made by unpaired *t*-test, and more than two groups were made by one way ANOVA analysis. *P* values <0.05 were considered statistically significant.

通过对以上动物实验研究论文的材料和方法部分的分析, 我们简单总结一下撰写动物实验等基础研究论文材料和方法部分的要点。

首先介绍实验动物情况, 从以下几个方面进行描述: ①实验动物种系及来源、实验时的体重(必要时还要写上动物的年龄如几周、几个月或几年)、动物的喂养环境、饲养何种规格的食品(饮食不同对大多数实验影响都很大)、饮水状况(包括饮水来源, 是自由饮水还是限量饮水)、标本的采集方法和过程以及实验所需测量记录的过程和结果。因为即使同种系的动物, 年龄体重不同或喂养环境及饮食不同, 实验所得的某些结果也会有很大的不同, 为使别人能重复实验得出相似的结论, 所有这些状况都必须描述; ②详细描述在动物体内进行实验的全过程, 包括实验时动物的状态、是清醒还是麻醉状态、何种麻醉方式、实验中应用了何种药物等。动物实验时, 动物所处的状态对实验的结果有很大的影响, 清醒时和麻醉状态下的结果有时会有很大的差别; ③实验分组: 简单明了地叙述实验分组(有时采用示意图表达), 描述每组的实验步骤, 每组动物的实验例数。

其次是根据实验设计的特点进行描述。如上例, 我们描述了清除率的测定、细胞膜碎片制备的详细过程以及应用多种化学制剂的成分和配置方法、免疫杂交和免疫组化的具体操作过程、抗体特性标号等。

最后是统计学方法(statistical analysis), 采用何种统计方法处理数据。

材料和方法部分体现了研究的科学性, 主要目的是描述实验设计, 介绍研究选择的研究对象以及研究采用的方法步骤, 研究所需的材料和主要设备, 有时需要表明材料和设备的来源地和型号。提供足够详细的资料,以便其他的研究者可以重复这些实验。

　　写作时,凡是属于技术革新、发明创造等,均需详细阐述,并且需要将设计原理、实验步骤、操作要点、观察记录方法、仪器安装、药品配置过程以及必需的线路图和注意事项等加以说明。如果实验的方法为公认的方法,则只需写出实验要点。如果将前人的方法加以改进,则需要详细阐述改进部分。例如有关后尿道瓣膜患儿的尿动力学研究(Urodynamic investigation of valve bladder syndrome in children. Journal of Pediatric Urology. 2007,3:118-121)。因为许多学者对尿动力学检查并不熟悉,因此材料方法中就单独列出了检查方法的细节:
"Urodynamic studies: Slow-filling (10% of predicted bladder capacity in milliliter per minute,room temperature saline used as filling medium) cystometry with surface perineal electromyography(EMG) was performed using a Dan Tech Urodynamic Unit. All the children were encouraged to drink water or milk until voiding. Immediately after voiding,a double-lumen catheter(6 Fr) was introduced into the bladder through urethra with no local anesthesia for measuring the post-voiding residual (PVR) and performing a flow/pressure study …"

　　多数读者会跳过这个章节,因为从摘要中他们已经大概知道了研究方法,他们可能对实验资料没有兴趣。

　　一般而言,基础研究论文的材料和方法部分的书写比较复杂,而临床研究论文在这部分的书写就比较简单,例如我们发表的一篇儿科方面的临床研究文章,材料和方法如下(Chen Y, Acta Paediatr., 2012, 101(6):583-586):

Materials and Methods

Healthy newborns (11 males and 10 females) during their first 28 days of life at the First Affiliated Hospital of Zhengzhou University were included. Ten were full term [38.5 ± 1.3 gestational weeks, range 37~40; weighing (3.2 ± 0.4)kg at birth) and 11 preterm (32.7 ± 1.6 gestational weeks, range 29~36; weighing (1.8 ± 0.5)kg at birth]. None had any signs of urinary tract pathology or symptoms. All Apgar scores were above eight at 1-and 5-min assessments. The study protocol was approved by parents and the regional ethical committee and performed according to the Declaration of Helsinki.

　　该研究的内容为新生儿的排尿模式。由于研究对象为新生儿,因此上面内容的材料和方法部分首先要描述研究对象性别、年龄、出生、体重的情况,然后说明在什么地方进行的研究以及强调研究通过了当地伦理委员会的批准,这是国际医学伦理对临床实验的要求。紧接着下面将对研究的具体方法 12-h free voiding 和 the subjects were observed from 9 a.m. to 9 p.m. at day 1,4,7,14 and 28、研究的几个指标 voiding frequency(VF),voiding volume(VV), post-voiding residual volumes(PRV)进行具体描述介绍。最后就是统计方法的介绍。

All newborns were observed for 12 h by well-trained urologists according to International Children's Continence Society (ICCS) standards (8). The subjects were observed from 9 a.m. to 9 p.m. at day 1, 4, 7, 14 and 28, but the first-day observation was started first 12 h after birth after the i.v. fluid had been supplied or after beginning of breastfeeding. For the newborns, 1~2ml of water was supplied every hour beginning from 2 h, and breastfeeding began from 6~12 h after birth, if refused fluid was supplied i.v. instead, according the standard protocol (9). The 12-h observation was divided into three consecutive 4-h periods. For each shift, a specialist was in charge of observation to avoid work fatigue and mistakes. Diapers were weighed before and after voiding using a microelectronic balance (accuracy 0.1 g) (LD1102; Dragon, Shenyang, China). The post-void residual volume (PRV) was measured (diameter × width × thickness × 0.5) within 30 sec after voiding by B ultrasound (accuracy 0.3mm; LOGIQ400; GE, Fairfield, CT, USA). The voiding parameters were recorded (see Table S1 and Fig. 1). Student's *t*-test was used for statistics, with $p<0.05$ being considered significant.

该段落进一步详细描述了如何根据国际小儿尿控协会（ICCS）的规定对新生儿排尿方式进行观察,详细介绍了观察的步骤、参数和方法等。

英文论文书写时,写好材料和方法极其重要,因为研究方法是结果的基础。同时,同行审阅论文时,会仔细阅读材料和方法部分。如果对实验能否被重复有重大疑问,无论结果多么振奋人心,都会建议编辑部拒绝稿件。下面我们对材料和方法的书写进行详细的介绍。

一、材料

（一）材料的定义

材料和方法二者关系紧密、相辅相成,在方法的描述当中,会涉及很多的材料应用。材料的描述往往也会提及方法的设计,不可孤立的只写材料或者是只写方法,文章常常会将二者融汇在一起进行叙述,特别是在基础研究的论文中。一般将研究对象或使用东西泛称为材料,如临床研究的患者也可放在"材料"里。当然许多论文涉及患者时往往用"患者和方法"替代"材料和方法";动物实验中涉及的动物、细胞培养中的细胞株等也是泛指材料。

一般的 SCI 杂志在该章节的格式是 Materials and Methods,但也有的杂志只写 Methods。以临床为研究对象的文章多采用 Patients and Methods 或 Study design。所以投稿前,应仔细阅读目标杂志的投稿要求和写作格式。

（二）材料的内容

材料包括详细的技术说明、材料数量及来源或者材料的准备方法。甚至有必要列出所用试剂相关的化学和物理特性。试剂书写使用学名或者化学名称,例如:"Functional analysis of the cis-acting elements responsible for the induction of the Cyp6a8 and Cyp6g1 genes of Drosophila melanogaster by DDT, phenobarbital and caffeine."。尽量避免使用商品名,尤其是含有广告宣传的商品名,主要原因是商品名可能只被原产国熟悉,并不为众人所知,有的甚至具有强烈的广告色彩,这样也会降低文章的学术性。然而,如果需要强调某些特许专卖产品,就需要使用商品名,再加上生产厂商的名称,如果已被熟知,有时也可不加厂商名。商品名往往有注册商标,当用商品名时,应该用大写(例如:Teflon,Oxybutynin 等),以和学名相区别。

实验动物,植物和微生物应该进行精确的分类,通常以种、属和学名进行分类。应该列出其来源,描述其特征(年龄、性别、遗传学和生理学特性)。动物实验的操作必须符合实验所在国家和卫生部门制定的爱护和使用动物的规定,以防实验中有虐待动物的现象。例如:

Studies were performed on male Munich-Wistarrats（性别和种属）initially weighing 250 g（Møllegard Breeding Centre, Eiby, Denmark, 产 地）. Rats were maintained on a standard rodent diet（Altromin，Lage，Germany，标准食品的产地）with free access to water（自由饮用自来水）. All procedures conformed with the Danish national guidelines for the care and handling of animals and to the published guidelines from the National Institutes of Health. The animal protocols were approved by the board of the Institute of Clinical Medicine, University of Aarhus，according to the licenses for use of experimental animals issued by the Danish Ministry of Justice.（动物实验的操作过程符合相关国家卫生部门制定的标准，实验设计得到了奥胡斯大学临床研究所委员会的审核批准，该委员会对动物实验的应用许可是由丹麦司法部颁发的。）

　　为了防止虐待动物的现象发生，在欧洲许多国家，动物保护委员会的成员会不定期的到各个动物实验场所进行检查，如果发现违规和虐待动物现象，即使你的实验符合规定，但实验中动物遭受了很大的痛苦，他们会马上中止你的动物实验，甚至撤销你的动物实验许可，每个做动物实验的人必须经过动物实验的培训获得证书后，才可进行动物实验。

　　临床研究的对象是患者，首先应说明患者来源是选自住院还是门诊，然后必须将选择的病例的年龄、性别、职业、发病病因、病程、病理依据、分组标准、疾病的诊断分型标准、病情进展和疗效判断依据描写清楚。当然这些内容不用面面俱到，上述内容可根据研究的具体情况加以选择说明，并突出重点。下面是一篇消化内科的以临床青少年患者为研究对象的研究论文（Zaslavsky C，J Pediatr Gastroenterol Nutr. 1998 Aug；27（2）：138-42），研究采用颗粒法测定便秘患者肠道转运时间，在该篇文章中的材料和方法部分中，将材料和方法分开描述，对材料部分即研究对象的描述如下：

　　The population studied consisted of 13 adolescents（研究材料的患者研究例数），aged 12 to 18（患者年龄），with constipation, and 13 without constipation（临床表现）. Patients were seen at the Hospital de Clínicas de Porto Alegre and Hospital Materno Infantil Presidente Vargas, in Porto Alegre, Rio Grande do Sul, Brazil from November 1993 to November 1994（诊治的时期和地点）. The constipated adolescents had hard stools, difficulty in evacuating, less than three bowel movements a week, no evidence of palpable rectal mass, and a history of constipation of at least 1 year's duration. Adolescents with neurologic and metabolic diseases. Hirschsprung's disease, spinal and anal anomalies, surgery of the colon, mental retardation, and a history of drug abuse were excluded. The group of nonconstipated adolescents had no digestive complaints and had more than three bowel movements per week（入选和排除标准）. All of the adolescents and their parents gave their informed written consent after the initial interview. The protocol was approved by the Ethics Board of the Hospital de Clínicas de Porto Alegre.

　　上述材料详细地告诉了读者他们的研究材料（患者）包括研究例数、患者年龄、临床表现、诊治的时期和地点，因为他们进行的研究的对象是特发性或功能性便秘，所以某些能引起便秘的疾病就必须被排除。具体的实验（肠道转运时间测定）过程则在方法部分中描述。当然，在很多临床研究中，需要健康的志愿者作为对照组，上面研究中也描述了相应的对照组（13 without constipation）。

　　接下来我们将进一步举例介绍对临床研究中健康对照组的描述，下面是消化内科的一篇有关少量钡餐检查测定和成年便秘患者肠道转运时间测定文章的材料部分：

PATIENTS AND METHODS

Experiment protocols（该部分描述了实验分组和每组人员的性别、年龄、身体状况、诊治地点、收治时间）

Protocol 1. This study consisted of 8 healthy volunteers (male 6, female 2) aged 20 to 56 with average age 40±6.1. For self control, the upper 8 volunteers subjected to the examination of radio-opaque pellets and small barium in different time. (受试者既是实验对象也是对照组,即自我对照。)

Protocol 2. This study consisted of 2 groups of subjectives. Group 1 consisted of 30 healthy volunteers (male 8, female 22) aged 20 to 69 with average age 42.5±8.1. This nonconstipated volunteers had no digestive complaints and had more than three bowel movements a week (健康对照组的例数、性别和年龄分布等). Group 2 consisted of 50 patients with chronic functional constipation (male 11, female 39) aged 17 to 72 with average age 45.7±7.8. All the patients studied here were treated in the first affiliated hospital of Zhengzhou University, China from 2004 to 2008. The constipated patients had hard stools, difficulty in evacuating, less than three bowel movements a week, no evidence of palpable rectal mass, and a history of constipation at least 2 year's duration. Patients with neurologic, metabolic diseases, spinal and anal anomalies, surgery of the colon, mental retardation, and a history of drug abuse were excluded.

All protocols were approved by the Ethics Board of the First affiliated Hospital of Zhengzhou University, China.

由于临床研究多是针对临床上的患者,因此常常需要伦理委员会的批准和患者的知情同意。从上面的消化内科的三个例子中,我们可以看到在临床研究的材料最后部分都阐明了实验通过当地伦理委员会的批准以及患者签署了知情同意书。

对初学者来说,面对一大堆资料,最困难的是怎样罗列这些材料,下面是另外一个例子,描述在临床上进行的对儿童患者的研究:

Sixteen children, aged 1 to 6.5 years (mean 3.2±1.8), with VBS were evaluated in the Pediatric Urodynamic Center of the First Affiliated Hospital of Zhengzhou University, China, from July 2002 to December 2004. Seven boys, aged 1e1.9 years (mean 1.6±0.3years), were in group 1 and nine boys, aged 2.9e6.5 years (mean 4.5±1.2 years), were in group 2.

以人为研究对象的论文,其材料部分有时表述为研究设计。下例是有关新生儿的研究,对孕期、出生体重和年龄进行了如下描述(Guilfoy VM, J Pediatr. 2008 Nov; 153(5): 612-5):

Study design

This study was designed to determine total energy expenditure and body composition in a group of ELBW (birth weight less than 1 000g) infants nearing discharge on full volume enteral feedings of fortified breast milk or post-discharge formula (Neosure™) (n=10, birth weight 0.8±0.1kg, gestation 26±0.8wk, age at study 68±9d, post conceptional age 36±1wk) and compare them with healthy term newborns all receiving breast milk [n=14, birth weight (3.5±0.5)kg, gestation (39.0±1.4)wk, age at study (2.3±1) d]. Body composition and total energy expenditure were measured using the doubly labeled water method over a 7 day period.

1. 研究新的诊断方法的论文 要说明受试对象是否包括了各种分型的患者(病情程度、是否有合并症、疾病诊疗经过等),受试对象及健康对照者的来源(不同级别的医院某种疾病的患病率和就诊率常常不同),诊断标准的依据,正常值的界定,该新诊断方法如何具体实施等等。例如:"A total of 200 women with urinary incontinence and 20 with upper urinary tract disease and normal lower urinary tract function were included in this study. Urodynamic examinations were performed in all patients according to the recommendations of the International

Continence Society（ICS）."。

2. 研究疾病的临床经过及疗效观察 需要说明选择病例的标准，病例的一般资料（如性别、年龄、病情程度等），分组标准与样本分配的方法（配伍、配对情况或完全随机），观察的疗效指标和判定疗效的标准。例如："Women attended a research clinic where they completed a standardized 1 hour pad test and were examined. Women were assessed preoperatively and postoperatively at 6 months, 1 year and 2 years. Main outcome measures success was determined by a negative 1 hour pad test（gain of <1 g）and no desire for further treatment for stress urinary incontinence."。

有时候，一些临床研究常常合并有实验室基础研究，这时候材料就包括了临床的标本（患者或者血样、尿等）和实验室的标本（小鼠、培养细胞、培养组织等），这时就需要对材料连同各自所需的实验方法分别描述。下面是一篇妇产科的有关多囊卵巢综合征卵巢颗粒细胞表达过氧化物酶 -4 的文章，我们可以看看作者是如何进行分别描述的[Meng Y, PLoS One. 2013 Oct 3;8（10）]：

Subjects

The ovarian samples of fifteen women were collected during transsexual operation and used as controls. The hormonal treatment was withdrawed at least 3 months in those transsexual patients before operation. The ovarian samples of fifteen PCOS patients were collected during surgical treatment. The diagnosis of PCOS was according to the revised Rotterdam European Society of Human Reproduction and Embryology/American Society for Reproductive Medicine Criteria. All PCOS women had oligomenorrhea or amenorrhea (eight or fewer spontaneous menses per year), clinical (hirsutism), and/or biochemical (elevated free androgen index) evidence of hyper and rogenism and polycystic ovaries by ultrasound scanning. This study was approved by the Institutional Ethics Committee of The First Affiliated Hospital of Nanjing Medical University. All volunteers gave the signed consent forms.

Five samples of PCOS ovaries and five samples of control group were fixed in 4% Paraformaldehyde for 24 h, stored in 70% ethanol, and dehydrated and embedded in paraffin. The paraffin-embedded samples were used for pathology diagnosis and immunohistochemical staining. Ten fresh ovarian tissues of PCOS and control group, respectively, were snap frozen and stored in liquid nitrogen until five of them were used for RNA extraction and qRT-PCR, while the other five samples were used for protein extraction and Western blot analysis. The Western blot and qRT-PCR experiments were repeated four times.

前面描述了临床研究部分所需要的卵巢标本情况和对标本实验的方法，然后下面描述基础研究部分所需要的从临床标本中分离提取的细胞和相应的方法。

Granulosa Cells were isolated from 16 women with PCOS undergoing *in vitro* fertilization and embryo transfer (IVF-ET) patients. 26 women with regular menstrual cycles were enrolled in control group, who were diagnosed as tubal or male factor infertility. The detailed medical history was taken. The volunteers were ≤32 years old, had body mass index ≤23kg/m², and had no history of other gynecological or medical disorders. All subjects were injected with a GnRH agonist-Lupride (Sun Pharmaceuticals, Mumbai, India) starting from mid-luteal phase. Once pituitary down-regulation was achieved after two weeks, they were injected with recombinant FSH (Gonal F, Serono, Geneva,

Switzerland). Follicular size was monitored regularly by ultrasound and serum estradiol assays. When there were three or more follicles with mean diameter ≥17mm, hCG (Pregnyl, Organon, The Netherlands) was administered subcutaneously. At 34~36 h following the administration of hCG, follicle size was estimated under ultrasound and then oocytes were aspirated. Follicular fluid of small follicles [(SFs,<12mm)] and large follicles [(LFs, ≥16mm)] from the same patient were collected in separate tubes. SFs and LFs were separately represented for immature and mature follicles.

二、方法

方法（method）包括实验方法以及统计学方法。

（一）实验方法

包括动物模型的制备和感染接种方式，手术及标本的制备方法，实验记录方法，观察步骤，记录指标；病例的记录方法、观察指标、诊断依据，治疗方法和疗效判定；药物的剂型、剂量、服用方法和疗程等。若为手术则应说明手术名称、手术具体术式、麻醉方法等。对存在创新及改进的地方，应作详细的介绍，以便他人重复实验。

分析病因学的研究论文要尽量详细地说明所用的研究设计方法（如临床随机对照试验、队列研究等）。例如：

This was a cross-sectional, case-control study using a structured self-administered questionnaire. To identify the unadjusted associations of each potential risk factor with prevalence of UI, univariate logistic regression analyses were used. A multiple logistic regression model was then constructed with only those variables that were significantly associated with the UI（$p<0.05$）in the univariate analyses. Multivariate logistic regression analysis was used to determine adjusted odds ratios（OR）and 95% confidence intervals（CI）.［来自 Ham E et al. Risk factors for female urinary incontinence among middle-aged Korean women. J Womens Health（Larchmt）. 2009, 18 (11):1801-1806］

研究治疗方法的论文，如手术，应说明手术名称、手术具体术式、麻醉方法等。若为药物治疗则应注明药物名称、生产厂家、剂型、剂量、给药途径与操作方法、疗程和疗效判定标准，中草药除上述以外，还应注明药物产地与制剂的方法。例如：

With the aid of a computerized randomization schedule, patients were randomized to the following groups: A-placebo; B-bethanechol, in a 10mg oral dose every 8 h; C-cisapride, in a 10mg dose every 8 h; D-bethanechol combined with cisapride, in the same doses above. All medication was provided in capsules, which were identical in appearance. Identification was only made by a standardized code. Randomization was only revealed at the end of the study, controlled by an independent investigator. All medication was administered during 30 consecutive days, starting from the first postoperative day.（来自 Alberto P. The effects of bethanechol and cisapride on urodynamic parameters in patients undergoing radical hysterectomy for cervical cancer. A randomized, double-blind, placebo-controlled study. Int Urogynecol J. 2006, 17:248-252）

如果进行的是临床病例回顾性分析，在方法部分也可如此描述，下面的例子是对颅脑外伤后颅内压增加的回顾性研究方法部分的描述［选自 Guerra SD, J Pediatr（Rio J）. 2010 Jan-

Feb;86（1）:73-9］:

Retrospective cohort study, with data collected from September 1998 through August 2003, including patients aged 0 to 16 who suffered severe head injuries, Glasgow score <9, and submitted to intracranial pressure (ICP) monitoring (n=132). Intracranial hypertension (IH) was defined as an episode of ICP > 20mmHg requiring treatment, while refractory IH was ICP over 25mmHg requiring barbiturates or decompressive craniectomy. Univariate analysis was followed by multivariate analysis; variables were considered significant if $p<0.05$.

下面是另一个回顾性研究论文例子,是有关急腹症剖腹探查回顾性研究的论文。它在对研究对象（材料和方法）方面的叙述不能将材料和方法分开［选自 Abantanga FA' Ann Afr Med. 2009 Oct-Dec;8（4）:236-42］:

From January 2001 to December 2005, all consecutive children aged >1 year but <15 years undergoing laparotomy for an acute intra-abdominal condition were prospectively enrolled in the study. Patient characteristics, diagnoses, postoperative complications, morbidity and mortality rate were all evaluated. Komfo Anokye Teaching Hospital serves the whole of Ashanti Region of Ghana, with a population of about 4.7 million, of which 41.9% are children below the age of 15 years. Referrals are also received from other parts of the country.

Descriptive statistics were produced using SPSS version 10.0 for windows where appropriate. A P value <0.05 was considered statistically significant.

在上述材料部分我们举了两个便秘患者肠道转运时间测定方法的例子来说明材料部分描述,在方法部分我们将再举这两个例子来说明方法部分是如何描述的:

（青少年颗粒法测定肠道转运时间）The radio-opaque markers were introduced through polyethylene catheters produced by the Biomedical Engineering Department at Hospital de Clínicas de Porto Alegre（not available for commercial use in Brazil）. The physical characteristics of the markers were: specific weight between 1.20 and 1.35, mass between 20 and 40mg, and length between 3 and 6mm. Twenty markers were placed in each gelatin capsule. The technique used to measure total and segmental colonic transit time has been described by Metcalf et al. [1] The adolescents swallowed one capsule a day for 3 days, and on the fourth day, a plain abdominal radiograph was taken. Abdominal radiographic films were obtained by a high-kilovoltage fast-film technique, to reduce radiation exposure（estimated surface exposure, 0.08 mrad per film）. The numbers of markers present in this radiograph was counted, and previously determined bony landmarks were used to locate each colonic segment …

在以上内容中描述了测定的方法和实验中实验对象所注意的事项。下面是用成人钡餐法测定肠道转运时间文章的方法部分,它描述了实验的方法、操作过程以及观察指标:

Experimental procedure

The method we used for radio-opaque pellets examination was same as described before[7]. The small amount of barium was made by 40g barium dissolved in 8ml water which formed a sticky paste. After the paste was taken, objectives followed with abdominal X-ray to check the location of barium, therefore to determine the transit times in different segments of gastrointestinal tract until the barium evacuated totally. During the examination, bowel movement was recorded.

All the volunteers and patients were advised not to alter their diets and not to ingest foods that might alter bowel motility. Stop using tranquilizer, cathartics and any medication which might interfere in the bower movement 2 days before the measurements were performed.

（二）统计学方法

统计学分析是必要的,但是应该归类分析数据,而不是统计数字。普通的统计方法可以直接使用;高级的或者不常使用的统计方法可能要求有文献引证。统计学方法应该包括使用的统计软件及版本、统计方法、检验标准等。像上面所举例提到的材料和方法中的描述,最后部分都是对统计学方法的叙述。例如:

Statistical analysis: Analysis of variance（ANOVA）was applied initially to study each group's continuous variables, followed by theTukey multiple comparison test. We used the chi-squaretest to compare data between study groups. Simple linearregression was used to evaluate the relationship betweenthe length of the vaginal cuff and parametrial volume andurodynamic parameters. In all tests, we used SPSS software. The statistical significance level was set at a<0.05.（来自:Alberto P. The effects of bethanechol and cisapride on urodynamic parametersin patients undergoing radical hysterectomy for cervical cancer. A randomized, double-blind, placebo-controlled study. Int Urogynecol J. 2006, 17:248-252）

另一个例子选自作者发表在 *Pediatr Nephrol* 杂志上（Wang G, Pediatr Nephrol. 2009 Aug；24（8）:1487-500）的文章对统计学方法的描述:"Values are presented as means ± standard error. Comparison between groups was made by unpaired t test. One way analysis of variance (ANOVA) analysis was used for comparison in more than two groups. P values <0.05 were considered to be statistically significant."。

总之,对方法的描述应该尽量精确。作者必须能够在方法中明确地表述清楚诸如"怎样做"以及"做多少"这类问题,而不能让审稿人或者是读者提出这样的问题。

三、材料方法中的参考文献

在描述研究方法时,应该给出充足的资料并尽可能详细描述实验方法,以便让读者或其他研究者重复这些实验。只有你的实验方法和结果能被别人重复出来才能得到大家的认可。如果方法是创新或者是改进的,必须提供所有需要的细节。但是,如果这种方法先前已经在一个规范的杂志上发表了,只需要给出参考文献书目就可以了。但是如果采用此方法的文章以中文发表在国内的杂志上,那再写 SCI 文章时对此方法还是应该完整描述。

有时候虽然方法已经用过,但是还是需要对原方法做一个简单的定义,举个例子,描述"cells were broken by ultrasonic treatment as previously described (9)"就比"cells were broken as previously described (9)"要好。

有时候就算以往的方法已经用过,并标上了相应参考文献,但是由于使用的机器类型不一样,个别操作步骤也不一样,因此还是有必要再重复描述一遍。下面是一篇发表在杂志 *Neurourology and Urodynamics* 上的文章,尽管以往的研究有关尿动力检测的方法步骤都有描述,但是不同地方使用的仪器型号不一致,因此需要再简单总结一下。

Urodynamic testing

Multichannel UDS investigations were performed using the DUET Logic Urodynamic Instrument (Medtronic, Skovlunde, Denmark) in accordance with ICS protocol (15). Symptoms and urodynamic parameters were recorded using standardized ICS terminology (3). Conventional filling cystometry was performed with patients in the supine position. Standard UDS was performed while the bladder was filled at a constant rate of 50mL/min using a normal saline solution at room temperature. VLPP was measured by increasing the total infused volume of sterile water to 200mL while the patient was seated and then asking the patient to perform a Valsalva maneuver until urine loss could be directly observed. The initial VLPP measurement was recorded before the measurement was repeated to verify the initial finding. If urine leakage was not observed with the Valsalva maneuver, the patient was asked to cough.

另外有一些基础实验的描述方法,如 Westernblot,PCR 等,虽然操作步骤差不多,但是每一个实验用到的抗体、引物等不一样,因此在附上了参考文献后,仍然需要再次简单描述一下。下面是一个发表在 *Biochemical and Biophysical Research Communications* 杂志上的例子。

The protein expression was checked on SDS-PAGE. The previously published protocol for purification of Flavivirus ED3s was followed [9] and [10]. In case of both proteins, cells were lysed by sonication. Where, both samples were subjected to 6 cycles of 30 s ON and OFF at50% power (Misonixsonicator) until the pellets were homogeneous. The sonicated cells were centrifuged at 4℃ for 1 h at 10 000 rpm to pellet the IBs. For DENV2-EDIII, the supernatant was discarded and pellet was resuspended in 40ml denaturing buffer [20mM Tris-HCl pH 8.0, 200mM NaCl, 1mM EDTA, 6 M Guanidine HCl and 5% (v/v) glycerol] using a rotating mixer or slow rocking at 4℃ for about 12-24 h until pellet is homogenous. The resuspended solution was centrifuged at 8 000rpm for 1 h (at 4℃) to pellet the insoluble fraction and the supernatant containing the denatured IBs. CD44-HABD protein was expressed as IBs and purified as described in Banerji et al. [11].

四、常用句型、语法和格式

在材料和方法中,从文献中摘抄一些常见句型举例如下,供参考。

1. … defines the definition of enuresis, and argues for its importance.

2. … devoted to the basic aspects of the investion decision making logic.

3. … gives the background of the research which includes …

4. … discusses some argument with and approaches to, natural language understanding.

5. … explains how flexibility which often … can be expressed in terms of …

6. … discusses the aspects of bladder control theory that are used in the …

7. … describes the diagnostic method itself in a general way, including the … and also discusses how to evaluate tis performance.

8. … describes a new measure of …

9. … is a fine description of fuzzy formulation of human decision …

10. … And … show experimental studies for verifying the proposed model.

11. … discusses a prevalence of enuresis based different risk factors in different countries.

12. … gives a specific example of severe enuresis.

13. … is the experimental study to make a ureteral obstruction model in rat.

14. … contains a discussion of the implication of the results of …

15. Section X applies this parameter measure to the analysis of xx and illustrate its use on experimental data.

16. Section X presents the primary results of the research: a survey of enuresis …

17. Section X contains some conclusions plus some ideas for further investigation work.

18. Section X illustrates the animal model with an example.

19. Various ways of justification and the reasons for their choice are discussed very briefly in Section 3.

20. In … are presented the block diagram expression of a whole model of …

21. In … we shall list a collection of basic assumptions which a … scheme must satisfy.

22. In … is analyzed the inference process through the two kinds of inference experiments … This Section …

23. In this section, the characteristics and environment under which … is designed are described.

24. We will provide in this section basic terminologies and notations which are necessary for the understanding of subsequent results.

25. The next section describes the detail method that goes into the clinical implicatin.

26. However, it is cumbersome for this purpose and in practical applications the formulae were rearranged and simplified as discussed in the following sections.

27. The three components will be described in the next 3 section, and an example of xx analysis of a computer information system will then illustrate their use.

28. We can interpret the results of study I and II as in the following sections.

29. The next section summarizes the method in a from that is useful for arguments based on …

在选定某个句型以后,仔细审查句式和语法。确保语法和标点符号正确;在引言和讨论部分,即使存在少许语法错误的情况下,通用概念的含义仍然是明了的。然而,在材料和方法部分,精确和特殊项目的英语的准确使用是必需的。

由于材料和方法部分通常给出简短的、不相关联的信息,写作有时候变得有伸缩性;相关的必要细节可能被遗漏。最常见的错误是只陈述了动作而不陈述发出动作的主体。如:"To determine its respiratory quotient,the organism was …"唯一陈述的关于这个活动的主体是"the organism"。有一个类似的句子"Having completed the study,the bacteria were of no further interest."会让人怀疑这些细菌"completed the study"。

"Blood samples were taken from 48 informed and consenting patients … the subjects ranged in age from 6 months to 22 years"(Pediatr. Res. 6:26,1972)。这句话从语法上没有问题,但是写法会让读者对 6 个月大的婴儿能表达他们的同意感到困惑。

当然,在底稿和校正过的稿件中都要查找拼写错误:"We rely on theatrical calculations to give the lifetime of a star on the main sequence(Annu. Rev. Astron. Astrophys. 7:100,1963)."。

中国人写英文论文,多半是先写好了汉语论文,然后进行翻译。最容易出现的错误是汉语式英语,因为你要按照每一句的字面进行翻译,就免不了出现上述错误。材料和方法部分,更是容易犯错误。审稿人阅读你的文章时,不能理解你所表达的意思,即使你的实验很有意义,也会很快退回你的稿件。所以建议在翻译论文之前,熟读论文,充分了解论文要表达的意思,有些地方意译即可,不需要逐字逐句的进行翻译。另外可多阅读一些与论文内容有关的英文文章,找出那些试验方法与你论文近似的文章作为参考,再进行该部分的写作。总之,熟能生巧,阅读多了,就会很自然地用正确的方法进行书写。

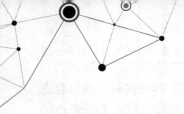

第 7 章
如何写作结果

Chapter 7
How to Write a Result

结果（result）是作者实验得出的数据，是结论的依据，是论著写作和学术价值的核心。结果的好坏代表着论文的学术水平或技术创新的程度。结果需要客观阐述研究成果并加以总结，是结论和实际应用的依据。研究结果应紧密围绕研究的主题并用文字或图表等显示，从而逻辑严谨、层次清晰地呈现出来。

一、写作要求

结果是对实验进行的总体描述。但是，结果内容的写作，不仅仅是将研究过程中得到的各种原始数据进行简单罗列，而是将这些原始数据，经过仔细审查、反复核对后，经过归纳分析和必要的统计学处理，从而可以支持相应的结论，然后用相对应的图片、柱状图、折线图等配以文字表述，将实验结果真实、准确、清楚地进行表达。要准确地表达必要的实验数据，摒弃不必要的部分。写作过程中需要注意以下几个方面：实验结果需要展示有科学意义的数据或图片；实验结果中不能夹杂其他人的数据；仅客观描述实验结果，不对研究结果进行评价、解释、分析和推理；实验结果不需要具体运算过程，只列出经过加工提炼或经统计学处理的数值即可；尽量采用图表、照片等方式辅以文字表述直观表示；同一数据在结果中不可以多次出现。

如果是按照"材料与方法"相对应展示结果时内容过多，可以将结果部分分成小段落并加上小标题，从而使层次分明。实验得出的数据应能支持有关文献的分析，从而说明事物的内在联系和客观规律。

二、结果中的数据描述

数据必须是真实的，不能伪造和篡改。作者需提供翔实全面的数据，把实验中得到的数据提供给读者，不要故意隐瞒或遗漏某些重要数据。一般情况下，杂志社不会因数据不够丰富翔实而直接拒稿，但肯定会因怀疑数据真实性而直接拒收。

把数据直接从实验室笔记上简单转移到底稿中是不可行的。最重要的是在论文中报告有代表性的数据，而不是重复的数据。实验可以多次重复，但数据并不需要全部罗列。选择出代表性的数据或对已有数据进行总结即可。早在 20 世纪，美国科学发展协会的主席 John Wesley Poweu 就阐述了同样的观念。用他的话说："愚人收集材料，智者挑选材料。"

实验取得的原始资料或数据需进行统计学处理和样本分析，并归纳出有规律的信息学统计资料。常用的统计指标有率和构成比（百分比）。小样本资料不宜计算百分比。使用百分比时，分母要交代清楚。原始资料或数据按照其性质，一般分为定量资料（计量资料）、定性资料（计数资料）和混合资料。

定量资料可以直接进行统计学分析。当资料为近似正态（或对称）分布时，可用算术均数 ± 标准差描述（或 $\bar{x} \pm SD$）。在"±"后直接写具体数值而无标准误（SE）或标准差（SD）符号表示，如 10.4 ± 1.3，容易引起混淆。因此，论文表格显示统计数据时一般都会在表格标题注明（$\bar{x} \pm SD$）或（$\bar{x} \pm SM$）。配对 t 检验，应给出差数的均数及标准误（或标准差）。当资料为偏态时，应采用中位数 M 和四分位数间距 QR 来描述，而不宜用均数和标准差。用非参数统计分析方法处理的资料，数据的中心位置用中位数表示，散布范围（如 95% 的散布范围）用百分位数表示。此外，若对原始数据进行了变量转换，则原始数据的均数及标准差不能很好地反映数据的中心位置及其散布范围，不必将其列出。在没有变异指标或精确性指标的情况下，不宜单独使用均数。

定性资料不能直接进行统计学分析，一般先将其分类整理成列表形式后，再选用假设检验、对数线性模型分析、Logistic 概率模型回归分析等统计学方法进行分析。在进行统计学处理时，遇到的资料可能大多是混合型的，即定性资料和定量资料混在一起。根据需要，可把定性指标作为分组标志，把定量指标作为观测结果，采用定量资料的秩和检验、差别分析等方法进行数据处理。此外，还可把定性资料数量化后看作定量资料，反之，可把定量资料离散化看作定性资料，并分别选用相应的统计分析方法来处理数据。

三、描述方法

（一）文字叙述

结果部分通常需要对实验进行简单概括，将论文"梗概"呈现给读者，然后将最有价值的实验数据进行总结。对数据应认真分析，去粗取精，不要认为越多越好而全部写到论文中。数据的取舍要有客观标准，不要按主观意愿随意取舍。简单的结果可以用文字直接描述或用很少的数据表示，复杂的结果或数据较多时，建议使用图表文字相结合的方式来表达，图表可以更加详细、完整地展现实验结果，配以文字指出图表中的重要特性或趋势。文字部分应避免对图表中数据的简单重复阐述和使用，而应该对图表中数据的意义、趋势及相关推论等应加以着重叙述。例如作者发表在欧洲泌尿杂志中 "An Epidemiological Study of Primary Nocturnal Enuresis in Chinese Children and Adolescents" 一文结果起始部分的概括性描述："A total of 11 799 children aged 5-18 years were investigated and 10 383 questionnaires were returned, giving a response rate of 88%. Finally, 10 088（85.5%）provided enough data for statistical analysis. The overall prevalence of PNE was 4.07%, ranging from 11.83% in 5-year-old group to 1.21% in 15-year-old group, and the prevalence stabilized to approximately 1% in the group older than 15 years."。

（二）图表应用

图表便于读者直观了解研究结果，是表达研究结果的重要手段。现代论文撰写提倡用图表来显示结果，有时显示原始数据，如个体值的散布情况，或相关和回归分析的散点图。

图或表要具有自明性,即图、表本身给出的信息就能表达清楚要说明的问题。决定同一组数据用表或用图表达,要看哪一种方式能更好地表达结果,但不能既用表又用图重复反映相同的数据。

1. **图的应用**　图的立体感强,能形象直观地展现出论文中各变量的关系,可以更好地将不同结果进行比较,有利于展现研究事物的特殊性和变化规律。如那些变化趋势明显的数据宜选用曲线图辅以文字表达,图文并茂,易于读者理解。选用图表展示研究结果还能够大大节省篇幅,有的内容用文字很难讲清楚,而用图表示可使结果一目了然。优质、漂亮的图在行家眼里可以是立体的、动态的,给人以一种真实感和形象的表现力。统计图的种类很多,可根据资料的类型和目的选用。

图通常可分为原始图和统计图。原始图包括病人照片、标本照片、显微照片、记录图、仪器设备外观照片及示意图。统计图包括条图、散布图、圆图、百分条图、线图、直方图和统计地图等。对定性资料可选用圆图、条图等;对定量资料可选用半对数线图、直方图(或多边图)、普通线图、散布图等。

考虑到版面费和出版社的支出费用以及排版难易度,编辑部对文中的附图有一定限制。因此,建议作者在供图时,尽量用最少的图提供最多的信息,必要时一些图用表格代替。具体用几幅图最好,不同的杂志有不同的要求,如 *NEJM* 要求图表最多不超过 5 个。图片太多显得啰嗦和累赘,杂志和读者都不喜欢。图片格式要求每个杂志不同,用 tif 格式较多,不推荐用 bmp 或 jpg 格式。不管什么格式,要求图要足够清晰(要求达到一定的像素)。黑白图片可免费,彩色图片需要收费,而且价格不菲。

以下系列图发表在 "Ureter obstruction alters expression of renal acid-base transport proteins in rat kidney" 中[Am J Physiol Renal Physiol. 2008;295(2):F497-506](图 7-1、图 7-2)。

作者通过这些图片向读者清晰展示了各个信号在不同组中的区别,同时附上了免疫组化图片,使得数字的变化区别与分布的变化相结合,更直接地介绍了结果。同时请注意在每张附图下作者附上图注,对文章中的结果部分内容也是一种补充。

印迹得出的条带一定要与统计数据相结合才更有说服力,单纯的条带差异已经不能满足编辑的要求,多数会被退回。

Fig. 2. Semiquantitative immunoblotting of membrane fractions of cortex plus outer stripe of outer medulla (C+OSOM), inner stripe of outer medulla (ISOM) from BUO and sham-operated rats. *A* and *C*: immunoblots were reacted with affinity-purified anti-type 3 Na$^+$/H$^+$ exchanger (NHE3) antibody and revealed a single ~87-kDa band. *B* and *D*: densitometric analysis (corrected according to densitometry of Commassie blue-stained gels and loading fraction of C+OSOM and ISOM) of all samples from BUO and sham-operated controls revealed a significant decrease in NHE3 levels to 21 ± 4% in the C+OSOM and to 27 ± 2% in the ISOM in obstructed kidneys (*$P < 0.05$). *E*: immunoblots were reacted with affinity-purified type 1 bumetanide-sensitive Na$^+$-K$^+$-2Cl$^-$ cotransporter (NKCC2) antibody and revealed a strong, broad band of 146- to 176-kDa molecular mass centered at ~161 kDa. *F*: densitometric analysis revealed a marked decrease from 100 ± 15% in sham-operated controls to 3 ± 1% in obstructed kidneys (*$P < 0.05$).

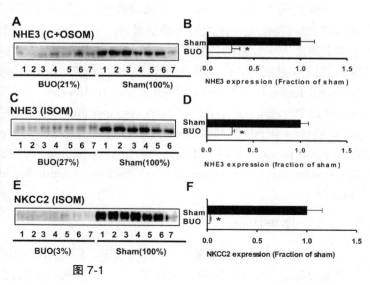

图 7-1

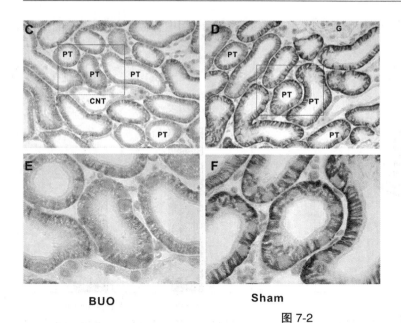

Fig. 3. Semiquantitative immunoblotting of membrane fractions of C+OSOM from BUO and sham-operated rats. *A*: immunoblots were reacted with anti-electrogenic Na⁺/HCO₃⁻ cotransporter (NBC1) and revealed a single ~140-kDa band. *B*: densitometric analysis revealed a marked decrease in the expression levels of NBC1 from 100 ± 4% in sham-operated controls to 71 ± 5% in obstructed kidneys (*$P < 0.05$). Immunocytochemical analysis of NBC1 in the proximal tubule (PT) from sham-operated rats (*D* and *F*) and 24-h BUO rats (*C* and *E*) is shown. The labeling of NBC1 was seen in the basolateral plasma membrane of the PT. NBC1 labeling in PT cells in BUO rats was much weaker compared with control rats. G, glomerulus; CNT, connecting tubule. Magnification: ×250 (*C* and *D*), ×630 (*E* and *F*).

图 7-2

上面这图片（图 7-2）需要注意的是都需要附注上放大倍数和染色方法，使读者能够读懂图片而不至于混淆。

散点图多用于描述统计数据的整体分布情况，并可用于尝试描述其趋势变化和回归相关关系（图 7-3）。

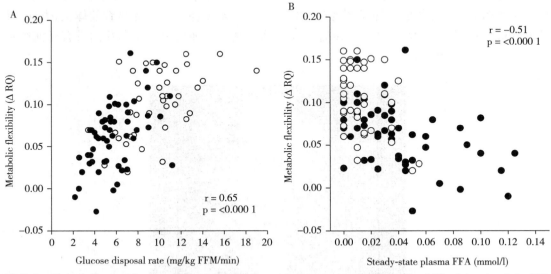

图 7-3　Correlation analysis in the whole study group between metabolic flexibility (steady-state RQ-fasting RQ) and glucose disposal rate（A）（type 2 diabetes: r=0.52, p<0.000 1; obese without type 2 diabetes: r=0.52, p=0.000 7）

根据图中数据关系将散点图制出，读者可以较为清晰地了解实验对象所测数据的分布情况，并在下方统计分析得出了相关系数等统计数据。

　　柱状图也是我们很早接触的统计图,虽然较为常用,实际应用中也需要注意各方面细节(图 7-4)。

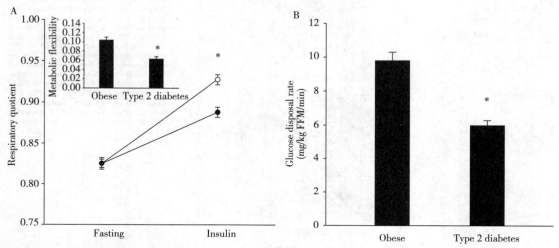

图 7-4　A: Respiratory quotient under fasting and insulin-stimulated conditions in obese with type 2 diabetes (·,n=59) and obese without type 2 diabetes (,n=42); inset: metabolic flexibility in both groups. B: Glucose disposal rate in both groups. Data are means ± SE. *P<0.05

　　请注意柱状图中上面的"T"在这里表示标准误,而并不是我们常用的标准差。这两个统计概念虽然很相似,但却完全不同,需要明确区分并正确使用。

　　另外还有一些图在科研论文中相对少见,但也是十分重要的,现一一举例(图 7-5)。这是一张 MRI 图片,类似的影像学图片列举在文中时一定要注意介绍受检者的体位,方向,并且最好标注标尺,并在需要注意的位置标注明确。避免单纯给出一张图片而没有任何解释说明,让读者一头雾水。

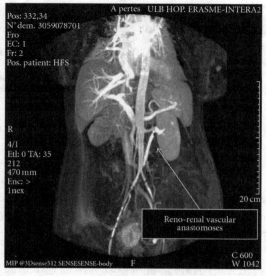

图 7-5　MRI angiography image after kidney transplantation in orthotopic position

2. 表的应用　表比文字表述更简明,表达更精确,它将大量数据系列化,便于读者阅读、比较和分析,是一种规范的科学语言。表格务求精练、简明、突出重点、栏目正确、数据准确、科学性强等特征。狭义统计表指仅显示统计结果的统计表,广义统计表还包括登记表、调查表等,本书的表指的是狭义的统计表。现代书刊中统计表格多排成三线表,表内少用或不用纵线,取消端线及斜线。

在文章"Development of nocturnal urinary control in chinese children younger than 8 years old"中结果部分共有三张表格,其中一张较为复杂(图 7-6):

TABLE III. *Influencing factors of children without NUC attainment*

Factor	Infants (1–3 yr)	Preschool (4–6 yr)	Primary School (7–8 yr)	Total (%)	Chi square	P Value
Gender					0.363	0.834
Male	156	141	49	346 (54.92)		
Female	130	110	44	284 (45.08)		
Frequency of nocturnal bed wetting*†					53.488	0.000‡
>1/p night	41	15	4	60 (9.52)		
1/p night	54	28	15	97 (15.40)		
4–6/p wk	21	12	4	37 (5.87)		
2–3/p wk	49	24	8	81 (12.86)		
1/p wk	28	27	5	60 (9.52)		
<1/p wk	92	145	57	294 (46.83)		
Associated daytime symptoms*†					7.683	0.02‡
Yes	28	43	17	88 (13.97)		
No	258	208	76	542 (86.03)		
Inhabitation					0.075	0.963
Rural	164	141	53	358 (56.83)		
Urban	122	110	40	272 (43.17)		
Arousal dysfunction*†					19.433	0.000‡
Yes	217	150	54	421 (66.83)		
No	69	101	39	209 (33.17)		
Family history*†					10.863	0.004‡
Yes	18	34	15	67 (10.63)		
No	268	217	78	563 (89.37)		
Treatment of the children without NUC					41.886	0.000‡
Wait for maturity	145	107	47	299 (47.46)		
Fluid restriction	3	28	11	42 (6.67)		
Waking to void	120	91	20	231 (36.67)		
Fluid restriction combined with waking to void	12	20	11	43 (6.83)		
Professional management	6	5	4	15 (2.38)		

KEY: NUC = nocturnal urinary control.
* P < 0.05, chi-square test between infant group and preschool group.
† P < 0.05, chi-square test between infant group and primary school group.
‡ P < 0.05, chi-square test among 3 groups.

图 7-6

作者结合表格在文中同样进行了分析描述:"The prevalence of the children attaining NUC in the cross-sectional and retrospective surveys is shown in I and II, respectively. The data showed that the prevalence of NUC in the cross-sectional survey was greater before age 4 and lower after age 5 than that in the retrospective investigation. In the cross-sectional survey, a significant trend was noted for an increasing attainment of NUC between 1 and 8 years of age (chi-square=106.687, $P<0.05$ for boys and chi-square=112.424, $P<0.05$ for girls). The influencing factors of the children without NUC attainment are shown in Table III."。

四、注意事项

（一）如实描述结果

语言表述上应做到"真实、准确"。真实就是不能掺杂丝毫虚假,需要客观如实地描述实际结果,与预期结果一致的要展现,和预期结果相矛盾的也要如实书写。不要片面地认为与预想结果或文献上的报道不一致的就是实验失败而认为没有价值;只要确认实验设计和实验方法科学无误、实验材料满足要求、操作过程无失当之处,那么这种不一致的结果有可能是新的发现,甚至有可能会否定前人的结论从而提出一个新论点。准确就是不要有错误,错误很大程度上都是工作粗疏所致,实验数据一定要反复验算,并且需要统计学处理。

结果应避免冗长空洞,力求简明扼要。Mitchell（1968）引用爱因斯坦曾经说过的话,"如果你要公开叙述事实真相,就把体面留给裁缝（If you are out to describe the truth, leave elegance to the tailor）。"论文前面的部分（引言,材料和方法）是用来说明为什么以及怎样得到结果的;论文后面的部分（讨论）是用来说明结果意味着什么。所以很明显整个论文的好坏都是以结果为基础。因此,必须十分清晰地显示结果。最常见的错误是语句全部重复那些已经通过图表显示的检查结果。更糟糕的是文中显示图表中已经出现的全部数据。为了强调一些重要的结果,也可以在文中重复图或表中列出的数据。对有些结果,即使文中不列出图表中的数据,也应该叙述这些结果的变化趋势,不可以简单只描述为结果见图或表。因为有些表和图包含了较多的信息,所以应该有侧重地描述一些结果。

为了简洁、清楚,最好不要将图表的序号用于段落的主题句,正确做法是直接概括出图表的结论,图表序号放在说明句子后面的括号中。例如:"Figure 1 shows the relationship between A and B"不如"A was Significantly higher than B at all time points of measurement (Figure 1)"。

（二）正确的时态应用

1. **指出结果在哪些图表中列出展现,常采用一般现在时** 如:① The common pathogen of urinary system is staphylococcus aureus;② The present study shows the variation in the temperature of the samples over time。

2. **叙述或总结研究结果的内容为过去的事实通常采用过去时** 如:① Based on these criteria, a cross-sectional study of PNE were performed in 2006 estimating the overall PNE prevalence in Chinese children and adolescents aged 5 to 18 years to be 4.07%, this was considerably lower than reported in Western countries, and we postulated it was related to cultural and economic differences between China and the West; ② In the past, the incidence of cervical spondylosis was more common in the elderly。

3. **对研究结果进行说明或由其得出一般性推论时,多采用一般现在时** 如:① The higher incidence of enuresis may be due to more and more popular using of disposable diaper in infants nowadays; ② The increased incidence of cervical spondylosis in office workers may be due to sedentary behaviour。

4. **不同结果之间或实验数据与理论模型之间进行比较时,多采用一般现在时** 如:

① These results agree well with the findings of previous study；② These experimental data and conclusions are consistent with those of previous studies。

如实验所得结果作为论证假说的论据不够充分,或尚无足够的文献资料对假说加以旁证,没有必要对结果广泛、详尽地讨论,或是实验结果与讨论的联系非常密切,即在讨论部分总是有必要结合结果的内容时,论文不必设单独的"讨论"一节,也可把"结果"和"讨论"合并为"结果与讨论"。

五、结果中常用的表达方式

1. 关系:

Compared to group 1, group 2 …

There was (were) (no) significant difference(s) or (No) significant difference(s) was found (observed) between … and …

… (did not) statistically differ in …

Compared with …

Among the 1 000 cases with … , 55% were … and 45% were …

There were good (linear) correlations between … and …

… showed no strong correlation between … and …

… correlated positively with …

A negative correlation (relationship) was found between … and …

… was closely related to …

2. 陈述:

… is shown in table 1

In the cross-sectional survey, a significant trend was noted for an increasing attainment of NUC

This paper (article, report) describes (reports, presents, discusses, analyze, evaluate, compare, describe) …

A case (study) is reported in which …

The results showed (demonstrated) that …

It was found that … 或 We found that …

It was observed that … 或 We observed that …

3. 增加或减少:

… decreased by (40%) …

… (a 70%) reduction in …

There was a (15%) elevation in …

… resulted in (a marked) increase in …

… was lowered from … to …

六、结果部分常见错误

医学科技论文书写结果时,常见的错误是统计学方法应用不到位或概念不清楚。应用统计学指标时常出现不同的问题。例如不考虑数据是否呈正态分布或近似正态分布,计量资料采用均数 ± 标准差描述;细胞实验或分子生物学实验(如 western blot、real time PCR、ELISA 等)数据用均数 ± 标准差表示,但其样本量或例数(n)却未在"结果"或"材料方法"中进行交代;将计数资料统计指标率和构成比(百分比)相混淆,构成比被误用为率来表述事物发生的强度;分母太小时,根本无法保证率或构成比的可靠性,却仍采用计算相对数比较结果。

　　"三线"表绘制不规范是论文结果撰写中的另一类常见错误。正确的"三线"表数值结果位数要对齐,避免出现交错换行的现象。不同类型数据(如均数、标准误)要有标目,表中需要列出相应的例数 n。大量统计结果的表达需要运用统计图或统计表,笔者审稿时发现很多科技论文的统计图表都有或多或少的问题,例如:①图形类别的选择不符合资料性质;②无图例或标目;③横轴或纵轴相等距离的尺度却并不代表等差数据(算术尺度)或等比数据(对数尺度);④条图的横轴刻度用算术刻度、纵轴不用 0 作为起点、排列顺序杂乱无章(正常应按自然顺序或指标大小排序);⑤圆图起点不设在 12 时或 9 时位置,排列顺序杂乱无章(正常应按各部分比例大小或自然顺序顺时针排列,其他项在最后);⑥统计表主辞和宾辞混淆或倒置,表的标目不明确,表中缺失数据、无数据或数据为"0"时留有空白,表中存在斜线或竖线,表中同一指标小数位数(精度)取舍不一致、小数点(位)不对齐等。如何在医学科技论文写作中使用好"三线"表应该引起大家的重视。

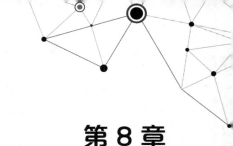

第 8 章
如何写作讨论

Chapter 8
How to Write the Discussion

讨论(discussion)是论文的精华和核心部分,它客观地回答了引言所提出的问题,是对研究结果认识的升华。在讨论中作者通过对研究结果的综合、分析和科学推论,阐明所研究课题的内在联系和发展规律,从更深的层次和更广的角度丰富和提高对研究结果的认识。讨论也是文章中难度最大的部分,最能体现作者理论水平的高低、学术素养以及专业知识的深和广度。很多文章被退稿不是因为原始数据不可靠或者意义不大,而是因为讨论没有写好。因此,讨论的重点在解释和推断研究结果,并能够体现作者的结果对某种观点是支持还是反对、是否发现了新的问题等。因此,撰写讨论部分时要尽量做到直接、明确,使审稿人和读者对论文的核心内容更加明了。

"讨论"的内容以精简为原则,尽可能避免华丽词汇,正如 Ralph Waldo Emerson 指出的那样:"it is the fault of our rhetoric that we cannot strongly state one fact without seeming to belie some other"。为了讲清楚主要的论点,已经谈过的内容在这一章节应该不予重复。

讨论很重要,因为:① Discussion is harder to define; ② The hardest section to write; ③ Papers often be rejected because of a faulty discussion。

讨论内容一般包括:① What do your results mean; ② Use the Discussion section to: A. Interpret the results in light of what was already known about? B. Point out the significance of the results for the reasons of doing the work; C. Place them in the context of other work; ③ Discuss the work of other researchers-consistent with theirs; ④ Explain to the reader what are the findings mean; ⑤ Demonstrate whether the data support original hypothesis-why or why not.

一、写作要求

(一)内容要求

讨论部分主要包括以下内容:

1. 有关本课题的研究背景、研究的最新进展及拟解决的问题。简要地概述本课题在国内外的研究背景和近况,以及本研究得出的结论和结果与国内外相同领域的先进水平相比居于什么地位,做此研究有什么创新之处,能够解决什么问题。科学研究的规律一般是按照"假说—推理—新假说—新推理"的方式进行,严格按照发现问题、提出问题、分析问题、解决问题这一程序进行。在论文中,就体现在前言中提出问题,在结论中回答问题,在讨论部分阐述问题是否得到解决,如研究实验是否成功,假说是否得到验证,诊断标准是否正确,治疗方法是否奏效等。当然,回答这些问题不能简单的停留在是与否,而是从深层次客观的阐述其缘由。因此必须将得到的感性资料、结果与相关理论知识相联系,然后从中揭示某一现象或事实的规律和本质。

下面收集一些文献中例子进行举例说明:

例1　CLINICAL STUDY OF URIC ACID UROLITHIASIS

Yii-Her Chou, Wei-Ming Li, Ching-Chia Li, et al

DISCUSSION 部分

The prevalence of uric acid urolithiasis varies in different geographical areas and countries, e.g. 5%~10% in the US, 17%~25% in Germany, 4% in Sweden, and up to 40% in Israel. The apparent geographic variations indicate that genetic, dietary, and environmental factors may have important roles in the formation of uricacid stones.

本段的意义:在不同国家地区,尿酸性结石的发病率不同,这与不同地域的基因、饮食及环境因素有很大的关系,说明了课题研究近况和背景。

Gout is an ancient disease and its association with uric acid stones has long been recognized. Uric acids tones are formed from dehydration, excessive sweating, intestinal alkali loss, and purine overload or overproduction. Idio pathic uric acid Nephrolithiasis may also develop despite the absence of the above causes. People with uric acid stones may have normouricemia in some situations, since it is believed that uric acid urolithiasis is due to defects in urinary acidification and excretion of urates.

本段意义为:痛风是一个古老的疾病,很久以前人们就认识到了它与尿酸结石的关系。尿酸结石由脱水、过量出汗、肠道碱丢失及嘌呤过多引起。特发的尿酸性肾结石可因其他原因发生。有尿酸结石的人一般都有高尿酸血症,因为尿酸性结石被认为是由尿酸化和尿酸盐排出引起的。本段亦说明了尿酸性结石发生的因素,为论文的进一步深入提供背景依据。

An increasing percentage of the population is affected by obesity and the metabolic syndrome, a condition that is metabolically characterized by insulin resistance and clinically defined by abdominal obesity, dyslipidemia, elevated blood pressure, and elevated fasting glucose. It is reported that patients with recurrenturic acid stones manifest clinical and metabolic abnormalities consistent with the metabolic syndrome. Lower urinary pH increases concentrations ofthe sparingly soluble undissociated uric acid, which directly promotes the formation of uric acid stones. Because of the overlapping clinical features between gouty diathesis and the metabolic syndrome, the relationship of the defective biologic activity of insulin andurinary acidification has been studied. It is suggested that the renal manifestation of insulin resistance maybe low urinary ammonium and pH. This defect can result in increased risks of uric acid stone formationdespite normouricosuria.

现代社会的糖尿病、高血压人群越来越庞大,复发性的尿结石病同这些病一样也表现出了代谢异常引起的代谢综合征。pH降低使尿酸沉积,形成结石。因为痛风和糖尿病均表现出代谢综合征,因此胰岛素的生物活性在其中的作用引起人们的关注。有人认为胰岛素活性降低可能引起 pH 下降,进一步导致尿结石的形成。本段介绍了国际学术界推测的一些可能的痛风诱因,简要的概述国内外对本课题的研究近况。

Our data show that patients with uric acid urolithiasis were mostly older males with high BMI, multiple stone presentation, lower urinary pH, and higher serum uric acid level. Acidic urine is a prerequisite for uric acid stone formation and growth. Management with urinary alkalization for stone dissolution and prevention of recurrence should be effective. Low purine diet ingestion to decrease hyperuricemia and lifestyle modification to reduce the incidence of overweight or obesity can also be helpful.

我们的研究显示大部分尿酸结石患者大多为高 BMI 的老年男性,伴有多发结石、低尿 pH 及高血清尿酸。酸性的尿液是形成结石的第一步。碱化尿液、低嘌呤饮食、改变生活习惯及减轻体重均可降低结石的发生率。此段提出了作者的观点,说明研究能够在以前的基础上解决什么问题。

例 2 "终末型逼尿肌过度活跃患者的尿动力学表现"(文建国等,中华泌尿外科杂志, 2005 年 6 月第 26 卷第 6 期)。

讨论部分首先写明选题的原因和拟解决的问题,以及能够达到什么目的。接下来进一步讨论本研究结果与国内外其他研究结果的异同点。讨论中提及 "Miller 等对 79 例逼尿肌功能过度活跃者研究发现……", "Dorkin 等对下尿路梗阻伴有逼尿肌过度活跃导致排尿的 79 例男性患者研究发现……", "验证了上述分析"以及"本研究结果发现神经性和梗阻性终末型逼尿肌过度活跃导致排尿的最大逼尿肌收缩压和最大尿流率时逼尿肌压力接近于正常对照组,但膀胱多不能完全排空,且梗阻性终末型逼尿肌过度活跃膀胱排空效率显著低于神经性终末型逼尿肌过度活跃,这提示了……"等,即清晰表明了被研究与其他研究的相同点,也突出了本研究的创新点。最后进行小结,突出研究的中心问题。

2. 阐明本研究选题的背景和目的。并根据研究目的,对自己的研究结果进行具体阐述分析,重点阐述该项研究的创新性及其在临床实践中的意义。

举例说明:

例 1 Comparison between ultrasound and noncontrast helical computed tomography for identification of acute ureterolithiasis in a teaching hospital setting.

Escola Paulista de Medicina

One advantage of our study was the short time interval between the US and CT examinations, with an average interval of four hours. This was a limitation in previous studies, in which CT and US were obtained with longer intervals between them. Shorter intervals minimize the likelihood that the stone could have passed through prior to the second examination. Varanelli et al. investigated the relationship between duration of the flank pain and frequency of secondary signs of ureteral obstruction on unenhanced helical CT. Their study demonstrated that all the secondary signs, except nephromegaly, showed significantly increased frequency as the duration offlank pain increased. In our data, there was nostatistical significance between the duration of pain and the frequency of identification of secondary signs.

本段强调了本研究的创新性与先进性,其对相关领域的研究有较为重要的意义。首先说明了之前研究的局限性,因为之前的研究 US 和 CT 的间隔时间过长,导致了准确率的下降。然后引用了相关的文章,与我们的研究结果相对比,既体现了我们研究的先进性和必要性,又使文章的讨论显得内容饱满。

例 2 Melamine Related Bilateral Renal Calculi in 50 Children: Single Center Experience in Clinical Diagnosis and Treatment. Wen JG, Li ZZ, Zhang H, et al J Urol. 2010; 183 (4):1533-7.

In the present study calculous diameter in children with renal failure was significantly greater than in those with normal renal function, indicating that renal failure may more likely occur in the presence of larger stones … In the present study all clinical symptoms resolved following conservative treatment, and the calculi elimination rate was 42% (21 of 50 patients) at discharge from the hospital. Since melamine related urinary stones are amenable to conservative treatment, we used hemodialysis, which maintained stable renal function and allowed the majority of patients to recover without intervention …

同样,本段讨论首先回顾了目前对这类疾病的认识。对于有肾衰竭的儿童,其结石的直径明显大于无肾衰儿童结石的直径。之后介绍了作者研究中的结果和结论,通过保守治疗结石溶解率约 42%。通过回顾和讨论,让读者一目了然,既了解了目前的研究背景,又突出了本研究的创新和亮点,使重点更加突出。

例 3　Switala J R, Hendricks M, Davidson A. Serum ferritin is a cost-effective laboratory marker for hemophagocytic lymphohistiocytosis in the developing world[J]. Journal of pediatric hematology/oncology, 2012, 34 (3): e89-e92.

The diagnosis of HLH in resource-constrained environmentsis made more difficult by reliance on laboratory criteria, which are often unavailable or limited. New proposed modifications to the diagnostic criteria (Table 2) will help to reduce this reliance, as they are some what less laboratory focused compared with the current criteria (Table 1). However, the onus is still on the clinician toactively make the diagnosis and pursue treatment early on.

The costs related to specific investigations are often not considered by the user. Cost considerations often move local, national, or institutional groups to relook at diagnostic and treatment criteria, to balance what is best for the patient against what is affordable for a service provider. South Africa, although arguably more fortunate than most other African countries, is not exempt to these pressures and we have had to make institutional alterations to the treatment guidelines for patients with HLH because of the costs of tests (cyclosporine levels) and drugs (cyclosporine, in particular). Furthermore these "hard" costs do not include hidden expenses pertaining to access, transport, and accommodation for poor patients, especially those expenses required to attend outpatient clinics several times a week. Table 4 has a list of the costs of the laboratory tests typically involved in the diagnosis and follow-up of HLH. Because the disease is a dynamic process, investigations may need to be repeated before criteria are met and a diagnosis is made. Laboratory facilities may be limited in some hospitals and some tests may not be available at all (eg, soluble IL-2 receptor levels and NKC activity). This then raises the question as to what the most cost-effective and clinically instructive strategy is. In our series, hyperferritinemia was a consistently reliable finding (93%) compared with either serum fibrinogen or triglycerides, which were elevated in only half of the patients. This finding is supported by other studies in which a ferritin level>500 mcg/L was found in 100% of patients with HLH.

本讨论的开头部分介绍了研究的背景,提出了本研究的初衷:按照 HLH 的诊断标准,HLH 的诊断过程需要的成本很高,包括检查费用及隐性的交通住宿及定期门诊复查的费用。因为 HLH 是一个动态变化的过程,从诊断前到确诊时的一段时间里,需要对患者进行不断的监测。而有些地方的医院设施存在一些缺陷不能进行相关的实验室检查(如 sIL-2 受体水平及 NK 细胞活性的检测），在这种情况下，找到一个既经济又简便的监测 HLH 的指标就迫在眉睫了。从而引出本文的研究对象铁蛋白，指出本研究患者的高水平铁蛋白的发生率并以先前研究为佐证，引出下面的问题。

3. 比较本研究结果与其他研究结果的异同。与国内外相关研究结果比较，分析其不同点及造成此种差异的原因，客观公正的评价自己和他人的研究结果，提出自己的想法和意见，对本研究的发现及创新点予以重点描述。涉及支持创新点的研究结果要详细说明。

举例说明：

例 1　Renal screening in children after exposure to low dose melamine in Hong Kong: cross sectional study

Hugh S Lam, Pak C Ng, Winnie C W Chu, et al

DISCUSSION 部分

… Comparison with other studies

The pattern of complications detected in the territory wide screening in the Hong Kong Special Administrative Region was similar to that of our cohort. Of 17 667 children screened at all special assessment centers up to 5 November 2008, only 10 (0.06%) had renal stones (≥4mm) detected. Echogenic foci closely related to the renal papillae are unusual findings on ultrasonography in asymptomatic children. In a report on 196 cases of microlithiasis in children, all but 13presented with abdominal or genitourinary symptoms.10 A large proportion also had urinary abnormalities, including haematuria (61%) and hypercalcuria (38%). In our children with renal deposits, only one had haematuria, but all had a normal urinary calcium: creatinine ratio. These hyperechoic lesionswere noted to have less acoustic shadowing than usual renal stones. The features of these suspected melamine related renal deposits on ultrasonography resemble gallbladder sludge rather than calcified stones.11 Even including these seven children with possible renal deposits, only a small percentage (0.2%) of children exposed to relatively low dose melamine were affected. None of our children developed acute renal failure or urinary tract obstruction, or required treatment. However, the high prevalence of abnormalities in urine is unusual. It is possible that a large proportion was false positive, as suggested by the small number of children with red blood cells in urine confirmed by microscopy. As reagent strips can be more sensitive than microscopy, 12 however, some of these children may genuinely have had mild haematuria. Results from a screening programme in Japan showed that in 6 197 school aged children, dipstick alone detected occult blood in 4.1% and protein in 2.1%.13 The proportion of children with haematuria detected by reagent strip testing was slightly higher in our cohort (6.6%). Using a multilevel screening algorithm in a larger cohort (23 121 Japanese children), haematuria was detected in 0.7% and proteinuria in less than0.01%.14 The proportion of children with haematuria confirmed by microscopy in Hong Kong is similar to that in Japan.

本段通过与其他研究结果的对比，来显示研究的异同点，并分析其可能原因。通过与香港的结果对比，显示了两个研究成果的相似性，但仍有不同。在作者研究的 17 667 例儿童中，仅有 10 例发现了肾结石。有 196 例微小结石的儿童，仅有 13 例有腹部或会阴部症状。对于其他的研究，有很大一部分其他的并发症，包括血尿和高钙尿症，但在作者的研究中仅有 1 例有血尿。通过作者与其他研究的对比，可以很明显地突出研究的特异性，从中得到新的信息,通过分析更容易获取结论,也更令人信服。

例2　Expression of AQP1-4 in hydronephrotic kidney in children

Wen JG, Li ZZ, Zhang H, et al

DISCUSSION 部分

… The majority of studies have involved experimental animal models which have provided fundamental understanding on the biophysical properties of aquaporins. Moreover, these animal studies have been pivotal for examining the localization of these transporters to the different segments of the nephron. From a very limited number of studies the localization of AQP1 have been confirmed and extended in detailed studies using normal and diseased human adult kidney samples. However, there are yet no reports on renal aquaporin expression and distribution in kidneys from children …

本段是另外一个通过对比来显示文章创新性的例子。首先描述了大部分实验通过动物模型提供了解水蛋白生物性质的基础,并通过动物实验确定了这些转运工具在肾脏中的位置。此外,文献报道只有有限的成人肾脏研究 AQP1,但是没有儿童肾脏水蛋白的表达及分布研究。通过回顾文献研究概况,作者将自己的实验目的表达得很清楚,或者说使其更加突出,让人一目了然。

例3　Yu J T, Wang C Y, Yang Y, et al. Lymphoma-associated hemophagocytic lymphohistiocytosis: experience in adults from a single institution[J]. Annals of hematology, 2013, 92(11):1529-1536.

Compared with patients from previous studies, however, the survival time in our cohort seemed longer. Takahashi etal. report a case series comprising 26 patients with lymphoma-associated HLH, with a median survival time of only 83 days. Another study conducted by Tong et al. shows that the median survival time of patients with Tcell lymphoma-associated HLH is only 40 days. Increased awareness of lymphoma-associated HLH, more aggressive chemotherapy, and better supportive care could all have contributed to the better survival among our study patients. However, the role of allogeneic HSCT in patients with lymphoma-associated HLH needed to be addressed as well.

Currently, only a few studies have examined the role of allogeneic HSCT in lymphoma patients presenting with HLH. Here, we report the cases of two patients with T cell lymphoma who did not only achieved complete remission but also obtained long-term survival from allogeneic HSCT. We hypothesized that allogeneic HSCT could provide sufficientgraft-versus-lymphoma effect to patients with T cell lymphoma associated HLH. Unfortunately, our study could not identify the graft-versus-lymphoma effect in patients with B cell lymphoma-associated HLH because only one patient in the B cell lymphoma group received this treatment. Furthermore, this patient eventually died of lymphoma relapse. Notably, neither grade 4 acute graft-versus-host diseases nor extensive chronic graft-versus-host diseases were observed in these three patients, suggesting that allogeneic HSCT could be a feasible and safe treatment strategy for lymphoma-associated HLH. The role of autologous HSCT on lymphoma associated HLH, however, was not investigated in this study because none of the patients in our cohort had received this treatment. Since Shimazaki et al. have demonstrated that high-dose chemotherapy followed by autologous HSCT can provide survival benefits, autologous HSCT should also be considered in patients with lymphoma-associated HLH.

本例说明了此研究结果与先前其他研究者的病例研究结果相比，队列中的患者具有更高的生存期，作者将较高的生存期归功于对淋巴瘤合并噬血细胞综合征早期的诊断、更强的化疗方案及有效的支持治疗。突出了本研究队列的干预措施对于改善疾病预后所作的贡献。最后特别提出了造血干细胞移植（HSCT）在改善患者生存方面的作用和价值，这也是本研究较先前研究的一个创新点。然而，作者在讨论最后又补充"Unfortunately, our study could not identify the graft-versus-lymphoma effect in patients with B cell lymphoma-associated HLH because only one patient in the B cell lymphoma group received this treatment." 及 "The role of autologous HSCT on lymphoma associated HLH, however, was not investigated in this study because none of the patients in our cohort had received this treatment."，既提出了本研究创新的方面，又提出了本研究所不能解决的问题，为后人进一步探索指出了方向。

4. 对本研究所得结果进行补充说明或解释，对结果进行分析探讨，对可能原因、机制提出见解，并阐明观点。指出结果可能存在的误差以及教训，提出在调查研究过程中的经验体会。

举例说明：

Yu J T, Wang C Y, Yang Y, et al. Lymphoma-associated hemophagocytic lymphohistiocytosis: experience in adults from a single institution [J]. Annals of hematology, 2013, 92 (11):1529-1536.

Survival of patients with lymphoma-associated HLH remained dismal in our study; the median overall survival time was only 231 ± 101.5 days. Notably, we observed a trend toward a higher survival time in patients with B cell compared with those with T cell lymphoma-associated HLH, even though HLH could be associated with poor treatment response in patients with B cell lymphoma but not necessarily in those with T cell lymphoma. However, the survival time difference was not statistically significant (330 ± 192.0 days versus 96 ± 37.4 days; p=0.198). Our results showed that improved survival in patients with B cell lymphoma-associated HLH might be due to both higher treatment response rate and rituximab application. In our study, both complete remission and use of rituximab provided survival benefit by reducing the hazard ratio to 0.08 (p=0.029 and p=0.045, respectively) in patients with B cell lymphoma-associated HLH. This result could be further supported by a study from Pfreundschuh et al., showing that rituximab can improve both disease-free and overall survival in patients with diffuse large B cell lymphoma.

One of the possible reasons for inferior survival in patients with T cell lymphoma-associated HLH is more profound cytokine storm. In our cohort, patients with T cell lymphoma had significantly higher serum ferritin levels than those in the B cell lymphoma group [$11,525.6 \pm 2,568.5$ versus ($3,790.6 \pm 823.7$) ng/ml; p=0.043]. Ferritin is one of the most important biomarkers predicting systemic inflammation; consequently, hyperferritinemia may indirectly suggest elevated cytokine activation. Moreover, hyperferritinemia might further result in activating an iron-independent signaling cascade that enhances hepatic proinflammatory mediators through the NFκB signaling pathway. This activated pathway potentially worsens organ damage in lymphoma-associated HLH patients, which might be associated with inferior survival outcome.

本例先提出研究结果显示了 B 细胞淋巴瘤组比 T 细胞淋巴瘤组的生存期稍长，但是此差异无统计学上的意义。虽然无统计学意义，但作者进一步讨论了 B 细胞淋巴瘤合并噬血综合征具有较长生存期的原因，是由于有较高的 CR 率及靶向药物美罗华的使用。并且再一次分析说明了 T 细胞淋巴瘤组预后差的可能原因,即更严重的细胞因子的释放,并以铁蛋白为例进一步说明了高水平炎症因子对预后的不利影响,对其可能的机制加以阐述。

5. 指出本研究的缺陷及进一步研究的方向、展望、建议及设想。任何科研活动都不可能是尽善尽美的,但许多问题、缺陷、遗憾可能是在走过一个完整研究历程之后才能意识到,因而有必要在讨论部分对设计上的缺陷、操作上的失误、讨论中的未尽事宜和有待进一步探讨的问题做一提示,这样不仅不会降低论文的学术价值,反而是科学性和可信性的具体体现,对他人的指导意义更大。对本研究的缺陷及局限性进行实事求是的评价、分析和解释,说明相互矛盾的结果和结论,说明本文未能解决的问题,提出今后研究的方向与问题。

举例说明:

Renal screening in children after exposure to low dose melamine in Hong Kong: cross sectional study

Hugh S Lam, Pak C Ng, Winnie C W Chu, et al

DISCUSSION 部分

… Strengths and limitations of study

The catchment area of our centre includes the northern areas of Hong Kong closest to the border with the mainland. Our cohort therefore includes a large mobile population that travels often and regularly between the Hong Kong Special Administrative Region and the mainland. A large population of the children is born in Hong Kong but live across the border. Children seen at our centre would therefore be expected to be at highest risk of exposure to melamine tainted milk products within Hong Kong, but probably of lower risk compared with infants and children living on the mainland. To date our centre has screened the largest number of children in Hong Kong.

A limitation of our analyses is the absence of are liable biomarker of melamine exposure. In view of the short plasma half life of melamine (three hours), blood concentrations are unreliable. The concentration of melamine in urine is also an unhelpful marker as levels decrease rapidly after exposure stops. As all our children had stopped consuming the contaminated milk products for some time before assessment, the concentrations of melamine in both blood and urine are unhelpful. In view of the large number of children seen at our centre, a detailed history of consumption of melamine tainted milk products was not systematically recorded and was only rechecked if abnormalities found on ultrasonography were confirmed. Furthermore, as different batches of the same brand of milk product could be contaminated to varying degrees. It was not possible to accurately calculate exposure tomelamine. There was also no easy way to avoid overestimation of children's consumption of contaminated products by anxious parents. Despite these problems, dietary history and parental perceived risk of exposure are the only surrogate measures of melamine exposure available and we are therefore subject to misclassification bias.

如前所述,任何实验都不可能尽善尽美。正确认识实验的不足,才能合理地解释实验的结果,得出合适的结论。第一段描述了因为实验研究的对象主要是香港北面与大陆交接地带人口流动性很大,因此这些孩子更容易暴露于三聚氰胺奶制品的危险下。第二段说明了另一个偏倚因素,由于三聚氰胺没有特定的生物标记物,其半衰期又很短,患儿的暴露病史也未有详细的记载,因此判断指标仅通过超声诊断来确定。而且,不同批次牛奶三聚氰胺的含量也不同。作者又进一步说明了已经将这些因素考虑,并采取了进一步措施减少偏倚,使文章的结果结论更加可信。

6. 讨论的最后需要进行小结。讨论在结束时一定要有明确的结论,从自己的结果出发,对自己的研究目的作出"是什么"或者"是怎么样"的论断,发现了什么就是什么。要避免含混不清的词语,例如"可能"(possible)、"也许"(perhaps)、"大概"(probably)、"或许"(maybe)、"好像"(likely)等。如果对结论没有把握,那就证明你需要更多的实验来证实你的结论而不是进行推论。

举例说明:

例 1　Renal screening in children after exposure to low dose melamine in Hong Kong: cross sectional study

Hugh S Lam, Pak C Ng, Winnie C W Chu, et al

DISCUSSION 部分

… Conclusions and policy implications

The data from our cohort suggest that large scale and urgent screening programmes may not be informative or cost effective in regions outside of the mainland of China. Evidence to show that urgent massive screening after exposure to low dose melamine will lead to any health benefits is lacking. It is possible that hyperechoic lesions at the renal papillae may be associated with exposure to low dose melamine—that is, levels below 0.63mg/kg/day, but the clinical significance of these lesions is uncertain at this stage and long term follow-up is mandatory. In view of the lack of evidence to guide the government initially, and the large number of severely affected children on the mainland, a largescale, territory-wide urgent screening programme was probably justifiable. In light of results of our screening programme, it may now be acceptable to arrange renal assessments for select groups on routine clinical service to avoid stressing the already overworked public health system of Hong Kong. The use of reagent strip testing of urine as the primary means of identifying haematuria may lead to a large number of false positive results, 12 resulting in unnecessary anxiety for children and their parents. We believe, however, that reagent strip testing remains a valuable tool for identifying people for further confirmatory testing by microscopy of urine in screening programmes handling large numbers of patients in a short period. Arranging microscopy as soon as possible after a positive reagent strip result would help minimise anxiety for children and their parents. We postulate that the difference in prevalence and severity of renal complications between our children and their counterparts on the mainland can be explained by the difference in levels of exposure to melamine. The severe acute complications observed on the mainland seem unlikely to occur elsewhere. Further medium and long term follow-up studies of these children are warranted to assess more comprehensively the public health impact of consuming milk products contaminated with melamine.

本段基于之前的数据及讨论,给出了合理的结论。文章认为,根据作者已统计的数据显示,对低剂量接触三聚氰胺儿童进行筛查是不可取的。尽管低剂量的三聚氰胺即可导致肾乳头损伤,但这些在临床上并不明显,仍有待长期进一步的观察。之后作者又进一步提出了自己观点。基于数据及分析的推断结论,才是文章的核心部分。

例 2　UROLITHIASIS IN CHILDREN

PETER-MARTIN BRAUN, CHRISTOPH SEIF, KLAUS-PETER JÜNEMANN, PETER ALKEN

DISCUSSION 部分

… Infant stone patients must be followed over a prolonged period in order to assess the safety and effectiveness of the treatment strategy. Sonographic and/or X-ray monitoring of the respective kidney should be performed at least 2 weeks and 3 months after ESWL. Any remaining stubborn residual fragments are then disintegrated in repeated ESWL treatment.

A meta phylaxis for metabolic disturbances and a long-term antibiosis for chronic infection are recommended in an attempt to avoid residual stones. Any existing infrarenal obstruction must first be cleared. In order to achieve the most beneficial success rates under low complications, it is advisable to perform this type of ESWL in centers that claim the experience necessary for ESWL, and endo urological measures in children.

本段文字既明确的说明了结论,同时又给出了合理的建议,使文章的结果很具有实用价值。对新生儿结石,必须经过长时间的随访以保证安全。至少 2 周后随访肾脏情况,并于 ESWL 后 3 个月随访,行 X 线和超声的检测。如果有遗留,则需再次 ESWL 治疗。为了使术后并发症最少,治疗效果最佳,减少手术后结石的残余,需要使用药物纠正代谢异常,对有慢性感染征象时需应用抗生素治疗。本段用词恰当,表达了明确的信息,令人信服。

一个好的讨论应满足如下条件:

(1)陈述文章结果的原理、关系以及推广性。要牢记一个好的讨论是在讨论结果而不是复述结果。

(2)指出任何研究中的特例和研究的缺点,提出悬而未决的问题及提出未来的研究方向。掩盖或者蒙混不合适的数据均不可取。

(3)指出自己研究和前人研究的相同点,不同点。

(4)不要拘谨,讨论一切自己研究的理论意义,或者任何可能的实际应用。

(5)尽可能清楚地表达自己的结论。

(6)为每个结论总结足够的证据。

文章的讨论可以涉及以上的内容,但不是每一篇文章都需要面面俱到地讨论这六方面的问题,要因文制宜,言之有物。更重要的是,讨论要紧扣文章的研究结果,突出自己的新发现、新观点。不要把讨论写成小综述。更不可抄袭某些专著和教科书的内容。同时,讨论不能报喜不报忧,不能隐瞒真相。

(二)写作格式要求

1. 标题式　以三个或三个以上小标题的形式分别讨论几个问题或几个方面。这种方法使文章显得层次分明、思路清晰,避免了因为面面俱到使讨论变的笼统、离题和分散,同时使讨论部分更加紧扣主题、突出重点,特别有益于初学者的写作训练。例如:

例 1　"晚期妊娠妇女下泌尿道尿控的特点"(文建国,中华妇产科杂志,2006 年 11 月第 41 卷第 11 期),其讨论部分"一、妊娠期尿动力学检查的意义","二、晚期妊娠自由尿流率的变化","三、晚期妊娠膀胱功能的变化","四、晚期妊娠静态尿道压力的变化"这四个小标题展开,重点一目了然。

例 2　"Family and segregation studies: 411 Chinese children with primary nocturnal enuresis" [Pediatrics International（2007）49,618-622（王庆伟,文建国等）],其讨论部分是以如下三个小标题的形式叙述:"PNE has a significant family tendency：PNE is a common, genetically complex and heterogeneous disorder. Genetic factors are of great importance in the etiology of PNE, while environmental factors (both somatic and psychosocial) exert major modulatory effects on the phenotype …";"Coexistence of different modes of inheritance has been found in PNE: Segregation analyses strive to identify the specific mode of inheritance by statistical analysis of pedigrees of a condition. They are a prerequisite for linkage analyses, which require a hypothesis as to the mode of genetic transmission. In the study involving comprehensive screening of 430 Danish families Eiberg et al. identified 11 families with PNE type 1 in at least two generations or more …"; "Family history is a useful predictor of marked PNE：A family history of PNE proved to be the strongest predictor for the age of attaining dryness in a study of children fromNew Zealand. 23 In children with at least two first-degree relatives with a history of PNE, the development of nocturnal bladder control was delayed by 1.5 years. In another cross sectional epidemiological study, the risk of enuresis was five fold to seven fold higher if one parent had a history of enuresis. If both parents were affected, the risk ratio was 11.3 as compared to healthy families …"。

2. 无标题式　以自然段落按一定逻辑顺序展开,国内外医学论文多采用这种方法。整个讨论中无任何小标题,一气呵成。例如:

例 1　"终末型逼尿肌过度活跃患者的尿动力学表现"（王庆伟,文建国等,中华泌尿外科杂志,2005 年 6 月第 26 卷第 6 期）。讨论部分共分 5 段。第一段对逼尿肌过度活动做总体解释。第二段、等三段、第四段分别介绍其他相关研究和本研究之间的相同点和不同点。第五段最后总结说明本研究的中心思想,逻辑清晰,思路明确。如:

OAB 和逼尿肌功能过度活跃是 ICS 2002 年推荐的新标准化术语,前者主要以……Miller 等[5]对 79 例逼尿肌功能过度活跃者研究发现,膀胱容量、感觉、逼尿肌收缩性等尿动力学参数中功能性膀胱容量是判断逼尿肌过度活跃严重程度最适宜的客观指标……

膀胱顺应性主要是指逼尿肌主动舒张以适应不断增加充盈体积的能力,其下降主要病理改变是逼尿肌纤维肥大,胶原沉积和纤维化。本组神经性及梗阻性患者期相型及终末型逼尿肌过度活跃患者膀胱顺应性均显著低于正常对照组,提示长期逼尿肌过度活跃可能会造成……

Miller 等[5]研究发现,逼尿肌无抑制收缩压越高,急迫性尿失禁发生频率越低,多伴有良好的尿道闭合功能,而逼尿肌无抑制收缩压低的患者多伴有……

综上所述,终末型逼尿肌过度活跃患者膀胱多为小容量和高度敏感性膀胱。逼尿肌无抑制收缩力……

例 2　"Is it possible to use urodynamic variables to predict upper urinary tract dilatation in children with neurogenic bladder-sphincter dysfunction?"（王庆伟,文建国等）讨论部分共有八段内容,虽然没有小标题也能条理清晰。如:

NBSD constitutes a significant proportion of clinical paediatric problems, and understanding its spectrum has always been a difficult task for urologists. The reasons are that, on the one hand, the dynamics and disturbances of the lower urinary tract of children differ from those in adults, most NBSD in children being due to abnormal spinal column development or myelodysplasia; on the other hand, there are continuous changes and development in NBSD with growth and maturation, particularly duringthe first few years of life. In addition, VUR is more likely in children with NBSD, as the anti-reflux mechanism of the vesico-uretericjunction is not mature in children, which contributes to UUTD …

本段为讨论的起始部分,首先提出了问题,"神经源性膀胱功能障碍临床常见,是泌尿外科难题",借此引出了要讨论的方向,并说明了导致这个问题有两方面的原因,并分别阐述。

Ghoniem et al. and Kurzrock and Polse, respectively, studied the urodynamic changes in 61 children with myelomeningocele and 90 with spina bifida, and found that there was close relationship between low BC and UUTD. The present findings were similar, showing that the BC of groups 1-3 was significantly smaller than that of the control group, indicating that a poor BC was a risk factor for UUTD. A lower BC could result in high intravesical pressure, which might damage the detrusor musculature support at the vesico-ureteric junction that is crucial for the normal anti-reflux mechanism …

Earlier, in 1965, Smith found that most bladder dysfunction in myelomeningocele was ACD and associated with UUTD; ACD is common in children with NBSD. In a review of 188 children with myelomeningocele, Schulman and Van Gool reported that the ACD accounted for 38% of children with NBSD. In the present study, the incidence of ACD in groups 1-3 was significantly higher than in the control group, indicating that ACD was indeed one of risk factors for UUTD. The children with ACD would void mainly by increasing their abdominal pressure, but could not completely empty the bladder, thus producing a high PVR and causing persistently high intravesical pressure during the storage phase. Such increased intravesical pressure might accelerate VUR and UUTD …

McGuire et al. studied the clinical progress of 42 myelodysplastic patients by urodynamics tests and followed the patients for a mean of 7.1 years. There was close relationship between UUT deterioration and intravesical pressure on urethral leakage of$>40cmH_2O$. Kurzrock and Polse found a significant difference in DLPP between a group with VUR and UUT deterioration and a group with no VUR and UUT deterioration. This is consistent with the present results …

Stark found that 40% of children with myelomeningocele had detrusor hyperactivity, and studies by Willemsen and Nijman and Soyguret al. showed that DOA was related to VUR and renal damage. The current study showed that 39%(40 of 103) of the children with NBSD presented with UUTD and 46% (45 of 97) with NBSD had no UUTD, but there was no significant difference in NDOA between the control and groups 1-3 …

对于第一段提出的问题,作者首先进行了文献回顾。"Ghoniem、Kurzrock 和 Polse 分别研究了脑脊膜膨出及脊柱裂患儿的尿动力情况,其研究结果显示了低膀胱顺应性与上尿道扩张的关系。最近的研究也发现了相似的结果……早在 1965 年,Smith 发现大部分的脑脊膜膨出患者膀胱功能障碍都是逼尿肌无力合并上尿路狭窄……McGuire 等研究随访了 42 例脑脊膜膨出患者,时长 7.1 年,发现上尿路病变和膀胱内压大于 $40cmH_2O$ 有密切关系……。Kurzrock 和 Polse 的研究也具有相似的结果……Stark 等研究发现 40% 的脑脊膜膨出儿童逼尿肌高功能,Willemsen,Nijman 和 Soygur 等的研究显示 DOA 和 VUR 及膀胱损伤有关……",作者本阶段回顾了多个研究结果,这些文献提供了较为详细的研究背景和方向,为作者阐述研究的创新性提供了依据。

Research on the relationship between bladder capacity and UUTD is limited [29]; in the present study, although there was no significant difference in MCC among the control and three subgroups, there were significant differences in RSCC, RUCC and RRRCC. The RSCC of groups 2 and 3 were, respectively, significantly lower than that of control and group 1, while the RUCC and RRRCC significantly increased with the severity of UUTD from group 1 to 2 …

There are fewer studies on the effects of several urodynamic variables on UUTD. Only one predicted UUTD by using a URS based on the LPP, compliance and DSD, and it had the highest sensitivity (89%) but the lowest positive predictive value (61%), using a risk score of 1. The present study used the ACD to substitute for DSD as one URS because we consider it is not only a very important variable of bladder voiding function, but it is also more closely related to UUTD, as observed previously …

回顾了这些研究,作者阐述自己研究的创新性,使其更具有说服力。很多研究对相同问题的不同方面进行了阐述,但作者具有新的独特的衔接,即是作者研究的闪光点。在本节,作者认为尽管有很多的研究,但膀胱的容积与上尿路扩张的关系仍需进一步研究。

In conclusion, a low BC, increased DLPP and ACD are good urodynamic factors to predict UUTD in children with NBSD, and these three factors reciprocally increase the occurrence and grades of UUTD. The grades of UUTD are compatible with increase RUCC and RRRCC. AURS of ≥2 is the urodynamic criterion for an accurate diagnosis of UUTD, with a sensitivity and specificity of 68% and 82%, respectively …

最后作者对研究做了总结,通过合理地推断得出结论。

通过以上两个例子,我们可以看出,即使是对于无标题的写作格式,依然可以很整齐。段落依据严谨的思维模式和顺序,按照提出问题、回顾研究现状、描述研究结果、阐述自己观点、分析并得出结论的模式,可以使逻辑清晰,易于阅读。

(三)讨论的字数标准

讨论应该在紧扣本文观察研究结果的前提下严谨立论。文字字数应该限制在全文的1/3 以内。不需要面面俱到、空泛的讨论以及超越限度的引申,但对于作者的新发现和新认识要着重表述。

例如:杂志 *The Journal of Urology* 对稿件字数的要求为:"Manuscript does not exceed 2 500 words for Original Article. Manuscript does not exceed 3 000 words for Research Article. Manuscript does not exceed 500 words for Letter to the Editor. Manuscript does not exceed 1 000 words for Opposing Views."。著名血液学杂志 *Leukemia* 对稿件字数及结果讨论部分的要求为:"Original Articles: Article: 4 500 words max, excluding abstract, references, figures and tables; Reviews: Article: 6 000 words max, excluding abstract, references, figures and tables; Concise Reviews: Article: 4 000 words max, excluding abstract, references, figures and tables; Letters to the Editor: 1 500 words max excluding, references, figures and tables. Results and Discussion: The Results section should briefly present the experimental data in text, tables or figures. Tables and figures should not be described extensively in the text, either. The discussion should focus on the interpretation and the significance of the findings with concise objective comments that describe their relation to other work in the area. It should not repeat information in the results. The final paragraph should highlight the main conclusion(s), and provide some indication of the direction future research should take."。

二、讨论的写作特点

（一）明确相互联系，充分思考可分析的研究结果

任何研究都不可能孤立的存在，都与前人、他人的研究存在着千丝万缕的联系。因此，我们不应该孤立的就事论事，应该在更为广阔而深远的背景下讨论研究和其结果。纵向与横向多角度的比较现在的和过去的、自己的与他人的研究结果，进而突出研究中取得的新进展、新结论以及发现的新事物、新现象。创新是科学研究的价值所在。理论上重复做别人已经解决的科学问题是没有意义的。但在现今世界的医学研究中，只有极少数的研究探索到了无人发现的领域，绝大多数研究充其量只是提供了部分证据来判断某一假说是否正确。简单地说，讨论的主要目的就是揭示观察指标间的关系，为了说明这一点，在此讲一个关于生物学家训练跳蚤的故事。

跳蚤被训练数月后，能够对生物学家的某些命令做出回应。其中最令人鼓舞的是每次只要生物学家大声说出指令："跳!"，训练过的跳蚤就会跳起来。这个教授准备将这项重大的发现发表在期刊上以供后人阅读。但是，作为一个真正的科学家，他决定更进一步的实验：找到与反应有关的器官结构。在这个试验中，他每次切断一条跳蚤的腿，跳蚤在听到指令后仍然继续跳跃。但是随着切断的腿越来越多，跳蚤的反应越来越不明显。最终，当所有的腿都被切断后，跳蚤一动不动了，对一次又一次的命令没有了任何反应。

这个教授最终决定发表他的文章，他开始动笔细心地描述前几个月的实验，他准备了一个可以震惊科学界的结论：当所有跳蚤的腿被切除后，跳蚤就完全失去了听力能力。这个故事说明研究者思考了观察指标之间可能存在的关系。但是，这个实验并不能完全证实上述教授的结论。

Claude Bishop 也讲了一个相似的故事："一个老师为了向学生们说明酒精的危害，于是设计了一个简单的实验。他准备了两个瓶子，一个装水，一个装杜松子酒，在每一个瓶子里放了一只蠕虫。水中的蠕虫自由地游来游去，而杜松子酒里的蠕虫很快就死了。""这个实验证明了什么?"他问，坐在后排的小约翰回答说："这证明如果你喝杜松子酒就不会得蠕虫病!"这个故事提示我们应该思考观察指标之间可能存在的关系。但是这个实验显然不足以证明喝杜松子酒就不会得蠕虫病的结论。

许多论文"讨论"部分存在的问题主要有：只是简单叙述了实验过程和实验结果，也就是罗列实验数据、描述实验现象；讨论过程中对"摘要"和"引言"中的内容多次应用，却忽略了作者本人对实验结果的分析；在讨论过程中虽然引用了大量国内外的文献，却没有整合和分析这些文献的观点，也没有表达自己的新观点；没有客观评价自己的研究结果，刻意避开研究的局限性，甚至是自吹自擂。笔者认为在讨论的过程中作者要明确地提出自己的观点：肯定什么，否定什么及自己的理由。对研究结果进行充分的发掘利用，了解结果之间的相互联系，作者本身思维逻辑性的好坏以及对相关知识的全面理解和熟练掌握运用的程度就会体现在讨论的过程中。举例说明：Mounier N, Heutte N, Thieblemont C, et al. Ten-year relative survival and causes of death in elderly patients treated with R-CHOP or CHOP in the GELA LNH-

985 trial [J]. Clinical Lymphoma Myeloma and Leukemia, 2012, 12 (3):151-154.

Overall this study showed that even after 10 years of survival, elderly lymphoma patients aged 60-80 years at diagnosis were still at greater risk of death than was the general population. The leading cause of death was not DLBCL but second cancers, especially of the lungs, and vascular diseases. Rituximab did not seem to add any significant long-term toxicity to the chemotherapy.

There is an increased risk of lung cancer after lymphoma, with most studies showing that this risk increases 2-3 times more than in the general population. It appears to be higher in male survivors of Non-Hodgkin lymphoma (NHL), possibly because of the higher prevalence of smoking among men; however, the contribution of tobacco history to the treatment-related risk of lung cancer after DLBCL could not be directly assessed in the present study. The chemotherapy regimens that have been associated with the risk of lung cancer include CHOP and doxorubicin, cyclophosphamide, vindesine, bleomycin, and prednisone (ACVBP). Mudie et al. reported that the relative risk (RR) of lung cancer rose significantly in a CHOP subcohort but not in patients given chlorambucil. At present, the incidence of second malignancies after lymphoma treatment using rituximab combined with chemotherapy is a matter of debate. In the present study, we failed to detect any impact of the rituximab given in combination with CHOP, but a longer follow-up is ongoing to confirm this. In addition, differing immunologic alterations, treatment such as high-dose alkylating agents, genetic susceptibilities, and other risk factors (eg, viral infections, tobacco use) may contribute to the patterns of second malignancy risk.

Doxorubicin, a key component of chemotherapy regimens in the treatment of DLBCL, is classically associated with heart failure. In a retrospective study conducted by the European Organisation for Research and Treatment of Cancer (EORTC) that included 974 patients with NHL treated with 6 or more cycles of doxorubicin-based chemotherapy, the cumulative incidence of cardiovascular disease was estimated at 22% at 10 years. The estimated RR of congestive heart failure was elevated at 5.4. The RR of stroke was also elevated at 1.8, but the RR of coronary artery disease, estimated at 1.2, matched that of the general population. Overall the risk of cardiovascular disease increased with the dosage of doxorubicin, increasing age, previous heart disease, and the presence of comorbidities, diabetes, and hypertension. As expected, the present study of patients aged 60-80 years showed that about 5% of the long-term survivors died of cardiovascular disease. Half of them also had preexisting hypertension. We noted with interest that rituximab seemed to have no effect on the risk.

本文是对使用 R-CHOP 和 CHOP 方案的老年淋巴瘤患者 10 年生存的分析研究。作者简单地概括了研究的发现后（第一段），就开始围绕 "The leading cause of death was not DLBCL but second cancers, especially of the lungs, and vascular diseases." 这一发现从继发性肺癌及淋巴瘤对心血管系统的影响等问题进行探讨。并且提出了 "At present, the incidence of second malignancies after lymphoma treatment using rituximab combined with chemotherapy is a matter of debate." 这一争议及 "We noted with interest that rituximab seemed to have no effect on the risk." 这一推断。

（二）参考阅读大量相关文献

最能体现作者参考文献量的多少以及对这一学术问题理解和掌握程度的就是讨论部分。因此，作者应该投入足够的时间和精力高度重视讨论的写作。不仅使作者的学术水平可以充分展现，同时读者对于相关问题的认识也得到进一步提高。科学、客观的讨论对于一篇兼具实用价值、科学价值、创造价值的医学论文至关重要。只有在搜集阅读大量参考文献的基础上将这些文献和自己所做的研究相结合，才能将讨论部分写好并且更加有深度，更加令人信服。

在搜集论文相关的文献资料时，应该特别注意搜集以下内容的文献：①沿用前人方法的，或在前人的研究基础上进一步发展改进的；②在理论上支持本文所述观点的；③自己文章所述与前人研究所得结论不同，需要加以解释说明的；④本文所研究的问题仍然存在争议或者正在探讨中的。搜集到这些资料后，编上序号，以便撰写文章时使用。

以下的三种现象不应该出现在引用文献的过程中：①为了证明自己的阅读量大而引用国外文献，甚至在没有看到原文的情况下二次引用；②自己认为不重要，或是没有发现，但是为了突出自己研究的"创新"和"价值"故意回避，没有引用或是没有系统地引用文献；③没有把自身的研究与引用的相关文献相结合，造成了讨论过程中的论文分割，使得作者的研究结果不能被读者深入地理解。

（三）选择要深入讨论的问题

讨论可以很好的体现作者学术研究的深度和广度。对于提出的问题作者的研究深入到了什么样的程度就是深度，从不同角度来研究解释得到的实验结果就是广度。如果讨论内容较多，可以选择分为几个题目单独讨论。要想把讨论写好，有下面两个重要步骤：

1. 选择有价值的结果进行深入讨论。一般来说，可根据以下几点来判断：如果你的研究结果具有创新性，还没有出现在其他研究中，那这个研究结果就具有重点讨论的价值；部分结果和前人的研究没有明显的差异，就没有深入讨论的价值，只需一笔带过就好。

2. 突显与他人不同的特点及自身研究的创新性，要与他人的研究有差异，不管差异的大小，有差异即是创新。我们摘录一段近期投往《新英格兰医学杂志》文章的部分讨论："Our present study indicates that poor height increase may be related to the insufficient calcium supply. Bonjour et al found that calcium supplementation had a possible positive effect on skeletal growth. Calcium-enriched foods significantly increased bone mass accrual with a preferential effect seen in the appendicular skeleton. Whether the lower body height related to insufficient calcium supplement or consumption of toxic milk powder warrants further investigation."。上述三个句子就是最常见的表述顺序。

（四）多层次多角度讨论选中问题

大多数情况下会选择 2 个以上的问题，因此要分层次分别描述清楚。一般来说，中间描述最重要的问题，开头和末尾描述不太重要的问题。开头是铺垫，末尾是总结，中间的重要问题可以将评审人和读者的情绪带至高潮。这样才是恰当的顺序。不管问题大小，重要性如何，都应该深入讨论问题的不同角度：首先要体现自身研究的创新性需要与类似的结果作对比；其次要从理论原理、实验设计、分析方法以及借鉴的分析方法等多种角度系统阐述是怎样得到这样的结果。重要的是深入阐述清楚所提出的问题,切忌使读者感觉意犹未尽。

(五)保持和结果的一致性

讨论是对结果的逻辑扩展,是从理论上分析和综合实验和观察得到结果,丰富和提高了对实验结果在广度和深度上的认识。需阐明论证研究得到的结果,同时作为理论上的依据为文章的结论服务。讨论部分的主线应该是自己的研究,然后把自己研究的结果与他人的相关研究结果进行对比,最后引出研究的结论。

探讨"研究结果"的意义是这部分的首要任务,为了给进一步的实践提供依据,需要把研究结果从感性认识层面上升到理性认识层面。讨论中要以结果为基础,进行合理分析,找出结果之间内在的联系,肯定最后的结论。必须做到有理有据。若有需要,应该以谦虚谨慎和客观公正的态度对自身研究进行评价。此外切忌离题发挥或重复他人的观点。

如果按讨论的内容进行推导,得出的结论与实验的结果相反,说明你的讨论思路是完全错误的或你的实验彻底的失败了,这种情形千万不能出现。所以讨论的描述和表达一定要足够的精确。由于中英文语言习惯的不同,在投稿之前应该尽可能避免表达不准确造成误解。

(六)结尾突出文章的重要性

结果的意义未被讨论或者仅仅有较少的讨论很常见。如果读者在读完讨论后还在问:"那又怎样?"。那就表明读者对结果的意义没有认识到。因此,通常讨论的结尾都应该总结科研的重要性,提出自己的结论。结论应该准确、完整、鲜明。结论的提出是作者将观察到的现象,实验结果所得到的数据,通过综合分析,构成若干观点和论点,然后将数据贯穿起来,经综合分析,构成总体论点。正如 Anderson 和 Thistle 总结的那样:"最终,好的文章就如音乐一样,都应该适时有一个高潮,很多文章因为虎头蛇尾而失去了它的价值。"("Finally, good writing, like good music, has a fitting climax. Many a paper loses much of its effect because the clear stream of the discussion ends in a swampy delta.")因此,结尾一定要突出文章的重点,使读者读过之后感觉重点鲜明。例如:

In conclusion, a low BC, increased DLPP and ACD are good urodynamic factors to predict UUTD in children with NBSD, and these three factors reciprocally increase the occurrence and grades of UUTD. The grades of UUTD are compatible with increase RUCC and RRRCC. AURS of ≥2 is the urodynamic criterion for an accurate diagnosis of UUTD, with a sensitivity and specificity of 68% and 82%, respectively. Even for the children with neurogenic damage and normal urodynamic findings, a close follow-up is important for the early diagnosis and timely treatment, as well as preventing progressive UUTD.

该段对研究进行的总结突出了文章的目的性、实用性。"总之,膀胱低顺应性,逼尿肌漏尿点压增高,无抑制性收缩是预测神经源性膀胱逼尿肌功能障碍患儿上尿路扩张较好的尿动力学参数,并且这三个参数相互影响,可增加上尿路扩张的风险。"通过对实验数据分析讨论,最终给予一个结论,并将结论应用于临床,与实践相结合,画龙点睛,这才是所有科研的终极目的。

三、综述中常用语法和句型举例

（一）时态应用举例

一般现在时、一般将来时和一般过去时是英文科研论文中使用最多的三种时态。科研写作的基本功就是准确的使用谓语动词的时态，在撰写英文科技论文的过程中，如使用了错误的时态，常常会改变文章所要表达的意思，从而使评审人与读者产生误解。为避免错误，首先要掌握三个基本要点：

1. **一般现在时**　主要用于描述客观存在的不受时间限制的事实，以及描述写论文之时发生或存在的感觉、状态、关系等，还有表达致谢的时候等。值得注意的是，出于尊重，凡是他人已经发表的研究成果作为"previously established knowledge"，在引述时普遍都用一般现在时。

2. **一般过去时**　用于描述写论文中作者自己所做的工作。例如对自己获得的材料、方法和结果的描述。

3. **一般将来时**　用于描述发生在撰写论文之后的动作和存在的状态。例如展望未来的研究方向。

例如：通常使用过去时来回顾研究目的。如："In this study, the effects of two different learning methods were investigated."。如果作者觉得所描述结果的有效性只局限于本次特定的研究，常常用过去时表达；相反，如果用现在时表达，则表示具有普遍的意义。如："In the first series of trials, the experimental values were all lower than the theoretical predictions. The experimental and theoretical values for the yields agree well."。通常使用现在时来阐述由结果得出的推论。使用现在时的理由不只是在讨论自己研究的结果而是说明作者得出的结论或推论具普遍有效的意义，并且研究结果与得出的结论或推论之间产生的逻辑关系是客观存在的不受时间限制的事实。如："The data reported here suggest (These findings support the hypothesis, Our data provide evidence) that the reaction rate may be determined by the amount of oxygen available."。总之，要严格选择讨论的内容，根据实验结果，按照逻辑推理的顺序，逐项进行分析，然后归纳、总结，由感性认识到理性认识，由表及里，由现象到本质，由主观到客观，做出正确的判断和推理，得出准确的结论。

（二）常用的句型举例

1. It is suggested that … 我们建议……，我们认为……

2. We conclude that … 我们的结论是……

it is concluded that … 结论是……

3. The results show … （研究）结果表明……

the data show that … 本资料表明……

4. This study indicates that … 本研究指出……

these findings indicate that … 这些发现指出……

5. This case illustrates that … 本例说明……

It is illustrated that … 这就说明……

6. These results demonstrate that … 这些研究结果证明……

7. This study confirms (that) … 本研究证实……

Data fail to confirm … 本资料未能证实……

8. We feel that … 我们认为……

The authors feel that … 作者认为……

9. We believe that … 我们认为……

On the bases of the authors' experience, . they believe(that)… 根据作者的经验,他们认为……

10. We consider … 我们认为……

11. This case points out … 本例指出……

12. The authors therefore proposes that … 因而作者的建议（认为）……

It is proposed that … 我们建议（认为）……

13. We recommend that …（be）我们建议……

It is recommended that …（be）我们建议……

14. These results support … 这些结果支持……

15. It is thought that … 我们认为……

16. It is suspected that … 我们怀疑……

17. In my opinion … 我们的意见是……

Our opinion is that … 我们的意见是……

The authors are of the opinion that 作者的意见是……

18. To the author's knowledge … 就作者所知……

19. In our experience … 根据我们的经验……

例如：

1. It is proposed that nonspecific ulcers of the colon should be managed conservatively.
我们建议,非特异性结肠溃疡应保守治疗。

2. We recommend that serum prolactin be measured when evaluating these patients and their families.
在评价这些患者及家属时,我们建议测定血清催乳素。

3. The report suggests that fibromuscular dysplasia of the renal arteries is acquired and may not be present from birth.
本报告认为该肾动脉肌纤维发育异常是后天性的,可能不是先天性的。

4. It is proposed that an increased conversion of carbohydrate to fat occurs during the period of rapid weight loss when relative excess of carbohydrate to amino acid results from an imbalance in the intestinal absorption of carbohydrate and protein.
此时由于肠道吸收碳水化合物和蛋白质不平衡,以致碳水化合物比氨基酸量相对过剩,因此向脂肪转化增多。

（三）常见语法错误举例

1. 把名词用作形容词

不用：ATP formation; reaction product.

而用：formation of ATP; product of the reaction.

2. 单词 "this" 后面一般要跟名词

不用：This is a fast reaction; This leads us to conclude.

而用：This reaction is fast; This observation leads us to conclude.

3. 描述实验结果统一使用过去时态

不用：Addition of water gives product.

而用：Addition of water gave product.

4. 尽可能使用主动语态

不用：It was observed that the solution turned red.

而用：the solution turned red or we observed that the solution turned red.

5. 对比句要书写完整

不用：The yield was higher using bromine.

而用：The yield was higher using bromine than chlorine.

6. 错误用词

不用：This phenomenon was in accordance with that seen in P. aeruginosa.

而用：This observation was in accordance with that seen in P. aeruginosa. ("phenomenon" usually means something very unusual.)

7. 单复数误用

不用：There are increasing evidences that …

而用：There is increasing evidence that … (the noun "evidence" is never pluralized by adding "s")

8. 指代不明

不用：An important finding of this study was that …

而用：An important finding of the present study was that …

9. 中式英语

不用：A lot of new problems and questions have been pointed out. Those force the researchers turn to new attempts both in theory and in methodology.

而用：A lot of new problems have arisen. All this forces the researchers to turn to new attempts both in ideology and in methodology.

总之，a good discussion will typically cover:

1）Relate the results to the original objectives;

2）Explain principles, relationships, and generalizations that can be supported by the results;

3）Discuss the theoretical implications and any possible applications of your work;

4）Address any exceptions that qualify the findings, or difficulties that point to areas for further investigation;

5）Explain how the results relate to previous findings, whether in support, contradiction, or simply as added data;

6）Give particular attention to the problem, question, or hypothesis presented in the introduction;

7）Present conclusions, supported by a summary of the evidence; State your conclusions as clear as possible; 是 ummarize your evidence for each conclusion;

8）Conclusions may merit a separate subheading or, rarely, a separate section.

注意讨论不要：

1）Repeat results;

2）Introduce new results;

3）Pretend to have solved everything;

4）Finish with throwaway sentences;

5）Try to walk around every possibility (speculate, over discuss).

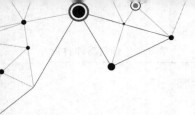

第9章
致谢和参考文献

Chapter 9
How to Write the Acknowledgments and References

致谢指作者对该研究和论文完成过程中得到的任何帮助的人、单位、组织和基金团体等表达感谢。致谢也是一种礼貌,正如 Ralph Waldo Emerson 说的那样:"Life is not so short but that there is always time enough for courtesy."。英文致谢词一般放在论文讨论和结论之后。英文致谢有很多模式,如:① This study was supported by grants from the National Natural Science Foundation; ② I sincerely appreciate my supervisor, Mr. Wen, for his instructive advice and useful suggestions on my thesis.

参考文献,顾名思义,就是参考过文献,也就是撰写科研论文或著作过程中参考过的论文、著作、发表的报告、指南等。GB/T 7714—2015《信息与文献 参考文献著录规则》将文后参考文献定义为"为撰写或编辑论文和著作而引用的有关文献信息资源"。在注释中若已注明了征引过的文献,那么文后参考文献中就不需要再列出了。参考文献有两种方式,一种为对正文中某一内容作进一步解释或补充说明的文字,列于当页脚,即脚注;一种放在文章末尾,致谢之后。

下面我们将分别对致谢和参考文献进行介绍。

第一节 致 谢

致谢是在某项研究中,在选题、构思或论文撰写方面曾给予指导和建议,除作者本人外对观察或实验具有重要贡献的人员,或者对仅参加部分工作的人员或给予过信息、资源、技术、经费及物质帮助的团体或个人表达谢意。此项应视具体情况而定,并非是每篇论文所必需的部分,只在很必要时使用。据调查,英文科技期刊中有致谢的文章的比例很高,一般在50% 以上。

一、致谢的范围

ICMJE(International Committee of Medical Journal Editors)对致谢范围的规定如下:

All contributors who do not meet the criteria for authorship should be listed in an acknowledgments section. Examples of those who might be acknowledged include a person who provided purely technical help, writing assistance, or a department chair who provided only general support. Editors should ask corresponding authors to declare whether they had assistance with study design, data collection, data analysis, or manuscript preparation. If such assistance was available, the authors should disclose the identity of the individuals who provided this assistance and the entity that supported it in the published article. Financial and material support should also be acknowledged.

Groups of persons who have contributed materially to the paper but whose contributions do not justify authorship may be listed under such headings as "clinical investigators" or "participating investigators, " and their function or contribution should be described—for example, "served as scientific advisors, " "critically reviewed the study proposal, " "collected data, " or "provided and cared for study patients." Because readers may infer their endorsement of the data and conclusions, these persons must give written permission to be acknowledged.

一般致谢对象包括：对论文的设计、选题、撰写、修改等方面给予指导或提出建设性意见的人；对观察和实验过程有过重要贡献的人；给予物质资助的单位、团体或个人；提供过资料、实验材料、实验仪器或给予其他帮助的人；为论文提供图片、图表、数据的人；提供某些有价值信息但又不能够成为作者的人（详见第 3 章）。致谢中应尽量指出致谢对象的具体帮助与贡献。

根据致谢的对象，可以分为下面三种：

（1）对单位致谢：即对研究提供资助的单位。如：① the author acknowledges the support of the Swedish Medical Research Council and the Medical Faculty, Goteborg University；② the research was supported by zhengzhou university.

（2）对个人的致谢：包括参与讨论或提供意见者、非商业性的材料提供者、提供技术协助的人员及文书人员等。如：① We thank Dr. J. Corcos, Department of Urology, McGill University, Montreal, Quebec, Canada, and Prof. Robert Levin, Albany College of Pharmacy, Albany, NY, USA, for their critical revision of this manuscript；② We thank John J. Mekalanos, Department of Microbiology, Harvard Medical School, Boston, Mass. for the generous gift of plasmids pGP704, pVMy and pSC 18.1 and V. cholerae JJM43；Costa Georgopoulos, Department of Medicine, University of Geneva, Geneva, Switzerland, for kindly providing E. coli CG2685 and CG5621.

（3）对基金支持的致谢：即经费的来源。如：① This research was supported in part by 43525-02 from the National Natural Science Fund Committee, P.R. China.　② This work was supported by grant R01 AI 30 010 from the National Institute of Health and in part by US. PHS Grant DE11549.

二、致谢在文中的位置

致谢一般单独成段，置于结论和参考文献之间，多数杂志都遵循如下顺序：Abstract, Introduction, Results, Discussion, Conclusion, Acknowledgement, References。但致谢也可以脚注的形式置于论文首页的下方，如 *Medical Hypothesis*，它要求在首页（Title Page）进行致谢。

The title page should give the following information: ① title of article; ② initials and name of each author, with highest academic degree(s); ③ name and address of the department or institution to which the work should be attributed; ④ name, address, telephone and fax numbers and E-mail address of the author responsible for correspondence and to whom requests for offprint should be sent; ⑤ sources of support in the form of grants.

因此,在撰写论文的致谢部分时,要按照期刊的具体要求,放在相应的位置。

三、致谢书写的注意事项

1. 态度要谦恭　致谢最重要的是谦恭的态度,它遵循任何其他文明生活领域的规则,同样也适合科技论文的写作。这好比借了邻居一样东西,会说声谢谢;朋友给你提供一个方便,也会记得说声谢谢。这些日常生活的礼貌规则同样应该用于科学界,如果你的同事给该课题提供了各种方便,你应该表示感谢。当使用书面形式表示感谢时,就形成了科技论文的致谢。

2. 谢辞要谨慎　要感谢别人提供了帮助。首先应该斟酌好要表达的致辞。否则,就会显得太随意,很难让人感觉到足够的诚意。对于致谢的对象称呼,可直书其名,也可加上尊称,如教授、博士等。一般排序的依据是贡献的大小,而不是年龄、地位。对于致谢的对象需要事先征得对方同意,随便向外面公布没有征得同意的致谢是很冒失的,这将会危及你们的友谊或者长期合作的机会。有时不合适的感谢不如不致谢,如果你很看重朋友或者同事提供的建议,你应该很慎重地以一种取悦于他们而不是冒犯他们的方式对他们进行感谢。

3. 用词要恰当　表示感谢常用的词语有"thank""appreciate""acknowledge"等,要避免添加诸如"wish""hope""would like to"等词语,否则会导致缺乏诚意,引起误会。例如:"I wish to thank Professor Wen"言外之意是 Professor Wen 不是特别值得感谢,这样不但违背作者意愿,也显得词汇冗余,直接用"I thank Professor Wen"更显得简洁和真诚。

4. 遵从期刊的习惯　参阅拟投稿期刊的"作者须知(information/instruction for authors)"和已发表在该刊上论文的致谢部分,应特别注意期刊对于致谢部分形式和表达的要求。对于基金资助的致谢信息尤为值得注意,部分期刊要求将其写到"致谢"中,而有的期刊则要求将其写到论文首页的脚注中。

5. 避免不符合规定的致谢　书写致谢时应该避免混淆作者和被致谢者的权利,将被致谢人放在作者的位置上;以名人或者知名专家包装自己的论文,将未曾参与研究甚至未曾阅读论文的知名专家写在致谢中。此外,如果只是对关于一种想法、建议或者解释表达感谢,你应该很明确地表达出来。如果你太笼统地表达感谢的意思的话,那么你的朋友可能感觉不到你的诚意。

四、致谢常用的英文句式

1. The author thanks/acknowledges/is grateful to/is indebted to ... 作者感谢……

2. ... is/are appreciated/thanked/acknowledged ... 应该感谢……

3. The financial support of ... is appreciated/thanked/acknowledged 感谢……提供的经济支持

4. ... provided financial support for this work/study/research, for which the author greatly appreciates. ……为本研究提供了经济支持,作者深表谢意

5. ... is appreciated for his/her advice/suggestions/encouragement/comments 感谢……的建议 / 提议 / 鼓励 / 评论

6. Thanks to .../Thanks are due to ... 感谢……

7. This paper is being presented with the kind permission of … 感谢……允许论文的发表

8. The author acknowledges the facilities made available by … 感谢……提供设备支持

五、致谢的表达举例

1. 论文后的致谢

（1）I would like to extend my sincere gratitude to my supervisor, Mr. Wen, for his instructive advice and useful suggestions on my thesis. 该句主要表达了对导师 Mr. Wen 给予论文的宝贵指导意见真诚的感谢。

（2）High tribute shall be paid to Mr. Chen, whose profound knowledge of English triggers my love for this beautiful language. 该句表达了对老师激发自己学习兴趣的感谢。

以上两例主要表达了对个人的谢意。

（3）I am deeply indebted to all the other tutors and teachers in Translation Studies for their direct and indirect help to me. 该句主要对导师和其他老师给予直接或者间接的帮助表示致谢。

（4）Special thanks should go to my friends who have put considerable time and effort into their comments on the draft. 该句主要对朋友表示致谢。

（5）I am indebted to my teachers for their continuous support and encouragement.

以上 3 个的例子表示对团体的致谢。

（6）This study was supported by grants from the National Natural Science Foundation. 该句表达了对基金的致谢。

（7）We are indebted to our principal collaborators at the First Affiliated Hospital of Zhengzhou University, JianguoWen and Zhenzhen Li, for their assistance with manuscript preparation/for providing expert technical assistance. 该句表达了对个人技术、方法等的致谢。

2. 论著或者综述后的致谢

（1）The authors acknowledge the contribution of the people with mesothelioma or asbestos related lung cancer and their family members who contributed their precious time, energy and reflections to this study.〔Lee SF, O'Connor MM, Chapman Y, Hamilton V, Francis K. A very public death: dying of mesothelioma and asbestos-related lung cancer (M/ARLC) in the Latrobe Valley, Victoria, Australia. Rural Remote Health. 2009 Jul-Sep;9 (3):1183.〕该句表达了对参与研究的患者及其家属的致谢。

（2）The authors would like to thank the general practitioners and nurses who responded to the questionnaire.〔Balcou-Debussche M, Debussche X. Type 2 diabetes patient education in Reunion Island: perceptions and needs of professionals in advance of the initiation of a primary care management network Diabetes Metab. 2008;34 (4 Pt 1):375-8.〕该句表达了对问卷参与对象和执行对象的致谢。

（3）The authors thank Ann A. Hohmann, Ph.D., M.P.H., for her mentorship, encouragement, and long-standing dedication to mental health services research. They also thank Howard Waitzkin for his helpful feedback on earlier versions of the manuscript.〔Robins CS, Ware NC, dosReis S, Willging CE, Chung JY, Lewis-Fernández R. Dialogues on mixed-methods and mental health services research: anticipating challenges, building solutions. Psychiatr Serv. 2008;59 (7):727-31.〕

该句表达了对研究提供帮助的团队和个人的致谢。

（4）The symposium was supported by funding from the Canadian Institutes of Health Research, Public Health Agency of Canada, Canadian International Development Agency and the International Development Research Centre. Dr Wilson is supported by the Canadian Institutes of Health Research.［Wilson K, McDougall C, Fidler DP, Lazar H. Strategies for implementing the new International Health Regulations in federal countries. Bull World Health Organ. 2008;86 (3):215-20.］该句表达了对研究项目和研究人员提供基金来源的组织的致谢。

（5）We are grateful to local residents, Area Chiefs and Assistant Chiefs, faith-based leaders and schoolteachers in Kilifi, staff at KEMRI and the District Health Management Team in Kilifi district for their active participation in this work.［Marsh V, Kamuya D, Rowa Y, Gikonyo C, Molyneux S. Beginning community engagement at a busy biomedical research programme: experiences from the KEMRI CGMRC-Wellcome Trust Research Programme, Kilifi, Kenya. Soc Sci Med. 2008;67 (5):721-33.］该句表达了对提供帮助的个人、组织、参与研究人员的致谢。

（6）I thank Annett Lösch and especially Benjamin Waters for their help in translating the language. I would like to thank the four reviewers for helpful comments. (Schicktanz S. Why the way we consider the body matters-reflections on four bioethical perspectives on the human body. Philos Ethics Humanit Med. 2007;2:30.) 该句表达了对论文翻译者、审稿专家的致谢。

（7）I am greatly indebted to Mr Wen, for his valuable instructions as well as his careful reading of the manuscript. 该句表达了对文章初稿审核的 Mr. Wen 的致谢。

第二节　参考文献

参考文献（references）是作者用以指明引用论据和数据的出处，或为提供读者参阅、查找和直接引用的文献，是科技论文不可或缺的组成部分。在科研论文中，必须注明对前人资料、数据及观点的引用或参考，如果没有列出参考文献就使用前人的材料，则会被认定为抄袭行为。

一、引用参考文献的原则

首先，参考文献应该是已经在国内外公开发表的文献。未发表的资料、文摘、论文，以及发表于内部交流的刊物上的文章或其他参考资料，都不允许作为参考文献引用，在国内外学术会议上交流的论文，因为交流范围较小，而且很难被别人查阅，所以虽然也是一种发表形式，但一般也不要著录。已定稿但是尚未印刷的论文可列在参考文献中，但是必须标明其状态。例如："Wen JG, Li ZZ, Wang Y, et al. Bilateral Renal Melamine Related Calculus in 50 Children: A Single Centre Experience in Clinical Diagnosis and Treatment. J Urol, accepted."。

其次，在论文提交前或印刷前应认真核对参考文献和原始文章，仔细核查每条参考文献的细节。作为参考文献必须经过亲自阅读。如果作者由于条件不具备只阅读过摘要，未阅读原文的文献，除少数特别重要者外，一般不允许作为参考文献。对科研工作有所启示或重要贡献的以及直接引用的文献应该被著录，切忌列入无关文献。

最后，随着互联网的发展，网页内容也可以出现在参考文献中。例：最近 *New England*

Journal of Medicine 杂志上发表的有关结石研究的文章 "Melamine and the Global Implications of Food Contamination"，就引用了网络的内容作为文章的参考文献："Melamine contamination in China. Rockville, MD: Food and Drug Administration, December 6, 2008. (Accessed December 6, 2008, at http://www.fda.gov/oc/opacom/hottopics/melamine.html#update)"。但是网络资源缺乏稳定性，研究者应尽量提供可靠的文献，以便读者查阅。

二、参考文献的格式

不同杂志对参考文献的格式要求差别很大。有人曾总结 52 种期刊中有 32 种不同的参考文献模式。一些杂志要求显示文献的题目，一些则不需要；一些会强调起迄页码，而其他的仅需标明起始页。而这些要求都可以在各杂志的稿约中找到非常细致的要求，例如 *New England Journal of Medicine* 对参考文献的要求是参考文献双倍行距，连续编号（包括正文和图表）；参考文献少于 6 位作者的，全部列出作者，多于 6 位作者的，列出前 3 位后加一个 et al.。举例如下。

References must be double-spaced and numbered consecutively as they are cited. References first cited in a table or figure legend should be numbered so that they will be in sequence with references cited in the text at the point where the table or figure is first mentioned. List all authors when there are six or fewer; when there are seven or more, list the first three, followed by "et al." The following are sample references:

（1）Shapiro AMJ, Lakey JRT, Ryan EA, et al. Islet transplantation in seven patients with type 1 diabetes mellitus using a glucocorticoid-free immunosuppressive regimen. N Engl J Med 2000; 343:230-8.

（2）Goadsby PJ. Pathophysiology of headache. In: Silberstein SD, Lipton RB, Dalessio DJ, eds. Wolff's headache and other head pain. 7th ed. Oxford, England: Oxford University Press, 2001:57-72.

（3）Kuczmarski RJ, Ogden CL, Grammer-Strawn LM, et al. CDC growth charts: United States. Advance data from vital and health statistics. No. 314. Hyattsville, Md.: National Center for Health Statistics, 2000. (DHHS publication no. (PHS) 2000-12500-0431.)

（4）U.S. positions on selected issues at the third negotiating session of the Framework Convention on Tobacco Control. Washington, D.C.: Committee on Government Reform, 2002. (Accessed March 4, 2002, at http://www.house.gov/reform/min/inves_tobacco/index_accord.htm.)

杂志还指出参考文献不能引用个人交流、未发表的数据或者文章。如果这些材料很重要，可以在正文中提及，如：

Numbered references to personal communications, unpublished data, or manuscripts either "in preparation" or "submitted for publication" are unacceptable. If essential, such material can be incorporated at the appropriate place in the text.

准备撰写论文时最好将详尽的参考文献资料或者文献的核心内容全部存入电脑文档。这样，在写稿时，如果需要就可以直接提取所需要的资料。即使准备投稿的杂志对参考文献格式要求比较简单（比如：没有要求文献题目），但最好还是以完整的格式罗列参考文献。这是因为：①所投稿件可能会被退稿，在改投其他杂志时参考文献的格式需要改变；②在以后写论文或者综述时，很可能需要重复使用相同的参考文献。

现在许多电脑软件程序能自动将参考文献规范成一系列格式。比如，EndNote 这个程序能规范 *Science*，*Nature* 以及许多杂志的参考文献格式。一般来说，按下设定键，参考文献格式就能改为自己需要的样式。如果稿件被拒，直接改变一下设置，就可以将参考文献改为另一杂志需要的格式。EndNote 不仅能修改最后参考文献的格式，也可修改正文中引证的格式。

另一种用以编辑参考文献的软件 reference manager，能自动从互联网文献资料库中（如 PubMed）获取所需要的参考文献。应用该软件避免了修改论文时产生的参考文献错位等错误的出现，比较适合于参考文献较多的论著或者综述。

参考文献的格式很多，但仅有三种格式常用："名称和年度"；"按字母表中的顺序"或"按正文中的编号"。

1. 名称和年度系统（Name and Year System）（著者——出版年制）

名称和年度系统（常常指的是哈佛系统）已经流行很多年，并被很多杂志和著作应用。此系统最大的优点是对读者便利。因为文献不需编号，可以轻易地添减。不论参考文献的列表修改多少次，"Smith and Jones（1990）"仍然是精确如初。如果 "Smith and Jones（1990）"需要引用两次或更多次，只需将第一次列为 "Smith and Jones（1990a）"第二次列为 "Smith and Jones（1990b）"，问题就迎刃而解了。但该系统给编辑带来些不便：当在一句话或一段话中（引言中多见）引用大量参考文献时，有时需要跳过几行的文献才能衔接上正文。

因为有些论文是由许多作者共同完成的，许多杂志应用的名称和年度系统有一系列规则。最有代表性的是，在应用其中一两个作者的名字的引用文献时，比如："Smith（1990）"，"Smith and Jones（1990）"，但如果文章有三个作者，第一次被引用时是全部被列出："Smith，Jones，and McGillicuddy（1990）"。再次引用这文献时将缩减为 "Smith et al.（1990）"当一篇文献有四个作者或更多时，即使第一次提到，也应被引为 "Smith et al.（1990）"。在参考文献部分，很多杂志更希望列出全部作者（不管多少），而其他的杂志仅列出前三位作者，之后以 "et al."省略。这都是不同的杂志稿约的要求，"*Biomedical Journals* 的投稿统一要求"（国际医学期刊编辑委员会，1993）的标准是：列出全部作者，六个以上的以 "et al."省略。（Interna-tional Committee of Medical Journal Editors，1993）says: List all authors，but if the number exceeds six，give six followed by et al.）。

例：

Day，R.A. 1994. How to write and publish a scientific paper. 4th ed. Phoenix: Oryx Press.

Huth，E.J. 1986. Guidelines on authorship of medical papers. Ann. Intern. Med. 104:269-274.

Sproul，J.，H. Klaaren，and F. Mannarino. 1993. Surgical teatment of Freiberg's infraction in athletes. Am. J. Sports Med. 21:381-384.

参考文献中出现的中括号及其中的字母分别代表不同的参考文献类型，常见的有[M]、[J]和[C]分别代表专著、期刊文章和论文集；[D]、[P]和[S]分别代表学位论文、专利和标准；[N]、[R]、[G]和[Z]代表报纸文章、报告、资料汇编和其他文献。

2. 按字母表排序系统（Alphabet-Number System）

字母表排序系统是按字母表中的顺序来排列参考文献，是在名称和年度系统的基础上修改得到的。

当你在正文中引用文献时，必须清楚名称和年份哪个更重要。如果他们都不重要（事实常常如此），那就仅用参考文献的编号 "Pretyrosine is quantitatively converted to phenylalanine under these conditions（13）"。如果你想显示研究者的名字，可在正文中这样表述 "The role of the carotid sinus in the regulation of respiration was discovered by Heymans（13）"。但如果你想强调时间，可表述为 "Streptomycin was Inst used in the treatment of tuberculosis in 1945（13）"。

按字母表排序参考文献举例如下。

（1）Day, R. A. 1994. How to write and publish a scientific paper. 4th ed. Phoenix: Oryx Press.

（2）Huth, E. J. 1986. Guidelines on authorship of medical papers. Ann. Intern. Med. 104:269-274.

（3）Sproul, J., H. Klaaren, and F. Mannarino. 1993. Surgical treatment of Freiberg's infraction in athletes. Am. J. Sports Med. 21:381-384.

3. 引文次序系统（Citation Order System）（顺序编码制）

引文次序系统以文献出现在论文中的顺序来为参考文献排序。该系统按照论文中引用的文献出现的先后顺序，参考文献编号[1][2][3]……在正文中引用的位置用上角标的形式标上序号。对于篇幅很长、参考文献较多的论文来说，顺序引用系统并不适用，尤其在增添或删去文献会增加繁重的重编序号的工作量。而且因为不按字母排序的陈列文献会导致同一作者的不同文献被分割开来。Microsoft Word 的文字编辑能解决这个问题，在正文中应用参考文献时，使用"插入 - 引用 - 尾注"系统，作者可以将所有参考文献按次序系统罗列到文章结尾。在删除或者移动原文的过程中，参考文献的顺序也会自动调整。如果在全文中多次引用同一参考文献时，可以应用"插入—引用—交叉引用"方法。

例：

（1）Huth EJ. Guidelines on authorship of medical papers. Ann Intern Med 1986; 104:269-74.

（2）Sproul J, Klaaren II, Mannarino F. Surgical treatment of Freiberg's infraction in athletes. Am J Sports Med 1993; 21:381-4.

（3）Day RA. How to write and publish a scientific paper. 4th ed. Phoenix: Oryx Press. 1994.

多篇文献被引用时，只需在一个方括号内全部列出各篇文献的序号、中间加逗号，当出现连续序号时，应注明起迄序号，以范围号隔开；与正文平排的，每个文献序号都要加方括号。例：①遥相关研究[2-4,7]指出，两种相反的流型……；②在解释同位素懈 $^{18}O/^{16}O$ 比率变化方面存在某些困难（[5]、[7]-[9]）。

4. 杂志缩写

尽管不同的期刊风格各有不同，但参考文献方面近年渐渐规范化，比如期刊缩写。几乎所有的主要杂志和次要杂志都采用被广泛采纳的缩写标准（美国国立标准学会，1969）。遵循缩写规则，作者可以缩写很多期刊名称，甚至不熟悉的期刊。知道这些很有用：比如说，所有的"ology"词被缩写为"l."（"Bacteriology"缩写为"Bacteriol."，"Physiology"缩写为"Physiol."）但是也存在一些例外情况，如 *Science*，*Biochemistry* 就从不缩写。如果你不知道某参考文献期刊的缩写形式，可以在 Pubmed 系统搜出该文章，在文章摘要的最上面 Pubmed 会显示该期刊最正规和通用的缩写格式。

5. 常见格式举例

以期刊已发表论著为参考文献，常见有以下格式：

（1）出版年放在杂志名后，如：Wen J G, Yeung CK, Djurhuus JC. Cystometry techniques in female infants and children. Int Urogynecol J Pelvic Floor Dysfunct, 2000, 11：1032112.

（2）出版年放在作者后，如：Serati M, Ghezzi F, Cattoni E et al (2012) Tension-free vaginal tape for the treatment of urodynamic stress incontinence: efficacy and adverse effects at 10-year follow-up. Eur Urol 61:939-946.

以教科书、参考书内容为参考文献:

Yeates, W. K.: Bladder function in normal micturition. In: Bladder Control and Enuresis. Edited by I. Kolvin, R. C. MacKeith and S. R. Meadow. Philadelphia: Lippincott, chapt. 3, pp.28-36, 1973.

以网页内容作为参考文献:

Melamine contamination in China. Rockville, MD: Food and Drug Administration, December 6, 2008. (Accessed December 6, 2008, at http://www.fda.gov/oc/opacom/hottopics/melamine.html#update)

6. 参考文献表

(1) 参考文献表加居中标题——"References",并列入全书目录中。

(2) 参考文献著录项目、著录格式。

参考文献表的著录格式,可按顺序编码制,也可按"著者—出版年"制,一篇文章或一本书只能选用其中的一种。

1) 顺序编码制:参考文献表中要按正文注明的序号加上方括号依次列出各篇文献。著录项目及其格式如下:

A. 专著

编著者、书名(含副书名)、版本(第 1 版省略)、出版地、出版者、出版年份。

(如果有需要,文献末尾可列出页码,前面加实心句号。中译本,需要在书名之后写上翻译者姓名。)

B. 论文集(或多著者书籍)

著者、文章名、论文集编者(其前加"见:"或"In:")、论文集名、出版地、出版者、出版年、文章的起讫页码。

C. 刊物

著者、文章名、刊物名称、卷或年(期)、文章的起讫页码。

D. 报纸

著者、文章名、报纸名称、年 - 月 - 日(版次)。

(参考文献第一行顶格排,转行齐文字排。)

例如:

[1] 冯端等 . 金属物理学:第一卷　结构与缺陷 . 北京:科学出版社,1987.108.

[2] 库克 M. 天体微波激射 . 周震浦等译 . 北京:科学出版社,1984.98.

[3] 李叫森 . 横断山区自然资源的开发与保护 . 见:中国青藏高原研究会编 . 中同青藏高原研究会第一届讨论会文选 . 北京:科学出版社,1992.64-71.

[4] Abell B C. Nucleic acid content of microsomes. Nature, 1956(135):7-9.

[5] 张揆一 . 一篇错译文章引起的风波 . 新闻出版报,1994-02-16(3).

2)"著者 - 出版年"制

A. 只要文中标注了著者姓名和出版年份的,其文献一定要列入参考文献表中。

B. 参考文献表先按语种分类排列,不需要排序号,按照中文、日文、西文、俄文、其他文种的顺序排列。然后,中文按汉语拼音字母顺序或是第一著者姓氏笔画顺序排列,日文必须按第一作者的姓氏笔画顺序排列,西文和俄文按第一作者姓氏首字母顺序排列。

　　C. 参考文献表中,当一个著者有单独署名的文献还有作为第一作者与他人合著的多篇文献时,其单独署名的文献按照出版年份的先后排列在前面,然后排他与另一著者合著的文献,最后排他与多人合著的文献。

　　D. 著录项目与顺序编码制大致相同,只有一点不同的是出版年需要排于编著者之后并加实心句号。

　　参考文献第一行顶格排,第二行之后缩进两格排。例如:

Anon.1981. Coffee drinking and cancer of the pancreas. Br. Med. J., 283:628.

Bryan K.1969 Climate and the ocean circulation: [1]the ocean model. Mon. Wea. Rev., 97:806-827.

Bryan K. Cox M D.1968. A nonlinear model of an ocean driven by wind and differential heating. J. Aunos. Sci, 25:945-967.

Ross J. Radiative transfer in plant conmmnities. In: Monteith JL, ed. Vegetation and the Atmosphere. Vol. London: Academic Press.1975.13-52.

Spar J.1973a. Transequaterial effects of sea-surface temperature anomalies in a global general circulation model. Mon. Wea. Rev., 101:554-563.

Spar J.1973b. Some effects of surface anomalies in a global general circulation model. Mon. Wea. Rev., 101:91-100.

　　(3) 编著者姓名以姓前名后的方式列出:名可以用大写的首字母代替,字母后不需要缩写点;如果作者的名字用首字母无法识别时,则应该用全名。

　　文献编著者少于三个时,可全部列出;若超过三个,则只列出前三个,其后用“等”这类的字来概括。

　　以机构和团体署名的文献,则编著者应为机构或团体的全称,若用简称或缩写,有时会造成混淆。

　　(4) 有些文献的编著者不明,编者项需要注明“佚名”或类似的词(如 Anon.)。如果是使用顺序编码制的参考文献可直接著录题名,省略此项。

　　(5) 著录英文文献时,应当以文献本身所属文中的习惯使用大写字母。

　　(6) 英文期刊刊名可使用全称,也可使用惯用缩写刊名(词与词之间空一格,缩写词是否加缩写点全书应保持一致)。不缩写单个词的刊名。期刊名称全书统一排正体或者排斜体。

　　(7) 期刊不需标“卷”或类似的词(如 Vol 或 V,ToM 或 T,Bd……),只需加上卷号。卷号全书统一使用白体或者黑体;如果是分卷、册的图书,则应该加“卷”“册”或类似的词(外文缩写词不必加缩写点,首字母全书统一大小写均可)。

　　(8) 参考文献中一律用阿拉伯数字表示版次、页码、期、卷、出版年等。版次中第一版不必列出,所以中文版次著录依次为“第 2 版”“第 3 版”……,同理西文文献版次著录以此为2nd ed., 3rd ed.,或类似的词。

　　(9) 引用非英文文献时,应该著录其能查阅到的英文格式。

　　(10) 如果引用的参考文献有多个语种的译本,无论是原版还是译本,文中标注和参考文献表中只需著录作者论文中引用的语种即可。例如:引用的文献有中译本,而作者引用的却是原版,则参考文献表中不必译出,只需著录原文即可;若引用的文献是中译本,则不必附原文,只需著录中译本再加上译者姓名即可。

　　(11) 参考文献表中,如果上下两条的编著者或出处相同时,不能用破折号、同一出处、同上或其他类似的词代替,应分别列出。

(12)一篇文献如果有多个出版地,只著录一个主要出版地即可;如果出版地不明,宜在出版地项的位置写"出版地不详"或类似的词(如 s.1.)并用方括号括注。

(13)一篇文献如果有多个出版者时,只著录一个主要出版者位置显要的即可;如果出版者不明,在出版者项的位置写"出版者不详"或类似的词(如 s.n.)并用方括号括注。

(14)翻译书一般有较多的参考文献,不必拘泥于上述的格式,可直接用原书照相制版。

(15)文献著录用的标点符号。

逗号(,)用于多名作者的姓名之间,出版者、期刊名和年、期或卷之间。

冒号(:)用于"见"或"In"之后,期号之后、出版社之后、副书名之前。

括号[( )]用于期号或者报纸的版次。

实心句号(.)用于其他项目之后,不加在末项。

三、著录参考文献常见的问题

1. 引文量偏低 文后参考文献的数量不仅体现了学术研究动向和理论知识来源的线索,同时展现了作者在科学研究过程中吸收知识的能力。目前,据中国科学技术信息研究所统计调查,总体来讲,我国科技期刊的引文量较低,我国科技论文在 1988—1992 年期间的平均引文数只有 5~6 篇;而 SCI 收录的论文在相同时期的平均引文数为 21.25~23.69 篇。导致我国引文数量偏少的重要原因有:作者版权意识差,有意无意地忽略本应著录的参考文献;研究问题的起点低,作者的文献阅读量小。部分期刊以限定每篇文章的引文数量的方式来压缩文章篇幅,这是错误的。

2. 引文时限较长 即对近期文献的引用量较少,导致论文的可信度下降。其原因可能为:作者难以获得新文献;作者缺乏查新意识,只注重已有资料;作者间接引用了很多前人引用过的文献。

3. 不规范的参考文献著录 作者不能按《文后参考文献著录规则》的标准规范执行,尤其是期刊的出版标识不完整,如无代表性的范例。

4. 出现间接引用(转引)问题 参考文献著录规则禁止参考文献的间接引用,这属于极为不良的现象。有些文献虽然直接影响对论题的阐述,却因为一些原因无法查阅到最早的原始文献,就只能通过其他评述文献转引;有的是作者在参考文献中加入了没有直接阅读过的文献,只是为了表明自己文献阅读量大、阅读面广。作者应该树立正确客观的科学态度,审稿人和编辑部应该逐条认真核实参考文献,才能杜绝此类现象发生。

5. 编造参考文献 有些作者为了增加文章参考文献的质量,可能会编造参考文献或引用的文章与作者的结果没有任何联系。这是绝对要杜绝的现象。

四、参考文献的位置

有些作者出于习惯错误地把所有参考文献全部放在段落、句子或者题目之后的末尾。以实际的情况为依据,在最准确最恰当的位置注明参考文献的出处才是正确的做法。引文最好放到句中引用它的关键点上。"We have examined a digital method of spread-spectrum modulation for multiple-access satellite communication and for digital mobile radiotelephony[1,2]",

引用文献更清楚则需要将句子重新排列 "We have examined a digital method of spread-spectrum modulation for use with Smith's development of multiple-access communication[1] and with Brown's technique of digital mobile radiotelephony[2]."。如果句子提及作者指出或作者认为等内容,则需要把参考文献的序号直接标在作者的后面。

　　总之,因为参考文献格式不一,各个杂志采用不同的系统,目前没有统一的标准,因此投稿前仔细阅读拟投稿杂志的投稿须知是十分重要的。

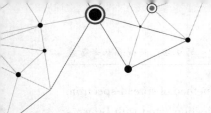

第 10 章
如何写作表格和插图

Chapter 10
How to Write the Tables and Figures

表格和插图（table and figure）是医学论文内容的重要表达形式。规范绘制的插图和合理设计的表格可以代替冗长复杂的文字叙述,将大量的数据资料以更加直观的方式清晰地呈现出来,而且还可以起到美化版面、节省空间的作用。表格表达的内容常是论文的核心和灵魂,正如 Peter Morgan 指出的那样:"A tabular presentation of data is often the heart or,better,the brain,of a scientific paper."。有的读者习惯先看图表数据来决定整篇论文是否值得阅读,因此图表的重要性可见一斑。

第一节 表   格

表格（table）是医学论文的重要组成部分,是统计资料的另一种呈现形式。表格对于数据资料的表达能力往往优于其他形式的描述,易于读者领会及分析。数据资料经过归纳及整理后以表格的形式呈现出来更容易表现出科学性及规律性,在医学论文中适当的采用表格可以将研究结果简明地展示出来。由于表格特殊的表现形式,读者可以更直观地对统计数据进行分析、计算、比较及查错。设计、编排合理的表格可以简化文字叙述,使科研文章思路清晰,结构紧凑,版面美观。

（一）表格的基本要求

科研论文统计表格的编排有三线表、卡线表、无线表及系统表等多种形式。其中三线表是国内外都推荐使用的形式,也是当前的医学科研论文写作中最常见的表格形式。通常一个表只有 3 条线,即顶线、底线和栏目线,组成要素包括表序、表题、表头、表身、表注,具有科学、合理、简洁、可读性强等优点。下面以三线表为例进行概述。

1. 表序和表题 表序及表题是表格的基本组成部分,两者之间无标点符号,中间空两格。按照表格在文中出现的顺序对表格进行编号即为表序,通常使用阿拉伯数字从"1"开始,按顺序编排,如"表 1""表 2"等,也有个别用罗马数字编号:Ⅰ、Ⅱ、Ⅲ等。表题要准确得体、简短精练。多采用短语形式,避免使用句子,但必要时需注明时间和地点。跟论文的标题一样,表题也要避免使用例如"计算结果""对照表"等没有明确指代对象的词语。因为缺乏特指性的表题不能使读者快速了解表格内容。表序和表题通常位于表身上方（图 10-1）,表序和表题的总长度以不超过表身宽度为宜,若表序及表题宽度超过表身宽度则需要换行书写。表序及表题的字号一般选用小五号黑体字,与正文及表身字体相区别。

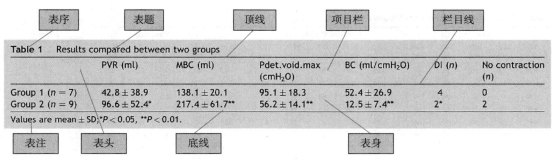

图 10-1　三线表的构成要素

2. 表项　表项由项目栏组成,是表格中具体项目的名称和类别。处理项位于项目栏左侧第一列,观测内容及结果项位于表身上方第一行,两者位置不能颠倒。项目栏中通常要放置多个"栏目",且不能在左上角画斜线标目。若栏目中的项由量的名称组成,其表示方法与插图中标目的表示方法相同;若表格内各栏目单位均相同时可将单位省略,标示于表格顶线上方右端。共用单位标注时只写本身符号,不用再写"单位"二字;相同栏目需要合并在一起,避免重复加注。

当表格的横向项目与竖向项目数相差较大时,或者宽度过宽或者长度过长时,为了美观或节省版面,可以进行转换处理,通过横表分段或者竖表转栏来解决。

3. 表身　表身是表格的主体部分,也是核心部分,包含表格内的大部分信息。表身内的数据资料用阿拉伯数字表示,单位及百分号等一律归并在栏目中。相邻栏内的内容相同时需分别写出,不能使用"〃"或"同上""同左"等字样表示。若表身中项目或数据空缺应使用"空白"表示,不能用"—"或"/"表示。表格中的内容必须完整、准确,且尽量不与文章正文内容重复。相同统计指标的精确位数需保持一致,小数点上下对齐。表格设计以三条横线或四条横线为宜,不宜过多,以保持表格整洁。表格设计禁用斜线条及竖线条。

4. 辅助线　在表格设计中,若项目类型较多,可根据需要在三线表的项目栏或表身添加横向辅助线,但仍称作三线表。表格中的栏目可为单层次或多层次的。辅助线可用于区分项目层次,说明隶属关系。辅助线通常比主线稍短,添加于横栏目中。表身上的辅助线可使表格更加清晰。文献中类似表如图 10-2 所示。

5. 单位　在标明单位时,应该按照国家法定计量单位规定使用拉丁化斜体字母标明物理量的名称,并用整体字母标出物理量的单位。物理量的名称与单位之间用"/"连接,如气温 $t/℃$、气压 p/kPa 等。表中单位符号使用要规范,如 μg(微克)不能写成 ug,kg(千克)不能写成 Kg。或按照投稿杂志要求使用相关单位。

6. 表注　表注即对表格的文字说明。若表格中的内容需要文字注释可在表身底部左侧,表格底线上方添加备注栏。表注也可集中标示于表格底线下方。若表注多于 1 条,应按顺序编号,排列于表下(图 10-2)。当然有的表格无需注释,则没有表注。

(二) Word 中表格制作过程

1. 在工具栏中选"插入表格",选取表格的行数和列数,或者从"表格"中选"绘制表格",点"插入表格",选所需的行数和列数。

Table 3. The accuracy of $\triangle P_{det}$ in different filling stages predicting UUTD

In the early filling stage					In the middle filling stage					In the end filling stage				
$\triangle P_{det}$ (cm H$_2$O)	SEN (%)	SPE (%)	PPV (%)	NPV (%)	$\triangle P_{det}$ (cm H$_2$O)	SEN (%)	SPE (%)	PPV (%)	NPV (%)	$\triangle P_{det}$ (cm H$_2$O)	SEN (%)	SPE (%)	PPV (%)	NPV (%)
>20	23	99	94	66	>40	10	98	77	62	>40	49	89	75	72
>15	51	94	85	74	>35	28	97	86	67	>35	59	84	71	75
>10	67	84	74	79	>30	39	94	81	70	>30	67	81	70	79
>8ª⁾	82	73	67	86	>25	58	89	78	76	>25ª⁾	85	77	71	89
>6	85	60	59	86	>23	72	87	79	82	>23	87	73	68	89
>4	87	52	55	86	>20ª⁾	85	82	76	89	>20	90	65	63	91
-	-	-	-	-	>18	87	77	72	90	>18	90	64	63	91
-	-	-	-	-	>16	90	74	70	92	>16	90	59	59	90

$\triangle P_{det}$, detrusor pressure; UUTD, upper urinary tract dilatation; SEN, sensitivity; SPE, specificity; PPV, positive predictive value; NPV, negative predictive value.
ª⁾The accuracy is high.

→ 顶线
→ 辅助线
→ 栏目线
→ 底线

图 10-2　三线表的辅助线和脚注标识

2. 填写横纵标题和数据,必要时填写单位。一些需要的 *、# 等也加上。
3. 自动套用表格,选择"简明型"。
4. 必要时点右键,修改边框和底线。
5. 写上表序和表题。
6. 如有表注,需加上。

(三)表格适用范围及范例

在科研论文书写当中,对实验数据的描述,可以有多种方式,如:文字叙述、表格、图表以及图片表达。表格的应用可以使某些实验结果的表达简单明了,一目了然。如表 10-1,在正文中只需简单叙述为双侧输尿管梗阻(BUO)后 24 小时血气分析的结果。读者即可一目了然的理解实验结果。表 10-2 同样可以看出两项研究中病例基本资料数据的比较情况。

但是,并非所有的实验结果均需要用表格表达。所以,在讨论如何制作表格之前要先审查是否需要制定表格。

表 10-1　BUO 后 24 小时血气分析的结果

	BUO 24h(n=7)	Sham(n=7)
Plasma pH	7.44 ± 0.01*	7.53 ± 0.01
Plasma HCO$_3^-$, mM	22.3 ± 0.39*	27.7 ± 0.52
Plasma total CO$_2$, mM	23.3 ± 0.38*	28.7 ± 0.55
Plasma ABEc, mM	−0.7 ± 0.49*	5.5 ± 0.39
Plasma SBEc, mM	−1.3 ± 0.46*	4.8 ± 0.44
Plasma SBCc, mM	23.9 ± 0.42*	29.4 ± 0.37

Values are means ± SE. BUO 24h, bilateral ureteral obstruction; Sham, sham-operated rats.

* $P<0.05$ compared with sham.

表 10-2　患者和肿瘤特点

Variable	Patients	
	Study A（%）	Study B（%）
Age		
≤60	33.1	31.2
61-70	34.3	37.6
71-80	26.6	28.3
>80	6.0	2.9
Gender		
Male	78.7	70.8
Female	21.3	29.2
No. tumors		
1	56.4	49.2
2-3	32.2	26.9
>3	11.4	23.9
Tumor size（cm）		
<3	80.4	54.2
≥3	19.6	45.8
T category		
Ta	55.9	19.4
T1	44.1	80.6
Grade		
G1	43.2	15.2
G2	43.9	57.9
G3	12.9	26.9

　　一般遵循如下原则:如果你所表达的数据不多,可在正文中用文字描述,通常不需要制定表格。此外,在实验记录中的大量数据常没有必要都在文本中加以说明。其次,和正文相比,出版表格的费用是非常高的,出版费用也是制定表格时应该考虑的问题。

　　如果结果文字太多可能会显得冗长,表格应用就显得尤为重要。它可以使读者很清晰地捕捉到你所表达这些结果的意义,显示出不同的变量对实验结果的影响,或各个实验组之间的结果差异(表 10-3)。

表 10-3　小鼠单侧输尿管梗阻前 24 小时血浆生化的改变

	UUO-A（n=6）	UUO-R（n=8）	Sham-A（n=6）	Sham（n=7）
P_{pH}	$7.36 \pm 0.05^{*¤\&}$	7.49 ± 0.01	7.48 ± 0.02	7.48 ± 0.01
$P_{HCO_3^-}$, mmol/L	$19 \pm 3.6^{*¤\&}$	29 ± 0.4	31 ± 1.7	29 ± 0.2
$P_{Total\ CO_2}$ mmol/L	$20 \pm 3.7^{*¤\&}$	30 ± 0.4	32 ± 1.7	30 ± 0.3
$P_{anion\ gap}$ mmol/L	$12.2 \pm 0.4^{*¤\&}$	10.5 ± 0.4	$9.0 \pm 0.5^{*}$	10.5 ± 0.3
P_{CO_2} kPa	14.5 ± 0.39	13.7 ± 0.39	14.5 ± 0.69	13.4 ± 0.38
P_{O_2} kPa	$4.4 \pm 0.47^{¤}$	5.2 ± 0.14	5.5 ± 0.19	5.3 ± 0.19
P_{Cl}, mmol/L	$108 \pm 3.2^{*¤\&}$	100 ± 0.4	100 ± 1.3	101 ± 0.3
P_{Na}, mmol/L	140 ± 0.3	140 ± 0.3	139 ± 0.2	140 ± 0.4
P_{K}, mmol/L	4.0 ± 0.2	4.4 ± 0.2	4.1 ± 0.1	4.0 ± 0.1
$P_{creatinine}$, μmol/L	$46 \pm 7.4^{*}$	$35 \pm 1.2^{*}$	$34 \pm 3.0^{*}$	25 ± 0.7
Pcreatinine, μmol/L	$46 \pm 7.4^{*}$	$35 \pm 1.2^{*}$	$34 \pm 3.0^{*}$	25 ± 0.7
Purea, mmol/L	$6.4 \pm 0.5^{*}$	$5.8 \pm 0.2^{*}$	$6.0 \pm 0.2^{*}$	4.4 ± 0.2

Values are means ± SD. n, number of rats; UUO-R: release of UUO for 4 days; Shamsham-operated rats; UUO-A: UUO-R rats with acid loading; Sham-A: Sham rats with acid loading; Plasma $_{anion\ gap}$, anion gap=Na^+-(Cl^-+HCO_3^-); PCO2, plasma partial pressure of CO_2; PO2, plasma partial pressure of O_2; $P_{creatinine}$, plasma creatinine; P_{urea}, plasma urea; P_{osm}: plasma osmolality; *$P<0.05$ compared with sham; $^\&P<0.05$ UUO-A vs. RUO-R; $^¤P<0.05$ UUO-A vs. Sham-A.

前面已经提到,并非所有的实验结果均需要用表格形式。表 10-4 和表 10-5 是呈交给杂志的许多不恰当的或无效图表的代表。

表 10-4 是错误的,因为表中两栏给出的是标准条件,而不是变量和数据。如果在试验中,温度是一个变量,它可以有自己的专栏,然而如果所有的实验在相同的温度下进行的,那么这个单一的信息应该在材料方法或者作为表格的脚注给出,而没有必要列表显示。表格中的数据应以一种容易被读者理解的方式展现在正文中。此表格的结果可以简单地理解为:培养基的通风对蓝色链球菌的增长是非常重要的。在室温下(24℃),静止的培养基里没有明显的增长,然而在震动的培养基下会出现明显的增长。

表 10-4　曝气对链霉素链霉菌生长的影响
(Effect of aeration on growth of Streptomycin coelicolor)

Temp (℃)	No. of expt	Aeration of growth Medium	Growth[a]
24	5		78
24	5	-	0

[a] As determined by optical density (Klett units)

[b] Symbols:+, 500-ml Erlenmeyer flasks were aerated by having a graduate student blow into the bottles for 15 min out of each hour;-, identical test conditions, except that the aeration was provided by an elderly professor

表 10-5　温度对橡木（Quercus）幼苗生长的影响

温度（℃）	Growth in 48h
−50	0
−40	0
−30	0
−20	0
−10	0
0	0
10	0
20	7
30	8
40	1
50	0
60	0
70	0
80	0
90	0
100	0

Each individual seedling was maintained in an individual round pot, 10cm in diameter and 100 in high, in a rich growth medium containing 50% Michigan peat and 50% dried horse manure

　　表 10-5 没有不变数据专栏，它看起来像个正确图表，自变量（温度）看起来也是合理的，但是因变量（增长）却有个可疑的 0 数字。当表格包括大量数字 0 时（不论使用任何计量单位时），或者当使用百分数时出现大量数字 100 时，表格数据易受到质疑。但有时为了特殊要求，或为了更加详细的提供实验结果，也需要列出为 100 的百分数，如表 10-6（Table 10-6）。那是因为表 10-6 列举的数据是半定量免疫杂交的结果，实验组细胞膜通道蛋白调节的变化是以 SHAM 组为基数（即 100%）的情况下所占的比例，读者可清楚地了解你的实验结果是在设定对照组的平均值为 100% 时，实验组通道蛋白的调节改变。更重要的是标准误（means ± SE）反映了测定蛋白通道所用的抗体品质不同，或你所工作的实验室技术操作规范和熟练程度。由于前两列和后两列是在不同的胶板上进行的杂交试验，所以每个实验组均有一个 SHAM 作为基数。

Table 10-6　Expression of key renal acid-base transporters in obstructed and non-obstructed kidneys from UUO-R and Sham operated rats (Protocol 2)

	OBS-R(n=8)	SHAM(n=7)	Non-OBS(n=8)	SHAM(n=7)
OSOM+C				
NHE3	$65 \pm 5\%^*$	$100 \pm 4\%$	$95 \pm 5\%$	$100 \pm 5\%$
NBC1	$46 \pm 7\%^*$	$100 \pm 4\%$	$112 \pm 9\%$	$100 \pm 6\%$
Pendrin	$106 \pm 2\%$	$100 \pm 5\%$	$121 \pm 17\%$	$100 \pm 5\%$
ISOM				
NHE3	$63 \pm 9\%^*$	$100 \pm 7\%$	$118 \pm 35\%$	$100 \pm 13\%$
NBCn1	$52 \pm 11\%^*$	$100 \pm 6\%$	$103 \pm 15\%$	$100 \pm 11\%$
NKCC2	$23 \pm 11\%^*$	$100 \pm 3\%$	$97 \pm 20\%$	$100 \pm 14\%$
H^+-ATPase	$54 \pm 9\%^*$	$100 \pm 6\%$	$100 \pm 9\%$	$100 \pm 4\%$
IM				
H^+-ATPase	$53 \pm 11\%^*$	$100 \pm 10\%$	$130 \pm 15\%$	$100 \pm 12\%$

Values are means ± SE; n=number of rats; OBS-R: 4 days release of obstructed kidneys; Non-OBS: contralateral non-obstructed kidneys; SHAM: kidney from sham-operated rats; C+OSOM: cortex plus outer stripe of outer medulla; ISOM: inner stripe of outer medulla; IM: inner medulla; *P<0.05 compared with SHAM

　　除了 0 和 100 等数字,要尽量避免一些"+"或者"−"等符号。表 10-7(Table 10-7)是经常出现在论文中的一个典型错误,很明显它并不能提供太多信息。这个图表所要告诉我们的是 S. griseus,S. coelicok,S. everycolor 和 S. Rainbowenski 生长需要有氧环境,而 S. nocolor 和 greenicus 等在无氧环境下才能生存。它所能表达的内容用一句话就可以描述,而不需要绘制这样的表格。

Table 10-7　Oxygen requirements of various species of Streptomyces

Organism	Growth under aerobic conditions[a]	Growth under anaerobic conditions
Streptomyces griseus	+	−
S. coelicolor	+	−
S. nocolor	−	+
S. everycolor	+	−
S. greenicus	−	+
S. rainbowenski	+	−

[a] In this experiment, the cultures were aerated by a shaking machine (New Brunswick shaking Co Scientific NI)

　　有作者认为所有数据都必须放到表格中,下面的表 10-8 就是个例子。该表格(在表格的脚注处)所得的结论没有统计学意义,这样就把一些相对不重要的实验数据弄得小题大做。如果这些数据值得发表,但是不需要列表显示,用下面的一句话就可以表达清楚:

即 Nocilin（14%）和 Potassiu（26%）死亡率的差别是没有统计学意义的。但是有些结果虽然没有统计学意义，但为了加强其他结果变化的意义，还是需要列出来的，如表 10-3 的血浆钠、钾以及血浆渗透压并没有统计学上的意义，但它们为血浆生化变化的重要指标，把它们列入表内，可以更清楚地给读者提供泌尿系梗阻后血浆生化指标的变化。然而，为表 10-8（Table 10-8）中列出的数据单独列表显然没有必要。

Table 10-8　Bacteriological failure rates

Nocillin	K Penicillin
5/35（14）[a]	9/34（26）

[a] Results expressed as number of failures/total, which is then converted to a percentage (within parentheses). *P*=0.21

另外，常见的无效表格之一是简单地罗列单词，表 10-9（Table 10-9）是个代表性例子。这种信息可以很容易地在文本中表达。一个专业文字编辑者会删去这种表格而把数据融入文本中。如果表格信息大部分或者全部已经出现在文本中，会出现明显的重复现象。过于繁杂的表格反而会不利于重点信息的传递，过于简单的表格可直接使用文字叙述。总之，作者首先需要明确要传递的信息，然后选择合适的表达方式进行表达。

Table 10-9　Adverse effects of nicklccillin in 24 adult patients

No. of patients	Side effect
14	Diarrhea
5	Eosinophilia（>5eos/mm^3）
2	Metallic taste"
1	Yeast vaginitis'1
1	Mild rise in urea nitrogen
1	Hematuria（8-10rbc/hpf）

上面表 10-4 至表 10-9 提供了许多典型的例子，告诉我们各种不需要列成表的资料。现在，让我们看看需要列成表格的资料。

在决定列表后，你应该给自己提出一个问题：怎样安排这些数据？ 一个表格有左右列和上下行，该如何安排？ 你可以水平或者垂直方向罗列一些数据，列表前应仔细斟酌哪些数据应该纵向表达，哪些数据应该横向表达，有条理地组织数据。

如表 10-10（Table 10-10）和表 10-11（Table 10-11）表达的信息是一样的，只是表 10-10 是横向而表 10-11 是纵向。为了使读者更容易抓住信息，而且安排的更紧凑印刷费用又不高，表 10-11 是首选。这种优点显而易见。从减少印刷成本来看，横向排列由于元素的多样性所有的列肯定是宽或是深的，而纵向排列来看，一些列可以是窄的而且不用转行。因此，表 10-11 比表 10-10 看起来更小，尽管它们包含相同的信息。文字在表的左边，数字（或小数点）在表的右边。例如表 10-11 可以说明这一点。

Table 10-10　Characteristics of antibiotic-producing Streptomyces

Determination	S. fluoricolor	S. griseus	S. coelicolor	S. nocolor
Optimal growth temp（℃）	−10	24	28	92
Color of mycelium	Tan	Gray	Red	Purple
Antibiotic produced	Fluoricillinmycin	Streptomycin	Rholmondelay[a]	Nomycin
Yield of antibiotic（mg/ml）	4 108	78	2	0

[a] Pronounced "Runley"by the British

Table 10-11　Characteristics of antibiotic-producing Streptomyces

Organism	Optimal growth temp (℃)	Color of mycelium	Antibiotic produced	antibiotic (mg/ml)
S. Jluoricolor	−10	Tan	Fluoricillinmycin	4 108
S. griseus	24	Gray	Streptomycin	78
S. coelicolor	28	Red	Rholmondelay[a]	2
S. nocolor	92	Purple	Nomycin	0

[a] Where the flying fishes play

　　表 10-12（Table 10-12）是一个精心设计的表（从细菌学的操作指南到作者），它是纵向而不是横向。清晰的标题使我们更容易理解数据的含义。它有说明性脚注，但不重复过多实验细节。请注意区别：它能恰当地提供足够信息，使数据的意义更容易理解而不用参考原文。

表 10-12　肌酐亚胺酶在新生隐球菌和孢子的诱导作用 [a,b]

	C. neoformans NIH12		C. bacillisporus NIH191	
	Total enzyme	Spact（U/mg of protein）	Total enzyme	Spact（U/mg of protein）
Ammonia	0.58	0.32	0.50	0.28
Glutamic acid	5.36	1.48	2.18	0.61
Aspartic acid	2.72	0.15	1.47	0.06
Arginine	3.58	2.18	3.38	2.19
Creatinine	97.30	58.40	104.00	58.30

[a] The inoculum was grown in glucose broth with ammonium sulfate, washed twice, and then transferred into the media with the N sources listed above

[b] Enzyme units in cell extract obtained from ca.1010 cells

　　这里需要提醒注意的是，三线表只有三个水平的行间线，但没有纵向的列间线。偶尔可以使用横跨间线（就像表 10-12 中的 NIH12 和 NIH191 即辅助线）。一般不用垂直间线，因为它们很难在大多数图形系统中插入。
　　有时为了排版的需要，也可以横行列表（应用较少），如表 10-13。

表 10-13　BUO 对大白鼠血浆渗透压及电解质的影响

	Na（mmol/L）	K（mmol/L）	Cl（mmol/L）	Crea（μmol/L）	Urea（mmol/L）	Osom（mosmol）
BUO（n=7）	138.9 ± 0.3*	5.4 ± 0.2*	96 ± 0.6*	372 ± 5.3*	40.7 ± 1.4*	338 ± 3.0*
Sham（n=7）	141.0 ± 0.3	4.0 ± 0.1	101 ± 0.6	30 ± 2.8	5.8 ± 0.2	300 ± 0.6

表中以均值 ± 标准差表示；Na:血钠浓度；K 血钾浓度；Cl 血氯浓度；Crea 血肌酐浓度；Urea 血尿素氮浓度；Osom 血浆渗透压；n:动物数目；* 与对照组相比 $P<0.01$

此外,对于表内的内容注意以下几点:确定适当的计量单位,将数字位数限制在 1~4 位数以内;若需使用"+""–""*"等符号做标记,需要分别在表格下方注明含义;认真核对数据,避免有误。

（四）注意事项

1. 标题中的指数　在标题中尽可能避免使用指数。这样经常造成混乱,因为一些刊物使用正指数和负指数表达同样的意思。例如:细菌学杂志使用"每分钟 $\times 10^3$"是指每分钟数千倍,而生物化学杂志使用"每分钟 $\times 10^{-3}$"是指同样的意思。如果标题（或者图表）里无法避免使用这些标签,应在脚注里说明以消除歧义。

2. 页边指示标记　论文中的所有表格应按出现顺序编排序号,并在正文中引用处标明序号。若全文中只有一个表格则示以"表 1"。例如,在页边上简单地写上表 3 并画上圈。这是个很好的核对过程,以确定你已经在文本中依次引用每一个表格。然而,这个过程主要是提供一些标志,为了使排序者在页码校正过程中知道在文本中插入表格的位置。如果你没有标示出位置,编辑者将会这样做。然而,编辑者可能会忘记表格的第一引用处,那么此表格将会放置在远离首次提及文本的地方。此外,在文中你可能想提前写上表的相关引用,然后再出现此表,只有通过页边注释,编辑者和排序者才能知道你想在文中什么地方出现此表。

3. 题目、脚注和缩写　表题应能简洁明了地表达表格内容,过于笼统或烦琐的表题均不利于表格主题内容的传递,影响表题自明性。注意表中脚注,如在表内使用缩略词,要在表下注明全部或者大部分定义。以后表格如应用同样的缩略词可以使用更简单的脚注:即参见前表的缩写。

为了节省表中的空间,鼓励在文中使用某些固定的缩写,能够恰当地设计表格,这对设计照相制版的表格特别有用。出现在一栏标题中第一个单词,应该大写首字母（如:Temp）或全部用大写字母（如:BUO）。

需要强调的是在确定表格最后形式之前,请务必阅读你准备选投杂志的投稿须知。杂志社可能建议更好地设计及能接受的表格形式,表格尺寸,以及其他要求。此外,大多数期刊坚持表格应该在单独一页中打印,表格或者图形应该放在手稿的末尾处,而且表格不应该以照片形式递呈。

总之,科研论文中的表格要求简单明了、层次清楚、有自明性。表格的结构要简单、整齐;内容安排要逻辑严谨,层次清楚。目前大多数学术期刊均要求将表题、标目、注释等内容使用中、英文标示,以便国际学术交流。在科研论文中合理地使用表格可简化文字叙述,并获得文字叙述难以达到的表达效果,使文章结构清晰,篇幅紧凑。随着计算机技术的广泛应用和电子版投稿的普及,过去照相制版技术容易出现的排版错误得到了纠正。这更强调我们注重投稿时表格的设计,避免出现错误表格。

第二节 插　　图

插图(figures)是科技论文的重要组成部分,它可以代替文字叙述,更加直观地表达特定的信息,使文章内容更加丰富。插图的表达形式非常重要,可以对插图本身的科学性或可读性产生影响,同时也会关系到版式的整体效果。因此,在应用插图时需要保证图稿的科学性,还应兼顾插图的表达形式。当文稿需要用插图来表示时,需考虑以下四个方面:①图形要符合表达需要且形式恰当;②该图形能清楚展现想要表达的数据信息;③适合图形的标题;④精确简短、让读者易懂的图注。

医学科研论文中常用的插图类型主要有:折线图(表示系列数据的变化趋势)、直方图(表示相关变量之间的对比关系)、饼状图(表示研究对象中各组分的含量关系及相关变化)、绘图(包括素描、组织图、流程图等,常用来展示研究对象的结构)、照片(展示研究对象的外观、形态等),等。在选用插图时需根据科研资料的类型及变化特点来匹配特定类型的插图。以期更加直观、准确地呈现出研究结果。

下面将介绍医学英文科研论文中最常见的线条图和照片图,说明如何准备插图。线条图易于呈现数据的变化趋势,有助于读者直观地了解事物的变化趋势。照片图易于呈现出实物外观,有时还可作为客观证据。两者均常用于科技论文写作。

(一)线条图

线条图以线段的走向表示一项指标(纵坐标)随另外一项指标(横坐标)变化的情况,是科技论文常用的统计图。线条图包含图序、图题、标目、标值、坐标轴、图注 6 个部分。线条图的设计要符合统计学及规范化的要求,整体图形要简明、完整、清晰。线条图整体轮廓以矩形为宜,高度与宽度比例应保持在 5∶7 左右。图中文字说明要简明扼要,必要时可用数码或代号表示,并附以图注。横坐标及纵坐标要标明指标名称及单位,并附以图例及图例说明,下面以图 10-3 为例说明。

1. 图序和图题　插图的序号即为图序,应按照在文中出现顺序用阿拉伯数字编排。插图的题目即为图题,需满足能直观、准确、简练地表达插图内容的要求。图题一般选用名词性词组或以名词性词组为中心语的偏正词组表述。图题的表述举例如下。

简单模糊的表述:"Graph of Relevant Data."。

过于烦琐的表述:"Outcome of Multifactorial Analysis of Relationship Between Symptoms, Chronology of Appearance, Diagnostic Signs, Blood Work Constants From The Literature, Health Outcome, and Other Parameters For Selected Group of Fifteen Adult Ostriches."。

比较恰当的表述:"Multifactorial Analysis of Health Records of Fifteen Adult Ostriches."。

2. 标目　标目是说明坐标轴意义的项目,由标目名称和相应的单位构成。单位符号应该使用国际期刊标准规定的正体字母标注。

3. 标值　标值是规定坐标轴数值的尺度,位于坐标轴外侧。标值的数值一般不超过 3 位数,小数点后不多于 1 位,如将 60 000m 改为 60km,6 000g 改为 6kg,0.006g 改为 6mg 等。

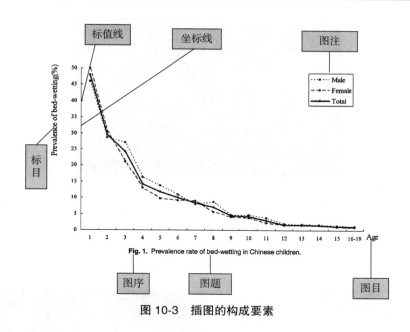

图 10-3　插图的构成要素

标值应规整化,如将实际测得的非规整数如 0.31、0.58、0.86 等改为 0.3、0.6、0.9 等。不能直接使用不规则的实测数值作为标值。

4. **坐标轴**　横轴表示某一连续量,纵轴表示事物现象发生的水平。数据点画在组段中间位置,相邻的数据点用直线相连,无数据的组段用虚线相连,线段不能任意延长。同一张线图上尽量避免画太多条曲线。当有两条或两条以上曲线在同一张线图上时,须用不同颜色或不同的线条形式加以区分,并附图例加以说明。值得注意的是,纵轴坐标可以不从 0 开始。因为标值的大小已经明示了增量的方向,所以在给出标值时不需要再使用箭头标志重复标示。

5. **图注**　图注说明语可以放置于图内或图外的适当位置,满足简洁准确、表述规范的要求即可。选取图注符号的形状和类型时务必保持版式清晰,易于阅读。我们在阅读科技论文时经常可以看到例如"▲""#""1""!",或"×""+""|""−"等类型的符号,这些符号形状相似,在视觉上不容易区分,严重降低插图的可读性及实用性。因此在实际的论文写作中需尽量使用"■""□""●""○""""等易于区分的符号。

6. **适当运用同类曲线的重叠**　当有两条以上曲线具有同一参变量时可以将这些曲线绘制在同一函数图上。两条纵坐标轴分居同一横坐标轴两端。注意:两纵坐标的标目和标值要分别标注。

(二)照片图

照片图也是一种重要的插图形式,多用于影像学研究、病理诊断研究等方面,例如 CT 与 MRI 扫描图片,超声诊断图片,电子显微镜下图片等。照片图需要有良好的清晰度及对比度,易于观察。科技论文中的照片图需要用电脑添加必要的标注文字、数字或符号,以增加直观性、美观性及协调性。提交论文时需还需提供电子照片,且多用 EPS、JPG、TIF 和 PSD 等图片格式保存。针对无法用电脑编辑加工的图片需要另附纸绘图标示,不应在图片上直接写画。实物图涉及大小者,需附以比例尺标明缩放比例。下面是常见的照片图举例(图 10-4~ 图 10-6)。

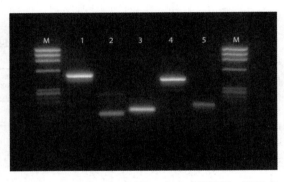

Fig. 1. Gel electrophoresis of PCR products of (1) TGF-α (540 bp); (2) EGF (103 bp); (3) HB-EGF (126 bp); (4) EGFR (454 bp), and (5) ribosomal RNA (151 bp). Marker DNA (M) is composed ΦX174 DNA digested with *Hae*III. The nine upper bands with the size of 1353, 1078, 872, 603, 310, 282–271, 234, 194 and 118 can be seen.

图 10-4　PCR 试验中凝胶电泳图

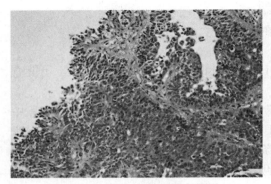

图 10-5　尿路上皮肿瘤病理图

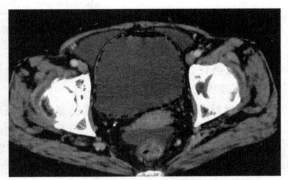

图 10-6　盆腔 CT 扫描图

（三）插图适用范围及范例

插图的基本要求是：①精确、简明；②要有图序和图题，图题要确切，有较好的说明性和专指性；③线条粗细要分明；④图标尽可能置于图中空白处，但要注意美观；⑤图的大小，图中字体的大小要适当；⑥图中插字应与文中字母正斜体一致。

下面图 10-7 所示一名患有瓣膜膀胱综合征的 6 岁儿童行尿动力学检查结果。图中左侧标目分列出检查指标膀胱压、尿道压、腹压、肌电图等，并按照不同标目设置不同的标值，图示中不同颜色线条很清晰表明相应压力曲线，图中箭头表明本图主要说明部分"间断性逼尿肌收缩"，整张图既全面展示尿动力学整体检查结果图像，也能重点反映出其不同之处，相对文字描述来说能更全面简洁表达。

同样，下图 10-8 把免疫印迹结果、数值表达结果和图题以横向相对应排列，很清晰显示出不完全尿路梗阻动物在术后不同时间和相应的假手术组动物的比较，从图片和数值上都可以准确反映出得出的结果，也很好地符合插图的要求。

对于由多张分图组成的同一张大图，各分图要用（a），（b），（c）等分别标注，且主图题和分图题要分开书写。图注和分图题等说明文字应放在主图题下方（图 10-9）。

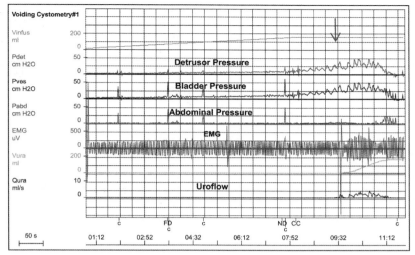

Figure 1 Pressure/flow/EMG study in a 6-year-old boy with VBS. Intermittent detrusor contraction was observed during voiding (arrow).

图 10-7　尿动力学检查结果图示

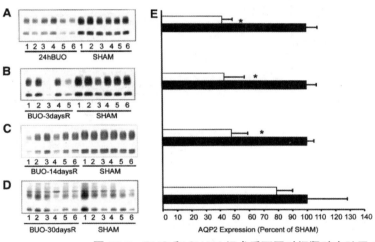

Fig. 4. Semiquantitative immunoblotting of membrane fractions of inner medulla (IM). A-D: immunoblots were reacted with anti-aquaporin-2 (anti-AQP2) and reveal 28-kDa the 35- to 45-kDa AQP2 bands, representing nonglycosylated and glycosylated forms of AQP2 after 24 h of BUO (A); 3 days after release of BUO (B); 14 days after release of BUO (C); and 30 days after release of BUO (D). E: densitometric analysis of all samples from BUO and sham-operated rats (corrected according to loading) reveal a persisted decrease in AQP2 expression in rats with BUO and 3 and 14 days after release of BUO (24-hBUO: 42 ± 7 vs. $100 \pm 6\%$; BUO-3daysR: 43 ± 14 vs. $100 \pm 7\%$; BUO-14daysR: 48 ± 11 vs. $100 \pm 5\%$, *$P < 0.05$), but 30 days after release of BUO, AQP2 levels did not differ significantly from sham operated.

图 10-8　BUO 和 SHAM 组术后不同时间肾脏内髓层 AQP2 的表达

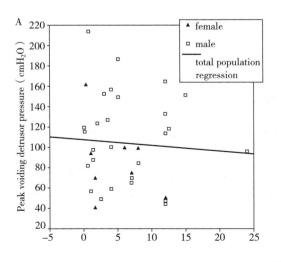
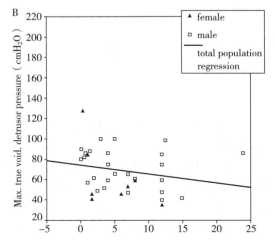

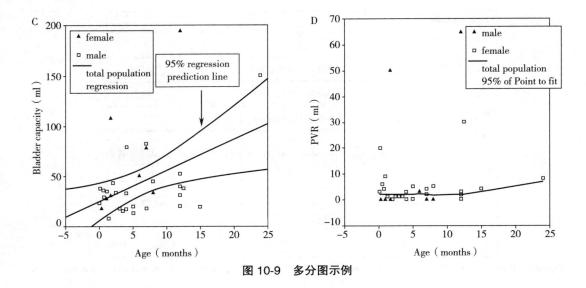

图 10-9 多分图示例

对于临床诊断试验的诊断与评价，多用 ROC 曲线（受试者工作特征曲线）来进行诊断分析，曲线下的面积越大，则诊断价值越高（图 10-10）。

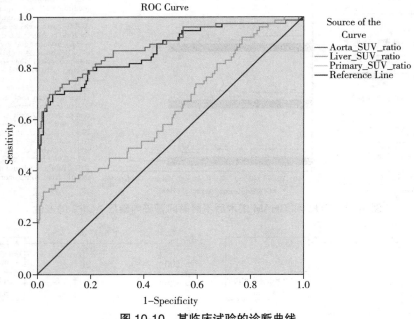

图 10-10 某临床试验的诊断曲线

在肿瘤疾病随访中，由于删失值的存在，多用生存分析方法进行研究，图 10-11 所示为 Kaplan-Meier 曲线。

对于某些临床外科手术方式的创新与改进，也可以在正文中通过插图或其他照片给予更清楚地说明，图 10-12 显示膀胱全切术方面的研究。此外，一些杂志也需要相关手术视频等作为佐证。

图示表达的选择要依据数据类型和表达需求来决定。SPSS、SAS、Stata 等统计软件和

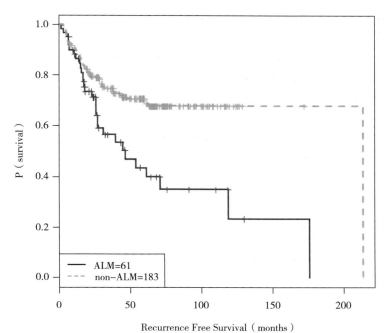

图 10-11　随访研究中生存分析曲线

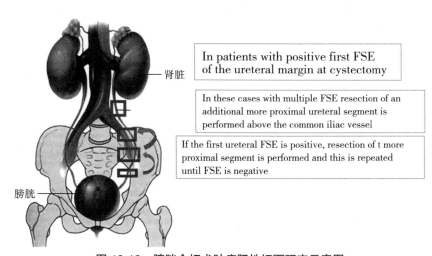

图 10-12　膀胱全切术肿瘤阳性切面研究示意图

Sigma plot 等绘图软件能提供很多不同种类的图形,其他诸如饼状图、箱式图,垂状图等不再一一赘述。

　　总之,对与图表的使用需要按需而定。表格可以更有条理的方式呈现统计数据,图形可以增加数据的变化规律及趋势的可视性。表格和图片的绘制需遵循简洁、清楚、重点突出的原则;插图及文章正文中的符号、单位、数值等要遵循一致性原则。此外在投稿时还应根据具体期刊要求遵循个性化原则。因此在投稿前还应认真阅读目标期刊的作者须知,定稿后保持插图及表格整洁、清晰。

　　最后,推荐 *American Journal of Public Health* 附表的审核清单,供参考。

Checklist for Preparing Tables

1. Each table stands alone; readers need not refer to the text for understanding.

2. The titles fully explain the data displayed; they are comprehensible apart from the text.

3. Displays are brief and clear with a minimum of statistical abbreviations.

4. Where appropriate, tables provide measures of uncertainty along with point estimates (e.g., standard deviations with means).

5. All but universal abbreviations are spelled out, except where explained in footnotes.

6. Overall sample sizes (N's) are presented at the top of each table or column. Percentages alone appear within individual cells if the N's can be reconstructed, except where numbers are small.

7. Confidence intervals are provided rather than beta coefficients and p values (e.g., for logistic regression analyses).

8. Redundancy is eliminated between text and tables.

9. Only results essential to the main thesis are presented.

10. Appendices available upon request from the author or deposited with the National Auxiliary Publication Service (NAPS) can contain additional results and supplementary material. (Information on NAPS is available from AJPH.) An appropriate footnote will be added to the text.

11. Once a paper is accepted, authors must obtain permission forthe use of tables and parts of tables copyrighted elsewhere. The permission letter, in which the publisher grants the specific use requested, must be sent to the Journal office.

第 11 章
综述写作

Chapter 11
How to Write a Review Article

一、概述

1. 综述的定义 综述(review)是作者大量查阅已发表的文献,以其为原始素材进行归纳整理撰写成文,也称文献综述。综述的目的是简要回顾一个特定主题的最新进展,总结当前知识现状,通过讨论最新研究成果,使读者对该主题有更全面深入的理解。正如《新英格兰医学杂志》要求的那样:"The purpose of a review paper is to succinctly review recent progress in a particular topic. Overall, the paper summarizes the current state of knowledge of the topic. It creates an understanding of the topic for the reader by discussing the findings presented in recent research papers."。

综述,顾名思义,是"综"与"述"的结合。综,就是对大量已发表文献资料进行归纳整理并综合分析,将查阅的大量文献简明扼要、层次分明、逻辑清晰地展现给读者。述,即评述,要对所写的专题内容有自己独到的见解,力求做到全面性、深入性和系统性。综述是教学、科研和生产中非常重要的参考资料,它把该领域、该专题及其分支学科的新技术、新发现、新进展等全面系统地呈现给读者,使对该领域、该专题感兴趣的读者用较少的时间和精力就可以获益匪浅。

2. 综述写作前需注意的问题 综述不是对参考文献等材料的简单罗列,而是对自己大量阅读和收集的材料进行归纳、总结并做出评论,进而从文献资料总结出重要结论的过程。当然,在确定要写综述之前,需要仔细阅读投稿杂志的稿约,确定杂志的要求。一些杂志对参考文献的要求比较严格,而另一些更关心文章的完整性。

例如《新英格兰医学杂志》规定:"Review articles are usually solicited by the editors, but we will consider unsolicited material. Please contact the editorial office before writing a review article for the Journal. All review articles undergo the same peer-review and editorial process as original research reports. They should be written for the general physician, not specialists. Consequently, they may include material that might be considered too introductory for specialists in the field being covered."。

《欧洲泌尿外科》杂志(*European Urology*)则要求所发表的 Review Articles 需要以 systematic reviews(包括 meta-analyses)为主,但是在投稿前需要与编辑部沟通并获得认可方可投稿,如未联系贸然投稿一般是不会接收的。该杂志要求是:"European Urology aims at publishing mainly systematic reviews (and, whenever appropriate). These are reviews that systematically find, select, critique, and synthesize evidence relevant to well defined questions about diagnosis, therapy, and prognosis. Manuscripts reporting systematic review and meta-analysis should comply with the PRISMA statement. Such review articles are in principle solicited by the editorial board. Authors who would like to submit unsolicited systematic review articles should first write to the editorial office describing the content of the review article they wish to submit. Review articles should not be submitted in full without prior approval from the editors."。

Neurology and Urodynamic 的要求更加明确:"Review articles will be solicited by a panel of editors, or may be submitted directly to the editor by the author. They are designed to provide an up-to-date review of the most modern and reasonable approach to a particular topic by a recognized expert in the field. They represent the authors' editorial point of view rather than a litany of dogma or an exhaustive compilation of all prior work in that field. These should not exceed 3 000 words and 50 references."。

但如果向一些主要以综述为主的杂志,如 *Nature Reviews* 系列杂志,投稿综述稿件时就不必提前与编辑部联系,但是仍需要符合杂志社对于稿件的要求。例如:"Review articles in the Nature Reviews clinical titles provide authoritative overviews of a field or topic. They provide information on the background as well as the latest advances related to the given topic, and place all presented information in the context of the rest of the field. Nature Reviews clinical content is targeted towards readers from a postgraduate level and upwards, including practicing doctors, researchers and academics, and should be accessible to readers working in any medical discipline."。*Nature Reviews* 编辑部的要求很高,稿件除了有必要的背景介绍和最新进展之外,还需要介绍与之相关的研究进展。

3. 综述的类型 按照搜集的原始文献资料数量、组织写作形式的不同,可将综述分为归纳性综述、普通性综述和评论性综述三类。

(1)归纳性综述:作者将查阅的文献归纳整理,并按一定的逻辑关系进行分类排列,使它们构成互相关联、条理清晰、文理贯通、系统严谨的学术论文。它能在一定程度上反映出某一专题或某一领域当前研究的进展。

(2)普通性综述:具有一定学术水平的作者,在查阅较多文献的基础上撰写的学术论文,其逻辑性较强、系统性较好,文中作者有自己的观点或对学术争论有倾向性。普通性综述对从事该领域研究的读者具有较好的参考价值和指导意义。

(3)评论性综述:是指在该领域具有较高造诣且具备较高学术水平的作者,在查阅大量文献的基础上,对原始文献归纳整理、综合分析,所撰写的可以体现该领域当前研究现状及未来发展趋势的评论性学术论文。该类综述有很强的逻辑性,能体现作者更多的见解及评论。对读者有普遍的指导及导向作用。

按照综述内容的不同《新英格兰医学杂志》将综述的类型分为:Clinical Practice,Clinical Therapeutics,Current Concepts,Drug Therapy,Mechanisms of Disease,Medical Progress(临床规培、临床治疗、当前观点、药物治疗、疾病机制、医学进展)。

1) Clinical Practice

Articles are evidence-based reviews of topics relevant to practicing physicians, both primary care providers and specialists. Articles in this series should include the following sections: the clinical problem, strategies and evidence, areas of uncertainty, guidelines from professional societies, and the authors' conclusions and recommendations.

2）Clinical Therapeutics

Articles are evidence-based reviews of topics relevant to practicing physicians. The series focuses on clinically oriented information about specific forms of therapy, including drugs, devices, and procedures. Each article in the series begins with a clinical vignette describing a patient with a specified condition for whom the treatment under discussion has been recommended. This vignette is followed by a definition of the clinical problem, a description of the pathophysiology and how the therapy works, clinical evidence, clinical use (including costs), adverse effects, areas of uncertainty, guidelines, and recommendations.

3）Current Concepts

Articles focus on clinical topics, including those in specialty areas but of wide interest.

4）Drug Therapy

Articles detail the pharmacology and use of specific drugs or classes of drugs, or the various drugs used to treat particular diseases.

5）Mechanisms of Disease

Articles discuss the cellular and molecular mechanisms of diseases or categories of diseases.

6）Medical Progress

Articles provide comprehensive, scholarly overviews of important clinical subjects, with the principal (but not exclusive) focus on developments during the past five years. Each article details how the perception of a disease, disease category, diagnostic approach, or therapeutic intervention has evolved in recent years.

4. 综述和研究性论文的区别 综述和研究性论文的格式不同。综述的书写格式比较多样化，通常不需要按照常规的研究型论文所需的 IMRAD 模式，而是直接将多方面的研究结果汇总并分析。但是也有不少综述是按照 IMRAD 模式写作，例如：在方法中介绍在哪些数据库中进行检索，检索的范围和主题词有哪些，纳入和排除的标准是什么，等等。综述和一般科技论文一样具有题目、作者署名、摘要、关键词、前言、主体、结论和参考文献等几个部分，参考文献是撰写综述的基础，一般参考文献引用数量和一般科技论文有所区别。

二者在结构内容上也存在差异。研究性论文需要详细介绍研究方法和展示实验结果，使读者认同其研究方法的科学性，相信实验结果可靠性；而综述主要目的是让读者，尤其是初学者，对该领域有一定的全面性了解。综述要指出该领域研究背景、研究现状、争论焦点等，有些综述还需要阐述作者的评论性意见，表明作者的学术倾向、评论优劣、预测发展趋势和应用前景等。撰写综述前拟定提纲不失为明智之举，提纲会有助于组织你的文章格式，这是非常重要的。如果你的综述的结构合适，综述在总体上会被很好地界定并且各个部分都会在逻辑上很好地组织起来并相互配合。此外，在你开始写之前，最好能确定综述杂志编辑（或者是也发表综述的基础杂志）是否会对拟撰写的综述感兴趣。也许，编辑会希望限制或者扩展所提交的综述范围或者添加或删除某些副标题。

5. 综述的特殊性 综述不是原创的文章，但是，综述可以包含一些作者尚未发表的科研成果。综述的目的是总结、回顾和分析已经发表的文章并将作者自己的观点融入其中。综述篇幅没有统一标准，参考文献不同杂志要求不同。英文综述投稿难度相对较大，参考文献相对较多，有时可以达到 200 多篇，字数要求也比中文综述要多。综述字数及文献等要求可查阅拟投稿杂志是否有明确规定，如未明确规定，可以参考该杂志已经发表过的综述。

综述的选题和内容可以相当广泛,这点与研究性论文不同。文献的回顾非常重要。真正优秀的综述绝不是简单的文献注释,应为出版的文献提供重要的评价并依据已经发表的文献总结出重要的结论。在格式上,综述与写好的学术报告和毕业论文没有太大的区别。

医学综述的特点是要有综合性、评述性和先进性。①综合性:综述需要对查阅的大量文献资料归纳整理并综合分析,既要以某一领域研究发展为纵线,反映该领域当前的研究进展,又要将同一时期国内外不同课题组的研究成果进行横向归纳总结,力求做到全面深入;②评述性:综述需要作者有自己的观点和见解,否则"综"而不"述"只能称为手册或讲座,而不是综述。综述需要体现作者自己的观点和见解,要对综合整理过的文献资料进行分析评价,反映出作者的态度和学术倾向;③先进性:综述绝不仅仅是对学科发展历史的简单罗列,而是要搜集掌握国内外最新的研究成果,了解最新动态,将该领域当前的研究现状和未来趋势及进展及时呈现给读者。

二、综述的书写格式

综述一般包括题目、作者、正文和参考文献等部分。许多杂志发表综述要求摘要和关键词。其中正文部分包含前言、主体和总结。

有不少杂志编辑部对于格式的要求十分详细,例如 *European Urology* 综述要求如下。

Abstract

Provide a structured abstract no longer than 300 words with the following sections: Context, Objective, Evidence Acquisition, Evidence Synthesis, Conclusion and Patient Summary.

Context: Include one or two sentences describing the clinical question or issue and its importance in clinical practice or public health.

Objective: State the precise primary objective of the review. Indicate whether the review emphasizes factors such as cause, diagnosis, prognosis, therapy, or prevention and include information about the specific population, intervention, exposure, and tests or outcomes that are being reviewed.

Evidence Acquisition: Describe the data sources used, including the search strategies, years searched, and other sources of material, such as subsequent reference searches of retrieved articles. Methods used for quality assessment and inclusion of identified articles should be explained.

Evidence Synthesis: The major findings of the review of the clinical issue or topic should be addressed in an evidence-based, objective, and balanced fashion, with the highest quality evidence available receiving the greatest emphasis.

Conclusions: The conclusions should clearly answer the questions posed if applicable, be based on available evidence, and emphasize how clinicians should apply current knowledge.

Text

The text of the manuscript should be divided as follows: Introduction, Evidence Acquisition, Evidence Synthesis, Conclusions.

Maximum word count is 4 000, including the abstract but not including the references, tables, figures, or legends.

Number of references should be limited to 50.

Take Home Message

Two or three sentences (no more than 40 words) summarizing the main message expressed in the article must be uploaded as a separate file.

针对文章全文甚至某部分都严格地限制了篇幅,同时不像一些杂志要求综述文章参考文献多多益善,而是限制了参考文献综述不超过 50 条。

Nature Reviews 系列杂志要求更为严苛,甚至包括参考文献的数目上限。例如:

Reviews text

All text should be written in Microsoft® Word.

Authorship

All authors are expected to have been involved at least in the research, writing and/or substantial reviewing of the draft manuscript and will be asked to declare their contribution.

Word limit

The length of the main text of the article should be according to the scope agreed with the journal team, and will depend on the nature of the article.

Language

Readers struggle with jargon-laden language or concepts, even in disciplines close to their own. Overuse of abbreviations or acronyms can also make text difficult to read and understand. Authors should, therefore, use plain language to explain concepts, and write as many terms as possible in full while adhering to the word limit. Advice on acceptable abbreviations can be sought from the journal team.

Title

The title should be 80 characters maximum, including spaces, without abbreviations.

Abstract

The unstructured Abstract of 200 words maximum should summarize the main points of the article. All information mentioned in the Abstract must be addressed somewhere in the main article. The Abstract should not contain references or display item citations.

Main text

Introduction

This section should introduce the article topic to readers who are not experts in the field. It should provide background information, supported by references, and explain why the Review is timely. The final paragraph should outline the rationale and organization of the article and explain what it aims to achieve.

Main headings and subheadings

Bold main headings should be used to break up the text. They should be 38 characters maximum, including spaces. Secondary (bold) and tertiary (italic) subheadings may be used to further organize text. They should be 45 characters maximum, including spaces. All headings should be on a separate line from each other and from the following text.

Conclusions

The final section should include the word "conclusions" in the main heading. The text should be a brief summary of the main points of the article with comments on the implications of the latest work and on possible future research directions.

Key points

You should provide a list of 4-6 brief (30 words or fewer) bullet points highlighting the main messages of the Review.

Display items

Reviews should contain display items to explain specific points made in the main text or the background science. These items should be cited within the main text. Each item must have its own concise and self-contained caption that includes a general title and more-specific explanations of certain features, and alphabetically listed definitions of any abbreviations. Wherever possible, these should be original items. If you wish to reuse items from previously published or copyrighted material, you must indicate clearly in the legend whether permission is needed from an individual or publisher. Footnotes may be used sparingly.

Boxes

Boxes should be provided as part of the main article Word document. These are useful tools for explaining basic concepts to non-specialized readers, presenting lists such as disorders to exclude in a differential diagnosis, etc. Boxes should contain only one column of text (maximum 300 words).

Figures

Figures may include photographs, slides, scan images, graphs and/or drawn schematics. Please see our artwork guidelines for instructions on how to prepare your figures for submission and publication.

Tables

Tables should be provided as part of the main article Word document. They should be clear and as simple as possible, contain at least 2 columns of data, and fit on one portrait oriented A4 page, with all text no smaller than 9-pt font.

References

References should be limited to a maximum of 35 per 1,000 words of article text, and lists should be as up to date as possible; authors should generally avoid referring extensively to their own published work. They should be cited with sequential, superscript numbers in the text and should be listed in number order at the end of the article. Any references applicable only to display items (i.e. not cited in the main text) should be cited in the legend and added to the end of the list. The following formats cover the most commonly used reference types:

1. Author, A. B. & Author, B. C. Title of the article. Nat. Cell Biol. 6, 123-131 (2001).

2. Author, A. B. et al. Title of the article. Nat. Struct. Mol. Biol. 7, 101-109 (2003).

3. Author, A. B., Author, C. D., Author, Z. X. & Author, B. C. Title of the article. EMBO J. 25, 3454-3461 (2006).

4. Author, A. B. in Title of Book (ed. Surname, I. N.) 75-98 (Publisher, year).

5. Author, A. B. Title of the article. Website title [online], complete URL (year).

If a reference has six or more authors, only the first author should be listed followed by et al. The Nature Reviews reference style can now be obtained for Endnote. Do not cite manuscripts in preparation or submitted papers that have not definitely been accepted for publication. Meeting abstracts and presentations may be included in some instances. Citations to personal communications and authors' own unpublished data should be kept to a minimum; written permission from the correspondent must be provided to accompany citations of personal communications.

Review criteria

You should provide details of how the research for the content of the Review was performed.

Online features

Supplementary information

Articles may be accompanied online by supplementary information at the editor's discretion, but such items should be kept to a minimum and must be directly relevant to the article. Supplementary information is not edited, so should be provided in a format suitable for converting to PDF for publication. Items should be cited in the main article—for example "(Supplementary Figure 1online)". The modification of supplementary information after a paper has been published requires a formal correction, so authors are encouraged to check their supplementary information carefully. Each supplementary item should have its own separate reference list.

Author biographies

For each listed author we require a brief biography (approximately 100 words) to be published online. This may include details of his or her current and past roles, training and research, as well as society memberships and other interests. Only an author's main affiliation will appear in print.

从这些规范要求可以看出一些国际性期刊对于综述审核极其严格。

1. **题目和摘要** 一篇综述是否能够被编辑选择发表很大程度上依赖于综述的选题。编辑实际上也是根据科研发展动向和读者关心的内容作为文章发表的依据。醒目的题目会让编辑和读者一看就有阅读的欲望,而不是直接忽视这篇文章。

综述一般不写摘要,但杂志要求可能有所不同。例如《美国外科杂志》(*The American Journal of Surgery*)则要求综述必须写摘要,而且对摘要的内容也做了明确的限定:"Review article abstracts should be labeled: Background, Data Sources, Conclusions. Review articles and surgical pharmacology articles must not exceed 25 pages or contain more than 100 references."。

根据不同的杂志要求,有些杂志需要在综述正文之前提供简短的摘要,以点出本综述的主要内容。与研究性论著文章不同的是,综述的摘要通常不需要很长,多数也不需要写出结论而只是需要明确本次综述的主要问题。例如,刊登于 2012 年《欧洲泌尿外科》杂志的一篇综述,其摘要如下:

CONTEXT:

Advances in basic research will enhance prognosis, diagnosis, and treatment of renal cancer patients.

OBJECTIVE:

To discuss advances in our understanding of the molecular basis of renal cancer, targeted therapies, renal cancer and immunity, and genetic factors and renal cell carcinoma (RCC).

EVIDENCE ACQUISITION:

Data on recently published (2005-2011) basic science papers were reviewed.

EVIDENCE SYNTHESIS:

Advances in basic research have shown that renal cancers can be subdivided based on specific genetic profiles. Now that this molecular basis has been established, it is becoming clear that additional events play a major role in the development of renal cancer. For example, aberrant chromatin remodeling appears to be a main driving force behind tumour progression in clear cell RCC. A large number of potential biomarkers have emerged using various high-throughput platforms, but adequate biomarkers for RCC are still lacking. To bring the potential biomarkers and biomarker profiles to the clinical arena is a major challenge for the field. The introduction of tyrosine kinase inhibitors (TKIs) for therapy has shifted the interest away from immunologic approaches. Nevertheless, a wealth of evidence supports immunotherapy for RCC. Interestingly, studies are now appearing that suggest a combination of TKI and immunotherapy may be beneficial. Thus far, little attention has been paid to patient-specific differences. With high-throughput methods becoming cheaper and with the advances in sequencing possibilities, this situation is expected to change rapidly.

CONCLUSIONS:

Great strides have been made in the understanding of molecular mechanisms of RCC. This has led this field to the enviable position of having a range of molecularly targeted therapies. Large sequencing efforts are now revealing more and more genes responsible for tumour development and progression, offering new targets for therapy. It is foreseen that through integration of high-throughput platforms, personalized cancer treatment for RCC patients will become possible.

这篇摘要与传统论著的摘要明显不同,第一部分为背景介绍(context),随后是综述的目的,第三部分和第四部分比较特殊,是本综述的资料来源以及总结内容,最后是结论。整篇摘要中没有像论著文章一样提出具体的统计数据,而是将当前的研究动态一一列出并整合。

综述的摘要也可以写得短小精悍,例如:

With diabetes mellitus (DM) reaching epidemic proportions, the identification of voiding dysfunction as a common and burdensome complication of this disease is critical. Research into diabetic voiding dysfunction significantly lags behind other complications of DM, such as retinopathy and nephropathy. Recent studies have revealed that DM predisposes patients to a wide range of lower urinary tract dysfunction, from the classic diabetic cystopathy of incomplete emptying to urgency incontinence. In this review, we discuss the current concepts of diabetic voiding dysfunction with a critical analysis of the available evidence.

(CurrUrol Rep. 2011 Dec; 12 (6): 419-26. doi:10.1007/s11934-011-0214-0. Bladder dysfunction in patients with diabetes. Gomez CS1, Kanagarajah P, Gousse AE.)

这篇文章以糖尿病患者的下尿路功能障碍为主线进行综述,摘要中只是介绍有关排尿障碍的研究远远落后于糖尿病肾脏和眼睛并发症的研究,把本综述的主要内容引出摘要就结束了。这是另外一种综述文章摘要的书写形式,摘要中仅将综述的主线内容说明即可,而不需要列出综述的主要内容和讨论方向。不过,综述摘要具体的格式需要结合编辑部的要求来撰写。

2. 前言 与一般科技论文一样,前言又称引言,是将读者导入论文主题的部分,主要叙述综述的目的和作用,概述主题的有关概念和定义,简述所选择主题的历史背景、发展过程、现状、争论焦点、应用价值和实践意义,同时还可限定综述的范围,提出综述写作的目的,使读者对综述的主题有一个初步的印象。例如:

Congenital hydronephrosis is a common manifestation often associated with malformation of the urinary tract. It is often detected incidentally by ultrasound and represents 50% of all abnormalities found prenatally. The incidence of detectable urinary tract dilation in utero has been reported to be 1% to 1.4% of all fetuses and confirmed postnatally in 0.65%. In children and adolescents, 25% of cases are diagnosed within the first year of life and 50% are recognized before the age of 5 years. Obstruction of the urinary tract is an important cause of renal insufficiency in infancy. In the pediatric population, obstruction at the pelvic ureteral junction (PUJ) is a common cause of hydronephrosis, and the obstruction is mostly partial and congenital. However, pelvic calyceal dilation or hydronephrosis is not indicative of urethral obstruction. The hydronephrosis seen on an intravenous urography merely reflects previous events but neither defines obstruction nor indicates the potential for progressive renal deterioration. A safe, but not clinically useful, dentition of obstruction is that if surgery is not carried out, then deterioration of the renal function will occur. Currently, the diagnosis is based either on the kidney's response to diuretic stimulus, e.g., a diuretic renogram, or on an antegrade pressure perfusion study (Whitaker test), even though both techniques do still provide false positive or negative results. The etiology of PUJ obstruction is still obscure. Obstructive hydronephrosis can be produced by lesions extrinsic, intrinsic, or unrelated to the anatomically precise PUJ segment. The most common type of extrinsic obstruction is caused by an aberrant or accessory renal artery or early branching vessel to the lower pole of the kidney. Intrinsic factors such as abnormal muscle orientation, absence of smooth muscle, and an excess of collagen in the PUJ have been proposed. However, it remains unclear whether these changes reflect the cause or are merely a histological consequence of obstruction. In the absence of obvious extrinsic factors, the PUJ obstruction has been hypothesized to be caused by a functional disturbance in the ability of the renal pelvis to initiate, form, or conduct peristaltic waves across the PUJ.（来自：Jian GuoWen. Partial Unilateral Urethral Obstruction in Rats. Neurourology and Urodynamics. 2002.21:231-250.）

这一段前言内容丰富，从提出先天性输尿管梗阻的临床危害开始，围绕输尿管部分梗阻的动物模型的建立，提出现有一些模型有一定不足之处，从而引出本文的主体。

最近笔者投稿的一篇综述，前言如下：

With the introduction of ultrasound monitoring during pregnancy, an increasing number of congenital abnormalities, such as spinal bifida or urinary dilatation, can be found before or early after birth. The parents of newborns with these congenital abnormalities often question their consequences for bladder function. However, the development of bladder function and voiding patterns in fetuses, newborns and infants is far from defined, and it remains difficult to predict bladder dysfunction at that age. In addition, there are no accepted diagnostic procedures or treatment methods for fetuses, newborns or infants with bladder dysfunction.

This review provides insight into the bladder function development process and its urodynamic evaluation in fetuses, newborns and infants less than 2 years old. First, we summarize the characteristics of bladder function development from fetal life to infancy, including embryological knowledge of bladder development, nerve distribution in the lower urinary tract, the micturition reflex, voiding patterns and the maturation of bladder function, based on evidence from animal models and human studies. Second, the role of the urodynamic evaluation of bladder dysfunction is reviewed. This includes indications for urodynamic studies (UDS), techniques and approaches for performing urodynamic examinations comfortably in infants and the interpretation of urodynamic parameters. Finally, the importance of performing invasive UDS in pediatric patients with functional lower urinary tract symptoms (LUTs), sphincter disorders, and different types of voiding dysfunctions are delineated.

这一段前言从小儿膀胱功能异常临床多见开始引入,提出小儿膀胱功能异常的评价标准尚未建立,影响临床诊断治疗这一现状。最后提出本文主要针对 2 岁以内小儿下尿路功能发育成熟的进展及其尿动力学评估进行综述。将有关的研究围绕 2 岁以内小儿下尿路功能这条主线展开,主要内容描述清晰,可读性较强。

前言的重要性在于其对读者的影响,读者会根据他们在开头几段所读到的东西而决定是否继续读下去。一篇综述的每个主要部分的首段也会影响读者,他们会根据在首段所读到的内容决定是阅读、浏览或者是跳过该部分。

3. **主体**　综述主体部分的篇幅范围特别大,短者 5 000 字左右,长者可达几万字,其叙述方式灵活多样,没有必须遵循的固定模式,常由作者根据综述的内容,自行设计。一般可根据主体部分的内容多寡分成几个大部分,每部分标上简短而醒目的小标题。部分的划分标准也多种多样,有的按年代,有的按问题,有的按不同论点,有的按发展阶段。然而,不管采用何种方式,都应该包括历史发展、现状评述和发展前景预测三方面的内容。

(1)历史发展:按时间顺序,简述该主题的来龙去脉,发展概况及各阶段的研究水平。

示例　Hydronephrosis is a radiographic diagnosis. In the past few decades, demonstration of hydronephrosis was presumptive evidence for obstruction, even though proof of the obstruction was frequently lacking. The widespread use of obstetric ultrasonography has led to the recognition of a much larger group of neonates with dilated urinary tracts, which has changed the distribution of causes of urinary tract dilation. In addition, many infants have asymptomatic urinary tract dilation. Modern methods of measuring renal function and imaging modalities have challenged the older concepts of pediatric urethral obstruction and its surgical management, creating a dilemma for the pediatric urologist. At present, the postnatal management, operative, and non-operative follow up of antenatally detected hydronephrosis are much debated(来自:Jian Guo Wen. Partial Unilateral Urethral Obstruction in Rats. Neurourology and Urodynamics. 2002.21:231-250.)

(2)现状评述:重点是论述当前国内外的研究现状,着重评述哪些问题已经解决,哪些问题还没有解决,提出可能的解决途径;目前存在的争论焦点,比较各种观点的异同并做出理论解释,表明作者的观点;详细介绍有创造性和发展前途的理论和假说,并引出论据,指出可能的发展趋势。

示例　Regulatory authorities, such as the US Food and Drug Administration (FDA), were quick to take up the term overactive bladder in a therapeutic area where most patients with symptoms suggestive of an overactive detrusor (urgency, urge incontinence, frequency, and nocturia) are treated without a definitive diagnosis, often in primary care. This is thought, by most, to be entirely appropriate. However, the definitive diagnosis of an overactive detrusor can only be made by urodynamic studies, although there is an appropriate reluctance to subject patients to an invasive test unless itis absolutely necessary. Many in the urodynamic community, including many ICS members, argued that the term detrusor overactivity had enduring value and that it should not be discarded. Therefore, it was retained.(Abrams P. Describing bladder storage function: overactive bladder syndrome and detrusor overactivity. Urology. 2003; 62 (5 Suppl 2) 28-37; discussion 40-2.)

（3）发展前景预测：通过纵横对比，确定该主题的研究水平，指出存在的问题，提出可能的发展趋势，指明研究方向，提示研究的捷径。

示例　Some criticism has been voiced that pleads for a less simplistic categorization of lower urinary tract dysfunction. Mattiason19 has written a very interesting discussion article in which he argues that observations alone are not sufficient, but that anatomy, physiology, and pathology need to be related to urodynamic observations. He argues, as other shave done, that the term detrusor overactivity neglects other important parts of the lower urinary tract, namely the urethra and pelvic floor. He argues that detrusor overactivity may be the result of urethral and/or pelvic floor dysfunction, and he could well be correct. However, with the current state of knowledge, the ICS subcommittee on terminology believed that it should standardize what it could describe. It is to be hoped that further research will clarify the situation and perhaps lead to additional investigational tests that can be precisely described and to new definitions and, perhaps, new classifications for lower urinary tract dysfunction. (Abrams P. Describing bladder storage function: overactive bladder syndrome and detrusor overactivity. Urology. 2003; 62 (5 Suppl 2) 28-37; discussion 40-2.)

4. **总结**　总结部分又称为结论、小结或结语。书写总结时，可以根据主体部分的论述，提出几条语言简明、含义确切的意见和建议；也可以对主体部分的主要内容作出扼要的概括，并提出作者自己的见解，表明作者赞成什么，反对什么；对于篇幅较小的综述，可以不单独列出总结，仅在主体各部分内容论述完后，用几句话对全文进行高度概括。应明确说明该综述所获得的结果只适用于一定的范围，而不能无限延伸，即该结论只适用于所收集的研究中研究对象情况一致的人群。具体说明该研究领域尚存在的问题和不足，指出需要进一步研究的方向，而不能仅笼统地说"目前尚存在分歧，需要进一步研究"。

结论的重要性：因为综述是广大的读者涉及的一个广泛的主题，所以"结论"应该是值得认真思考或下功夫去写作的重要部分。这对于高科技的、先进的、还令人费解的主题尤其重要。

5. **参考文献**　参考文献是综述的原始素材，也是综述的基础。因此，拥有足够的参考文献显得格外重要。列明参考文献是对被引证作者劳动成果的尊重，不但可以表明作者引用的资料有其科学依据，而且可以为读者提供研究该主题时查找相关文献的线索。应列出综述所引用的全部文章、观点、统计学分析方法的出处，文献引用格式应参考拟投稿杂志的稿约。以前有些杂志对参考文献的数量有所限制，但目前的观点认为，所有相关的参考文献均应列出来。

综述的参考文献数量要求较论著多，至少四五十篇，个别数百篇，但综述的参考文献需以最新最近的文献为主体（尤其是近五年）。最好也有几篇本学科最古老的参考文献。

三、综述的写作步骤和注意事项

（一）综述的写作步骤

1. **选题**　如何选题才能构思一篇高质量的综述呢？多数作者选择综述作为开始科研

写作的第一篇文章,并以此作为学习相关领域知识的方法。首先在自己日常工作所熟知的范围之中查找有哪些困惑,有哪些经验能够与其他同事交流,随后针对这些困惑和经验需要在网络上查询近期是否已有此方面相关的综述发表。其次在决定开始综述写作之际,需要阅读大量相关文献,首先要将自己变成此方面的专家才能有权威有能力写作该方面的综述。片面的文献阅读会严重影响写作阶段的全面性。

确定写作方向之后,作者多数也会初步确定投稿的方向,这时需要根据自己可能投稿的杂志有针对性地选择相应期刊的综述作为参考,根据已经发表综述的描述方法将自己综述的轮廓勾勒出来。综述的选题应遵循以下几个原则:

（1）选择的专题或领域:应是近年来进展甚快、内容新颖、知识尚未普及而研究报告积累甚多的主题;或研究结论不一致有争论的主题或是新发现和新技术有应用价值的主题。

（2）选题与作者的关系:应选择与作者从事的专业密切相关的主题;或是与作者从事专业交叉的边缘学科的主题;或是作者即将进行探索与研究的主题;或是与作者从事专业关系不大,但乐于探索的主题;或是科学情报工作者作为研究成果的主题。

（3）题目要具体、明确,范围不宜过大。切忌无的放矢,泛泛而谈。

（4）选题必须有所创新,具有实用价值。

2. 搜集文献　题目确定后,需要查阅和积累有关文献资料,这是写好综述的基础。因而,要求搜集的文献越多、越全越好。对初学者来说,一般首先搜集有权威性的参考书,如专著、教科书、学术论文集等。教科书叙述比较全面,提出的观点为多数人所公认;专著集中讨论某一专题的发展现状、有关问题及展望;学术论文集能反映一定时期的进展和成就,帮助作者把握住当代该领域的研究动向。其次是查找期刊及文献资料,把近期进展性资料,吸收过来,可使综述更有先进性,更具有指导意义。

3. 阅读和整理文献　阅读文献是写好综述的重要步骤。因此,在阅读文献时,必须领会文献的主要论点和论据,记录心得体会,摘录文献精髓,为撰写综述积累最佳的原始素材。阅读文献、记录心得体会的过程,实际上是消化和吸收文献精髓的过程。注意对文献进行整理、分类编排,使之系列化和条理化。最终对分类整理好的资料进行科学分析,结合作者的实践经验,写出体会,提出自己的观点。

4. 撰写成文　撰写综述之前,应先拟定写作大纲,决定先写什么,后写什么,哪些应重点阐明,哪些地方融进自己的观点,哪些地方可以省略或几笔带过。重点阐述处应适当分几个小标题。拟写提纲时开始可详细一点,然后边推敲边修改。提纲拟好后,就可动笔成文。按初步形成的文章框架,逐个问题展开阐述,写作中要注意说理透彻,既有论点又有论据,下笔一定要掌握重点,并注意反映作者的观点和倾向,对相反观点也应简要列出。对于某些推理或假说,要考虑到医学界专家所能接受的程度,可提出自己的看法,或作为问题提出来讨论,然后阐述存在问题和展望。

5. 修改定稿　初稿形成后,待"创作热"冷却再进行反复修改,包括以下几个方面:

（1）内容和主题的修改:对综述撰写的目的、意义是否明确,选题是否恰当,信息是否全面,周密等方面再进行检验、查核,并做出必要的修改。

（2）材料的修改:包括对材料进行增减或更换,突出新颖性,抓住研究热点,丰富综述的内容。

（3）结构的修改:主要是使综述的整体突出、层次分明、均衡衔接,同时也使篇幅符合规定要求。

（4）语言和文字的修改：文章的语言和文字要求语句准确、精练，力争"词无浪费、句无虚发、言简意赅、用词恰当"。并对错别字和标点符号进行校对和改正。

（二）撰写综述的注意事项

1. 综述内容应是前人未曾写过的。

2. 对于某些新知识领域、新技术，写作时可以追溯该主题的发展过程，适当增加一些基础知识内容，以便读者理解。对于人所共知或知之甚多的主题，应只写其新进展、新动向，不重复别人已综述过的前一阶段的研究状况。

3. 综述的素材来自前人的研究报告，必须忠实原文，不可断章取义，歪曲前人的观点。

4. 综述的撰写者必须对所写主题的基础知识、历史与发展过程、最新进展全面了解，或者作者本身也从事该主题的研究工作，是该主题的"专家"，否则容易出错。

5. 撰写综述时，搜集的文献资料尽可能齐全，切忌随便收集一些文献就动手撰写，更忌讳阅读了几篇资料，便拼凑成一篇所谓的综述。

6. 综述的原始素材应体现出一个"新"字，即必须有最新发表的文献，一般少将教科书、专著列为参考文献。

7. 文献综述结果要说清前人工作的不足，衬托出做进一步研究的必要性和价值。

8. 采用了文献中的观点和内容应注明来源，模型、图表、数据应注明出处，不要含糊不清。

9. 文献综述在逻辑上要合理，即做到由远而近，先引用关系较远的文献，最后才是关联最密切的文献。

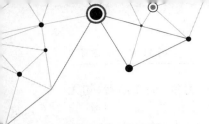

第12章
大会交流和壁展

Chapter 12
How to Prepare an Oral Presentation and Poster for a Conference

第一节　大会交流

大会交流（meeting presentation）包括口头发言、讨论和壁展等、是宣传展示自己科研成果的方式。一种科学思想、一项科研成果及新的科研方法等，只有通过会议的交流，才能得到承认和推广，才能真正转化为生产力和运用到临床实践中。学术会议作为学术交流的主要形式，在交流学术思想、了解学术发展动态、结识国际学者、提高我国学者在国际学术领域的知名度等方面起到了重要作用。每年世界各类学科的重大学术会议达一万次以上，这尚不包括区域性会议和一些学会的年度会议。当代科学工作者频繁参与国际、国内的学术活动，已成为时代发展的必然结果。

改革开放初期，我国学者出国和参加国际学术会议的数量很少，这对于当时多数年轻的学者来说是可望而不可及的事情。随着中国经济及科学文化事业蓬勃发展，我们不仅有经济实力也有一定的科研水平进行国内外的学术交流，很多学者不但可以参与由我国学术团体和部门组织召开的国际学术会议，而且有机会到国外参加国际学术会议。这使得我国科技工作者与国际同行进行交流的机会增多，从而促进了我国科技发展，也向世人展示了我们的科技成果。

一、学术会议的性质和要求

学术会议是短时间内的高层次、高水平、密集型科技信息活动，参加会议的学者一般要求会前提交论文或论文提要，会议的组织者根据与会者提交论文的内容和作者本人的要求，安排大会报告、分组报告或壁展等。由于会议日程紧张，发言和讨论都要严格控制时间。一般会议的发言时间为5~10分钟，发言后有2~5分钟的提问和学术讨论时间。发言者在10分钟内，将几年的研究成果清楚、明了、简洁、直观地介绍给与会者。参加会议的科学家一般都是各国的专家、学者、学科带头人，也有学术界的新秀、研究生、大学生等。与会者所提交的论文代表了各自最新的研究成果，是经过会议专业组织筛选出来的优秀论文。国内会议或者国际会议选中投稿者提交的论文作为大会发言或者壁展时会有邀请信，里面会具体告知发言时间、演讲幻灯或者壁展要求，与会者应该严格按照会议要求提前准备发言。

二、关注会议通知

了解某一学术会议的信息需留意会议的征文通知。学术会议征文通知会提前以各种形式告知与会者,一般都包括以下内容:首先是会议的名称、会议日期和地点;然后是主办和承办单位等;征文的主要部分说明会议的范围、主题以及对会议摘要的要求,比如摘要的格式、上交日期等;最后还包括会议联系人的信息,如地址、电话、电子信箱等。征文通知里还包括会议展望、摘要评审要求、会议的费用等。对于会议摘要,只要是在会议内容的范围内,一般都可以通过评审,应邀参加会议。

下面给出的是一个 ICS-2009 年的会议征文通知:

ICS e-News, 27 March 2009, Issue 13.

Abstract Submission for ICS 2009, San Francisco

Submit your abstracts for the opportunity to present your work at the ICS 2009 Annual Meeting in San Francisco. Visit the ICS Abstract Centre now to access the abstract submission guidelines, instructions and application form.

THE DEADLINE FOR SUBMISSION OF ABSTRACTS IS WEDNESDAY, 1 APRIL, 2009 AT 23:59:59 GMT+1 (UK DAYLIGHT SAVING > TIME).

Deadline for Expressions of Interest and Nominations for ICS Committees 1 April 2009. The following committees are specifically calling for interest in membership: · Ethics Committee · Publications and Communications Committee. Please send your nominations for the following ICS posts by 1, April 2009 · Continence Promotion Chair · Neurourology Chair.

In order to stand for a position as Chair you need to be nominated and seconded by two ICS members. Deadline for applications to host 2013 ICS ANNUAL MEETING are to be received at the ICS office by 1, April 2009.

For more information on any of these items please contact the ICS office click here. International Continence Society Educational Course in cooperation with the Thai Urological Association, 3-4 April 2009. Venue: Zign Hotel, Pattaya, Thailand.

The ICS is pleased to announce an Educational Course to be held in Thailand in collaboration with the Thai Urological Association (TUA). The ICS course will take place on the first days of the TUA's annual meeting. The TUA meeting will then continue from the end of the ICS course until 5 April. As well as using local Thai experts, the ICS will bring internationally renowned speakers to speak on topics that include: Neurourology, Good Urodynamic Practice, Overactive Bladder, LUTS, Dysfunction and Prolapse Surgery. All ICS members and non-members are welcome.

For further information, visit www.icsoffice.org. If you are interested in participating in any of the mentioned activities or have any questions, please do not hesitate to contact the ICS office on info@icsoffice.org.

ICS e-News, is a regular information service designed to keep you informed about all relevant events in a timely fashion.

Contributions and feedback are most welcome. If you wish to see this e-News as a PDF, please go to the News Section on the ICS website www.icsoffice.org.

International Continence Society, 19 Portland Square, Bristol BS2 8SJ, UK

Web: www.icsoffice.org. E-mail: info@icsoffice.org. Tel:+44 (0) 117 9444881. Fax:+44 (0) 117 9444882

此会议通知包括了会议投稿的截止时间,以及开会期间的行程安排和会议主题。还包括会议联系人的信息,以便投稿者如有不清楚的地方可以及时询问。

三、会议摘要的准备和投稿

绝大部分的国内和国际学术会议征文要求投论文摘要。不同的学术会议对会议论文摘要的要求不同,但一般都要包括研究目的、材料和方法、结果和结论,有时也会要求叙说研究的背景和对结果进行简要的分析。拟参加会议的人员应根据会议的具体要求,准备论文摘要的格式。论文摘要多通过会议网站投稿系统投稿,但也有学术会议接受电子邮件和普通的信件投稿。

会议摘要通常包括一些研究资料和主要的研究结果,但不包括已经发表的成果,不影响稍后整个研究论文的发表。有些国际会议会出版会议摘要。

会议摘要能帮助读者快速且准确判断会议发言的基本内容,从而帮助与会者决定是否需要参会以获得发言的更多内容。一篇好的会议摘要应满足下列要求:

1) 不带个人感情色彩,不指责他人,以提供资料、增进知识为主要目的。

2) 主题清晰明了,没有任何语法错误,数据准确,风格一致。

3) 提出研究背景和理由,这一叙述一般位于摘要的开端,简短地说明为什么做此项研究,此项研究的目的和意义何在。

4) 清楚地叙述研究目的或假设,即从这一研究中将得到的收获。

5) 简短但具体地列出研究方法,特别要强调不同于其他研究的地方。

6) 给出实验中所涉及物质的科学名称。

7) 简要地总结主要的研究结果。

8) 简洁地表述主要的结论或推荐意见,强调研究工作、结论或推荐意见的重要性。

9) 一般不要在摘要中引用参考文献。

10) 摘要篇幅通常应限制在 500~800 个单词之间。

下面所给出的是一个作者投 ICS 年会的会议征文摘要作为参考:

Uroflowmetry combined with ultrasonic residual urine: good approach to evaluate detrusor function for benign prostatic hyperplasia patients

Jian Guo Wen, An Feng Lou, Qing Wei Wang. Urodynamic Center, and Department of Pediatric Surgery, The First Affiliated Hospital of Zhengzhou University. Key-Disciplines Laboratory Clinical-Medicine Henan, Zhengzhou, 450052, China

Hypothesis/aims of study

To investigate the significance of uroflowmetry combined with ultrasonic residual urine in evaluation of detrusor function in the patients with benign prostatic hyperplasia (BPH).

Study design, materials and methods

Uroflowmetry combined with ultrasonic residual urine (UCURU) and invasive pressure-flow studies (IPFS) were performed in 150 cases with BPH. Detrusor function was divided into three groups, detrusor overactivity, underactivity and normal according to flow curve shape, maximum flow rate and residual urine. The results from both urodynamic studies were compared using X^2 test.

Results

In UCURU, ninety patients had detrusor overactivity, thirty-four patients detrusor underactivity and 26 detrusor normal. In IPFS, one hundred patients had detrusor overactivity 20 patients detrusor underactivity and 30 patients detrusor normal. There were no significant difference of detrusor activities diagnosis between UCURU and IPFS (P=1.109). The sensitivity, specificity, accuracy by UCURU were 75%, 70%, 73% in diagnosis of detrusor overactivity, 80%, 86% and 8%, detrusor underactivity, respectively.

Interpretation of results

IPFS recognized as an accurate assessment of detrusor function. But our study found that there were no significant difference of detrusor activities diagnosis between UCURU and IPFS. It suggests that UCURU can be used to evaluate the detrusor function in the patients with BPH. It is mainly reason that the three parameters of UCURU could complement each other and exclude the role of other interfering factors.

Concluding message

Compared with IPFS, UCURU is also a useful tool in evaluation of detrusor function in patient with BPH.

该摘要主要介绍作者评估自由尿流率联合残余尿量在诊断良性前列腺增生患者逼尿肌功能重要性的研究。其创新之处在于，以往诊断此病需要侵入性的压力流率检查，给患者造成痛苦，而该研究结果显示自由尿流率联合残余尿量同样可以准确地评估逼尿肌功能。

会议投稿成功后，会议组委会组织相关专家对论文摘要进行评审，对符合要求且优秀的论文摘要的作者，以会议组委会的名义发送邀请信。以 2009 年美国泌尿学会年会发出的邀请信为例显示邀请信的具体格式及内容要求：

Dear Dr. Wen,

I write to you on behalf of American Urological Association (AUA) Public Media Committee Chair Ira D. Sharlip, MD, and AUA Communications Manager Wendy W. Isett. We are pleased to inform you that your studies titled, "The Clinical Analysis of Double Renal Calculus in 50 Infants and Children Fed Melamine Contaminated Milk Powder" and "The Clinical Analysis of Urolithiasis in 165 Infants and Children with History of Feeding Melamine Contaminated Milk Power" were both selected as Newsworthy Abstracts for the AUA 2009 Annual Meeting Press Program. It is a great honor to have your abstracts chosen; fewer than 30 abstracts are selected for promotion in any given year.

As part of the 2009 Press Program, we invite you to present your abstracts at a special session for the media. This session will provide members of the media with additional information and valuable insight into your findings. Would you be available to participate in a 30-minute press conference during the date and time below?

#1060: Clinical Analysis of Double Renal Calculus in 50 Infants and Children Fed Melamine Contaminated Milk Powder

#1061: The Clinical Analysis of Urolithiasis in 165 Infants and Children with History of Feeding Melamine Contaminated Milk Power

Sunday, April 26, 2009

3:30-4:00 p.m.

Hyatt Regency McCormick Room CC23

Please respond to this e-mail by Friday, March 27, 2009 with your confirmation or availability to present your abstract during this scheduled time. We look forward to your participation.

If you have any questions or concerns, feel free to contact me.

Best Regards,

Dana

Dana L. Gugliuzza

Marketing & Communications Associate

American Urological Association

1000 Corporate Blvd. Linthicum, MD 21090

P: 410-689-4029

F: 410-689-3911

该邀请信是通知作者的两篇论文摘要,题目分别为 "The Clinical Analysis of Double Renal Calculus in 50 Infants and Children Fed Melamine Contaminated Milk Powder" 和 "The Clinical Analysis of Urolithiasis in 165 Infants and Children with History of Feeding Melamine Contaminated Milk Power",被美国泌尿外科年会选中。邀请信中会说明对摘要有什么具体安排,比如作为大会发言或者作为壁展等等,你可以按照邀请信中的安排做相应的准备,下面会有详细介绍。

四、学术会议注册

会议组委会在你投稿成功后会给你发送邀请函,然后你就可以考虑学术会议注册了。学术会议一般都要求注册,即交纳一定费用和进行正式登记。注册形式包括预注册和现场注册,预注册就是在会议开始之前交纳费用和进行正式登记,而现场注册是在到达会议场所后才交纳费用和进行登记。预注册有许多好处,比如预注册费一般比现场注册费用低,预注册可以事先预留希望参加学术活动及游览活动的位置等。如果你确定将参加此国际学术会议,最好按时进行预注册。如果你事先不能确定能否参加此国际学术会议,如不确定能否拿到会议所在国的签证,最后才确定参加会议,此种情况下最好选择现场注册。

大型学术会议一般都印发预注册手册,预注册手册中包括预注册的有关信息,专业参观及游览活动介绍,和研究生大学生活动、工作面试、伴侣活动、照顾孩子、住宿、交通等情况,同时附有相关的表格。

例如:图 12-1 是 2014 年里约热内卢 ICS 会议的注册费用,注册时间越提前,费用会越低。其中 ICS 会员或非会员,护士,物理治疗师和实习医生的注册费用都有区别。

五、准备大会发言和展示的内容

提交摘要和注册之后,关键的工作就是准备会议演讲和展示内容,即准备壁展(poster)或大会发言(oral presentation)。壁展的准备工作包括展板展示的内容选择、版面设计、展板制作等,另外练习怎样向读者简单明了地介绍展示的内容,思考一些读者可能提出的问题以及它们的答案。大会发言的准备工作包括内容的选择,直观教具(如幻灯片、多媒体)的制作,然后反复练习演讲。好的演讲首先要有好的内容,然后掌握一些生动演讲的技巧,关键是要反复练习。

Registration Fees

(In USD) Fees apply to payments received prior to the indicated deadlines.

Category	Early	Late	On Site
Available	Until 30 July	31 July-12 October	From 13 October
Full Participants-ICS Member*	600	700	800
Full Participants-Non-Member	800	900	995
Local fee for members only*	450	550	650
Nurses/Physiotherapists/Trainees-ICS Members*	350	435	535
Press	Free but pre-registration required		

图 12-1

1. 大会发言的目的和注意事项　大会发言应达到三个目的:①满足大会程序要求;②达到自己的目标;③符合听众的兴趣。演讲内容必须符合大会和听众的要求。听众阅读幻灯片的速度比发言者读幻灯片的速度快。因此,发言时要简明扼要,不能照本宣科。正如 John Wayne 指出的那样:"Talk low, talk slow, and don't say too much."。

听众的注意力集中时间是有限的,你必须非常清楚地组织你的演讲,突出重点。①分析听众已经知道了什么? 他们需要知道什么? 他们能够吸收多少信息? ②确定你希望交流的主要观点是什么? 围绕这一主要观点来建立起演讲内容;③选择有效的支持性资料,记住你的听众最多只能记住三至四个要点,以及二至三条支持这些要点的详细资料,所以只选择那些能使你的听众信服的资料;④选择适当的组织形式,你的支持性资料通常可用某一常见的方式来组织,比如问题与答案形式、比较和对照形式、以时间为序等。无论你选择什么形式,一旦选定,就从头到尾使用它;⑤准备一个提纲,只包括要点和主要的支持观点。除非当你感到内容太专业不能正确解释时,或对自己的英语水平不太自信时,才写出全文;⑥选择适当的直观教具,最常用的是幻灯片。

2. 幻灯片的准备　大会发言一般都要准备高质量的幻灯片(power point slides),它是黑暗的会议厅里唯一可见的东西,可对听众产生更强烈的影响。因此,准备优秀的幻灯片对会议的成功至关重要。

制作幻灯片时应注意如下几点:①保证所有幻灯片适用于科学报告,并与研究题目相关,不要包括可能冒犯任何听众的幻灯片;②屏幕上所显示的每一张幻灯片的内容在会议厅的后排也应看得清楚,一张幻灯片应只包含一个概念或观点,使听众容易跟随你的演讲;③不要将书页直接扫描成幻灯片,效果太差;④尽量减少文字。在一张幻灯片中,应只显示要点,文字少于 10 行;每一要点以新一行开头,避免使用重复句子,并且不超过 2 行;选择较大的字体,不要全部使用大写字母;保证文字的可读性,一般选择 24 或 26 号字体;⑤不要在同一图形中出现太多的曲线,不同的曲线使用不同的颜色;使用几个简单的图形而不用一个复杂的图形;⑥整个幻灯片避免使用太多的颜色,蓝色和黑色比红色或绿色更容易辨别,不要用红色作背景颜色;⑦幻灯片中不要出现拼写错误,一定要进行拼写检查,或请同事阅读草稿,帮助发现问题,提出改进意见。对于 10~15 分钟的大会发言,准备约 15~20 张幻灯片较合适。一般在幻灯片的右下角标出页码,这样有利于掌握讲课速度,按时讲完幻灯。

近年来,越来越多的会议要求使用会议统一的模板制作幻灯。如下图就是按照 2012 年亚太小儿泌尿年会(APAPU)要求制作的幻灯(图 12-2)。

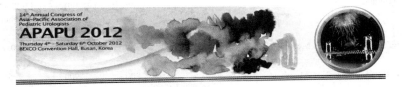

Pediatric Bladder Function Development and its Urodynamic Evaluation

Jian Guo Wen MD,Ph.D,Prof.
Pediatric Urodynamic Center,　First Affiliated Hospital of Zhengzhou University , China

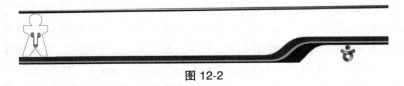

图 12-2

3. 大会发言前准备　在出席大会之前,一定要在同行面前反复练习你的演讲。练习可以帮助你掌控演讲的时间,还可以得到同行建议性的评论,当然更重要的是反复练习能让你更有信心。计划演讲 10 分钟至 12 分钟,留下几分钟来介绍自己和回答听众的问题。此外,应该到年会提供的练习厅进行幻灯片检查和演讲者练习,在那里你有机会再一次预演演讲。你还要清楚演讲会议厅位置,并且在会议开始前 30 分钟到达,向会议主持人介绍自己,并将幻灯片交给管理幻灯机的人,让自己熟悉会议厅,注意演讲台到屏幕的距离,知道屏幕指示仪和幻灯机遥控器的位置,知道怎样操作麦克风。

4. 演讲内容的准备　演讲内容一般由引言、主体、结论三部分组成,分别占整个发言的 10%~20%,65%~80% 和 10%~15%。

(1)引言:叙述你要做什么,从开始就要抓住听众的兴趣,开场白应该自信有力,绝不以道歉形式作为开始:"由于水平有限,下面的发言难免有错,请批评指正……",这类开场白在国际性演讲中是有害而无益的,使演讲开头就显得苍白无力。

记住,听众与演讲者建立起联系需要几秒钟的时间,所以开始不要介绍关键的信息。演讲者可以介绍一下自己的演讲内容或显示一张有题目的幻灯片,这样可以容许听众逐步进入状态,经过这一初始阶段,就应该引出主题:①解释演讲的结构;②列出研究工作的目的和目标;③解释这一主题使用的方法。

一定要让听众清楚你的基本问题和论点,必要时,可提供一些背景资料和定义一些关键的术语。总之,当开始演讲时,你就成了焦点,从开场白就别让听众失望。好的开始就是与听众建立起好的关系,直达要点,介绍自己的演讲目的和轮廓。

(2)主体:取决于演讲的类型,包括实验的主要结果及发现。除非需要解释实验资料,尽量不要叙述详细的方法步骤。

呈现总结性的统计结果而不是单一的结果,显示统计分析的最终结果和介绍结果的重要性,避免讲解琐碎的步骤。显示结果时应该一目了然,图形和曲线通常比表格更好,听众能更好地看出资料的趋向和联系,每个图应有一个短的题目,资料符号和趋向线应清楚地标示出来。

以适当的速度向听众讲述你的"故事",避免因为紧张使演讲速度过于急迫,应言简意赅,很好地组织直观教具,如果需要使用相同的图形两次,就应该准备两份,而不应在演讲中再次寻找同一幻灯片。保持演讲的主体结构尽可能简单,在每一个分支处进行标明,以便听众跟随你的结构和进展。

主体部分可能会涉及专业术语,必要时要进行解释,要尽量做到通俗易懂,深入浅出,逻辑清楚,让听众真正地明白你要传达的信息。

(3)结论:听众的注意力在演讲过程中一般会降低,但在接近结尾时又集中起来,此时,他们希望抓住结论性的评论或建议。在接近演讲的末尾,你可以作如下的提示:"作为结尾,我将显示……","现在我将进行总结……","在结论里,我推荐……"。此时,疲倦的听众会重新打起精神,你又唤起了他们的注意力。

结尾要具有说服力,不要让人们感到你没什么更多的东西可说,而只是想谢谢听众好心来出席你的演讲。因为演讲的结尾比开头给听众留下更强和更长久的印象,在结尾应总结出要点和显示这些结果是重要的,最好对演讲开头提出的问题进行明确的回答,前后呼应。另一种加强结尾的方式就是说明设计成果的局限性,指出哪些还需进一步研究和发展。这种诚实和直率的评论能帮助你渡过回答难题的危机。

5. 讨论阶段　如果演讲后有听众提问和评论,你就有机会加入一些省略的资料,澄清问题,还可以对反对意见进行答辩。进行演讲后,通常会有人提问,对付提问的最好方法就是事先作准备,考虑会被问到哪些问题,准备一些简短的答案,让朋友提出各种可以想到的难题,然后尽量解决。提问中,对于不知道答案的问题,也可以作一些科学上的猜测。

演讲后的讨论阶段可以显示出听众对演讲的反映和接受情况,提问题的数量可以揭示一些情况,如果没有人提任何问题,提示你的演讲可能效果欠佳,但也可能听众对它并不感兴趣或你用了太多的数据将听众说服了。大量的提问则提示你可能触动了某一"敏感的神经"(学术讨论的热点),令人兴奋的评论至少表明听众对演讲作出了反应。

问题的类型也可以揭示一些情况,如果询问者主要讨论文章的主要概念和结果,可以假定听众已经意识到你文章的要旨。相反,如果问题是一些不连贯的侧面观点,你应该考虑听众是否明白你的中心和真正的信息。

当问题看起来太复杂时,请提问者重新组织问题,有时你会发现一个看似不相关的问题最后变成重要的、有趣的、值得答复的问题。另一方面,不要害怕说你不知道答案:如果你不知道答案,就直接承认,听众会欣赏你的诚实。

对提问者要有礼貌。如果你想在演讲结束后才回答问题,可以说明。如果要回答的问题太长,会打断演讲,可要求提问者等到演讲的末尾再给予答复。任何情况下不要同提问者争执,争执只会使听众感到不舒服。如有不同意见,可建议会后讨论。会后,你可主动找提问者,其一表示对提问者的礼貌和友好;其二,讨论可以澄清一些问题并让你学到不少东西。

6. 演讲过程中注意事项
(1)语速要适中,宁慢毋快:适当变换语调(使用设问),吸引听众注意。
(2)开玩笑要谨慎:因为有可能你的听众无法领会你的幽默,更有可能你的玩笑会冒犯到某些人。如果真的要讲笑话,也要尽量简短。

(3) 向听众解释幻灯片上的内容时,不要一直背向听众,要与观众有交流。

(4) 尽量不要后退使用前面的幻灯片,如果需要,可以制作两张相同的幻灯片。

(5) 不要一字不漏地读出幻灯片上的内容,扼要说明即可。

在学术会议上发表演讲绝非易事,尤其是对首次登台的人更是如此,但是只要有充分的准备和练习,也一定可以有出色的表现,从而将自己的研究成果与更多的人交流分享。

第二节　壁　展

壁展(poster)指用来展示数据、描述实验的展板。近些年,不管国内还是国际会议,壁展变得非常普遍。随着网络和电子产品的发展,电子壁展开始成为现代学术会议的重要内容。壁展的发展主要是由于需要参加会议交流的研究论文逐渐增加,如何安排越来越多的论文报告,会议组委会面临巨大压力。因此,相应的改革应运而生,即充分利用壁展的方式扩大学术交流机会。一些大的年会即使有足够的会议室,安排许多同时开展的研讨会或分会也很困难,更棘手的是参加会议的科学家很难或根本不可能有机会参加其他的报告会。为解决以上面临的实际问题,以壁展方式展示研究成果就应运而生。

国际会议展示壁展都有自己的要求。例如国际尿控协会(ICS)会议的壁展展示包括两种,分别是演讲壁展和非演讲壁展。前者不但要在特定的会场进行口头发言,而且也要打印出壁展。口头演讲3分钟,演讲后有2~3分钟的现场讨论时间。非演讲壁展可以在壁展区域展示,作者在会议期间进行展示,但是没有安排特定的口头演讲和讨论时间。ICS会员可以从网站上查看这些壁展,而且可以从网站上下载这些摘要,但是这些摘要将不能发表在当时的ICS官方杂志之上。

一份设计完美的壁展不但会让你在国际会议或者国内会议上展示自己的研究结果,而且会获得壁展设计奖,这将是对你的付出很好的回报。

一、壁展的历程

出现壁展之前会议组委会因为会场的原因拒绝了大量的论文摘要,壁展出现后,组委会就可以告诉那些被拒绝的人,大会决定以壁展的形式展示他们的成果。在早期,壁展是被贴在会议酒店或中心的走廊里,但仍有很多作者,特别是那些想展示他们第一篇论文的毕业生,都很乐意他们的文章能以壁展的形式展览而不是完全被拒收。年轻一代的科学家其实更喜欢壁展的形式。

当今,壁展展览已经被很多会议接受且成为大会很有意义的一部分,一些大的学会年会专门为壁展展览准备了空间。甚至一些小的学会也鼓励壁展展览,因为很多科研工作者认为用壁展展示他们的科研成果比传统的10分钟演讲更有效。从此,21世纪的科学界,进入了一个科学展览的时代。

二、制作壁展前的准备

由于壁展成为很多学术会议的常规组成部分,壁展的制定规则变得更加严格。很多壁展要去适应既定的空间,因此必须详细说明其要求。因为壁展变得很常见,会议组委会就要提供标准和其他所需材料,这样与会的科学家就不用往大会城市运送或携带体积庞大的材料。

在了解会议组委会的明确要求之前,不要去准备壁展的制作。你需要知道展台的高度和宽度,也要知道把展示材料固定在展台上的方法,壁展的最小规格以及展览的顺序(通常是由左到右)。会议日程安排通常会提供这些信息。当今,会议组织者一般要求参会者上传设计好的壁展,由会议筹办方统一制作壁展。也有会议提供电子屏幕展示壁展,省去了制作壁展过程。

三、壁展的设计和准备

学术会议的主要目的就是交流信息,不论会议文章是以展板式展示(壁展)还是口头大会发言,都应记住,你的文章必须是经过仔细准备的,能清楚、简洁、有效地传递信息并抓住听众的注意力。那么,我们应该如何制作壁展呢?

1. **壁展计划** 你应把自己的注意力放在引言、方法、结果、讨论、总结以及文献等部分,精心设计各个部分。在一张普通的纸上作一个小尺度的展板草图,着重文章需要强调的要点,考虑标题、文字、曲线、图形、图解等,并将这些想法包括到草图中去。

常用展板的尺寸一般是 47.5 英寸高,91 英寸宽(约 120cm × 230cm)。展板的左上角留下 3 英寸 × 6 英寸(约 7.6cm × 15.2cm)的位置,在这里将放置组委会为你提供的一张卡片,卡片上写的是展板文章的编号。各个会议组委会提供的展板尺寸是不一样的,每年都可能有变化,因此,在开始准备展板前,应明确组委会提供的尺寸。

一般情况下组委会将为你提供展板,你必须按照展板的尺寸设计你的壁展。而且壁展的字体也是有要求的,标题将使用几号字体,内容使用几号字体可以使读者站在一定的距离很清晰地看到。所以壁展制作者在设计前一定要参照具体要求。下面是 ICS 国际会议所提供的展板以及展示的壁展(图 12-3)。

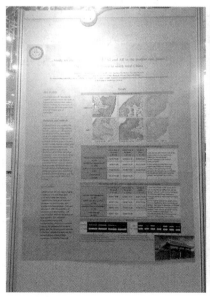
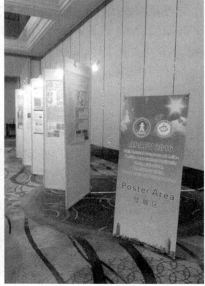

图 12-3

2. 壁展组织 在展板的左上角将放置一个展示文章的编号,从这里开始,文章应从上到下,从左到右放置。附有题目、作者、工作单位的大标题放在版面的顶部。用字母、数字或箭头向读者标出文章的顺序。文章摘要可以设计在一张大的壁展中,也可以是分布在几张小的壁展中,但要按顺序粘贴。

壁展的内容要简洁,集中于二至三个要点。组织壁展还应遵循导言格式,设计良好的壁展,文字应该很少,以留足够的空间来进行插图说明。用简单的曲线、图形、图示突出趋势和进行比较,在图形和表格的题标中标出关键的东西。一定要注意使用文字,使读者容易理解,事实上,要点概括通常比整段文章效果更好。尽可能少用缩写和首字母缩略词,避免太多的数据、文字、复杂的图形。记住,许多人在你不在场时,将阅读和研究你的展板文章,因此,文章传递的信息一定要清楚、简明。选择一种颜色作为展板的背景颜色,曲线、图形中应用适当的对比颜色。

题目应简短且能引人注意(如果可能的话),如果太长就不适合在展板上展览;题目应该在 10 尺(3m)之外就能看到,字体应该用粗黑体,30mm 高。作者的名字应该小一点(大约 20mm 高),正文应该用 4mm 高的字(24 号字适合于正文)。改变一下字体(如 Letraset 字体)是一个很好的选择,特别适用于标题。可以用标准(2'/4 英寸)加数器改变标题的字体,以达到整齐的目的。标题应放在壁展的顶部,最好用颜色或颜色线条突出你的题目、文章内标题、小标题。标题、小标题的字体比文章的字体至少大 25%,也可以用电脑程序来制作展示规格的字体。

壁展的内容应该是明确的、不需额外解释,能让不同的读者以他们自己的速度来阅读。壁展的文字内容短小、简洁、易读,尽量少使用完整的句子和段落,而应使用一句总结性的叙述。由大小写字母组成的文字比完全是大写字母的文字更容易阅读。用于小标题的字体应比正文字体大,比主标题的字体小,这类字体应是黑体或半黑体。

绪论应该简洁地描述一下问题,如果壁展在开头没有清晰地陈述(试验)目的,它就是一份失败的壁展。方法部分应尽量简短,或许只用一两句话就足以描述所使用的方法。结果在一篇文章中通常是最短的部分,但却是一个壁展的主要部分。讨论应尽量简洁,单独的结论可以用几个短句来表述,尽可能减少参考文献的数量。

壁展应有强调的部分,以便路过者能很容易分辨他们感兴趣的内容。如果是他们感兴趣的壁展,就会用充足的时间询问相关细节。包含更多细节信息的宣传册也是个很好的主意,这将会受到同行专家的好评。

四、总结

壁展的优势就是可以用各种各样的表述方式,也不会限制所使用的颜色,任何类型的照片、图表、图片、绘画、X 线片甚至卡通图片都可以使用。对于展示一个复杂实验的结果,壁展确实比口头表述要好。在壁展里,你可以很好地组织和强调几种思路,给阅读者了解实验现状,如果他们要求,可以进一步得到详细的资料,而口头表述对于大致了解单个结果或观点较好。

第13章
给编辑部的信、述评和个案报道

Chapter 13
How to Prepare a Letter to Editor, Editorials and Case Report

一、致编辑部的信

致编辑部的信（letters to the editor）通常是指对某一期刊近期刊登的科技论文的发表意见，类似科技论文发表后的同行评议，经该期刊编辑部审阅后，有意义的信件将会在该期刊上发表。致编辑部的信的格式一般为标准的信件格式，有以下几种类型：

1. 对期刊刊登的文章表示赞同。
2. 增加新的观点，扩大某篇论文的覆盖面。
3. 以新的、不同的视角讨论某一问题。
4. 对论文表示质疑或持有不一样的观点。
5. 对论文中的某点表示关注。
6. 向论文的作者分享自己的观点。
7. 有些期刊会将短小的研究报告或者案例报告以致编辑部信的形式刊登出来。
8. 如果编辑不能正式录用某篇论文，但觉得该论文有一定的意义，那么可能会考虑以致编辑部信的形式发表该论文的浓缩版本。

如果信件内容是对刊登的某篇论文发表的评论，论文的作者可以考虑对这封致编辑部的信做出回复，此回复也有可能被期刊发表出来。

信件的内容通常如下：①首先确定要评论的论文；②写这封信的理由，即为什么要写这封信；③提供证据；④小结；⑤参考文献。当然，在对某一期刊撰写致编辑部的信件以前，要查阅相应期刊的投稿须知，按照投稿须知的要求写信。如 *Journal of Urology* 投稿须知中提出："Letters to the Editor should be useful to urological practitioners. The length should not exceed 500 words. Only letters concerning articles published in the Journal within the last year are considered."（致编辑部的信首先要求对泌尿外科的从业者是有帮助的，信件不得超过 500 个字，信件评论的对象只能是针对本杂志一年以内刊登的文章）。再如 *European Journal of Obstetrics Gynecology* 投稿须知中提出："Letters to the Editor are limited to a maximum of 600 words (excluding references, names and addresses of the signers, and the phrase 'to the Editor'). Only one type of letter will be considered for publication: Letter to the Editor-Brief Communication giving a brief case presentation or short report of a pertinent clinical observation. Please use the correct format following the criteria: max 600 words, max 5 references, max 1 table or 1 figure, no abstract, no keywords, no headings. The information must be presented as a true Letter, e.g. starting with 'Dear Editor, we found that … etc.' Brief communications that do not meet this criteria will be returned to the author."。(致编辑部的信不得超过 600 个字,除外参考文献、写信人的名字、地址、和"致编辑"这些词语。只有以下类型的信件才会考虑发表:简短精练的论文评述或相关临床观察的短篇报道。按以下的标准格式:不得超过 600 个字、最多 5 篇参考文献、最多 1 个表格或者 1 个图表,不需要写摘要、关键字、标题。按照正式书信的形式呈现所要表达的信息,例如开头需写:"编辑部您好,我们发现……"。如果信件没有按照这样的格式书写将会被退回。)

下面,我们举例说明致编辑部的信的格式。

Dear Sir,

We have read the article published by Na et al. [1] with great interest. The conclusions reported by the authors was that treating hydrosalpinx prior to the IVF procedure is thought to improve the likelihood of successful IVF outcome. None of the cases experienced persisting pain need for surgery or hospitalization.

Recent studies have argued for sclerotherapy after aspirating a hydrosalpinx under ultrasound in hope of better success rate in IVF/ICSI cycles than that obtained without aspiration [2, 3]. To overcome the drawback of high recurrence rate associated with ultrasound-guided transvaginal aspiration of hydrosalpinges, ethanol sclerotherapy has been introduced as a new therapeutic option. Ethanol rapidly coagulates the active endothelial cells lining the cyst wall but penetrates the fibrous capsule slowly causing minimal local or systemic complications [4]. However, in an experimental controlled animal study, Atilgan et al. [5] shed lights on the possible damage level of adjacent ovarian reserve in rats after local ethanol application through inducing fibrosis and apoptosis. As yet, no data are available in the literature concerning its effect on the ovarian reserve in human as well as its long-term sequelae especially in women suffering from infertility.

Here we report the laparoscopic findings of five patients who had undergone ethanol sclerotherapy for hydrosalpinges before attempting IVF/ICSI. All patients were planned for laparoscopy before repeat IVF/ICSI cycles because of recurrence with persistant pelvic pain not resolved by analgesics. All women had a medical record of a prior diagnostic laparoscopy before first IVF/ICSI trial reporting no adnexal adhesions. The most distressing finding was that all patients had severe and unusual pelvic adhesions surround the ovaries. The adhesions were thick, string-like, and the majority of which were adhered to the Douglas pouch and the lateral pelvic wall. Interestingly, in two cases, there were thick adhesions between the rectum and the intestine, which might have been caused by the leakage of injected ethanol.

It has been suggested that adhesion formation could occur after transvaginal aspiration alone [3]. However, the findings described here show that all the cases undergoing ethanol injection for hydrosalpinx had severe and unfamiliar thick ovarian adhesions. Although the exact mechanism of extensive adhesions after leaked ethanol sclerotherapy are unknown, one may infer that chemical irritation of the visceral peritoneum together with the fact that the ovary is sensitive to noxious chemicals, potential damage might remain to be excluded. Furthermore, the possible toxicity of injected ethanol to ova located in the surrounding ovarian cortex together with the actively dividing oocytes has not been completely excluded.

Based on these findings, ethanol sclerotherapy for hydrosalpinx before IVF/ICSI cycles, despite being less invasive when compared with surgery, seems to be a traumatic and harmful therapy and should be used cautiously. Further randomized trials are required to confirm these data.

Reference

1. Atilgan R, Ozkan ZS, Kuloglu T, Kocaman N, Baspinar M, Can B, et al. Impact of intracystic ethanol instillation on ovarian cyst diameter and adjacent ovarian tissue. Eur J Obstet Gynecol Reprod Biol. 2014; 174:133-136.

2. Jiang H, Pei H, Zhang WX, Wang XM. A prospective clinical study of interventional ultrasound sclerotherapy on women with hydrosalpinx before in vitro fertilization and embryo transfer. Fertil Steril. 2010; 94:2854-2856.

3. Kafali H, Yurtseven S, Atmaca F, Ozardali I. Management of non-neoplastic ovarian cysts with sclerotherapy. Int J Gynaecol Obstet. 2003; 81:41-45.

4. Na ED, Cha DH, Cho JH, Kim MK. Comparison of IVF-ET outcomes in patients with hydrosalpinx pretreated with either sclerotherapy or laparoscopic salpingectomy. Clin Exp Reprod Med. 2012; 39:182-186.

5. Zhang WX, Jiang H, Wang XM, Wang L. Pregnancy and perinatal outcomes of interventional ultrasound sclerotherapy with 98% ethanol on women with hydrosalpinx before in vitro fertilization and embryo transfer. Am J Obstet Gynecol. 2014; 210:250. e1-250. e5.

上述信件的主要内容,首先提出所阅读的论文,讲述论文的基本内容。论文指出试管婴儿之前行输卵管积水治疗能有效提高试管婴儿的成功率。然后本封信在本篇论文的基础上讨论了在试管婴儿之前,用酒精注射乙醇硬化治疗输卵管积水,虽然可能提高试管婴儿的成功率,但可能存在酒精泄露造成或加重盆腔粘连的风险。酒精注射治疗输卵管积水相对于手术治疗尽管有创伤小的优点,但仍然是一个存在创伤和有害的治疗,应该谨慎应用它,确认这些资料还需要做进一步的随机实验。

随着电子时代的来临,越来越多的期刊要求以电子邮件或者在线投稿的方式提交致编辑部的信。另外,致编辑部的信有以下几点需要注意:①期刊一般都有严格的长度限制,所以应该措辞简练,最好着重于阐述一点,并紧紧围绕这一观点展开描述;②遵循科技论文的写作思想,做到有理有据;③注意语气和态度,对已经刊登的论文提出批评意见,作者应该采用谦虚礼貌的口吻。在回复批评自己论文的致编辑部的信时,不管收到信件时心情如何,在作出回复时都要心平气和。

如果致编辑部的信是对已刊登论文发表评论,一般要求在论文刊登后不久就应该向编辑部投稿。有些期刊明确规定了致编辑部信的有效评论期,过了这个有效评论期后,编辑部就不再考虑接受任何有关该论文的信件。这就要求读者对刊登的论文做出快速回应,而这种快速回应将是未来医学科技论文进步的关键。致编辑部的信能给予作者更多的灵感,成为科学论文的有益补充,也会对医学的交流和进步做出贡献,值得鼓励和推动。

二、述评

述评(editorials),即对书籍、杂志或其他出版物发行的有关科技论文的评论性文章。其中书评,其对象为"书",是评论或介绍书籍的文章。而社论是指有些期刊会邀请科技人员撰写的评论性的意见。但两者评论的原则大体上是相同的,均为实事求是和真知灼见地分析书籍与论文的组织形式和内容的文章,进一步对创作的思想性、学术性、知识性和艺术性进行更深层次的挖掘及探求,在作者、读者和出版商之间构建信息交流的渠道。美国著名书评家钟斯 Llewellyn Jones 在《书评写作法》一书中说:"书籍 book 与箱子 box 两词都出自印欧语系同一语根,此种机缘巧合,颇有暗示性。箱子有盖子 cover,书籍有封面 cover;箱里可以有内容 contents,书籍亦同。"

　　述评的内容一般应包括以下方面:①生动的开场白,用一两个简短的语段介绍作者的姓名、论文题目等基本信息;②阐明写作目的和主题;③指出评论书籍或论文的优缺点,并提供证据;④指出评论论文的科研成果意义。具体的写作要求,可以查看投稿期刊中的读者须知。例如 *Clinical Oncology* 读者须知中提出:"Editorials must be no more than 1 500 words in length and relate to articles published in the Journal, or to issues of relevance for the readership. Editorials are normally solicited by the Editor and Assistant Editor, and authors should discuss other proposals with the Editor prior to submission."。(述评不得超过 1 500 字,内容必须和本刊刊登的论文相关或者是与读者有关的问题。述评通常是收到编辑或助理编辑的邀请而书写的,但作者需要和之前发表论文的编辑讨论其他的建议。)

　　下面,我们将给予几篇述评的示例。

　　示例 1:

Editorial comment

This is the editorial comment for the article of "Abnormal Sleep Architecture and Refractory Nocturnal Enuresis". Children with refractory NE were generally believed to have too deep sleep and decreased arousability since they do not wake up in response to a full bladder [1]. Recently the classic deep sleep theory was questioned and interaction between bladder overactivity, and cortical arousability was found (reference 6 in article). These authors present evidence for a disrupted sleep architecture present evidence for a disrupted sleep architecture in children with a high incidence of PLMs during sleep and increased cortical arousability leading to awakening. This provides additional evidence of increasing arousability in children with refractory NE. However, the weakness of the study is that they had no control data and the number of observed children in the younger group in limited. Therefore, to further evaluate cortical arousability function in enuretic children a different methodology is necessary in the future.

Reference

1. Nevéus T: Diagnosis and management of nocturnal enuresis. Curr Opin Pediatr. 2009; 21:199.

　　本篇述评围绕着"难治性夜尿儿童的异常睡眠特征"这篇文章展开,首先介绍了论文的主要研究内容,并对上述研究成果给予肯定。同时用谦虚的口吻提出论文的不足之处,即没有设置对照组,较小年龄观察组的病人数有限。最后,评论者提出对未来的展望。

　　示例 2:

Editorial comment

This article is a retrospective account of the experience of 1 center in treating bilateral stone disease in patients exposed to melamine tainted formula. The take home messages are that stones occurring in these infants are radiolucent (made primarily of uric acid), and can be treated conservatively with hydration and urine alkalization. A debate would probably emerge regarding the group that presented with renal failure and apparent bilateral obstruction. Eight of 9 patients were treated with hemodialysis instead of ureteral stenting, which the authors imply is an advantage. Many institutions, including ours, would have opted for stenting to relieve the obstruction, followed by conservative treatment until the stones resolved. Hemodialysis would have been reserved for those patients whose renal insufficiency persisted despite relief of the obstruction. Prompt diagnosis, medical support and conservative management work most of the time but sometimes surgical intervention is warranted. This article is timely in that there has been much dramatic and zealous speculation in the news media regarding the urinary consequences of melamine exposure in children. Unfortunately the report does little to tie the occurrence of stone disease to melamine exposure in any other than a circumstantial way. The study is an observational account of 50 patients, and while there certainly appears to be a link, there are still few scientific epidemiological data or mechanistic explanations that infant ingestion of melamine tainted formula results in kidney stones. As a result, the findings must be interpreted with some caution.

本篇述评是我们发表的一篇关于"我中心 50 例和三聚氰胺奶粉有关的婴儿双侧肾结石患者的临床诊断和治疗"的英文论文。首先对本论文的基本内容做一些简单的介绍,接着提出质疑的问题,问题与肾衰竭和双侧输尿管梗阻的这组有关。论文的作者提出 9 例患者采用血液透析代替输尿管支架治疗,并暗示这是一个治疗的优势。而我们许多研究机构,包括我们中心,更多的是选择输尿管支架首先解除梗阻,接下来再行保守治疗至结石消除。血液透析一般用于那些尽管梗阻解除但是肾功能不全持续存在的患者。最后肯定了这篇文章的价值,但是强调三聚氰胺引发的肾结石的研究较少,对临床的发现仍然缺乏科学的流行病学数据和机制。

以下是我们的回复:

Reply by authors

We agree with stenting to relieve obstruction in the common stone case. However, hemodialysis was performed according to the regimen issued by the Ministry of Health, China. A good treatment effect was achieved for the patients with melamine stones and acute renal failure. In addition, not all patients with renal failure had significant ureteral obstruction and for those patients hemodialysis is appropriate. Furthermore, the patients at our center chose hemodialysis for renal insufficiency rather than stenting after knowing that these 2 methods have a similar treatment effect. Finally although we agree that more proof is needed, many facts have been provided that demonstrated a close association between the consumption of melamine tainted powdered milk and urinary stones. A series of articles have been published on this topic (reference 6 in article).[1], [2] Recently Guan et al reported significant evidence demonstrating that the outbreak of urinary stones in young children in late 2008 in China was related to the consumption of melamine tainted formula.

Reference

1. www.who.int/foodsafety/fs_management/infosan_events/en/index3.html. Accessed January 11, 2010.

2. Ding J: Childhood urinary stones induced by melamine-tainted formula: how much we know, how much we don't know. Kidney Int. 2009; 75:780.

作者的回复:首先我们同意在普通的肾结石患者中输尿管支架是解除梗阻的主要方法。但是,血液透析方法的应用是根据中国卫生部发布的治疗方案实施的,它对三聚氰胺产生的肾结石和肾功能不全者产生良好的效果。另外,不是所有肾功能不全的患者都有明显的输尿管梗阻症状,对于这些患者,血液透析是合适的治疗方法。再者,我中心的患者在得知两种方法有相似的治疗效果后,选择了血液透析而不是输尿管支架。最后,我们也表示在这个事件上需要更多的证据,越来越多的事实显示含有三聚氰胺的奶粉和肾结石的形成有着密切的联系。一系列关于三聚氰胺的文章已经发表,最近的一篇文献显示,有确切的证据表明2008年中国儿童肾结石的暴发和三聚氰胺有密切联系。

撰写一篇合格的述评,应注意以下几点:①认真阅读全文,在掌握全局的基础上写作,但可以就一篇论文的某一部分或者某一点进行评论;②客观公正,不带有个人感情色彩,体现客观性;③尽量运用评论性语言,注意语气和态度,强烈的个人观点和批评会疏远读者,而温和的个人理解会吸引读者;④保持主题的相关性。

好的述评可以为出版社和文章作者提供有价值的反馈,为医学论文起到画龙点睛的作用,并对有同样兴趣的读者提供有用的指导,在读者和作者之间架起互动的桥梁。

三、个案报道

个案报道(case report)是通过回顾性分析,对临床单个或几个病例的详细报告,对新发及罕见疾病、某些常见疾病的特殊临床表现,或某种诊治措施产生的某种结果等进行详细的描述、记录和评价。个案报道一般以下两种类型为基础:①单个病人身上某种罕见疾病的临床表现,这是最常见的个案报道发表类型;②对多个病人身上发现的某种特殊的疾病进行报道。

个案报告不同于科技论文中的"论著",但也有写作的基本格式要求,一般以下格式为基础(不同的杂志也有具体要求):①引言,引言中主要向读者介绍本文中的病例及交代为什么这个病例是罕见病例;②病例描述,这部分主要描述相关资料,包括病人的基本信息、主诉、临床表现及体征、各项检查结果、治疗方法及效果评价等;③文献综述,相关疾病的文献报告和情况说明;④讨论,说明疾病的独特性和罕见性,并比较与报道类似疾病其他文献的相同与不同之处,总结本篇报道的意义和用途;⑤结论,提供有利的证据,指导怎样将本篇个案报道的信息运用于临床;⑥参考文献,对于个案报道具体的写作要求,亦可以查看各个期刊中的读者须知。例如 *Ultrasound in Obstetrics and Gynecology* 投稿须知中提及:"Case reports should be structured into headed sections as follows: Title, Abstract, Case Report, Discussion, References. The main text should contain no more than 1 000 words and there should be a maximum of 4 images and 15 references."。(个案报道的结构如下:标题、摘要、个案报道、讨论、参考文献。正文不得超过1 000字、4幅图和15篇参考文献。)再如 *Journal of Surgical Oncology* 中提及:"Case Reports. Manuscripts for this section should have a complete review of the literature as well as long-term follow up when appropriate. Limit Case Report submissions to 5 double spaced pages and 10 references."。(这部分应该包括一个完整的综述和合适的长期随访时间,个案报道的手稿字数限制为5页、行间距为双倍行距和参考文献10篇。)

个案报道虽然在内容和字数上较"论著"简单,但发表一篇高质量的个案报道并不容易,它需要医生具有丰富的临床经验、善于发现问题、分析问题的思维和高超的临床病理书写技能。在临床工作当中,要时时用心,善于发现有价值的病例。如果着手开始写作,在积极查看相关文献的同时,要注意全面收集病例资料,越详细越好。个案报道基于临床研究的深入观察,不仅能引发新的研究热点,有时候还是人民认识疾病的最直接的手段。正因为如此,也最容易受到医师和其他读者的关注。年轻的医生也可以通过书写个案报道,培养敏锐的观察力和良好的习惯,锻炼严谨的临床诊疗思维,记录在临床上所观察到的病例和病案。

四、小结

致编辑部的信和述评要求读者在书写时:首先,要认真阅读被评论论文,在充分理解论文的基础上,加上自己的经验和理解进行书写。其次,写作的内容最好是针对论文中的某一点,围绕这一点展开论述。最后,书写这一类型的文章,要像书写科技论文一样使用缜密的语言,做到有理有据,逻辑严密。一篇好的个案报道完全可以写成论述,关键是要求临床医生在执业过程中要善于发现和总结自己在临床工作当中有价值的病例。

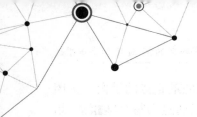

第 14 章
如何撰写医学学位论文

Chapter 14
How to Prepare a Medical Dissertation

医学学位论文（medical dissertation or thesis in medicine）是研究生对以获得学位为目的的医学科学研究工作的全面总结，代表获得学位应该具备的研究水平的重要学术文献资料，是申请和授予相应学位的基本依据。学位论文撰写是研究生培养过程的重要环节和基本训练内容，集中反映了一名研究生的基础理论和专业知识的扎实性和系统性，反映了研究生在本门学科中掌握知识的深度和广度，以及灵活运用基础理论解决实际问题的能力和基本实验技能，也是衡量研究生从事科学研究和独立承担专门技术工作的能力以及是否已达到研究生培养目标的依据。

学位制度起源于欧洲中世纪。公元 1180 年，巴黎大学授予了第一批神学博士学位。学位论文答辩制度是由德语国家首创的，以后各国相继效仿。凡经答辩通过的学位论文，一般都是具有独创性的研究成果，能显示论文作者的专业研究能力。由于各国教育制度规定授予学位的级别不同，学位论文也相应有学士学位论文、硕士（或副博士）学位论文、博士学位论文之分。其中博士学位论文具有较高的学术价值。

20 世纪中后期，世界上每年产生的博士和硕士学位论文约 10 万篇左右。学位论文除少数在答辩通过后发表或出版外，多数不公开发行，只有一份复本被保存在授予学位的大学的图书馆中以供阅览和复制服务。为充分发挥学位论文的参考作用，一些国家的大学图书馆将其制成缩微胶卷，编成目录、索引，并形成专门的学位论文数据库。其中有少数国家对学位论文进行集中管理，如英国学位论文统一存储在大不列颠图书馆，不外借，只对外提供原文的缩微胶片；日本的学位论文也由日本国立国会图书馆统一管理。1938 年起美国的大学缩微胶卷公司编辑出版《国际学位论文文摘》月刊，分 A 辑（人文与社会科学）、B 辑（科学与工程），1976 年增加 C 辑（欧洲学位论文，季刊）。

我国于 1979 年开始恢复学位制度。目前，我国的学位论文大部分存放在各个学校的图书馆供本校学生借阅。只有被评为优秀的学位论文才上传到网上，供不同学校学生查阅。根据《中华人民共和国学位条例》的规定，学位论文分为学士论文、硕士论文、博士论文三个等级。

学士论文是大学本科毕业生为获得学士学位和毕业资格所需要撰写的学术论文。临床医学学士多不要求撰写学士论文。这里我们不再介绍学士论文。下面分别介绍两种研究生学位论文，即硕士论文和博士论文的撰写过程。

第一节　如何撰写医学硕士论文

医学硕士论文（master's thesis in medicine）即攻读医学硕士学位研究生所要求撰写的论

文。它反映作者广泛而深入地掌握了专业基础知识,具有独立进行科研的能力,对所研究的题目有新的独到见解。论文的研究方向新颖,有较好的科学价值,有利于提高本专业学术水平。

医学硕士论文的写作应论证严谨、逻辑清晰、结构有条理。也就是说,在写作过程中,必须要清清楚楚地交代本研究所涉及的对象和方法以及所有实验结果,使得这个专业领域内的任何读者,都可以理解本实验并验证其研究成果。

在硕士论文研究开始前,首先需要撰写的是研究的开题报告。开题报告是学位论文工作的重要环节,是学位论文顺利进行的基础。学位论文开题报告的主要内容包括以下几个方面:

(1) 立论依据:是指所选课题的科学意义和应用前景研究现状分析,主要参考文献目录等。

(2) 课题研究内容、预期目的或成果:具体说明课题的主要研究内容,要重点解决的关键问题,课题所要达到的具体目标或课题要取得的具体成果。

(3) 拟采用的研究方法、实验对象、试验方案及可行性分析。

(4) 研究生本人与课题有关的理论学习、资料查阅及工作基础,包括:理论学习科目及自学情况、国内外文献资料综述、参与导师的科研课题的情况、实验、科研报告、撰写论文等。

进行开题报告工作的研究生必须由本人填写《研究生学位论文开题报告表》,由导师或指导小组签署论证意见,并随同研究生中期考核有关材料上报研究生培养处审核。

硕士研究生学位论文开题报告的要求:

(1) 字数应在 5 000 字以上。

(2) 阅读的主要参考文献应在 20 篇以上,其中外文文献应不少于 1/2。硕士研究生应着重查阅近年发表的中外期刊文章。技术标准、产品样本、网址网页等不列为参考文献。

(3) 由医学各学科组织开题报告评审组对硕士研究生的开题报告进行评议审查。评审组由教授或具有硕士生导师资格的副教授 3~5 人组成。

(4) 硕士研究生将本人撰写的学位论文开题报告书面材料提交指导教师审阅,经学科审核后提交给开题报告评审组。

(5) 硕士研究生的开题报告时间由各院系根据研究生工作进度情况确定,但距提交硕士学位论文的时间应不少于 8 个月。

完成医学硕士课题研究后,学位论文的撰写应在指导教师指导下独立完成。时间应在一年左右。论文的基本论点、结论和建议应有新见解,并对医学发展具有一定的理论意义和实际意义;对论文所涉及的各个主要问题,应具有坚实的理论基础;并能做出详细而深刻的解答。

硕士学位论文是一种科学技术论文,在撰写时应符合科学技术论文的一般规格和要求。字数一般不少于 3 万字(不含专业学位),插图可控制在 50~60 幅以内。

一、标题

论文的第一个主体就是标题(title),其基本功能是:①概括全文,标题应能准确地概括全文内容,一般要求提纲挈领,点明主题,做到文题相符;②吸引读者,读者往往"以题取文",论文题目应有吸引力,这样才能吸引人去读正文。一般情况下,看标题的读者远远多于读正文的读者；③便于检索，标题是检索论文的重要索引，好的论文标题有利于流通和传播。

标题的语言特点有：首先，标题一般只是文章的"标签""称呼"，不反映具体内容，一般不必用完整的句子；另外，多用名词、词组（英文更是如此）。

标题的写作要求是：①言简意赅，专家们建议一般不要超过 20 个字，如果不超过 15 个字更好。如果实在难以精练，可加副标题。但标题过短而令人费解也不可取；②避免太空洞、太广泛、太笼统的标题，如"对尿不湿的研究"就是一个既宽泛又空洞的标题，而"使用尿不湿对儿童和青少年遗尿的影响"就是一个符合实际的标题，突出了研究的目的和实验对象；③少用或不用问题型标题，在学术论文中，问题型标题一般不多见，因为疑问型标题编制索引也比较困难；④尽量少用非标准化的缩略语。例如化学结构式、数学公式、不太为同行所熟悉的符号、简称、缩写以及商品名称。英文标题还应尽量避免名词、动名词混用。

例如《北京大学医学部研究生学位论文书写格式及有关要求》规定："题目应准确概括整个论文的核心内容，简明扼要，让人一目了然。一般不宜超过 20 个字"；《上海交通大学研究生学位论文格式的统一要求》规定："论文题目不得超过 20 个汉字"。

二、摘要与关键词

（一）摘要

摘要（abstract）是学位论文内容的准确概括而不加诠释或评论的简短陈述。它是整个学位论文的精华。学位论文的摘要浓缩概括了学位论文研究工作的目的、课题、基本观点、主要内容、研究方法及结论等。

论文摘要可分为两类：概括型摘要和资讯型摘要。概括型摘要概括论文的主要论点、分析过程和结论，一般短小精悍，主要用于理论性较强的论文。资讯型摘要不但要概括综述论文的内容、要旨、重点，而且要概要地介绍论文采用的主要方法，列出有关的数据、试验结果。如果是创新方法，还要说明基本原理、操作步骤、采用的数据等关键资料，多用于技术性较强的论文。其长度应为全文的 1/30 左右。总体上说，概括型摘要比较宏观，文体正式，篇幅小；资讯型摘要比较微观，文体灵活，篇幅长。

摘要应具有独立性和自明性，摘要的内容应包含与论文同等量的主要信息，使读者通过读摘要就能获得必要的信息。论文摘要控制在一页内书写，格式应为文字。

摘要应短小精练，达到提纲挈领的作用，言简意赅，重点突出。

硕士学位论文摘要应该同时给出中、英两种文字的摘要，中、英文摘要内容要一致。摘要的字数以汉字计，硕士学位论文为 500~700 字。学位论文摘要一般采用陈述方式，用第三人称撰写。

论文摘要的文体比较固定，即：开头、展开、结尾。开头就是主题句，开门见山点出主题；展开段进一步阐明论文的内容、研究方法、分析过程及研究结果；结尾段是给全文做出结论，并指出结论的意义。论文摘要的内容完整性主要体现在研究的目的、研究的方法、研究的结果和研究的主要结论这四个方面。论文摘要可独立成篇，应避免过于简短，避免句子结构太呆板，避免使用非规范的缩略语，一般不用疑问句和感叹句。

英文摘要是用英文概括论文的主要内容，并非是中文摘要的逐字逐句的翻译。要语句通顺,语法正确,准确地反映论文的内容。

英文表达中能用短语表达的句子应尽量避免使用从句,更贴近地道的表达。同时应注意避免基本的语法错误,如 "The congenital hydronephrosis which are caused by partial ureteral obstruction (PUO) are common in clinical, there have about 1%~2%" 中的 "there be" 句型和 "have" 句型的混搭,应避免。修改后如下:"The congenital hydronephrosis due to urethral obstruction is common in clinical practice, occurred in 1%~2% of newborns."。

(二)关键词

关键词(key words)是指论文中最主要、最关键的、重复率最高的词或词组。关键词的功能在于使读者了解全篇主旨。也有利于全文检索。

我国的科技期刊要求,论文需标引 3~5 个关键词。应为美国国立医学图书馆编辑的最新版 *Index Medicus* 中医学主题词表(MeSH)内所列的词。如果最新版 MeSH 中尚无相应的词,处理办法有以下几种:①可选用直接相关的几个主题词进行组配;②可根据树状结构表选用最直接的上位主题词;③必要时,可采用习用的自由词并排列于最后。关键词中的缩写词应按 MeSH 还原为全称,如 "HBsAg" 应标引为 "乙型肝炎表面抗原"。每个英文关键词第一个字母大写,各词汇之间用分号 ";" 分隔。

三、正文

正文(text)要求论点正确、推理严谨、数据可靠、文字精练、条理分明、文字图表清晰整齐,各类单位、符号在论文中必须统一,外文字母必须注意大小写、正斜体。在论文的行文上,达到科技论文所必须具备的 "正确、准确、明确" 的要求。计算单位采用国务院颁布的《统一公制计量单位中文名称方案》中规定的名称。简化字采用正式公布过的,不能自造和误写。利用别人研究成果时必须附加说明。引用前人材料必须引证原著文字。

硕士论文的正文结构包括引言、材料方法及结果与讨论等部分。

(一)引言

引言也可以称为前言(introduction),是全篇论文的引子。主要包括以下几个方面的内容:①研究的出发点;②研究的主要问题及范围;③相关领域前人的研究成果、水平及存在的问题;④理论分析依据、研究设想。通常将文献综述作为前言的重要内容。综述用大量篇幅研究课题进行历史回顾,对前人的研究成果进行综合评述从而引出自己的课题。

(二)材料方法

研究对象一般资料应详细,纳入和排除标准要明确,是临床实验的要注明知情同意书,以及相关的伦理委员会的材料。下面是一篇硕士论文的部分材料内容:

1. 实验材料

1.1 实验动物及分组

SPF 级健康雄性 SD 幼鼠 30 只,购自郑州大学动物实验中心,年龄(8±1)周,体重(180±20)g,适应性喂养 1 周后,大鼠随机分为 3 组:CUUO 7d 组、14d 组及 sham 组。

1.2 主要试剂及仪器

Trizol 试剂	Invitrogen 公司
SuperRT cDNA 第一链合成试剂盒	北京康为世纪公司
UltraSYBR Mixture（With ROX）	北京康为世纪公司
MiRNA-101 及 U6 引物	上海捷瑞公司
α-SMA 大鼠多克隆抗体	Abcam 公司
预染蛋白 marker	上海威奥生物公司
脱脂奶粉	伊利公司
ECL 发光试剂盒	北京碧云天公司
显影底片、显影剂及定影剂	北京索来宝公司
超低温冰箱	美国 Thermo 公司
BP121S 型分析天平	龙腾电子有限公司
7500 Real time PCR 仪	美国 ABI 公司
DYY-Ⅲ水平电泳槽	北京六一实验仪器厂
……	

1.3 主要试剂配制

（1）30% 丙烯酰胺储存液

丙烯酰胺 　　　　　　　　29g

N,N'- 亚甲基双丙烯酰胺 　　1g

溶于 100ml 纯水中，滤纸过滤，棕色瓶中 4℃保存。

（2）10% SDS

SDS 　　　　　　　　10g

溶于 80ml 纯水中，用浓盐酸调 pH 至 7.2，加水至 100ml，室温保存。

（3）10% 过硫酸铵

过硫酸铵（AP） 　　　　1g

溶于 10ml 纯水中后，过滤后分装，–20℃冻存，一月内使用。

……

研究方法要描述到位，使实验结果具有可靠性；别人通过描述的实验方法能重复本研究。不可重复的实验难以让人信服，一般没有意义。研究方法的特点：侧重叙述，交待前因后果；注重说明，交待实验的软硬条件，把事物的形状、性质、特征、成因关系说清楚。记住研究需要使人受益，可促使后人进一步思考。写作要求：准确说明实验要求，如材料、环境等；清楚介绍实验设备，如性能、指标、规格等；细致描述实验方法，步骤、过程等；精确计算实验数据，说明使用的统计学软件和方法。

如下是同一篇硕士论文的部分方法内容：

材料和方法

2. 实验方法

2.1 总 RNA 的提取

1）引物设计

根据 GenBank 库中的大鼠 miRNA-101 和 GAPDH 的基因序列, 用 Primer 5.0 设计 miRNA-101 和 U6 引物, 由上海捷瑞公司合成。

2）荧光定量 PCR 反应

以上述生成的 cDNA 第一链 1ul 作为模板, 进行 miRNA-101 扩增反应, 同时以 U6 作内参, 反应体系如下:

试剂	体积
2×miRNA qPCR premix（With SYBR and ROX）	25μl
Forward primer（10μM）	1μl
Reverse primer（10μM）	1μl
miRNA 第一链 cDNA	1μl
RNase-Free Water	up to 50μl

PCR 反应条件:预变性（95℃ 15s）一个循环,变性（55℃ 30s）退火/延伸（72℃ 1min）共 40 个循环,并增加溶解曲线分析（95℃,15s,60℃,1min,95℃,15 s,60℃,15s）

……

2.2 Western blot 检测

2.2.1 蛋白质定量 采用 Bradford 法,即考马斯亮蓝 G-250 染色法。

（1）样品蛋白浓度的测定

①取 1.5ml 离心管若干个, 每管加入 1ml 4℃储存的考马斯亮蓝溶液。室温下放置 30min 后可用于测量蛋白浓度;②取一管考马斯亮蓝溶液加入 100μl 0.15mol/L 的 NaCl 溶液, 混匀后放置 2min 后可做为空白样品,将空白样品倒入比色杯,根据标准曲线程序,按 blank 测空白样品;③将空白样品弃之, 分别使用无水乙醇和无菌水, 清洗比色杯 3 次（每次 0.5ml）;④取一管考马斯亮蓝加入 0.15mol/L NaCl 溶液 95μl 和待测蛋白样品 5μl,混匀后静置 2min, 倒入比色杯中测量样品蛋白浓度。

2.2.2 western blot 检测步骤

1）预处理样本:蛋白提取液中加入上述上清液 1/4 体积的 5xSDS 上样缓冲液,充分混合后 37℃ 15min 变性,-20℃保存。

2）清洗玻璃板:使用洗衣粉轻轻擦洗玻璃板两面。接着使用自来水冲洗干净,再用蒸馏水冲洗后立在烤箱里晾干。

3）SDS-PAGE 凝胶的配制:7.5% 分离胶及 5% 浓缩胶首先配制 5ml 7.5% 分离胶,充分混匀后缓慢加入 1.0mm 的 Mini 垂直凝胶板中,避免产生气泡,影响蛋白的通过。纯水封闭后,室温放置 45min;此时,当分离胶凝固且与纯水形成清晰的界面时,倾去上层液体,用滤纸吸去残余液体;再配置 2ml 5% 浓缩胶,灌注上层,将清洗干净的 1.0mm 成型梳子缓慢插入浓缩胶中,其深度根据所加上样量决定,两面高低基本保持一致,室温 30min 后使用,加入蛋白上样量。

4）上样、电泳：每个插孔上样量 10~15μl，但均保持上样量一致，留下一孔加预染条带的蛋白 marker 5μl，稳压 90V 电泳，20min，当蛋白电泳至浓缩胶与分离胶界面时，再次调节电压至 120V，继续跑电泳约 1.5~2h。

3. 统计学方法

采用 SPSS 17.0 软件进行统计学分析。计量数据以 $\bar{x} \pm SD$ 表示，采用单因素方差分析及相关性分析进行数据处理，$P<0.05$ 为差异具有统计学意义。

（三）结果与讨论

浓缩观察事实，归纳实验发现，分析研究结果，指出争议问题，阐明作者观点，得出最后结论。特点：句式尽量简单，一目了然，常用图表加以分析，篇幅可长可短。要求：①结果和讨论是论文中的关键，是画龙点睛之笔，成败由此判断，不可轻视；②通常分题讨论，注意阐述分析结果，不要重复实验过程；③实验成功的部分是核心，要有评述；④实验失败的部分也可加以分析，引起同行考虑。总之，结果和讨论是作者通过实验，推理得出的最后见解，是整个论文的归宿，既要反映事物内在联系，又要鲜明准确。

下面是 *Pediatric Urology* 杂志一篇文章结果中的图表（图 14-1，图 14-2），其中表格是一种稍复杂的三线表，所有相关重要信息都要纳入。

Table 2. HR, RF, and EEG frequency in relation to voiding pattern in newborns with HIE

	Groups			
	Pre30	Pre5	Post5	*Post30*
Newborns with HIE				
HR (bpm) (%)	137 ± 9	139 ± 9 (1.4 ± 0.6)	144 ± 10 (5.1 ± 1.2)	*140 ± 9 (2.2 ± 0.8)*
RF (bpm) (%)	34 ± 5	32 ± 4 (−8.4 ± 1.8)	31 ± 5 (−9.1 ± 3.1)	*34 ± 4 (−2.1 ± 2.7)*
EEG frequency (Hz) (%)	*1.4 ± 0.1*	*1.4 ± 0.1 (0.0 ± 0.0)*	*1.4 ± 0.1 (0.0 ± 0.0)*	1.5 ± 0.1 (0.0 ± 0.0)

图 14-1

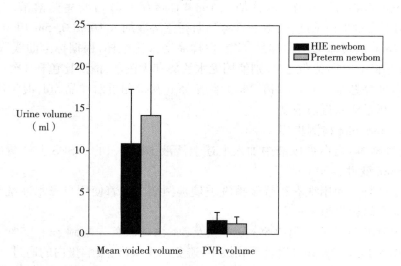

Figure 1. Comparison of mean voided volume and PVR volume between 21 HIE neonates and 19 preterm newborns.

图 14-2

（四）结论

结论必须完整、准确、鲜明,使人只要一看结论就能全面了解论文的意义、目的和工作内容;要突出与前人不同的新见解,认真阐述自己的创新性工作在本领域中的地位、作用和意义;严格区分申请人的成果与导师科研工作的界限。结论是理论分析和实验结果的逻辑发展,是整篇论文的归宿,结论是在理论分析、试验结果的基础上经过分析、推理、判断、归纳的过程而形成的总观点。

四、综述

综述是综合论述(summarize,review),是针对该论文的主题,对前人工作进行的总结。综述一般要求:①围绕论文论著研究主线进行;②一般代表性的方法,演算法应有年代、作者、主要成果的简单描述,主要成果指标对该研究方向发展的贡献,存在的主要问题;③最后引出哪些是需要解决的问题,如:自己的论文研究主题;④综述一般在 10~20 页。近年来学位论文前面一般安排"绪论",后面安排"综述"。

五、注释与参考文献

在写作论文的时候,经常需要引用资料。但是引用资料和抄袭又常容易使人混淆。

界定引用和抄袭最重要的标准就是在整体上是不是有自己的观点,有没有自己的立论,别人的文献是不是作为自己观点的一个补充和引证。如果没有形成自己的观点和判断,完全是把别人的东西搬过来,堆砌起来,这就难免会有抄袭之嫌。如果有自己的观点,资料是为你的观点服务,这就是合理的引注。

注释是指论文中直接引用的他人观点、方法、数据的文献出处。注释应以加方括号的数字以上标标出,如"文建国等[14]",统一编排在论文正文之后。若所在学科有特殊需要,也可适当采用脚注。

参考文献必须是学位申请人真正阅读和参考过的资料,按照学术论文、著作、会议论文、学位论文、电子文献、专利的顺序用阿拉伯数字统一进行编排。

参考文献的标注方式和参考文献表列法,可采用"顺序编码制"或"著者-出版年"制。确定采用某种方法后,在正文中的标注方法和列表中的写法是一一对应的。

按文章正文部分引用的文献出现的先后顺序连续编码,将序号置于方括号中、右上标。引用多篇文献时,只需将各篇文献的序号在方括号内全部列出,各序号间用逗号。连续序号可标注起讫序号。例如:张三[1]指出……,李四[2,3]认为……,形成了多种数学模型[7-9,11-13]……。同一文献在论文中被引用多次,只编 1 个序号,引文页码放在"[ ]"外,文献表中不再重复著录页码。例如:文建国等[4]15-17……,文建国等[4]55认为……。

六、附录

以下内容可放在附录之内:正文内过于冗长的公式推导;方便他人阅读所需的辅助性数学工具或表格;重复性数据和图表;论文使用的主要符号的意义和单位;程序说明和程序全文。

每个附录应有标题。附录的文字、表格、公式编排格式与正文相同。附录按正体大写字母编号,即附录 A,附录 B,……。只有一个附录时,也要编号,即附录 A。附录编号与附录标题之间空一个汉字符。例如:附录 A ×××统计数据。附录中图、表、数学表达式的编号,应与正文编号区分开,即在阿拉伯数码前冠以附录的编号,如图 A.1,表 B.2,式 C-3 等。

表中参数应标明量和单位的符号。建议采用三线表(必要时可加辅助线)。表单元格中的文字一般应居中,不宜左右居中的,可采取两端对齐的方式书写。表单元格中的文字采用 11pt 宋体字,单倍行距,段前 3 磅,段后 3 磅。表格尽量不跨页如表过大,一页内难以排版、需跨页时,需在第二页加表头,表序号前加"续"字。

七、个人简历、在学期间发表的学术论文与研究成果

个人简历包括出生年月日、获学士学位的学校及时间等;研究成果指申请学位期间参加的研究项目、获奖情况及申请的专利等;学术论文应已正式发表,未发表的只列已录用(有正式录用函)的论文。

攻读学位期间发表的学术论著:按发表学术论文、著作的时间顺序,列出本人在攻读学位期间发表或已录用的主要学术论著清单,著作及学术论文的书写格式与参考文献相同,包括题目、发表刊物(出版社)名称、卷册号、年月及署名位次。

八、致谢(后记)

致谢(acknowledgements)是作者对该论文的形成给予各类资助、指导和协助完成研究工作以及提供各种对论文工作有利条件的单位和个人表示的感谢。致谢应实事求是,语言要诚恳、恰当、简短,切忌浮夸之辞。

如:致谢

感谢参加论文评阅及答辩委员会的各位专家!

在即将结束硕士生活之际,我在这里衷心感谢导师 ××× 教授 3 年来对我学习、科研、生活各方面悉心的指导和无微不至的关怀。从治学到做人,从学习到工作,他的关爱伴随着我成长。他无私的品质、博大的胸襟、敏锐的洞察力、严谨的治学风格、孜孜不倦的追求精神和高尚的医德、精湛的医术,使我受益匪浅,激励我不断进步,是我终身学习的榜样。因此,能在求学和人生旅途上能遇到这样一位恩师,我感到自己非常幸运。同时,衷心感谢 ××× 科的 ××× 老师等全体科室人员在我学习过程中给予的大力支持。同时感谢 ××× 科和实验室的 ××× 等在我进行科研课题时给予的大力帮助。

衷心感谢我身边的同学:××× 等在生活方面给予的无微不至的关心、学习科研方面给予的热心帮助。

九、硕士论文其他要求

(一)论文打印与装订要求

为规范学位论文格式,提高学位论文质量,根据国家有关学位授予细则的规定,论文统

一用 A4 纸标准输出,双面印制,左侧装订。要求纸的四周留足空白边缘,每一面的上方(天头)和左侧(订口)应分别留边 25mm,下方(地脚)和右侧(切口)应分别留边 20mm。论文中各标题字用小三号黑体字打印,正文字体的大小为宋体四号或小四号,每页要有页眉,其上居中打印"××××大学硕士学位论文"字样。

(二)硕士学位论文的架构要求

精心设计的论文架构,主题突出,线索清晰,各章节之间的逻辑关系一目了然,且各章节在篇幅上保持一个大致的平衡。没有逻辑的混乱,也没有畸轻畸重之偏颇,这样的论文堪称构造完美且丰满。

1. **主题与线索**　硕士学位论文的撰写应该突出主题,各章节围绕主题展开。论文主题见之于论文标题,各章主题见之于各章标题,各节主题见之于各节标题。一般情况下,学位论文可以设计二级标题、章和节,或章和点。点通常用中文"一""二""三""四"来表达。篇幅大者,还可以设置三级标题:章、节和点。文中出现的所有标题必须在目录中标明。读者通过浏览论文目录从而对论文的学术水准做出自己的基本判断。实际上,在论文撰写过程中,作者反复推敲,用力最多的,也是论文目录,因为目录可以反映全文的主题与线索。

论文主题是硕士论文的中心论点。各章主题围绕论文主题展开,各节主题围绕各章主题展开。层次分明、逻辑关系清晰的章节目录,反映的是作者良好的学术素养。

2. **逻辑关系**　论文叙说的逻辑,从根本上讲,是在构造一个完整的论辩。将每一章中的每一个小节标题联系起来,构成本章完整的论辩,将每一章的标题联系起来,构成本书完整的论辩。作为一种分析策略,论文的作者和论文的读者,都不妨对自己的论文的每一节或每一章,进行一句话式的归纳,再将这几句话合在一起,检查其中的逻辑关系。这样的分析,通常会发现论文是否存在思维的混乱或逻辑的混乱。

3. **平衡原则**　论文构造应遵循平衡的原则,即论文核心各章篇幅应大致相等。每一章中,各节篇幅也应大致相等。论文结构的不完美,反映的是论文内容的不完美,结构的完美与内容的完美是统一的。如果出现这种情况,就要考虑合并或分拆,也要重新考虑章与章或节与节之间的逻辑关系。总之,在论文写作中,追求形式和内容的完美统一,是论文撰写的目标。

(三)硕士学位论文的基本原则和要求

1. **立论客观,具有独创性**　文章的基本观点必须来自具体材料的分析和研究,所提出的问题在本专业学科领域内有一定的理论意义或实际意义,并通过独立研究,提出了自己一定的认知和看法。

2. **论据翔实,富有确证性**　论文能够做到旁征博引,多方佐证,所用论据自己持何看法,有主证和旁证。论文中所用的材料应做到言必有据,准确可靠,精确无误。论文内容要求:主题明确,结构合理,论点鲜明,论证有力,行文流畅。

3. **论证严密,富有逻辑性**　作者提出问题、分析问题和解决问题,要符合客观事物的发展规律,判断与推理要言之有序,天衣无缝,才能使全篇论文形成一个有机的整体。

4. **体式明确,标注规范**　论文必须以论点的形成构成全文的结构格局,以多方论证的内容组成文章丰满的整体,以较深的理论分析辉映全篇。此外,论文的整体结构和标注要求规范得体,符合学术论文写作规范。

5. **语言准确、表达简明** 论文最基本的要求是读者能看懂。因此,要求文章想得清,说得明,想得深,说得透,做到深入浅出,言简意赅。

6. **研究成果的创新性和学术水平** ①有新见解,新观点,新发现;②在理论上有重要的补充和完善,或建立了新的理论体系;③研究新情况,总结新经验,解决了重要的新问题;④创造了新的研究方法。

7. **论文字数** 硕士学位论文正文篇幅在 2 万 ~3 万字,博士论文达到 5 万字左右。

8. **要求阅读与课题相关的参考文献量** 博士论文至少 100 篇,硕士论文至少 40 篇,其中外文文献要占 1/3 以上。

学位论文质量好坏固然取决于选题及科学研究的深度和广度,但根据大量实验及所取得的数据进行总结与提升也是极其重要的,扎实的理论基础,丰富的实践经验,敏锐的观察能力,宽泛的知识积累,深厚的文学功底,是写好学位论文的基本功。只有努力学习,勤于实践,才能逐步提高学位论文水平及研究生培养质量。

十、附录

（一）参考文献著录格式

A. 连续出版物

［序号］主要责任者.文献题名［J］.刊名,出版年份,卷号（期号）:起止页码

［1］袁庆龙,候文义.Ni-P 合金镀层组织形貌及显微硬度研究［J］.太原理工大学学报,2001,32（1）:51-53

B. 专著

［序号］主要责任者.文献题名［M］.出版地:出版者,出版年:页码

［2］刘国钧,郑如斯.中国书的故事［M］.北京:中国青年出版社,1979:115

C. 专著中析出的文献

［序号］析出责任者.析出题名［A］.见（英文用 In）:专著责任者.书名［M］,出版地:出版者,出版年:起止页码

［3］罗云.安全科学理论体系的发展及趋势探讨［A］.见:白春华,何学秋,吴宗之.21世纪安全科学与技术的发展趋势［M］.北京:科学出版社,2000:1-5

D. 学位论文

［序号］主要责任者.文献题名［D］.保存地:保存单位,年份

［4］张和生.地质力学系统理论［D］.太原:太原理工大学,1998

E. 专利文献

［序号］专利所有者.专利题名［P］.专利国别:专利号,发布日期

［5］姜锡洲.一种温热外敷药制备方案［P］.中国专利:881056078,1983-08-12

F. 国际、国家标准

［序号］标准代号,标准名称［S］.出版地:出版者,出版年

［6］GB/T 16159-1996.汉语拼音正词法基本规则［S］.北京:中国标准出版社,1996

G. 报纸文章

［序号］主要责任者.文献题名［N］.报纸名,出版年,月（日）:版次

［7］谢希德.创造学习的思路［N］.人民日报,1998,12（25）:10

H. 电子文献

［序号］主要责任者.电子文献题名［文献类型/载体类型］.电子文献的出版或可获得地址（电子文献地址用文字表述）,发表或更新日期/引用日期（任选）

［8］姚伯元.毕业设计（论文）规范化管理与培养学生综合素质［EB/OL］.中国高等教育网教学研究,2005-2-2

附:参考文献著录中的文献类别代码

普通图书:M;会议录:C;汇编:G;报纸:N;期刊:J;学位论文:D;报告:R;标准:S;专利:P;数据库:DB;计算机程序:CP;电子公告:EB。

（二）量和单位著录格式

要严格执行 GB 3100~3102—93（国家技术监督局 1993-12-27 发布,1994-07-01 实施）有关量和单位的规定。

量的符号一般为单个拉丁字母或希腊字母,并一律采用斜体（pH 例外）。为区别不同情况,可在量符号上附加角标。如:

A	—截面积,散热面积	Th	—弧柱温度
B	—磁感应强度	t	—时间
Br	—剩磁感应强度	tc	—触动时间
Bs	—饱和磁感应强度	td	—运动时间
C	—电容	U,u	—电压

在表达量值时,在公式、图、表和文字叙述中,一律使用单位的国际符号,且无例外地用正体。单位符号与数值间要留适当间隙。

第二节　如何撰写医学博士论文

医学博士论文（MD. PhD. thesis）是攻读医学博士学位研究生所撰写用于申请博士学位的论文。它要求博士研究生在博士生导师的指导下,能够自己选择独立的研究方向,开辟新的研究领域,掌握本学科有关领域的前沿理论知识,显示熟练的科学研究能力,在本学科有所创新,能够提供创造性的见解。博士论文要求具有较高的学术价值,对学科的发展具有重要的推动作用。

医学博士论文也是作者攻读医学博士期间研究成果的总结,是衡量作者是否达到博士水平的重要依据;医学博士学位论文,应表明作者具有独立从事医学科学研究工作的能力,并在科学或专门技术上做出创造性成果;反映作者在本学科上掌握了坚实宽广的基础理论和系统深入的专门知识,是标志最高层次学历教育水平的学术作品。是否有科研创新是博士和硕士论文的重要区别之一。博士论文国家图书馆、学校图书馆要长期保存。因此,论文

应选题新颖、适当,立论正确,分析透彻、推理严谨、论据(数据)可靠、图表清晰、文字简练、层次分明、引证、书写格式要符合规范。论文工作时间不少于二年,字数一般不少于5万字(不含临床医学专业学位)。

一、内容

1. 关于医学博士论文的选题 选一个好的题目,是写好学位论文的第一步,也是非常关键的一步。要选择自己特别关注、最感兴趣的问题,围绕一个专题展开全面、系统的论述,才有可能写出一篇较好的博士论文。博士论文的题目应达到以下几点:①博士学位论文应接触科学前沿,其基本观点、结论和建议应在学术上和对国家经济建设方面具有较大的理论意义和实用价值;②博士论文要反映作者查阅了大量的国内外文献资料,掌握了本领域的科学动态,对要研究的课题有全面的评述;③从博士学位论文的理论分析上,显示出作者具有坚实的理论基础和系统深入的专业知识;④博士学位论文要有创新、设计严密、实验严谨、数据真实可靠;⑤医学博士论文的题目要避免机械的雷同,如"×××蛋白在×××癌中的表达意义"此类题目,也许前期别人在本专业的研究是创新的,有开创性;但是生搬硬套用于自己的博士论文题目就显得俗套了。

博士生撰写学位论文,一般说来选题最好是经过了自己的思考,有感而发,有话想说,才能写好。但这也不是绝对的,如果博士生自己实在找不到一个好的选题,请老师帮助,老师也可以根据该生的具体情况,推荐一个较为合适的选题,但也要经过学生的仔细思考,认为适合自己,才可以确定。如果开始就由老师命题,又不是自己想写的研究方向,平时对它思考得不多,硬要去写不一定能写好。现在博士研究生多数需要承担导师的国家自然科学基金,研究方向已经确定,尽快阅读文献和标书,能够尽快适应课题,多能完成很好的博士论文。博士论文的题目不宜过小。太小的题目无法展开。但是题目也不能过大,避免显得博士研究过于空泛,而内容又不足以支撑过大的题目,例如"尿流动力学新技术和新参数在诊断下尿路功能障碍中的应用"题目范围就过大。该题目看起来好像对于尿流动力学技术和参数有了创新的研究,而且也用于了下尿路功能障碍的诊断。但是仔细研读题目就发现尿动力学新技术和新参数反应的内容很多,尿动力学技术在不断地发展,而且新的技术和参数会越来越多。该题目就显得十分空泛,没有把自己要突出的新技术和新参数反映出来,会让读者觉得有吹捧该研究"新"的嫌疑。因此还是要把自己研究具体的新方法和新参数在题目中显示。如"膀胱尿道同步测压和尿流加速度诊断下尿路功能障碍的应用研究"。这样既说明了具体的创新技术和参数,又说明了应用研究的领域,会让读者觉得是实实在在的创新应用研究。

2. 关于收集资料 确定了选题后,就要立即查文献和着手去收集资料,收集资料是个逐渐积累的过程,要尽量多浏览有关的专著、论文和报刊文章。从中吸取营养,或者找到灵感。资料的收集要随时留意,有时也许在偶然间会遇到很好的材料,就要留心把它记下来。撰写博士论文,还要特别要注重对外文资料的收集。要收集最新的资料,新的立法、新的观点、新的见解、新的数据。

收集外文资料至关重要。要尽可能看外文版的原文,因为翻译过来的资料总会或多或少地失真。当然,一个人很难懂得许多国家的语言,因此,当遇到有些问题自己无法解决时,可借助其他专家的帮助。尤其是选题与临床应用接近的研究,一定要多注意最新的欧洲或者美国,甚至各国发表的指南性综述(guideline)。这样会让博士生更加确定自己应该努力的方向。(Dillon BE1,Zimmern PE. When are urodynamics indicated in patients with stress urinary incontinence? Curr Urol Rep. 2012;13(5):379-84.)该综述是关于压力性尿失禁患者进行尿流动力学检查指征的综述,且作者针对的就是压力性尿失禁这一单纯的疾病,并没有将其他的尿失禁,或者混合尿失禁的类型纳入。这是一篇 Good UDS Practice Guidelines,所以对于尿流动力学研究方向的博士生来说,尤其是在压力性尿失禁亚方向有兴趣的话,该综述无疑就会有很大的指导作用。如果能将该综述翻译为中文,这就为自己以后博士学位论文的写作有较大帮助。

3. 围绕学位论文的选题,争取尽早陆续撰写和发表文章　确定好选题后,按照选题的内容,逐步展开研究。完成阶段性工作就可以开始思考写作思路,成熟一章,就可以把它写出来,先把它作为一篇论文送出去发表,力争在撰写学位论文的过程中逐步形成几篇相对独立的小论文。学位论文的写作过程,本身就是一个思考不断成熟、认识不断深化的过程。随着拥有的资料越来越充分,自己的思路也渐渐清晰,就要把已经梳理清楚,思考比较成熟的这部分形成书面的文字,进一步整理成可以发表的文章。这样既完成了博士论文的写作,又形成了在研期间的科研成果。

特别提醒切忌只是一味地堆积资料而不去疏理、运用。否则,资料收集了一大堆却迟迟不动手写作,到最后才去动手时,"灵感"早就消失了,那就很难写出一篇有灵性、有创意又能引人入胜的好文章。所以,在我们逐渐收集资料和整理资料的过程中一定要注意小节性总结,也许每一个小节写出来的短篇论著将成为博士学位论文的重要素材。

4. 注重理论联系实际　一篇好的博士论文,一定要注重理论联系实际。例如:临床医学的博士研究生进行的动物实验需要时刻提醒自己思考现在进行的实验对临床工作有何意义。反过来说,切忌搞成华而不实、"空对空"的抽象概念演绎。需要注意以下几点:

(1)博士论文中,应当引用一些必要的数据,作为对重要观点支撑引用的数据可以是综合的,也可以是局部的。数据的来源是广泛的,问题是自己要多留心收集这些数据。在引用数据时还应注意:必须对若干数据进行比对,有时可能会发现几个数据彼此有冲突,或者有较大的差异。遇到此类情况就要认真核对,去伪存真,不可在引用的几个数据之间发生明显的矛盾。数据的描述以及统计一定要遵循医学统计学所规定的统计方法,正确运用各种统计学方法,合理运用统计学术语,不可过分夸大某种统计方法所代表的含义。最好的办法是求助专业的统计师对自己的统计方法进行必要的指导。

(2)书写论文时,需要注意选择合适的量化词;关于一些问题的判断时,常常要用一些比较模糊的量化词,例如"极少""个别""少数""多数""大部分""绝大部分""很多""许多"等,尽量把握好分寸,避免选词不当而引起的表达错误。当然一些绝对性词语的应用也要注意,如"一定""肯定""绝对"等。比如在一些肿瘤的研究中,提到某药物绝对是靶向治疗××癌的新发现等,就很不恰当。

5. 关于对引文、脚注的要求　为了避免引文和脚注中经常出现的很多不该发生的错误,非常有必要提醒大家关注以下几点:

(1)引文应当尽量引用原著和第一手资料,保持其准确性;如医学博士论文中引用某些经典的理论依据或者诊断治疗原则时,就一定要从原著中摘引。如在尿动力学研究中提到的关于压力性尿失禁的漏尿点压分型,最经典的理论就是 Mcguie 提出的压力分型,当然有很多的作者在文章中都应用过该经典的分型。我们在论文的写作中就不能把其提到该理论的文章作为参考文献。这不仅在医学博士论文中适用,在其他的文学甚至历史学论文中也应该注意这些问题。如某篇论文引用某伟人的话,脚注却注明为转引某刊物发表的一篇论文而非原著,很容易明白其根本没有看过原著;这种不严谨的治学态度极易导致断章取义、以讹传讹现象的出现。

(2)引文不能断章取义,要忠于原著。如果需要引述的文字太多,可用省略号删节,切忌断章取义或更改原文。有的论文引述他人的论述十分不准确,与原文核对不符,甚至出现"强加于人"的表述,情节严重则需要承担法律责任。另外,如果为了准确的表达某些作者的意思,过分地引用原文,大片段落地摘抄也是大忌。所以博士生在写医学博士论文时要做到既不能扭曲原作者的意思,也不能长篇大论地摘抄。最好的办法就是在原文中标出自己想引用的观点或者方法等,然后用自己的语言和符合自己论文逻辑的表达方式来高度概括。

(3)完成论文后,需要仔细校对,包括正文和引注。同学间可以相互帮忙校对,排除错别字和一些其他低级错误;另外注意引文与文章主体的契合度,即引文要有力地、恰当地支持你的观点,增强说服力;相反如果引文与文章主体关系不大,宁可删除引文,不必画蛇添足。

6. 关于论文的开篇和结尾 论文的开篇很重要,论文的开篇应言简意赅,开门见山,说明自己的观点,让人眼前一亮,吸引读者继续看下去。一篇博士论文,开头通常包括绪论、写明选题的意义、研究目的、研究方法、有哪些创新、还有哪些疑难问题有待解决等。

博士论文分为若干章节,系统地、全面地逐层阐述作者的观点;但一般完成最后一章后不宜直接打住,为做到首尾呼应,通常有一段结束语与开篇呼应,对前面提出的问题,在文尾要有个交代,用总结性的文字将全文收场。一篇论文不仅要提出问题、分析问题,还要最终解决问题。结尾不要拖泥带水,要言尽意止。所以,在一篇合格的博士论文中,问题的提出,对问题的分析,解决问题的方法,得出的结论之间一定要有一些承上启下的段落或者句子出现。这样会显得有更好的连贯性和逻辑性,也符合科技论文的写作方式。医学博士论文的各个部分应该是环环相扣、主体突出的,让读者从头到尾都有想读下去、想去得到解决问题之道的感觉。医学博士论文"形"不能散,"神"也不能散,开篇和结尾要相互呼应,中间部分要作为强大的论据支撑。

7. 关于论文中语言文字的要求 写文章是以书面语言来表达作者想要说明的问题,不同于口头的陈述。相比口语化的表述书面语言要更为洗练,因此评价论文优劣的一个很重要的形式要素即为书面语言运用的好坏。在此强调以下几点:

(1)博士论文要善于运用不同的表达方式,文字要清爽、通畅,切忌病句连篇。相同的话,不同的人说,所用的语言就不同。文字的表述就显得灵活多变而不死板,而且是一种需要长期磨炼的硬功夫,博士生要想书写一篇好的论文,书面语言是必须要过关的。

(2)在表达问题时,还要注意选择合适的词汇,博士论文撰写时,要反复斟酌文字表述,选择恰当的词语来表述。

8. 关于论文的写作进度 做任何事情都要做到提前准备,机会是留给有准备的人的。以免突发情况冲击既定计划,因此选好博士论文题目后,及时进入状态,早思考,早准备,早动手,确保按期完成任务;根据学校要求的进度,制定详细计划,并严格执行,确保按期完成。

刚入学的一年级博士生应以学位论文作为学习的主线,尽早开始规划三年或四年的学习。选择一个自己感兴趣的专题作为主攻方向，不断地扩充自己的知识，围绕这个专题，根据自己的研究书写若干文章，争取获得更多的科研成果。随着对这一专题认识的不断深入，还可检验这个题目有没有写成毕业论文的意义。当然书写文章不限于学位论文的选题，可以撰写无数的小论文作为练笔，但学位论文的选题作为主线需要更多精力来深入钻研。

很多博士研究生反映，博士论文撰写很有难度，需要大量的时间和精力的投入，但"有志者事竟成，破釜沉舟，百二秦关终属楚"；只要努力，一份付出，一分收获，写出一篇有广度、深度、高度、厚度和力度的博士论文不是难事。

二、基本格式

（一）摘要

摘要是对论文研究内容和结果的高度概括。应包括对所研究问题的描述、研究目的、方法、结果和最终结论，重点是结果和结论。摘要应具有独立性和自明性，摘要的内容应包含与论文同等量的主要信息。即使不阅读全文，通过摘要就能获得必要的信息。摘要中切忌出现图片、图表、表格或其他插图材料。论文摘要是对整个论文的高度概括，应该囊括博士论文的必要和重要信息。要让读者在摘要中阅读到该论文的创新点，研究的目标和完成的情况，主要的实验方法，得出的重要结论。下面以一篇国家级优秀博士论文的摘要为例子说明（钱程：Fas 信号和 TLR 信号促进调节性树突状细胞负向调控 CD4⁺T 细胞反应及相关机制研究，2008，第二军医大学）。摘要摘录如下。

作为功能独特的专职性抗原提呈细胞（antigen-presenting cell，APC），树突状细胞（dendritic cell，DC）是目前发现的唯一能直接活化初始型（naïve）T 细胞的 APC，其在诱导 T 细胞免疫应答或免疫耐受的过程中发挥了十分重要的作用。DC 的功能与其不同的亚群和所处于的功能状态（非成熟、成熟）密切相关。……

鉴于目前尚未见 Fas 信号和 TLR 信号参与调节性 DC 的功能调控、特别是参与调节性DC 与 T 细胞相互调控的报道，我们在本研究中分两部分内容，分别研究了 Fas 信号和 TLR信号对调节性 DC（diffDC）的调控作用和相关机制，并在此基础上研究了 Fas 信号和 TLR 信号刺激后的 diffDC 与 T 细胞相互调控的意义。

（1）Fas 信号促进调节性树突状细胞 diffDC 分泌免疫调控因子及相关机制研究

结果发现，……

综上所述，在本部分实验中，我们发现 diffDC 高表达 Fas 但抵抗 Fas 信号诱导的凋亡。来源于基质细胞 ESSC 的 TGF-β 通过活化 ERK 而促进了 diffDC 高表达 Fas。Fas 信号可促进 diffDC 高分泌 IL-10 和 IP-10，其机制可能是通过 ERK 活化导致 GSK-3 失活从而上调 β-catenin 所介导。Fas 信号也可促进 diffDC 高分泌 IL-6，其机制可能是通过 ERK 活化诱导 STAT3 高度磷酸化有关。Fas/FasL 信号参与了 diffDC 和活化型 T 细胞的相互作用后诱导 diffDC 更高分泌 IL-10 和 IP-10，但是不参与 diffDC 更高分泌 IL-6 的过程。进一步研究表明，Fas 信号能够增强 diffDC 对于抗原特异性 T 细胞增殖的负向调节作用。我们的结果提示脾脏内活化的 T 细胞和 diffDC 间的"cross-talk"可能在免疫应答反应的后期促进 diffDC 更好地发挥免疫负向调节作用，从而有利于维持机体免疫功能的稳态。

（2）TLR 信号促进调节性树突状细胞 diffDC 趋化 Th1 细胞并抑制其增殖的相关机制研究

……

综上所述，在本部分实验中，我们发现 diffDC 在 TLR 激动剂刺激后可分泌更高水平的 IP-10，其机制是由于 TLR 激动剂诱导 diffDC 分泌 Ⅰ型干扰素（IFN-α/β），然后自分泌 Ⅰ型干扰素促进了 diffDC 的 IRF-3 表达和 STAT1 磷酸化，最终导致 TLR 激动剂促进 diffDC 高分泌 IP-10。进一步研究表明，diffDC 通过高分泌 IP-10 选择性地趋化 Th1 细胞并抑制 Th1 细胞的增殖，从而提出了调节性 DC 参与 T 细胞应答反应的负向调控的新方式新机制。

总之，我们的实验结果表明，脾脏基质细胞来源的 TGF-β 诱导的 ERK 活化促进了 diffDC 高表达 Fas。Fas 信号通过 ERK 所介导的 GSK-3 的失活而上调了 β-catenin 表达，从而诱导 diffDC 高分泌 IL-10 和 IP-10；活化型 T 细胞能够通过 FasL/Fas 促进 diffDC 高分泌 IL-10 和 IP-10……

摘要点评如下。

摘要第一段首先提到调节性 DC（regulatory DC）的定义。以及 DC 对于 T 细胞功能的研究取得了很大进展，但目前为止，对于调节性 DC 亚群和 T 细胞相互调控的方式和机制仍不十分清楚，有待于进一步深入研究。这相当于研究的背景和引言。第二段提到初步实验结果，发现以往均被认为终末分化细胞的成熟 DC，与脾基质细胞共培养后能够进一步增殖并分化为一类能够通过分泌 NO 而抑制 T 细胞增殖的新型调节性树突状细胞，从而提出了成熟 DC 并非是终末分化细胞的观点，其在完成了抗原递呈任务之后，在次级淋巴器官微环境的作用下，仍能够进一步增殖分化，发挥免疫负向调控功能。所以作者在该段落的末尾提及，对于调节性 DC（diffDC）如何识别危险信号、如何与 T 细胞相互精密调控、其发挥负向免疫调控的相关机制是什么我们并不十分清楚。起到承上启下的作用。第三、四段就很自然的表明了自己研究的方向和主要内容：我们在本研究中分两部分内容，分别研究了 Fas 信号和 TLR 信号对调节性 DC（diffDC）的调控作用和相关机制，并在此基础上研究了 Fas 信号和 TLR 信号刺激后的 diffDC 与 T 细胞相互调控的意义。然后分别叙述了两部分研究的主要内容，并在最后得出结论：Fas 信号和 TLR 信号能够通过不同的信号转导通路而促进调节性 DC 负向调控 CD4$^+$T 细胞反应，参与了调节性 DC 与 T 细胞的相互调控作用。本实验结果为今后进一步研究新型调节性 DC（diffDC）在维持机体免疫稳态中的生理作用，以及在病理状态下对免疫反应的负向调控提供了一定的实验基础，为探索肿瘤、自身耐受和自身免疫性疾病等的发生机制及免疫治疗的应用提供了新的研究途径。

这是摘要写作的常规模式。在介绍自己研究内容时使用了两个小标题：（1）Fas 信号促进调节性树突状细胞 diffDC 分泌免疫调控因子及相关机制研究；（2）TLR 信号促进调节性树突状细胞 diffDC 趋化 Th1 细胞并抑制其增殖的相关机制研究。既有并列，又有递进，且给人的感觉比较醒目，层次分明。

关键词是一些精练、简短的词或词组，能反映论文内容信息和主题概念，便于文献索引和检索，尽量采用本专业规范性的公知公用的词语。英文摘要与中文摘要的内容相对应，为中文摘要的英文译本。英文摘要超过 1 页时双面打印。页眉内容与每一部分的标题一致。

（二）论文格式

为规范学位论文格式，提高学位论文质量，根据国家和学校有关学位授予细则的规定，学位论文的基本格式如下：

1. 论文内容编排要求　学位论文基本结构包括前置部分、主体部分和结尾部分；前置部分包括封面、扉页、独创声明和论文使用授权书、目录；主体部分包括序或前言、中文摘要、英文摘要、论文正文、注释与参考文献、附录；结尾部分包括攻读学位期间取得的科研成果、致谢（后记）。各部分内容的编排要求如下。

前置部分：

（1）封面：一般根据学校提供的模板统一印制封面，不同内容印刷在相应规定位置，采用相应大小的字体和颜色，可印出校徽，一般用黑体字打印论文题目，用宋体字打印专业名称、姓名、导师姓名和职称、论文提交时间、学号、分类号及脊背处论文题目等其他内容。论文题目限制在 30 个汉字以内。

（2）扉页：论文扉页内容与封面一样，作者和导师姓名相应位置由本人签字用于学校存档。

（3）独创声明和论文使用授权书：独创声明意在表明所呈交论文为本人在导师指导下独立完成的成果，不存在剽窃和抄袭内容。论文使用授权书则表明作者了解学校有关保留和使用论文的规定，并授予相关使用权利，并由本人亲自签名。

（4）目录：目录是将论文内的章节标题集合排列，与论文内容所在页码一一对应，内容包括主体部分和结尾部分的相应内容。

主体部分：

（1）序或前言：学位论文的引言，一般是作者对本篇论文基本特征的简介，如说明研究工作缘起、背景、主旨、目的、意义、编写体例，以及资助、支持、协作经过等。这些内容也可以在正文引言（或绪论）中说明。

（2）中文摘要：摘要要体现独立性和自含性，在不阅读全文的情况下，就能获得论文的主要信息。摘要一般包括研究目的、研究方法、结果及结论等，要突出论文的创新或独到之处。硕士论文中文摘要字数在 500~600 之间，而博士论文在 800 字左右。摘要的最后需要列出 3~5 个关键词和论文分类号。

（3）英文摘要：英文摘要为中文摘要的译本，在内容与中文摘要保持基本一致的前提下，要做到语法正确，语句通顺，准确反映论文内容。

（4）论文正文：正文是学位论文的核心部分，占论文的主要篇幅，可以包括：调查对象、实验和观测方法、仪器设备、材料原料、实验和观测结果、计算方法和编程原理、数据资料、经过加工整理的图表、形成的论点和导出的结论等。格式规范根据学科的不同及研究课题的需要而定。论文中出现的符号、缩略词、公式和计量单位等须遵循国家的有关规定。内容要简练可读，层次分明，合乎逻辑，准确完备，客观真切，实事求是。

（5）注释与参考文献：注释为论文中的字、词或短语，需要进一步加以说明，而又没有具体的文献来源时，用注释。注释可作为脚注在页下分散著录，也可集中著录在"文后"。

参考文献为作者阅读和参考过的资料，按照学术论文、著作、会议论文、学位论文、电子文献、专利的顺序用阿拉伯数字统一进行编排。

（6）附录：附录为正文的补充部分，并不是必须项目，主要列入正文内未做详细表述或由于过分冗长而未列出的实验性图片、原始数据、测量问卷、公式推导等。附录可根据需要编排或省略。

结尾部分:

(1)攻读学位期间取得的科研成果:按时间顺序,一一列出本人在攻读学位期间发表或已经录用的主要学术论著,包括题目、刊物名称、卷册号、年月及署名位次。

(2)致谢(后记):致谢为实事求是地向提供各种有利条件的和给予各类资助、指导和协助完成研究工作的单位和个人表示感谢。

2. 论文打印与装订要求 一般统一用 A4 纸打印,双面或单面印制,左侧装订。要求纸的四周留足空白边缘,每一面的上方(天头)和左侧(订口)应分别留边 25mm,下方(地脚)和右侧(切口)应分别留边 20mm。论文中各标题字用小三号黑体字打印,正文字体的大小为宋体四号或小四号,每页要有页眉,其上居中打印"××××大学博士学位论文"字样。

三、撰写要求

实际上,学位论文的撰写在选题那一刻就已经开始了,从某个层面上来说,撰写论文的过程就是整个攻读学位的过程。写一篇好的论文,选题至关重要,需要具备以下三个特点:①先进性,论文选题着眼于本学科专业的热点,学位论文的起点应该定位于最前沿的问题;②前瞻性,即具有预测性,根据研究课题预测可能获得或者希望取得成果,也就是对科研的结果有基本预测;③创造性,研究方法较前人有重大改进,提出了新的概念,实验结果较前有重大突破,这些都属于创造。因此,做好选题从某种意义上来说,就已完成了论文工作的一半。

总体上来看,论文撰写是对整个研究工作的归纳与升华,是由外而内的分析过程,是运用数学分析诠释物理概念过程,也是用实验数据有力佐证理论的过程。一篇好的论文每个环节都要精雕细刻,掌握好学位论文的文体体例和语言特点对写好学位论文十分必要。在科技领域,自然科学研究者的工作是描写自然现象,分析其规律,并探索将这些规律应用于人类实践的方法,对各类成果进行描述和表达,这就是科研工作的特点,在论文中要严谨准确地表达思想,使用简洁精练的语言,推理要符合逻辑,不能引起歧意和误解。

一般学位论文具有比较固定的体系结构,包含一些主体项目,各个主体项目都有特定的作用,写作时有具体要求和一定的语言特点。以下阐述的要点,供初学者参考。

1. 标题 首先标题应具有创新性和前瞻性,要与自己的专业背景相契合,应具有实际意义或能看出对医学领域中实际存在的问题进行研究,能够为解决临床问题提供新的思路和方法;其次,应具有科学性和严谨性,应该充分考虑研究工作的可行性和可操作性;最后,应该符合学术和道德规范,避免抄袭、剽窃。标题的基本作用、语言特点和写作要求同硕士论文标题的要求。

2. 关键词 关键词的语言特点有:①名词多见,数量一般限制在 4~6 个,最多不超过 10 个;②出处明确,一般从标题或摘要中选取;③书写要求严格,包括书写、位置、称谓等必须符合规范,关键词间用逗号或分号隔开。还以上述论文为例,该摘要的关键词是:调节性树突状细胞、T 细胞、免疫微环境、Fas、TLR、信号传导、免疫调节。7 个关键词涵盖了研究内容的主线,名词和动词短语相结合。

3. 摘要 摘要的功能是:①摘要概括和浓缩了论文全部内容,是论文的缩影,便于读者了解全文的梗概;②摘要是扩大流通的媒介,为扩展论文的传播范围,可根据论文摘要编制索引资料或编入文摘刊物,极大地方便了检索。

4. **正文** 学位论文的正文一般结构比较固定,科技论文是论述客观事物及其规律的说理性文章。因此文体比较写实,十分注意语言的非形象性、准确性,保持叙述的客观性,不能带有感情色彩。论文应包括以下几个部分:

(1)研究背景:主要是起铺垫作用,需查阅足够的国内外相关专业文献,阐述相关铺垫知识,系统精练且和谐地引出论文的研究主题。

(2)研究对象、研究方法和研究结果:①研究对象一般资料应详细,纳入和排除标准要明确,是临床实验的要注明知情同意书,以及相关的伦理委员会的材料;②研究方法要描述详细到位,由此得出的实验结果的可靠性才能令人信服;并且研究方法要具有可重复性,不可重复性的实验,则意义有限;③研究结果,实事求是地详细描述实验结果,保持客观性,不能夸大不实,更不能弄虚作假。

(3)结果与讨论:结果浓缩了实验结果或观察事实,讨论则通过归纳实验中的发现,分析研究结果,提出具有争议问题,讨论不同的观点,并阐明自己观点,从而得出最终的结论。特点:句式简单,常用图或表格进行分析,一目了然,篇幅可长可短。

5. **综述** 研究论著前面或后面一般安排"综述"。医学博士论文附的综述可以是两篇,也可以是一篇。但是综述的目的是为了让读者更加明白课题研究的意义,了解该领域的研究进展。当然也可以说是为了让不太了解该领域的读者能够轻松地读懂整个论文。所以在博士论文的综述中要体现的就是基础性、全面性、前沿性,从而引导读者进入该领域的研究范畴。

6. **合理运用参考文献** 引用文献的目的是对自己的观点进行补充和引证,界定引用与抄袭的重要标准就是在整体上是否有自己的观点和立论。如果完全是把参考文献中的东西搬过来,堆砌起来,没有形成自己的观点和判断,这就有抄袭之嫌。

有关博士论文的标题、关键词、摘要、正文、综述和合理应用参考文献等要在满足硕士论文撰写要求的基础上更上一层楼。博士论文强调创新性,内容更丰富。撰写的基本要求详见本章第一节。

四、注意事项

医学博士论文的形式框架要做到丰满且全面。无论是摘要,还是正文的内容都要注意分成多个部分,每个部分都要有中心的思想突出。这样分别叙述各个部分的好处是可以让博士生在每一部分有的放矢地写作。即使在每个小部分没能及时完成,也可以随时在有灵感的时候进行补充。

1. **主题与线索** 和撰写硕士论文相似,博士论文更要突出主题,各章节要围绕主题展开。论文各节主题见之于各节标题,各章主题见之于各章标题,论文主题见之于论文标题。

以论文主题为中心,各章主题依次展开;以各章主题为中心,各节主题依次展开。据此做出逻辑关系清晰、层次分明的目录,能够很好地反映作者的学术素养。而医学博士论文的写作一般都是分成几个部分,每个部分下面都分成几个步骤,每个步骤环环相扣,直到最后得出总体的结论。比如对于肾癌的某个靶向基因到临床药物靶向治疗的研究。首先就是体外细胞培养的研究,然后是裸鼠成瘤的研究,最后进入药物靶向干预的体内研究。这样分的三个部分,从体外到体内,直到药物干预。既有很好的逻辑性,也有很深入的研究,也符合转化医学这一现代医学发展趋势。当然在每一个部分都可以取得很好的实验结果,都可以写成几个小论文。既保证了毕业所需要的发表论文数量,也保证了在大论文写作中内容丰富。

2. **逻辑关系**　博士论文面临更高层次的要求,无论是整体的结构还是内在的逻辑性都需要更好地梳理。不妨将自己论文的各节或各章归纳为一句话,再将这几句话合在一起,检讨其中的逻辑关系;这是一种十分高效的分析策略,很容易就会发现自己或论文作者逻辑的混乱或者思维的混乱。

3. **平衡原则**　论文核心各章篇幅应大致相等,论文结构的不完美能够反映出论文内容的瑕疵。内容的完美与结构的完美是一致的。

五、结语

虽然科学研究及选题的广度和深度最终决定学位论文质量的好坏,但是通过大量实验,并对所得实验数据进行总结与提升同样十分重要的;完成一篇优秀的学位论文需要深厚的文学功底,广泛的知识积累,敏锐的观察能力,扎实的理论基础和丰富的实践经验;因此我们需要投入足够的精力,刻苦学习,用于实践,不断提高学位论文的写作水平。

六、附录

(一)国际上博士培养的类型

目前国际上存在两种类型的医学博士学位,即专业学位和科研学位。科研学位是把培养的重点放在科研上,着重训练研究生的科学思维和科研能力,毕业后获得学术理论研究博士学位,如美、英的哲学博士学位(PhD)。专业学位重视临床能力的训练,目的是把研究生培养成为某一医学专业的专家,毕业后获得应用型博士学位,如美国的医学博士学位(MD)。尽管两者的培养侧重点有所不同,但最终目的都是为了培养高素质的医学人才。博士研究生培养模式是对不同教育类型或不同国度、院校、学科的研究生教育相比较而言的,以某些反映其总体特征的鲜明特点表现出来。如强调课程学习,实行严格的资格考试是以美国为代表的博士生培养模式,而以科研和撰写博士论文为主要任务则是德国博士生培养模式的特点。各国的医学教育制度与本国的国家制度和文化传统有着密切的关系,从不同国家的文化背景及属地关系来看,世界各国高等医学教育的学制主要有以下几种类型。

1. **德式学制**　大多数欧洲国家实行这一学制,实行理论教学、实验室训练和临床实践的渐进式教学,在博士生招生方面没有考试的要求,即所谓的"零考试制度"。通常以论文形式考查学生的专业水平和研究能力。学制为6年,在6年中要通过3次国家考试和论文答辩,毕业后授予医学博士学位。德式学制是一种典型的学徒式培养模式,主要特点是导师对研究生进行个别指导和培养,没有专门的管理机构,其师生之间的关系是师徒关系,研究生的招生、培养与科研、论文写作等方面的工作均由导师个人负责和指导。其博士培养主要特点:教学自由、学习自由、研究与教学相结合,以及强调临床与实践教学相结合。这样,不但公共基础课得以加强,基础知识较为扎实,实用性广,而且注意到了理论与实践的结合,使学生在医学实践中不断加强能力的培养。大多数欧洲国家实行这一学制,如丹麦、捷克、希腊、荷兰、葡萄牙、西班牙等。

2. 俄式学制　俄罗斯的医学教育均在各医学院校中进行,分基础教学和专业教学两个阶段,基础阶段又分为公共课和医学基础课两部分,而专业阶段又分为专业基础课和专业课两部分。公共课、医学基础课和专业基础课共约 3 个学年,专业课约占 3 个学年。每学期均举行考试,成绩合格者升入高一年级。医学系的第六年为选修期,学生可以从内科、外科或妇产科中任选,完成专科培训以后,经考试及格,授予 MD 学位。

3. 美式学制　美国现有医学院校中绝大多数为 4 年制医学院校。美国医学院校的学生在毕业时,获得 MD 学位。美国的医学教育有如下特点:一是理科大学本科毕业后方能进入医学院校学习,科研型博士招生不限制专业背景;二是各院校对招生人数都进行严格控制,为精英教育;三是重视学生动手能力和临床技能的培养;四是医学院毕业生必须在完成一年住院医师培训、并通过美国医师执照各阶段考试后,才能成为一名通科医师。如果要想成为专科医生,还必须再经过 3~5 年不等的专科医师培训,并通过全国各专科委员会的专科医师考试,方可成为一名专科医师。

4. 日式学制　在日本读医学学士学位需要 6 年的时间,博士学位需要 4 年时间才能获得。因为博士入学之前要求至少有两年以上的临床工作经验,所以入学后即可在担当住院医师工作的同时,逐步开展研究工作。相关人士的推荐在博士生的录取中起很大的作用,博士生进入科室后,先轮转半年,通过相互选择确定相应的学组,开始在高年资医师的指导下开展研究工作。毕业答辩分初审和终审两个阶段。初审评审组由非本科室的相关资深教授和专家组成,约 4~5 人,多数博士生可以顺利进入终审。终审评审组的组员与初审相同,不同的是本研究室的教授参加进来并担任评审组长。能够进入终审的博士生多数可顺利毕业。

5. 我国高等医学教育学制概况　我国医学学制有 3、5、6、7、8 年 5 种,是世界上学制层次最多的国家。国内目前的博士培养体系有两个模式:一是 8 年制硕博连读,另外就是传统的 3 年或 4 年博士研究生制度。具有医学或相关专业硕士学历、学位或具有同等学力者通过考试,由各招生单位组织实施博士生导师面试集体讨论筛选。实行单一导师制,要完成具有开拓性、先进性、理论与实践价值的论文,经院校学位委员会批准授予博士学位,其学位可分科研型和临床型。中国医学博士培养制度深受欧洲模式影响,具有典型德国模式的特点。近年来学习北美,博士培养制度又具有北美模式的某些特点。实行课程学习和学位论文研究并重的政策。但培养模式相对保守,课程学习的系统性不如美国,导师指导也比较单一,不同院校、不同导师培养的博士生差距往往较大。

(二)关于 MD 与 PhD 的区别

MD 和 PhD,都是学位的缩写。MD 是医学的专业学位,具有 MD 学位的人,可以参加医师执照考试。国内医学院校临床专业毕业后一般都可以称为医生(medical doctor),相当于欧美国家的 MD。如果攻读博士研究生后获得的博士学位则相当于欧美国家的 PhD。医学方面的 PhD 可以理解为科研型博士学位。PhD 是与"专业学位"相对应的理学学位。国内非医学专业的学生获得 PhD 学位后可以从事生理、生化、遗传等基础研究类工作,但是不能参加医师执照考试。在美国,医科是 4 年本科毕业后再考医学专业,考上后再学 4~5 年医学专业的同时考医师资格证(3-step)。毕业就是 MD,拿到 MD 之后还要经过 5~6 年的时间才有机会考上专科医生的执照。

MD 和 PhD 根本出发点是不同的,一个是职业教育学位,一个是学术研究学位。在很多领域,PhD 也称之为哲学博士。哲学博士(Doctor of Philosophy,简称 PhD、Ph.D. 或 D.Phil.),通常是学历架构中最高级的学衔。大学本科(学士)及 / 或研究院(硕士)毕业后,再进行数年的研修后,撰写论文并通过答辩,方获发哲学博士学位。PhD 的拥有人并不一定修读“哲学”。所谓哲学博士,是指拥有人对其知识范畴的理论、内容及发展等都相当熟悉,能独立进行研究,并在该范畴内对学术界有所建树。因此,哲学博士基本上可以授予任何学科的博士毕业生。

第 15 章
投稿与校对

Chapter 15
Submission and Proofing

第一节　如何准备底稿

一、准备论文底稿

如何准备底稿(prepare the manuscript)是投稿前必须考虑的问题。准备底稿其实也可以认为就是把写好的论文按照拟投递杂志的要求重新整理的过程,包括文章正文、相关图表、附录、投稿信等。

准备底稿的前期基础是根据研究目的制订研究计划,通过预实验验证研究的意义和可行性后,即可根据计划按部就班进行实验。实验过程中需要继续查阅文献,完善实验方法,优化技术流程,并同时开始撰写论文。实验完成以后,应该对相关数据进行总结分析,撰写科研底稿。

在底稿准备好前,仔细阅读将要投递杂志的"作者须知"栏。随着时代发展和技术革新,现在国内外杂志基本都网上投稿。投稿前,作者要仔细核对稿件中统计数据和各部分内容的表述是否准确,避免因笔误或打印错误导致稿件科学性、严谨性受到影响。论文相关课题若为基金资助项目或科技攻关项目的支持,需要在文稿首页下方写明项目全称和编号,并将基金资助证明复印件随投稿稿件一并上传;若论文课题已获国家级或省市级科技奖项,也要将获奖证书复印件随投稿附上。

国外杂志社通常提供更加完整详细的 Information for Authors。例如世界著名杂志 *The Lancet* 提供的 Information for Authors 多达 5 页。将投稿过程中所遇到的每一步细节都讲解清楚,包括对稿件的具体要求以及如何上传稿件等。同时,仔细阅读该杂志近期发行的刊物,尤其关注该杂志可能变化广泛的编辑风格,比如引用文献的类型、标题和副标题、摘要的长短和位置、表格和图解的设计、脚注的处理。

二、底稿分页

通常的做法是,底稿的每一章开头都另起新的一页。题目及作者的名字和地址在第一页,这页被称为首页(title page);摘要在第二页;引言从第三页开始。随后的每一章(材料方法和结果等)重新开始一页。图注单独列一页。列表和图解(以及图注)应放于底稿后,不能穿插于底稿中。但是投稿时编写的页码往往只是作者临时编写的页码,与文章正式发表时的页码完全不同。而论文最终发表时的页码是由编辑部排版完成的。

　　Microsoft Word 提供了简易的添加页码的方法,可使页码出现在页面顶部的页眉和底部的页脚区。

　　1. 为页面顶部的页眉和页面底部的页脚添加基础页码,选择"插入"菜单中的"页码"命令,在"位置"框中,选定将页码放置于页眉中还是页脚中。如果不希望页码出现在首页,可清除"首页显示页码"对话框。如有其他需求还可选择其他所需选项进行设置。

　　2. 添加页码和其他信息,如日期和时间,在"视图"菜单中选择"页眉和页脚"命令,在"页眉和页脚"工具栏上可以选择"在页眉和页脚间切换"命令进行切换,也可以直接选择"插入页码"。如有其他需求还可选择其他所需选项进行设置。

三、页边空白和标题

　　按照惯例和美观要求底稿需要足够宽的页边空白。上下各留一英寸(约 25mm),这在两边是最低限度。在修改底稿时需要用这个空间。副本的编辑和排序也需要用这个空间做必要的说明。另外,编辑和印刷过程中,最好用带有编号线的页面,它能轻易显示出有问题的位置。在此建议根据要求在 word 里面建立好一个模板,这样就不必每次都调节格式。

　　最后论文提交之前,仔细检查标题。所有标题必须居中,上下均留空间。

　　除了主标题之外,个别杂志也采用简短标题或书眉标题(running title)。这些应作为便于阅读的标志,以引导读者浏览全文。查阅投稿杂志最新出版的刊物,确定它用什么类型的标题。标题和简短标题应该是"标记",而不是句子。

　　避免三级(甚至四级)标题,论文层次太多也影响全文的整体性和逻辑性,除非该杂志指定这种用法。通常科研底稿用二级标题已足够,许多杂志不允许用更多级的标题类型。但文献综述例外,由于综述文章太长,往往要求刊物用三级或者四级标题。

四、电子版底稿

　　现在编辑电子底稿,最常用的是 Office 软件的 Microsoft Word(以下简称 Word)。需要熟悉 Word 的功能,在撰写和编辑长篇幅的科技论文时,才能避免不断地调整格式。

　　底稿包括两个层次的含义:内容与形式。内容是指底稿中表达作者思想的文字、图片、表格、公式等整篇文章的章节段落结构。形式则是指底稿的页面、边距、字体、字号等。相同内容可以有不同形式,如一篇底稿投稿到在不同的出版社可能要求不同的形式。不同内容可以使用相同形式,如同一期刊上发表的所有文章的形式都是相同的。

　　选择模板编写底稿可以提高效率,除了 Word 提供的标题、正文等标准模板外,还可以自定义模板。对于相同排版表现内容一定要使用相同模板,这样能大大减少工作量和出错机会。如果全文调整排版格式,只需修改相关模板一次即可。使用模板的另一个优点是 Word 可以自动生成目录和索引。一般情况下,撰写底稿时需要参考作者须知,里面会有清楚的格式要求。这样,在撰写底稿前,作者就可以根据要求对模板进行一番设定,方便编写底稿。在此笔者推荐一种有效的方法解决 Word 排版问题,就是第一次按照最常见最通用的杂志排版要求对标题、摘要、正文、表格、图片等进行排版后,将该 Word 文件保存作为模板。以后撰写论文,可以在此模板基础上撰写。例如可以在此模板上撰写摘要可以删除原来的摘要再进行撰写,也可以将写好的新的摘要粘贴在模板的摘要位置,注意选择"匹配目标格式"。

（一）使用交叉引用设置编号

设置编号或序号,推荐使用交叉引用。手动输入编号或序号可能给文章的修改带来很大不便。设置标题样式可以进行标题编号,设置题注的编号可以对表格和图形的编号。录入"参见第 × 章、如图 × 所示"等字样时,使用交叉引用,不要直接敲编号。这样做的好处是,当插入或删除内容时,所有的编号和引用都会自动更新,并可自动生成图、表目录。

（二）对齐

切忌用手动敲空格来对齐段落文字,所有的对齐都应该用标尺、制表位、对齐方式和段落的缩进等来进行,尽量通过其他方法来避免手动打空格。同理,不要用敲回车来调整段落间距。

（三）绘图技巧

底稿中会用到图形和表格。表格可以通过 Word 提供的工具编写。框图和流程图等图形的编辑,可以使用 Office 中绑定的 Microsoft Office Visio Professional。Visio 对象复制到 Word 的速度相对较慢,可以试试 Smard Draw,速度比 Word 快,操作更容易,功能也比 Visio 强大,使用也比 Visio 容易。当然,如果只是最简单的柱状图、折线图,也可直接运用 Excel 软件绘图。

（四）编辑数学公式

底稿中编辑数学公式,可以使用 Math Type 5.0,Word 中的公式编辑器就是 Math Type 3.0 版。安装 Math Type 软件后,Word 会增加 MathType 这个菜单项,其操作命令一目了然。Math Type 的自动编号和引用功能,有良好的对齐效果,还能自动更新编号。在 Word 正文中插入公式常见的一个问题是把上下行距都撑大了,影响全文视图效果,这个问题可以通过固定行距来修正。这里需要注意的是,当撰写底稿时采用 Math Type 5.0 编写的公式,在打印底稿时,一定要在装 Math Type 5.0 的计算机上打印,否则公式容易"失踪"。

（五）参考文献的编辑和管理

Word 没有提供管理参考文献的功能,但 Reference Manager 或者 Endnote 可与 Word 匹配得非常好,录入参考文献就像填表格一样输入相关信息,如篇名、作者、年份等。在正文中需要引用文献和插入标记,它会自动生成美观专业的参考文献列表,并且参考文献的引用编号也是自动生成和更新的。这可以保持格式上的一致、规范,减少出错机会,还可以防止正文中对参考文献的引用与参考文献列表之间的不匹配。从长远来说,一次输入的参考文献信息可以在今后其他文章中重复利用。另外,可以使用 Word 中菜单"引用"——"插入尾注"功能插入参考文献,序号自动排列。

（六）使用分节符

如果在一篇文档里要得到不同的页码格式、页眉、页脚如摘要、前言、方法、结果和结论等,可以插入分节符,并给每一节设置不同的格式。

（七）及时保存、多做备份

设置自动保存,间隔一小段时间就 Ctrl+S。每天的工作都进行备份。Word 具有版本管理的功能,即将一个文档的多个版本保存到一个文件里,并提供比较和合并功能。但保存几个版本后,文件变得很大,一旦一个版本损坏后,所有版本都会打不开。另外,插入的图片和公式最好单独保存到文件里另做备份,防止编辑的图片和公式都变成了大红叉。在此笔者推荐几个常用而有效的保存方法:①每天工作后将文件夹的文件名后面缀上当天日期,同时并删除前面不需要的文件夹;②经常将工作后的文件以邮件或微信形式发给合作伙伴,既方便大家互相沟通工作进展,也有利于保存数据和劳动成果;③在不同的电脑和硬盘备份,以防数据丢失。

（八）大纲视图与文档结构图

使用大纲视图撰写文章的提纲,对于调整章节顺序是比较方便。使用文档结构图撰写文章提纲,可以很方便地定位章节。

五、投稿前的细节检查

底稿投稿前要进行一些细节检查,防止一些小的拼写、标点、提行等错误,目前流行的是经典 28 个细节检查。作者在投稿前,根据下面的内容逐项审查,可以避免遗漏。下面摘抄英文杂志常用的 CHECKLIST,供参考。

CHECKLIST TO USE BEFORE SUBMITTING A PAPER TO A JOURNAL

Have you …?

1. spell checked the whole paper?

2. rewritten your paper at least three times?

3. stopped working on your paper for a day?

To see and hear your words better when you look at it again.

4. put your main point into your title?

5. put your most significant findings first? Your gold first?

6. made it easy for readers to tell from your title and your abstract what is new and important about your work?

7. made sure all your verbs and subjects match?

Plural verbs have plural subjects? Singular verbs have singular subjects?

8. spelled the same name exactly the same way throughout your paper?

NOT "Bragg … Brag"

BUT BRAGG every time!

9. asked a friend or a native English speaker to read your paper and tell you what's confusing or unclear?

10. changed nouns to adjectives when necessary?

NOT "three dimension ordered array"

BUT "three dimensional ordered array"

11.　used active verbs rather than passive verbs as much as possible?

NOT "The effects were investigated ..."

BUT "We investigated the effects"

12.　found a way to break a sentence that's much too long (over 4 lines) into two sentences?

13.　broken up a paragraph that is way too long into two paragraphs?

14.　tried to reduce your paper to its skeleton by making a one page outline of it?

Might help you see if your paper is organized in the best possible way.

15.　Made all equivalent items look the same?

NOT "scheme 1 ... Scheme 2"

BUT "Scheme 1 ... Scheme 2"

16.　removed all contractions, such as "can't" or "couldn't"? and changed them to "cannot" or "could not"?

17.　checked the columns of numbers in your Tables and made all the decimal points in the same column line up vertically?

18.　put a noun right after "this" or "these" every time you use one of those words?

19.　moved "however" away from the beginning of sentences to a spot later in a sentence where it sounds better?

20.　made all your abbreviations the same?

NOT 48 hrs 3 hours 2 h five h

BUT 48 h 3 h 2 h 5 h

21.　used strong definite words?

NOT "We have been interested in"

BUT "We have focused on"

22.　used parallel wording where you lead your readers to expect it?

NOT "not only for fabricating ... but also for reduction"

BUT "not only for fabricating ... but also for reducing ..."

OR "not only for the formation of ... but also for the elimination of ..."

Don't mix words ending in "ing" with "ion" words.

23.　proofread your paper 3 times? At least!

24.　read your paper aloud to yourself?

25.　Did you use "later" when you meant "latter"?

26.　looked for fruit in your figure captions?

A fig is a fruit you can eat, but "Fig." is the correct abbreviation for "Figure." Don't forget the period in the abbreviation.

27.　proofread your references? Made sure that a journal title, no matter how often it occurs, is always spelled the same way?

28.　followed the reference format for the journal you are submitting to?

六、修改和润色

一般而言,刚刚撰写完成的初稿都不能完全达到投稿要求的,因此需要进行修改和润色。下面介绍几种常用修改稿件方法。

(一)诵读法

诵读法是一种简便易行、效果显著的方法。初稿完成后,诵读几遍,一边读一边思考,把文意不接、语意不顺、缺字少词的地方,随手改过来。

(二)比较法

把自己的初稿和同类文章中的优秀范文对照、比较,反复揣摩,分析得失,然后加以修改。这样,在改好文章的同时,也领悟到了写作之道,提高了表达水平。这种方法适合于对各类公文的修改,初学写作者也可以试试。

(三)搁置法

初稿修改时,发现一时改不好或把握不足时,可以先搁置一段时间,等到头脑冷静、思路清晰开阔后,再拿出来看看,这时,一些问题就可能被发现。

(四)旁证法

修改稿件时,多听取各方面的意见,扬长避短,去粗取精,大有益处。"三人行,必有我师焉"。自己改不下去时,可以请旁人帮助修改;或听取他人修改意见后,自己再动手改。

改稿之法因文而异,因人不同,以上方法,也不是单一的,实践中往往综合运用。文稿撰写者必须高度重视修改这一环,通过自己反复推敲、加工,使文稿从内容到形式都达到精粹、完美的高度。对于一般作者,最重要的也是反复地锤炼文章和锻炼自己。

第二节　投　　稿

研究成果只有写成论文发表后,才能得到社会的承认和转化为生产力。也就是说,只有文章被发表在期刊上,其价值才能得到体现。投稿(submission)是发表文章的必备动作。不同的杂志影响力不同(影响因子不同),投稿前应该慎重考虑目标期刊,投稿时根据杂志社要求仔细、认真、耐心准备投稿稿件。从投稿到文章发表一般经过选择期刊、投稿、修回、接受发表等步骤,每一个步骤都非常重要,都要认真对待。

一、正确选择投稿期刊

生物医学外文期刊种类繁多,即使同一分支学科或同一临床专业也有许多期刊。每个期刊的办刊宗旨、专业范围、主题分配、栏目设置及各种类型文章发表比例各不相同。在选择投稿期刊之前,我们应该首先对备选期刊有一定的了解后才能做出正确的选择。因此应该认真阅读拟投杂志的投稿须知,了解期刊特点和涉及学科范围。了解期刊,除了关注它的影响因子外,还应包括以下几点。

（1）读刊头（masthead statement,通常放在期刊前面的文题页上）,以了解刊名、办刊宗旨、编辑委员会组成、编辑部成员、出版商及各联系地址等。

（2）浏览目录和栏目设置,以确定该刊物是否会发表你研究领域的文章,以及发表的比例有多大。注意栏目设置,确定拟投稿件的栏目,看拟投栏目文章的范例,对应投稿须知了解撰写论文具体的要求及格式。

（3）某些期刊在刊登文章时候,也会刊出投稿和接收日期（submitted and accepted dates）,作者可计算出底稿从投稿到出版的发表周期。

（4）注意广告数量,以间接判断期刊质量。一些广告公司都喜欢将金钱投到质量高、影响力大的期刊上。

（5）查找期刊发行量,通过 11 或 12 月份出版的杂志最后几页上的"所有权、管理和发行声明"查找期刊发行量。

（6）核查期刊是否刊出北美和欧洲以外国家的作者撰写的文章。有些期刊还刊登报道计划,作者可依此拟订自己的投稿计划。

对期刊有了一定了解以后,还需对自己研究内容进行评估。作者首先应确定期刊的征稿范围是否涵盖自己的论文主题,论文撰写格式是否与期刊要求一致。如果答案是"否",则应立即寻找其他可能的刊物或者修改论文撰写格式。无论拟投论文多优秀,但如果不在期刊征稿范围内,则不太可能被该刊物发表,如关于骨科的研究,哪怕再有价值和意义,也不可能发表在肾脏病学杂志。

通过上述对期刊的了解,我们可以判断期刊的学术位置。大部分科研工作者都希望自己的科研成果能够发表在学术水平高的期刊上。因为高水平的期刊有利于信息的国际间传播和广泛交流,对学术成果的认可具有权威性。

选择期刊的方法有很多,无论是哪种均应先列出一个简单的拟投期刊表,然后逐一进行比较筛选,作出选择。可以通过国外著名检索系统（数据库）评估期刊的学术质量和权威性,再逐一核对自己论文主题是否在期刊征稿范围内。目前常用的数据库有以下三种:

1. ISI 数据库　即美国科学信息研究所（Institute for Scientific Information,ISI）,是国际著名数据出版公司,其文献选自 4 000 余种自然科学期刊与 3 000 余种社会科学和人文科学期刊,主要出版物《科学引文索引》（*Science Citation Index*,SCI）、《科技会议录索引》（*Index to Scientific & Technical Proceedings*,ISTP）、《现刊目录》（*Current Contents*,CC）和《期刊引证报告》（*Journal Citation Report*,JCR）。ISI 已久负盛名,成为各国进行科学评估的重要数据依据,每年都会对入选期刊进行评价。通过出版 JCR,公布其数据库收录期刊的被引证数据——影响因子（Impact Factor,IF）、及时率（即当年被引证率）、半衰期等,并在不同学科的期刊按照以上数据进行排序,其中最常见和最重要的是 IF 的排序,下面将会专门讨论。

一般而言,IF 越大,表示期刊影响越大、越具有权威性,世界著名期刊的影响因子都很高。但影响因子不是一成不变的,而是动态变化的。影响因子与期刊发行量不一定呈正比,有些期刊总是发表重要论文,其影响因子很高,但发行量相对较小。ISI 每周出版的 CC 有助于作者了解哪些期刊发表与自己研究主题相关的文章。

如果想把论文投到自己研究领域以外的期刊,查阅该期刊发表其他领域文章的概率是多少时,可查阅 JCR 的"引用期刊表",该表列出其收录期刊的论文总被引用次数及被其他期刊引用的次数,由此可了解各期刊发表其他领域论文的情况。

2. **NLM 数据库**　即美国国立医学图书馆(National Library of Medicine,NLM),收录世界上近 4 000 种医学期刊,编制的医学文献分析和联机检索系统(Medical Literature Analysis and Retrieval System,MEDLINE)及其《医学索引》(Index Medicus,IM)是世界上最有权威的医学文献检索系统。目前分析医学期刊的国际地位和知名度常根据该系统评价为指标。MEDLINE 是 NLM 的主要数据库,创建于 1966 年,可以通过联机检索期刊上已发表的论文摘要,已实现全球资源共享。IM 创建于 1879 年,仅能通过主题和作者进行检索。国内大部分医学图书馆均有 IM 供读者查询参考。如果作者仅想查询与临床医学有关的英文期刊,可通过《医学索引节略本》(Abridged Index Medicus,AIM)检索,该索引收录约 200 种英文临床医学高质量期刊。

3. **文摘数据库**　是查找相关主题论文及评估期刊学术质量的重要工具,常用的有美国著名的《生物学文摘》(Biological Abstracts,BA)、《化学文摘》(Chemical Abstracts,CA)和荷兰《医学文摘》(Excerpta Medica,EM)等。

查找各专业论文及期刊可通过相关的专业索引或文摘检索,如美国《工程索引》(Engineering Index,EI)及其联机系统 COMPENDEX 收录有关生物工程方面的论文及其期刊;《心理学文摘》(Psychological Abstracts,PA)及其联机系统 PsycINFO 收录许多与医学有关主题的论文;《社会科学文摘》(Sociological Abstracts,SA)收录与社会医学、社会精神病学有关的论文及期刊。通过索引和文摘检索时,主要的数据服务系统收录的内容有重叠。据 1984 年 NLM 公布的资料,IM 收录的约 90% 论文也被 SCI 收录,其中有 50% 出现在 CA 中。因此,建议作者仅采用 IM 或 MEDLINE 搭配一种或一种以上非 NLM 刊物的其他检索服务系统。如检索有关社会医学的论文及期刊,可通过 IM 和 PA 或《社会科学引文索引》(Social Sciences Citation Index,SKI)或《社会科学文摘》(Sociological Abstracts,SA)。检索有关临床药学,可用 IM,《药学文摘》(Excerpta Medica)和《国际药物文摘》(International Pharmaceutical Abstracts,IPA)。

二、期刊的影响因子

如果有很多期刊均适合投稿,那么应该选择哪一个呢? 杂志的声望或 IF 是重要的考虑因素。未来事业的发展(晋升、学科和实验室评估等)不能仅仅依靠发表文章的数量。评审委员会更注重期刊的质量。多篇发表在"垃圾"期刊上的文章无法与一篇发表在知名期刊上的文章相提并论。

怎样区别期刊之间的不同呢? 这并非易事,期刊分很多等级。总体来说,可以通过一些文献研究做出合理的判断。中科院 JCR 期刊分区是选择投稿杂志的一个重要参考指标。当然,也可以了解最近出版的本专业领域的重要文章,明确他们的出处。如果研究领域的大部分文章都刊登在期刊 A、B 和 C,那么你应该将投稿的目标锁定在这三个期刊中。若期刊 D、E 和 F 只是发表了些无足轻重的文章,即使其再适合于自己的研究领域,也不能视为第一选择。

目前,医学界用于外文文献检索的主要工具是 PubMed,而用于中文文献的主要检索工具包括中国知网、万方数据资源系统、中国学位论文全文数据库及维普科技期刊全文数据库)。运用其可以确定哪些期刊被引用次数较多,包括数量和每篇发表文章平均引用次数(即影响因子)方面。影响因子是美国科学情报研究所(ISI)的期刊引证报告(JCR)中的一项数据。指的是某一特定期刊的所有文章在特定年份或时期被引用的频率,它的高低是目前衡量学术期刊影响力最重要的一个指标。由尤金·加菲得(Eugene Garfield)在 1960 年代创立,目前 IF 已成为判定期刊质量的重要依据。通过 The Institute for Scientific Information(ISI)的网站 Journal Citation Report 能查找各个杂志的影响因子。

目前有两种 SCI 分区:中科院分区和 JCR 分区。前者按刊物 3 年 IF 平均值,后者按当期(1 年)的 IF 进行分区。两者都是四个分区,中科院分区分别是 1 区、2 区、3 区、4 区,JCR 分别是 Q1、Q2、Q3、Q4。中科院的分区是金字塔结构,1 区是前 5% 的期刊,2 区是 6%~20%(含 20%)的期刊,3 区是 21%~50%(含 50%)的期刊,4 区是后 50% 的期刊。JCR 根据刊物 IF 的高至低平均划分为 4 个区,每个区含有该领域总量 25% 的期刊。中科院分区有大类和小类之分,而 JCR 分区只有小类。国内作者以中科院分区为准,如果没有特别要求以中科院分区小类为准,我们就默认以中科院分区大类标准为主。

三、期刊的发表周期

另一个需要考虑的因素是期刊发行的频率。月刊间隔的时间比季刊短。假如审稿时间相等,季刊则额外滞后 2~3 个月才能发表。由于出版滞后,加上编辑审稿的时间,很多月刊的滞后时间介于 4~7 个月,季刊可能会累积到 10 个月。并且很多期刊都存在积压现象,不管是月刊、双月刊还是季刊。某些杂志也设有"绿色通道",即能在短期内刊登已经接受发表的文章,但是,作者必须支付相对较多的费用。整体上,外国期刊强调研究的实效性、创新性,所以发表周期较短,甚至有的杂志在一个月内就可以发表,而国内期刊往往所需时间较长。但是随着我国医学事业和出版业的不断发展,尤其是网络投稿系统的发展,国内期刊的发表周期也大大缩短了。这样既为科研工作者或者临床医师节省了时间,也使我们的最新研究能够尽快与读者见面。

四、期刊的读者群

期刊声望、发行量及发行频率都是非常重要的。但是文章的读者群是谁呢?假如你正在报告一个生物化学方面的重要研究,你当然应该试着把文章刊登在该领域具有国际影响力的期刊上。有关病理学的研究最好发表在 The Journal of Pathology 上,而临床研究的文章则应该投稿到 The New England Journal of Medicine。综合性杂志的读者群往往较广,例如 Science 几乎涵盖各个科学学科。而比如 The Journal of Urology 杂志大多数读者是从事与泌尿外科专业相关的科研人员与临床医生。所以,每个期刊都有自己特定的读者群。

五、在线投稿

目前,各大杂志都已经实现在线投稿。

在线投稿的过程为进入该杂志主页,然后在"用户登录"栏进行注册,也叫作者登记。一般要求作者填写姓名、单位、地址,联系方式包括电话、传真和电子邮箱等信息。登记完成后,就根据系统提示依次输入文章信息和各部分内容,如题目、摘要、关键词、作者、正文、图表等。在输入每部分时,一定要通读该部分的有关要求,确认自己输入的文件是否符合要求,如按要求,原稿不能超过 20 页,但有的原稿长达 40 多页,甚至更长,这就需要缩减;有的刊物要求关键词 5~10 个,如果原稿只有 4 个,则必须补充到 5 个以上,10 个以下。输入完稿件内容和信息后,需要检查每部分内容输入的完整性,如果系统检查完整性没有问题,有的期刊可以选择将所有投稿部分生成 PDF 文件浏览投稿全貌,这样作者可以检查一下投稿内容是否完整,如有时作者在输入文件时过于匆忙,十个图只输入一半,生成 PDF 后仔细浏览,可以发现遗漏的图,这样就避免了不完整稿件投到编辑部导致不好的结论或评审结果。最后在检查完所有部分完整输入,生成的投稿完整时,不要忘了点击投稿发送键。否则,稿件只会存储在作者自己的文件夹中,而不是发到编辑部。原稿在网上成功投出后,作者的邮箱能立刻收到编辑部的回执。如果有问题,投稿网页会出现问题预警或解决问题的提示。如果作者不能根据提示解决问题或问题反复出现,可与杂志社网上投稿支持部门联系,寻求帮助。值得一提的是,部分著名杂志的网页上除有作者投稿须知外,还专门附有网上投稿的指导示范文件。作者初次投稿时,可以根据示范文件提示,一步一步投稿。总之,网上投稿并不难,关键是原稿要准备充分,投稿过程中根据网页提示按部就班,遇到疑问不要视而不见,不能单纯求快,否则欲速而不达。

在线投稿往往都需要作者有一个固定的邮箱,大都采用邮箱来注册,设置的密码应该是容易记忆且常用,按照网站的要求逐步填写作者,上传论文,一般在论文上传后都能直接在网站链接上找到生成的 PDF 格式的论文,以供作者审阅。

在最后提交(submit)前,随时可以修改文章的内容以及填写的其他数据。

六、投稿信

在每次投稿时应该附带给编辑写一封投稿信(Cover Letter)。Cover Letter 要求直截了当地向编辑说明投稿的背景,明确投稿的期刊,如果是第一次投稿,还需要详细指明通讯作者及其联系方式,语言要精练,词句要简明。在撰写 Cover Letter 还要明确以下问题:是原始底稿还是编辑要求修回的稿件(如果是修回稿件,编辑又是谁),或者是被审稿人或编辑写错了地址的稿件? 如果有多个作者,哪位是供稿作者,地址是什么? 地址是特别重要的,因为底稿上面显示的地址不一定是供稿作者的地址。在投稿信中或底稿首页应该注明供稿作者的电话和邮箱地址。

每个杂志的具体要求不一样,一般在杂志的 guide for authors 或 instruction for authors 会提到。如果没有说明具体要求,可按通用要求书写。下面是几个 Cover Letter 的例子。

示例 1:

From

Jian Guo Wen, MD, PhD, Professor

The Pediatric Urodynamic Center and Pediatric Surgery,

First Affiliated Hospital of Zhengzhou University

China

Email: × × × × × ×

2009-05-28

To

Dr Jan Adolfsson

Editor in Chief, Scandinavian Journal of Urology and Nephrology

Dear Editor, Dr. Adolfsson,

Thank you for your kind review of our manuscript entitled "Expression of renal aquaporins is downregulated in children with congenital hydronephrosis" (SJUN-2009-0145). It has been revised accordingly.

A list of abbreviations has been enclosed in the end of revised manuscript and "Abstract page 2 line 17-23 (Both RT-PCR and immunoblotting. …) of MATERIAL and METHODS in the old version has been moved to the RESULTS on new version of revised manuscript. We are sorry for our careless in preparing the first version of the manuscript. Hope the revised manuscript has fulfilled the requirement of the publication.

Thanks again for your kind help.

Sincerely yours,

Jian Guo Wen, MD

Zhen Zhen Li, MD

Represents of all coauthors

示例 2：

Dear editors:

This is our manuscript entitled "The effects of periventricular white matter injury (PWMI) on the bladder function of preterm infant" by Ya Lun Wang, Jian Guo Wen, Yu Ming Xu, et. This manuscript is submitted to be considered for publication as an "original article" in your journal.

All authors have read and approved the version of this article, and due care has been taken to ensure the integrity of the work. We certified this submission is original work and neither the entire paper nor any part of its content has been published or has been accepted elsewhere. This manuscript is not being submitted to any other journal.

In this manuscript we found the effects of PWMI on the voiding pattern of preterm infant is obvious indicating the cortex have participated in the voiding of preterm infant.

We believe this paper may be of particular interest to the readers of your journal as it refer to the effects of the brain injury of neonate on the voiding pattern conforming to the content requirement of your journal.

Thank you very much for your attention to our paper.

Sincerely yours.

Ya Lun Wang on behalf of the authors.

Corresponding author: Yu Ming Xu at the Department of Neurology and Jian Guo Wen at the Urodynamic Center of Children, the First Affiliated Hospital of Zhengzhou University, Zhengzhou 450052, China. Email: ××××××, phone number: ××××××××; fax number: ××××××;

下面再列举一个作者投稿到 *The Journal of urology* 的稿件修回时的 Cover Letter：

RE: JU-09-605R1

Dear Dr. Rushton:

Thank you very much for your comments and suggestion on my manuscript (JU-09-605R1)-on Bilateral Renal Melamine Related Calculus in 50 Children: A Single Centre Experience in Clinical Diagnosis and Treatment.

The article has been revised based on the appended critiques from your consultants and the answers have been attached.

A detailed explanation of the revisions following each comment made by the reviewers with an indication of where the changes have been made in the text has been provided. The details of the changes made to the revised text have been highlighted in bold type to help identify them. The re-revised manuscript has been revised again by Prof. S.B. Bauer, Department of Urology, Children's Hospital, Boston, USA and Prof. Corcos, Department of Urology, McGill University, Montreal, Canada. We appreciate very much their kind help.

The length of the text has been reduced to 2 240 words (not including Abstract part). The number of references has been limited to 17 and the first 3 authors have been listed for each reference.

The revised manuscript has been uploaded.

Sincerely yours,

Jian Guo Wen, MD, PhD, Professor

Department of Pediatric surgery

First affiliated hospital of Zhengzhou University

Zhengzhou, 450052; China

E-mail: × × × × × ×

第三节　校稿和预订

一、校稿过程

以下简要描述了文章被采纳后所经过的校对（proof reading）过程。

在校正拼音和语法错误时,底稿通常需要经过一个编辑过程。编辑将核对所有的缩写词、度量单位、标点符号和拼写,使其标准化,以便与杂志格式保持一致。如果底稿有任何不明确或者需要附加说明时,编辑可能会直接与你沟通。

编辑部将校样稿通过邮箱寄回作者,让作者核对文章所做的修改、检查排版错误、回答编辑提出的所有问题。最后,排版者将输入作者修改过的校样稿。这个版本即为出版后在杂志上看到的最终版本。

二、为什么把校样发送给作者

一旦底稿被采用,有些作者就会不再关注它;当收到校样时,他们也很少会留意,并认为论文不会再有任何错误。为什么要把校样发送给作者？一个重要的原因是检查排版类型的准确性。换句话说，你应该认真检查校样中的排版错误。无论你的底稿多么完美，只有发表才有意义。如果出版的文章有严重的错误，随后会产生各种各样的问题，至少损坏你的名声。这种损害是非常实际的，因为过多的错误会完全破坏读者对文章的理解。有时一个放错位置的小数点就能使一篇已经出版的论文变得毫无用处。

三、单词拼写错误

单词拼写错误虽然对理解文章影响不大，但是对作者的名誉影响不好，会令人笑话的。如果论文中提到"远（院）内感染"，读者明白你的意思，但会把它当成一个笑话，而你并不会认为其很好笑。

如果阅读校样时，你用平常阅读科研论文同样的方法和速度，那么你可能将会漏过 90% 的排字错误。

阅读校样最好的方法是：第一，阅读。第二，审核。正如我刚才所提到的那样，阅读将会漏过 90% 的排字错误，但是它能够发现遗漏的错误。如果印刷漏掉一行，那么阅读是发现这个错误唯一可行的方法。或者让两个人阅读校样，一个人大声朗读，同时，另一个人跟随他的节奏仔细核对底稿。

上文中提到了一个放错位置的小数点可能会导致严重的错误。校对时通常有一个惯例：认真仔细地检查每一个数字，尤其是要仔细核对表格，这很重要。原因有二：第一，在输入数字时错误经常发生，特别是表格性材料；第二，你是唯一能够发现这种错误的人。大多数拼写错误是在印刷人员的校对室或者杂志编辑部被发现的。但是，这些职业校对者是通过"目测"发现错误的；而他们无法知道"16"实际上应该是"61"。

四、标记修改处

当你在校样中发现某个错误时，这个错误被标记两次。一是在它发生错误的原位置，另一是在它旁边的页边空白部分。排版者就是通过页边空白标记来识别错误的。只在排版正文中提示的修改很容易被漏掉；旁批用来提醒人们注意它。

如果你清晰明了地标记出修改内容，那么这个恰当的修改是成功的。如果你采用已制定的校对标记，就能够减少误解的机会，为自己和所有相关者节省时间。标记是一种广泛用于所有出版业的语言。所以，如果你愿意花费时间去学习这种语言，你将能够运用它们去校对职业生涯中可能涉及的各种排版材料。

五、对校样的附加说明

本章的前半部分描述了将校样发送给作者是为了让他们检查排版的准确性。此外，校对阶段不是修订、改写、增加更多新资料或者做任何其他重大改变。不能对校样做太大变动有三大原因。

第一，道德理由。无论是校样还是校样中的改动都不是编辑一个人看的，除非这是一个人操作的小杂志，否则做出重大改动是不妥当的。在同行审阅后，校样是被编辑认可的底稿而且应该印刷出来,而不是一些包括没有被编辑和审稿人看过内容的其他新版本。

第二,打乱排版材料是不明智的,除非确实有必要。因为这样做可能会增加新的排字错误。如果在一行中插入一个单词,那么下面的许多行可能需要重新排版(保持均匀或者"合理的"页面)。

第三,修改的费用昂贵。你不能滥用出版社的时间(除非你是一个科学协会的忠实会员);另外,这样做很可能对你的修改付出一大笔费用。大多数杂志对作者一些合理的修改收取费用。如果你公然地对校样做过多改变,那些总编辑或者业务经理将迟早制裁你。

允许一定类型的添加校对。当一篇同样或相关主题的论文已经出版,而你的论文尚在校对中,这时添加就很需要了。如果有新的研究内容,你可能想改写论文的几个部分,但是必须抵制住这种诱惑,上文已经陈述了原因。你需要做的是在校对中准备一份短附录(只有几句话),描述新研究的大致性质,并提供参考文献书目。这样一来,附录就可以打印在结尾部分而不影响论文的主体。

六、增加参考文献

很常见,当出版一篇新论文时,你想增加参考文献,但是你不需要对正文做任何明显的改变,这与你既想增加一些语句又想增加一些新参考文献不同(下文显示杂志采用依编号、字母顺序排列目录的方法)。

如果你在校样中增加一个参考文献,不要给参考文献重编号。许多作者都会犯重编号的错误。这种错误是严重的,因为这样需要在参考文献和文章中做许多改动,无论引用参考文献的编码出现在哪里,都将涉及巨大的改动;文章中受影响的行列被重新输入时会产生新的错误;几乎可以肯定的是,你至少会遗漏其中一个参考文献。原来的旧编码也将出现在印刷版本中,使文献更混乱。

你应该做的是给新的参考文献增加一个编号"a"。如果这个参考文献按字母顺序排列介于文献 16 和 17 之间,用"16a"表示并加入其中。这样,剩下的目录编号就不必再做改动了。

当然,随着软件的发展,现在如果应用专业的参考文献软件例如 Endnote 等,可以完美地解决这个问题。任意添加文献,后面的参考文献编号可以自动修改。同时交叉引用或者投稿不同杂志社对参考文献要求不同的问题,该软件都可以很简单地完成。

七、校对图表

仔细检查校样图表特别重要。通常,原始底稿和原始图表随校样一起返回给作者。尽管杂志编辑部的校对者帮你寻找了排版错误,但你必须判断图表是否能有效地被复制。校样必须和原稿进行比较。

不知道说的什么意思?图表和其他线形图很少有问题,除非编辑认为它们的尺寸太小而难以辨认,或比例不匹配,但这种情况很少发生。

然而,照片有时也会出现问题,这应该是由作者自己来发现。与原稿相比,如果校样后照片整体颜色较暗,可能是因为感光过度所致;如果细节缺失,应该重新扫描印刷照片(不要忘了把原始图表和校样一起归还)。

如果校样比副本颜色淡，这可能由于曝光不足导致。然而，也可能是"印刷者"（指所有涉及印刷过程的所有工作者）有意将照片拍成这样。特别是缺少对比照片时，曝光不足比正常曝光能包含更多的细节。所以，比较曝光水平不是主要的，而要留意细节问题。

有时候照片的某一个区域会特别重要。如果是这样，而你对复制品不满意，可以通过旁批或用一个涂盖层告诉印刷者，印刷者就会把重点放在这部分上。

八、认真校对，减少抱怨

很多作者在自己的文章被出版后发现文章的某些地方仍存在瑕疵，比如抱怨图片的位置被印颠倒或者偏向一侧等。其实出现这些错误只能怪当初自己在校对时没有认真负责的去逐字逐段的修改，所以，如果你打算抱怨，那就请在校对时抱怨吧。无论你相信与否，你的抱怨很可能被杂志社慷慨地接受。交纳版面费的人知道，为确保出版质量，我们已经做了大量投入。我们需要把好质量关，不能让钱财浪费。

通过优秀的出版商雇用优秀的印刷工作人员，才能印刷出优秀的期刊。已出版的论文会刊出作者姓名，但这与出版商和印刷者的名声也息息相关。他们期待你与他们合作，从而出版更好的论文。

由于这些杂志的主编必须保证论文的印刷质量，所以他们绝不会以低价雇佣印刷者。约翰.罗斯金曾说过："世上的东西，总是有可以妥协的余地，价钱也并非不可动摇，于是只在乎价钱的人就成了商家的合法猎物。"毫无疑问，价格是保证印刷质量的重要指标，有好价格才有好质量。

第四节　如何订购杂志或文章单行本

正如 John K. Crum 指出的那样："Most authors will purchase between 100 and 300 copies of reprints for each article they publish, for 'professional self-advertising' for distribution to their colleagues upon demand."。这里简要介绍有关文章被采用发表后订购杂志或文章单行本的注意事项。

有一些期刊仍然通过"印刷期刊"程序生产抽印本。如果采用这个程序，你应及早确定你的订单。早期按照指示寄回样本和订购表格，不要等着正式订单，否则会打乱你自己的工作安排。试着找到一个采购订单号码，拿到采购订单号本身也可能出现延迟。

新的系统有一个巨大的优势：论文的出版可以随时随量。因此，如果你发表在这样的期刊，你根本不需要担心出版的论文数量。

典型的价格清单出示在表 15-1 中。

表 15-1

Pages	100	200	300	400	500	Additional 100's
4	$137	$156	$172	$189	$204	$15
8	211	235	258	276	297	19

续表

Pages	100	200	300	400	500	Additional 100's
12	294	325	355	381	407	24
16	390	427	463	497	531	31
20	488	532	576	615	652	37

第16章
投稿前审查和投稿后审稿

Chapter 16
How to Check and Review the Manuscripts Before and After the Submission

　　随着科研的国际化及研究生培养机制的发展,国内出现了越来越多的英文科研论文,并且在数量与质量方面都有了飞跃的提升。但是,与西方国家相比,医学领域的科研成果向国外期刊投稿的比例并不高,接收率则更低。究其原因,除了国内作者英文写作与表述能力较差之外,还与作者对国外期刊的投稿政策及标准并不了解有很大关系。往往有很多比较优秀的稿件,因不熟悉国外期刊的投稿范围和投稿程序导致拒稿,错失了最佳投稿时间,以致在与同行间的竞争中处于劣势。因此,医学工作者在掌握如何撰写英文科研论文的同时,也有必要了解如何进行英文科研论文投稿前的审查程序和投稿后的审稿过程。

第一节　投稿前审查

　　在选择期刊投稿之前,作者对稿件的自我判断尤为重要,严谨的作者不仅是自己所写论文领域的专家,也将对本人所写文章的创新性进行初步判断。本书作者作为十余种国内外杂志的特约审稿人,在审阅过程中发现很多文章存在写作格式及表述不准确、语法错误多等诸多不符合投稿要求的问题,这表明文章作者并没有充分认识到投稿前自我审稿的重要性。如果文章因为上述原因而降低其学术性,甚至导致退稿就很令人惋惜。虽然作者自我审稿不是第三方审稿,但是作者可从自我编审角度来尽力完善稿件,提高编辑和审稿专家的认知度,也为提高论文的刊用率打下基础。因此,我们有必要鼓励和引导作者进行自我审稿。

一、投稿须知

　　投稿前需要仔细阅读杂志的《投稿须知》部分。它通常位于杂志网站首页的突出位置,属于"author information"内容中的重要部分。我们首先需要通过杂志的"投稿须知"了解该杂志的研究目标和范围,从而确定自己所做的研究是否符合杂志的宗旨;其次需要了解该杂志的具体要求,包括伦理要求、格式要求、排版要求、插图及表格限制、需提供的附件等等内容,并根据要求对自己的文章进行修改,使其符合投稿所需条件。杂志要求动物实验和临床试验一定需要当地伦理委员会的批准和审核后方可进行,需要作者提供伦理委员会审核编号。作者充分准备好投稿所需的一切资料后,便可开始投稿过程了。

　　总之,投稿前的作者自我审查有助于完善论文的内容和形式,提高作者论文的水平,还有助于作者发现新问题,补充新证据。在文章写好后,我们不妨将其放置一周左右,然后再重新通读审视,这时,极有可能发现文章中原本存在的一些问题,如论证不力、表述不清、语法错误、错写漏写等。重新通读文章还可能因某种触动产生新的思考。作为作者,千万不能写完后马上投出,站在编辑的角度重新审视文稿是十分重要的,也是慢慢提高自己写作水平和逻辑思维水平的重要步骤。在自我审稿过程中,需要站在编辑角度对文章提出质疑,找到问题并加以修补和改正,力求作品臻于完美。

二、根据杂志要求自我审稿

在上一节中,我们已经初步了解杂志"投稿须知"的重要性,下面我们将结合实例为大家详细讲解如何按照杂志要求对自己的稿件进行审核和修改。

一般来说,在投稿 SCI 文章之前,作者需要先在相关杂志网页上下载"Information for Authors",了解杂志对所投稿件的相关要求,使作者在投稿前按照要求先自我审稿,以便符合杂志的审核规定。认真阅读和使用"作者须知",需要作者做到:

1. 读刊头(masthead statement)　刊头包含的信息有杂志的宗旨,内容,编辑部成员,出版商及联系地址等。

2. 浏览目录(table of contents)　注意查看杂志的发文意向,以推断自己投稿文章的接收概率。

3. 注意观察杂志接收的文章类型　如论著、综述、评论等。

4. 可在杂志主页上下载近期发表的文章全文,并据此对自己文章进行格式调整。

5. 可根据杂志已发表文章的投稿日期和发表日期间隔,从而推断出杂志通常的见刊周期有多久。

6. 查看杂志所刊发文章中是否囊括各个不同国家,有没有地域差别。

7. 是否收费,收费金额是否在自己承受范围之内。

现将一些英文杂志的"Information for Authors"的部分内容列举如下:

1.《柳叶刀》(*The Lancet*)

(1) 文章研究方向审核:下面是 *The Lancet* "作者须知"中关于论著研究方向的说明,需要作者在投稿前先审核自己文章内容是否符合杂志要求。

The Lancet priorities reports of original research that are likely to change clinical practice or thinking about a disease (*Lancet* 2000; 356:2-4). We invite submission of all clinical trials, whether phase I, II, or III (see *Lancet* 2006; 368:827-28). For phase I trials, we especially encourage those of a novel substance for a novel indication, if there is a strong or unexpected beneficial or adverse response, or a novel mechanism of action. Systematic reviews of randomised trials about diseases that have a major effect on human health also might warrant rapid peer review and publication. Global public-health and health-policy research are other areas of interest to *The Lancet*. We encourage the registration of all interventional trials, whether early or late phase, in a primary register that participates in WHO's International Clinical Trial Registry Platform (see *Lancet* 2007; 369:1909-11). We also encourage full public disclosure of the minimum 20-item trial registration dataset at the time of registration and before recruitment of the first participant (see *Lancet* 2006; 367:1631-35 and http://www.who.int/ictrp/dataset/en/index1.html). The registry must be independent of for-profit interest. Reports of randomised trials must conform to revised CONSORT guidelines, and should be submitted with their protocols. All reports of clinical trials must include a summary of previous research findings, and explain how this trial contributes to the sum of knowledge. The relation between existing and new evidence should be shown by direct reference to an existing systematic review and meta-analysis; if neither exists, authors are encouraged to do their own, or to describe the qualitative association between their research and previous findings (see *Lancet* 2005; 366:107). All reports of randomised trials should include a section entitled Randomisation and masking, within the Methods section.

- Cluster randomised trials must be reported according to CONSORT extended guidelines.
- Randomised trials that report harms must be described according to extended CONSORT guidelines.
- Studies of diagnostic accuracy must be reported according to STARD guidelines.
- Observational studies (cohort, case-control, or cross-sectional designs) must be reported according to the STROBE statement.
- Genetic association studies must be reported according to STREGA guidelines.
- Systematic reviews and meta-analyses must be reported according to PRISMA guidelines.

从以上要求可以看出,杂志将优先考虑刊登有可能改变临床实践或某种疾病观点的原创性研究(Lancet 2000;356:2-4)。杂志欢迎各种类型的临床试验研究,无论是Ⅰ期临床、Ⅱ期临床还是Ⅲ期临床研究(Lancet 2006;368:827-828)。对于Ⅰ期临床试验,如果存在强烈或意外的疗效或者存在新的有益或不良反应或新的作用机制,杂志将特别鼓励具有这些特性的文章的发表。对人类健康有重大影响疾病的随机试验的系统回顾性研究也可能进入快速的同行评审和发表渠道。全球公共卫生和卫生政策研究也是《柳叶刀》感兴趣的一个领域。杂志鼓励所有的介入性试验研究在世卫组织国际临床试验注册平台登记处进行注册,无论是早期还是晚期(Lancet 2007;369:1909-11)。杂志还鼓励在注册时和招募第一名受试者之前向社会完全公开披露最低的 20 项试验注册数据包(Lancet 2006;367:1631-35 和 http://www.who.int/ictrp/dataset/en/index1.html)。注册管理机构必须是非盈利机构。随机试验报告必须符合修订后的 CONSORT 指南,并应与其协议一起提交。所有的临床试验报告都必须包括对以前研究结果的总结,并解释该试验如何有助于提高知识。现有证据和新证据之间的关系应通过直接参考现有的系统评价和 meta 分析来显示;如果既没有系统评价也没有荟萃分析发表,那么杂志鼓励作者自己进行评价分析,或者描述自己的研究与以前的发现之间的定性关联(Lancet 2005;366:107)。所有随机试验报告都应在方法部分包括一节标题为"随机化和分组"的内容。

- 必须根据 CONSORT 扩展指南报告整群随机试验。
- 报告危害的随机试验必须根据扩展的 CONSORT 指南进行描述。
- 必须根据 STARD 指南报告诊断准确性的研究。
- 观察性研究(队列,病例对照或横断面设计)必须根据 STROBE 声明进行报告。
- 遗传关联研究必须根据 STREGA 指南报告。
- 必须根据 PRISMA 指南报告系统评价和 meta 分析。

(2)其他方面审核:作者同时还需对文章字数、结构、计量单位等方面进行全面审核。*Lancet* 中相关信息如下:

All Articles should, as relevant:

- Be up to 3 000 words with 30 references.

- Include an abstract (semistructured summary), with five paragraphs (Background, Methods, Findings, Interpretation, and Funding), not exceeding 300 words. Our electronic submission system will ask you to copy and paste this section at the "Submit Abstract" stage.

- For randomised trials, the abstract should adhere to CONSORT extensions: abstracts (see *Lancet* 2008; 371:281-83).

- For intervention studies, the abstract should include the primary outcome expressed as the difference between groups with a confidence interval on that difference (absolute differences are more useful than relative ones). Important secondary outcomes can be included as long as they are clearly marked as secondary.

- Use the SI system of units and the recommended international non-proprietary name (rINN) for drug names. Ensure that the dose, route, and frequency of administration of any drug you mention are correct.

- Use gene names approved by the Human Gene Organisation. Novel gene sequences should be deposited in a public database (GenBank, EMBL, or DDBJ), and the accession number provided. Authors of microarray papers should include in their submission the information recommended by the MIAME guidelines. Authors should also submit their experimental details to one of the publicly available databases: Array Express or GEO.

- Include any necessary additional data as part of your EES submission.

- All accepted Articles should include a link to the full study protocol published on the authors' institutional website (see *Lancet* 2009; 373:992).

从以上信息可以看出,所有文章应该:

- 最多不超过 3 000 个单词和 30 篇参考文献。

- 文章包含摘要(半结构摘要),长度不超过 300 字。电子提交系统会要求作者在"提交摘要"阶段复制并粘贴本节。

- 对于随机试验,摘要应符合 CONSORT 扩展:摘要(参见 Lancet 2008;371:281-83)的要求。

- 对于干预研究,摘要应包括主要结果,表现为组间差异(置信区间为差异)(绝对差异比相对差异更有用)。只要明确标记为次要,就可以包括重要的次要结果。

- 使用 SI 系统的单位和推荐的国际非专有名称(rINN)作为药物名称。确保提及的任何药物的给药剂量,途径和频率都是正确的。

- 使用人类基因组织批准的基因名称。新基因序列应存放在公共数据库(GenBank,EMBL 或 DDBJ)中,并提供登录号。微阵列论文的作者应在其提交的资料中包含 MIAME 指南推荐的信息。作者还应将其实验细节提交给公众可用的数据库之一:Array Express 或 GEO。

- 包含任何必要的附加数据,作为 EES 提交的一部分。

- 所有接受的文章应包括在作者机构网站上公布的完整研究协议的链接(参见 Lancet 2009;373:992)。

2. 美国《泌尿外科杂志》(*Journal of Urology*)

以下是美国《泌尿外科杂志》"作者须知"中对论著的要求。

Original, Research and Special Articles should be arranged as follows: Title Page, Abstract, Introduction, Materials and Methods, Results, Discussion, Conclusions, References, Tables, Legends. The title page should contain a concise, descriptive title, the names and affiliations of all authors, and a brief descriptive running head not to exceed 50 characters. One to five key words should be typed at the bottom of the title page. These words should be identical to the medical subject headings (MeSH) that appear in the Index Medicus of the National Library of Medicine. The abstract should not exceed 250 words and must conform to the following style: Purpose, Materials and Methods, Results and Conclusions.

从以上要求可以看出,论著需要按以下几部分来安排:扉页、摘要、引言、材料和方法、结果、讨论、结论、参考文献和图表。扉页中包括简明扼要的题目、所有作者的名字和单位,描述简洁,不超过 50 个单词。扉页的最下面为 1~5 个关键词,这些关键词需要与美国国家医学图书馆(National Library of Medicine)医学索引(Index Medicus)中的医学论文主题词(medical subject headings,MeSH)保持一致。摘要不应超过 250 个单词,并按照目的、材料和方法、结果和结论的形式撰写。

References should not exceed 30 readily available citations for all articles (except Review Articles). Self-citations should be kept to a minimum. References should be cited by superscript numbers as they appear in the text, and they should not be alphabetized. References should include the names and initials of the first 3 authors, the complete title, the abbreviated journal name according to the Index Medicus of the National Library of Medicine, the volume, the beginning page number and the year. References to book chapters should include names and initials of the first 3 chapter authors, chapter title, book title and edition, names and initials of the first 3 book editors, city of publisher, publisher, volume number, chapter number, page range and year. In addition to the above, references to electronic publications should include type of medium, availability statement and date of accession. The statistical methods should be indicated and referenced. Enough information should be presented to allow an independent critical assessment of the data.

除了综述外,所有文章引用的参考文献不应超过 30 个。自我引用不要太多。参考文献需要在合适的位置用数字进行上标,不按字母顺序进行排列。参考文献的格式包括前 3 位作者的姓名及缩写、题目全称、根据国家医学图书馆医学索引中的杂志名称缩写、卷、起始页及年份。书籍的参考文献格式为前 3 位作者的姓名及缩写、章的题目、书的题目及版本、前 3 位编辑的姓氏和名字首字母、出版地、出版商、卷、章、页码范围及年份。除了以上内容,电子出版物的参考文献还应包括媒介类型、实用性声明和接受日期。统计学方法应指明出处。参考文献应提供足够的信息保证数据进行独立的决定性评估。

Digital illustrations and tables should be kept to a necessary minimum and their information should not be duplicated in the text. No more than 10 illustrations should accompany the manuscript for clinical articles. Magnifications for photomicrographs should be supplied and graphs should be labeled clearly. Reference to illustrations, numbered with Arabic numerals, must be provided in the text. Blurry or unrecognizable illustrations are not acceptable. Visit http://rapidinspector.cadmus.com/zww for detailed instructions for digital art. The use of color is encouraged at no charge to the authors. Tables should be numbered and referred to in the text. In general, they should present summarized rather than individual raw data.

图表尽量要少,避免与文章内容重复。临床型文章不超过 10 张图,微观图需要提供放大倍数,且标示清楚。图表出现在文章中的位置应用阿拉伯数字标注清楚,模糊或难以辨认的图表不予接受。更多关于图表的详细说明,请登陆 http://rapidinspector.cadmus.com/zww 进行查询。彩图不再另行收费。表格应排序,并在文章恰当的位置标注清楚。一般来说,作者应提供概括好的数据而非原始数据。

第二节　投稿后审稿流程

一、内部评审

作者投稿之后,稿件会被上传并保存至杂志编辑部,编辑部将组织一名或以上由科学家组成的工作人员进行评审,初步审核稿件是否符合本刊宗旨。不合格的稿件将被退稿,合格稿件进入下一步的同行评审阶段。

以《柳叶刀》为例,该杂志对文章进行筛选的重要一环即是内部评审。编辑会对投稿文章的内容和质量进行初步把关,不少文章在这一环节中就铩羽而归。一旦无法通过内部评审,拒稿通常发生在一周内。

二、同行评审

如果文章通过了内部评审,接下来将会被编辑送出进行同行评议。参与评议的审稿人多为 2~3 人。正常情况下,所有在英文杂志上发表的文章都会经过同行评议过程,但是对于一些非研究类文章,如"correspondence"或者"comment",有些则不需经过同行评审即可决定结果。

1. **编辑部组织专家评审**　编辑部选择合适的审稿人对稿件进行审理。如何选择审稿人非常重要,下面列举《自然》(Nature)杂志对如何选择审稿人的说明:

Selecting peer-reviewers

Reviewer selection is critical to the publication process, and we base our choice on many factors, including expertise, reputation, specific recommendations and our own previous experience of a reviewer's characteristics. For instance, we avoid using people who are slow, careless, or do not provide reasoning for their views, whether harsh or lenient. We check with potential reviewers before sending them manuscripts to review. Reviewers should bear in mind that these messages contain confidential information, which should be treated as such.

从以上信息可以看出,审稿人的选择对于文章出版过程非常重要。编辑部会考虑审稿人多种因素,包括是否为专家、声望、具体建议及审稿人以往的审稿经历等。杂志社避免使用那些审稿不及时、不认真或不能提供审阅原因的审稿人,不管其审阅严厉还是宽松。编辑部会在给审稿人发送手稿之前和其进行联系,审稿人应该对文章涉及的内容严格保密,不能随意泄露。

编辑部将预审稿件分别发送给三位评审人,并告知受理审稿期限、上传网址、用户名和密码。审稿人需在规定时间内完成审稿,并上传审稿意见。

2. **审稿人审稿**　审稿人一般是所投稿件相关专业、领域的专家,其在收到编辑部发送的预审稿件及相关信息后,会及时进行阅稿并撰写审稿意见。

杂志审稿要求:有时,编辑部在告知审稿人进行审稿的同时,会将杂志的审稿要求一并发送给审稿人。下面是美国《泌尿外科杂志》邀请文建国教授审核一篇文章时所附的杂志审稿要求,如下:

GUIDELINES FOR ASSESSING SCIENTIFIC ARTICLES

1）Is the title specific and appropriate for literature search retrieval?

2）Does the abstract provide details regarding: Purpose, Materials and Methods, Results and Conclusions?

3）Are the objectives of the investigation clearly stated in the Introduction?

4）Are the methods described well enough to reproduce the experiment or study?

5）Is the followup adequately detailed?

6）Can the reader assess the results based on the data provided?

7）Are the conclusions supported by the data presented?

8）Is there a summary of the findings and implications of what was found?

9）Have the authors provided the reader with potential problems and limitations of their study?

10）Have the authors explained why and how their study differs from others already ublished?

11）Are the references complete, accurate and appropriately cited in the text, following Journal guidelines (number and format)?

通过以上信息,我们可以看出,科研论文审稿要求具体如下:

1）文题是否详尽,是否适合文献检索。

2）摘要是否提供了详细信息,包括:目的、材料和方法、结果及结论。

3）研究目的是否在引言中阐述清楚。

4）实验方法能否被继续重复实验或研究。

5）随访研究资料是否详细。

6）读者能否在所提供数据的基础上评估结果。

7）数据是否支持结论。

8）论文是否含有研究结果总结和所发现研究结果的提示。

9）作者是否给读者提供研究的潜在问题和局限性。

10）作者是否已经解释其研究为什么和如何不同于其他已发表的研究。

11）参考文献是否完整、准确,引用是否合适,是否遵照杂志的要求(数量、格式)?

3. **审稿人上传审稿意见**　审稿人撰写完审稿意见后,需及时将其上传至编辑部指定的网址上,并填写相关信息。现将美国《泌尿外科杂志》审稿人上传审稿意见流程举例如下:

（1）审稿人登录网址:http://ju.edmgr.com/,输入用户名和密码,点击"Reviewer Login"进入审稿人页面。

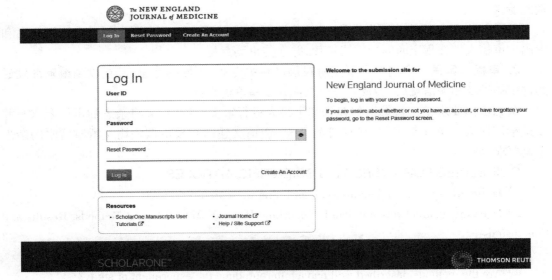

（2）按照步骤一一填写，这里就不再详细说明。

（3）查看审稿记录，详见下图。

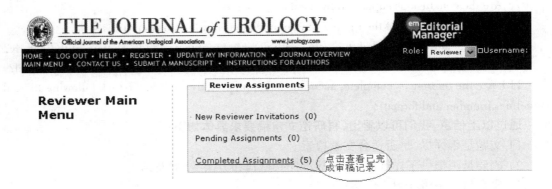

下图是一个美国《泌尿外科杂志》审稿记录。

Completed Reviewer Assignments for Jian Guo Wen, MD												
Page: 1 of 1 (5 total assignments)								Display 10 results per page.				
Action	My Reviewer Number	Manuscript Number	Article Type	Article Title	Status Date	Current Status	Final Disposition	Date Reviewer Invited	Date Reviewer Agreed	Date Review Due	Date Review Submitted	Days Take
Action Links	3	JU-10-31	Pediatric Article	Gender and Urinary PH Affect Melamine Kidney Stone Formation Risk	Jan 12, 2010	Under Review		Jan 12, 2010	Jan 13, 2010	Feb 02, 2010	Jan 22, 2010	10
Action Links	2	JU-08-1958	Pediatric Supplement	Evidence for Abnormal Sleep Architecture in Refractory Nocturnal Enuresis: A Pilot Study	May 18, 2009	Completed	Accept	Jan 05, 2009	Jan 05, 2009	Jan 26, 2009	Jan 10, 2009	5
Action Links	1	JU-08-1956	Pediatric Supplement	Effective Conservative Treatment of Hyperreflexic Neurogenic Bladder	Feb 12, 2009	Completed	Reject	Dec 30, 2008	Dec 30, 2008	Jan 20, 2009	Jan 10, 2009	11
				Intractable Voiding								

4. 编辑部致谢审稿人　编辑部为感谢审稿人对本刊所做出的审稿贡献,一般会致谢审稿人。下面是美国《泌尿外科杂志》为感谢文建国教授作为审稿人发来的致谢信。

Jan 20, 2010

Dear Dr. Wen:

On behalf of the Associate Editors, Section Editors, Assistant Editors and members of the Editorial Board, I would like to thank you for reviewing manuscripts for *The Journal of Urology*. We sincerely appreciate the time, expertise and advice that you provide to the editors and authors. We hope that we can continue to rely on your judgment in our efforts to maintain the integrity of The Journal of Urology as a truly peer-reviewed, scholarly publication.

Many thanks.

Sincerely yours,

William D. Steers, M.D.Editor

三、编辑部终审

原则上,若一篇文章三位审稿人的审稿意见中有两位或以上支持本文,则编辑部将告知作者按照审稿人意见进一步地修改,并回答审稿人提出的问题。但是,退修的稿件并不意味着文章最终能够接受发表,作者此时不能掉以轻心,应及时处理退修稿件,认真答复审稿人的问题。

退修稿修回后,编辑部将组织进行终审,决定文章是否接受发表。

四、作者校对

通过内部评审和同行评审的文稿将会发回作者以便校对。此时,作者应根据杂志要求对稿件进行详细审查,按照要求进行修改和确认。审核无误的稿件将会被接受发表。

快速审稿　有些情况下,稿件可以通过快速通道进行审稿。现将一些杂志的快速审稿通道举例如下:

(1)《柳叶刀》快速审稿通道

We offer fast-track peer review and publication of randomised controlled trials that we judge of importance to practice or research (see Fast-track publication).

从上述信息可了解到,杂志提供快速同行评审和公布随机对照试验,并认为这些试验对于实践或研究具有重要意义(快速出版物)。

For papers that are judged to warrant fast dissemination, which will usually be primary research (Articles), *The Lancet* will publish a peer-reviewed manuscript within 4 weeks of receipt. If you wish to discuss your proposed submission with an editor, please call one of the editorial offices in London (+44 [0] 20 7424 4943) or New York (+1 212 633 3667).

对于被认为需要快速传播的论文(通常为原创性研究),《柳叶刀》将在收到文稿后 4 周内对通过同行评审的文章进行发表。如果您想与编辑讨论您提交的内容,请致电伦敦编辑部(+44［0］20 7424 4943)或纽约编辑部(+1 212 633 3667)。

（2）美国《泌尿外科杂志》快速审稿通道

Rapid Review Manuscripts that contain important and timely information will be reviewed by 2 consultants and the editors within 72 hours of receipt, and authors will be notified of the disposition immediately thereafter. A $250 processing fee should be forwarded with the manuscript at the time of submission. Checks should be made payable to the American Urological Association. If the editors decide that the paper does not warrant rapid review, the fee will be returned to the authors, and they may elect to have the manuscript continue through the standard review process. Payment for rapid review guarantees only an expedited review and not acceptance.

通过上述信息得知，两位顾问和编辑在 72 小时内将会对重要稿件进行评审，作者很快将被告知稿件的处理情况。底稿上传的同时需要提前支付 250 美元的稿件快速处理费。如果编辑认为稿件不需要进行快速审稿，那么费用会退还给作者，同时稿件进入常规审稿程序。对快速审稿进行付费仅仅保证了稿件的快速审理，而非确保稿件一定会被接受发表。

第 17 章
医学英文论文写作常用语法及缩写词应用

Chapter 17
Grammar and Abbreviations in English Medical Scientific Writing

第一节　常见写作错误分析

一、写作要简单易懂

英语论文的写作要求简单易懂。然而,用英语写论文,对于母语不是英语的人来说,难度可能比较大。即使你的母语是英语,写作之前仍有必要读一读论文写作方面的书,因为你的很多读者的母语并不一定是英语。应该避免使用语法复杂的句子,以便非英语母语的人们感觉简单易懂。正如诗人 Arthur Kudner 所描述的那样:

Never fear big long words.

Big long words name little things.

All big things have little names.

Such as life and death, peace and war.

Or dawn, day, night, hope, love, home.

Learn to use little words in a big way.

It is hard to do.

But they say what you mean.

When you don't know what you mean.

Use big words—

That often fools little people.

虽然本书前面的章节已经勾勒出科学论文的写作大纲。但是,按照这个大纲不一定就能写出高质量的英语论文。必备的英文写作知识尤其是英文语法对成功撰写医学科研论文尤为重要。

二、避免英文论文写作常见语法错误

(一) 不一致

这里的不一致,不仅指主谓不一致,还包含数、时态及代词等的不一致。

例:When one have a car, he can do what he want to.(人一旦有了车,他就能想干什么就干

什么）。

剖析：one 是单数第三人称，因而本句的 have 应改为 has；同理，want 应改为 wants，本句是典型的主谓不一致。

改为：Once one has money, he can do what he wants（to do）。

（二）分裂不定式

分裂不定式即在 to 和动词之间放上一个副词或 please，所插入的副词常与不定式的动词原形连用，故分裂不定式要合乎习惯，不可滥用。

例：I want you to clearly read that last sentence.

剖析：clearly 在下面的句子中就不能放在 to 和 read 之间。然而在口语里，根据其所强调的位置，却经常把 to 和不定式分开，如：I want you to clearly understand what I'm telling you（我希望你清楚地理解我告诉你的事）。这样的副词还有 completely（完全地），fully（全部地），really（真地）和 truly（真实地）等；如：It's difficult to really understand the theory of relativity（真正理解相对论是不易的）。

改正：I want you to read that last sentence clearly.

（三）串句

串句即错误地将两个或两个以上的独立分句合写成一个句子，没有正确使用标点或者连词，忽略了英语语言中的逗号本身没有连接句子的功能这一原则。改正的方法是将逗号改为句号或者分号，或者使用适当的连词如 and、but、or、so 等，或者将其改成主从句。

例：The old man listened with a puzzled expression, he held an unlit cigar in his delicate finger.

剖析："一逗到底"是中文写作中的常见现象，但在英文中是不允许的，两个独立的句子之间应该用句号或者分号，或者连词。

改正：The old man listened with a puzzled expression with an unlit cigar in his delicate finger.

（四）破句

破句是指不完整的独立子句，常见有：从属连词导致的破句、ing 分词和不定式结构导致的破句、增添细节和缺少主语导致的破句。

例：Scientists report no human deaths due to excessive caffeine consumption. Although caffeine does cause convulsions and death in certain animals.

剖析：第一个句子是完整的，但是第二个 although 引导的让步从句缺少主句，是不完整的。修改方法很简单，将两个句子之间的句号改为逗号即可。

（五）修饰语错位

修饰语可以是单词、词组或从句。其在英语与汉语中的不同之处在于同一修饰语在句子的不同位置所表达的句子含义也不尽相同。如果修饰语放置不当，无法明确表达作者意愿，就可能导致歧义现象。避免修饰语错置的关键是使其尽可能靠近被修饰语，更要注意避免一词修饰多个句子成分而导致的歧义现象。

例：The old man bumped into the lamp post going to the clinic.

剖析：going to the clinic 从语义上看是修饰主语 the old man 的，但置于句尾导致表达不清楚。

改正：While going to the clinic, the old man bumped into the lamp post.

（六）悬垂修饰语

悬垂修饰语是指位于句首的修饰短语与后面的句子逻辑关系混乱。在修改时，一定要点明动作的发出者，将悬垂成分修饰的对象作为主句主语，或将悬垂修饰语丰富扩展成从句。

例：At the age of nine, my grandfather died.

剖析：这句中 at the age of ten 只点出十岁时，但没有说明"谁"十岁时。按一般推理不可能是 my grandfather，应该是 I。

改正：When I was nine, my grandfather died.

例：To do well in university, good grades are essential.

剖析：句中不定式短语 to do well in college 的逻辑主语不清楚。

改为：To do well in university, a student needs good grades.

（七）错误的平行结构

在写作时，为了不破坏两个（或两个以上）含义并列的成分（包括单词、词组、从句及句子）的平行结构，需要用相同的语法形式来表达。在修改错误的平行结构时，关键在于找到单词、词组、从句或句子的平行点，进而删去导致不平行的多余成分或添加缺少成分。

例：Many people choose high speed train because it is fast, offers convenience, and it is not very expensive.

剖析：fast 是形容词，offers convenience 为动词短语，it is not very expensive 则是一个句子，三者无法并列。

改正：Many people choose high speed train because it is fast, convenient, and inexpensive.

（八）词性误用

名词、介词用成动词；形容词用成副词等现象称为"词性误用"。

例：None can negative the importance of computer.

剖析：negative 系形容词，误作动词。

改为：None can deny the importance of computer.

（九）用词不当

中英文在词汇的运用上存在很多不完全对应的情况，因此在论文写作中需要谨慎选择词汇，避免用词不当，而这需要我们在日常学习中多多积累相关词汇，掌握准确的英文表达。

例：Reading can increase my words, rich my knowledge and enlarge my eyesight.

剖析：这句话可以明显看出是简单将中英文词汇对应起来，词汇的选择失误影响了句子的理解和整体效果。

改正：Reading can enlarge my vocabulary, enrich my knowledge and broaden my horizons.

（十）指代不清

指代不清是指代词与被指代的人或物关系混淆，或句子前后代词不统一。

例：Mary was friendly to my sister because she wanted her to be her bridesmaid.

（玛丽和我姐姐很要好，因为她要她做她的伴娘。）

读完上面这一句话，读者无法明确地判断两位姑娘中谁将结婚，谁将当伴娘。如果我们把易于引起误解的代词所指的对象加以明确，意思就一目了然了。这个句子可改为：

Mary was friendly to my sister because she wanted my sister to be her bridesmaid.

例：And we can also know the society by serving it yourself.

剖析：句中人称代词 we 和反身代词 yourself 指代不一致。

改为：We can also know society by serving it ourselves.

（十一）累赘

言以简洁为贵，写作要做到言简意赅。可以用单词的不用词组，可以用词组的不用从句，写句子无多余的词，写段落无多余的句子。这样写出来的才是精炼的文字。

如：In spite of the fact that he is lazy, I like him.

本句的 the fact that he is lazy 系同位语从句，我们按照上述"能用词组的不用从句"可以改为：In spite of his laziness, I like him.

再如：For the people who are diligent and kind, money is just the thing to be used to buy the thing they need.

剖析：整个句子可以大大简化。

改为：Diligent, caring people use money only to buy what they need.

（十二）语体不当

医学论文是正式的文体，因此在语言运用上要注意避免过于口语化的表达，尤其要避免使用俚语。

例：The experiment aims to get the DNA sequence.

剖析：get 是英语中使用频率非常高的一个词，除了可以表示"得到"，还可以表达"吃饭""买东西"等意思，但正因为此，这个词不够正式，不适合在论文中使用。

改正：The experiment aims to determine the DNA sequence.

总之，识别分裂不定式或修饰语或动名词错位并不容易，同时也很难发现比如时态、语态、标点符号、大小写等方面的错误。但是如果你适当注意句子构造就可以避免这些问题。"句法（syntax）"这个词涉及不同的单词组合成的成语、短语和句子的语法。

下面我们用 Robert Day 的十句话作为小结：

THE COMMANDMENTS OF GOOD WRITING

Each pronoun should agree with their antecedent.

Just between you and I, case is important.

A preposition is a poor word to end a sentence with.

Verbs have to agree with their subject.

Don't use no double negatives.

Remember to never split an infinitive.

Avoid cliches like the plague.

Join clauses good, like a conjunction should.

Do not use hyperbole; not one writer in a million can use it effectively.

About sentence fragments.

三、正确使用双重否定

双重否定句在英语中是一种格外特别的句型,具有一般否定句和肯定句所不能达到的表达效果。人们一般只把双重否定句理解为肯定语气从而忽略了其强调否定及委婉否定的功能。

(一)否定词 no/not 等 + 表示否定意义的形容词

例如:

He has no small reputation as a doctor. 他是名气很大的医生。

No way is impossible to professor. 教授面前无险路。

It is not uncommon for postgraduate to have friendly relationship with their supervisors.
研究生与导师建立友好关系并不罕见。

It is conflict and not unquestioning agreement that keeps freedom alive.
使自由保持活力的是冲突而不是绝对的一致。

Nothing is unnecessary. 没有什么是不必要的。

(二)否定词 no/not/never 等 +without…

例如:

No smoke without fire.［proverb］【谚】无火不起烟;无风不起浪。

We cannot succeed without your help. 没有你们的帮助,我们就不能成功。

They never meet without quarreling. 他们每次见面必吵架。

Nothing to be got without pains but poverty.[proverb]【谚】只有贫穷是可以不劳而获的。

(三)否定词 no/not/never/nobody/few 等 + 具有否定意义的动词或短语

例如:

There is no denying the truth. 真理是不能否认的。

The tart reply did not discomfort him. 那尖刻的回答并没有使他难过。

The Dole company says it is the biggest fruit packing company. Nobody disagrees.
多尔公司说它是世界上最大的水果罐头公司。没有人对此提出异议。

In spite of the increased debts, few fail to repay.
尽管借债越来越多,但很少有人不能偿还欠款。

(四)双重否定句在英语中不仅只限于以上三种类型,还有一些其他的形式

例如:

It is impossible not to do the work. 不做这件工作是不可能的(否定形容词在前,而否定词

在后,否定不定式)。

I'd review all the facts of the case and, not infrequently, wonder if I hadn't made a poor decision. 我会重温那位急诊患者的整个病情,常常怀疑自己做出了不妥的决定(否定词后接具有否定意义的副词)。

But it seemed no impossibility to Marconi. 但在马可尼看来,这不是不可能的(否定词后接具有否定意义的名词)。

There is no rule that has no exception. 任何规则都有例外(两个相同的否定词重复使用)。

英语中的多重否定是指在一个句子中同时出现两个甚至两个以上的否定词或者具有否定意义的词,以便达到特殊强调的效果,在非标准英语中,一般仍为否定含义。而在标准英语中则表达肯定含义,且具有特别强调效果。因此,在遇到此类含有多个否定词的语句时,要认真审读,正确判断其所要表达的真实含义,避免理解错误。在翻译为汉语时,一般译成双重否定式,有些情况下译成肯定式效果更佳。例如:

I won't trouble nobody about nothing no more. 我再也不在任何事情上麻烦任何人了。

在英语中,否定词可以否定整句,或否定一部分句子,或否定自己本身,不管何种情况,否定词都具有一定的否定范围。通常否定词处于句中被否定部分之前或之后,即被否定范围之内,但有时也会出现否定转移,即否定词处于句中被否定范围之外,与被否定部分隔开。当存在否定转移时,往往会导致读者对否定词所否定的对象判断错误,以至于错误理解、错误翻译句子。因此,需要注意避免此种情况的发生。例如:

He does not complain because there are a lot of difficulties in the work.

他并不因为工作中有太多的困难而抱怨(误:他不抱怨,因为工作中有太多的困难)。

四、正确区分单数和复数

如果用第一人称代词,根据需要应用单数和复数。不要用 editorial we 代替 I。仅有一个作者用 we 是不正确的。动词复数形式的应用在科学论文中是一个最常见的错误。例如:你应说 10 g was added,不是 10 g were added。原因是因为增加的是单纯数量。如果把 the 10 g were added 1 g at a time 叙述成 10 g were added 则是正确的。

单复数的难题同样存在于名词中。在科学论文写作中,这个问题尤其严重,特别是在生物学中,因为我们的词语大多来源于拉丁语,这些词的绝大多数保留着它们在拉丁语中复数的含义,作者应用这样的名词时应谨慎。这些词中有很多(e.g., data, media)已进入通俗的语言中。很多人习惯性运用 data is 的结构,而忽略了其真正的单数形式 datum。不幸的是,这不严谨的用法在科学领域之外普遍存在,甚至一些词典都已默认。例如,韦氏第十版新编大学词典叙述:"The use of data as if it were a singular noun is a common solecism",但是为规范起见,我们在论文写作中应把这类词看作复数,谓语动词应使用复数形式。

五、正确运用名词

科学论文写作中另一频繁出现的问题是过多应用抽象名词,而应用动词替换名词则可解决这一现象。如 "Examination of the patients was carried out" 应变为更直接的 "I examined the patients";"separation of the compounds was accomplished" 可改为 "the compounds were separated"；"transformation of the equations was achieved" 可变为 "the equations were transformed"。

　　数字规则：一位数的数字应用英语拼出来；两位或多位数应用阿拉伯数字表示。应该写 "three experiments" 或 "13 experiments"。例外的是：如果数字后跟测量单位时，要用阿拉伯数字表示，应该写 "3ml" 或 "13ml"。更加需要注意的是避免句子的开头是数字。例如：句子应该以 "Reagent A（3ml）was added" 开始，或 "Three milliliters of reagent A was added."。事实上，还有一个例外，如果一句子中包含一系列的数字，而且至少其中的一个是不止一位数的数字，那么所有的数字应用数码代替（例如："I gave water to 3 scientists, milk to 6 scientists, and beer to 11 scientists."）。

六、避免词语滥用

　　避免使用自相矛盾或冗长的词语。有些人这样描述：well-seasoned novice（做个经验老到的新手）；一报纸文章提到 young juveniles（年轻的青少年）；邮票和货币商人的商店上的标记意为 authentic replicas（真正的复制品）。如果还存在表达方式比 7 a.m. in the morning 更愚笨，那就是 viable alternative（可行的选择）。在科学论文写作中，某些词曾被成千上万次错用，其中一些存在严重的错误，比如，当涉及大规模或总计时会用到 amount 这个词，用它来衡量涉及单位的多少。"An amount of cash" 的表达是正确的，而 "An amount of coins" 则是错误的。又如，"and/or"，从你的写作词汇中摒弃掉这个屡遭谴责的蹩脚用法。

　　例如：fine of ＄25 and/or imprisonment for not more than 30 days

　　应改为：a fine of ＄25 or imprisonment for not more than 30 days, or both. 这是因为 or 这个词通常包括 and 的意思。

　　类似的例子有：

　　Case：这是在术语中最常见的一个词。"in this case" 意为 "here"；"in most cases" 意为 "usually"；"in all cases" 意为 "always"；"in no case" 意为 "never"。

　　It：这个词可以指除人以外的一切事物或动物，也可用于指性别不明的婴儿或用于确认某人的身份。"Is it a boy or a girl?"（是男孩还是女孩？）"There is a knock on the door. It must be the postman."（有人在敲门，一定是邮递员。）it 还可用于代替指示代词 this、that 以及复合不定代词 something、anything、nothing 等。如："What's this?" "It's a new machine."（"这是什么？" "是一种新机器。"）这个常见有用的代名词可能因先行词不清晰而难以理解。如 "Free information about VD. To get it, call 555~7 000"。

　　Like：经常被误用做连词，其实它仅可作介词用。like 作介词，意为 "像"、"和……一样"。例如："She looks like her mother." "The boy jumps like a monkey." "It looks like rain." "We don't need a man like him." 当需要连接词时，可用替代词 "as"。"Like I just said" 这句应以 "As" 开头。

　　Only: 将 "only" 这词放在句首、句尾或任何两词的中间，结果会有很大不同。Only 置于不定式之前时一般表示不理想或意想不到的结果。例如：

　　I went all the way to his home only to find him out at a meeting. 我径直到他家里去，不料发现他出去开会了。

　　Quite：这词经常用在科学论文写作中。如果发现它出现在你的初稿中，删除这词并再次读这句子。你将发现 quite 是完全不必要出现的词。

Which：尽管 which 和 that 经常被互换应用，但有时他们不能互换。which 是正当地用在非限制性定语从句中，引导的从句对剩下的句子来说不是必须的，that 则必须引导定语从句。检查以下两句 "CetB mutants, which are tolerant to colicin E2, also have an altered …"，"CetB mutants that are tolerant to colicin E2 also have an altered …" 注意意义上的本质不同。第一句话表明所有的 CetB 突变株对大肠杆菌 E2 都是耐受的，第二句表明只是其中的一部分 CetB 突变株对大肠杆菌 E2 是耐受的。

While：如果存在时间关系，正确的是运用 while；否则，最佳选择便是 whereas。"Nero fiddled while Rome burned" 是正确的。"Nero fiddled while I wrote a book on scientific writing" 则是错误的。

生活中词语误用会导致很多笑话，比如 thunderstruck 这个词，就有如下搞笑的 "经典" 表述："although I have never had the pleasure of meeting anyone who has been struck by thunder." 这句话中，Jimmy Durante 通过滑稽误用来创建他的戏剧风格，我们都很喜欢，但是里面的词语误用却很少被发现。

少数情况下，你可以有意误用词语，以增添你说话或写作的独特魅力。如："Tin is really nostalgic about the future." 有时候词语的误用也能闹出笑话来，这里有一个留学生的故事。他来到国外不久，校长邀请许多学生和全体老师相聚下午茶会，一些老师与外籍学生交谈。首先的问题是："Are you married?"，这同学回答："Oh, yes, I am most entrancingly married to one of the most exquisite belles of my country, who will soon be arriving here in the United States, ending our temporary bifurcation"。大学教师们疑惑的相互看着对方一会儿，然后进入下一个问题："Do you have children?" 那个学生回答 "No" 考虑了一会儿后，那学生决定对这个回答延伸一下，因此他说，"You see, my wife is inconceivable（不可思议的）"。这时，提问者开始想笑了，因此，那学生感觉自己失言了，他补充道，"Perhaps I should have said that my wife is impregnable（坚不可摧的）"。听到这样的解释，教师们开始大笑，那学生决定再试一次："I guess I should have said my wife is unbearable（难以忍受的）"。

七、避免使用委婉的词语和习语

在医学论文写作中，应避免应用委婉的词语和习语。The harsh reality of dying is not improved by substituting "passed away"。例如 "Some in the population suffered mortal consequences from the lead in the flour" 一些人因食用面粉而遭受致死性的后果，这句话应该说得更清楚些，同时删除委婉的说法 "Some people died as a result of eating bread made from the lead-contaminated flour"，一些人食用铅污染面粉做成的面包而死亡。mortal consequences 作为一考试的问题，大多数人不能简单地说出 died。一些创造性的新的答案是 "Get the dead out" 和 "Some were dead from the lead in the bread"。

八、慎用修辞

修辞是利用多种语言手段收到尽可能好的表达效果的一种语言活动。学术论文注重真实客观，文采其实并不重要。为了避免学术论文的 "矫揉造作"，要慎用修辞，甚至倡导 "零修辞"写作。在医学英文论文写作中,建议慎用明喻和暗喻,尽量不用。我们都见过复杂的隐喻,也深知含隐喻的句子理解起来很费力,比如:A virgin forest is a place where the hand of man has never set foot。微生物学家 L. Joe Berry 曾经说过:"Boy, I got shot down in flames before I ever got off the ground."。

九、其他细节

坦率地说,英语是门奇怪的语言。have(had)的过去式改为过去分词时只是重复,这不是很奇怪吗?"He had had a serious illness."。奇怪的是,可以在语法正确的句子中将 11 个 had 连起来。如果一人描述他老师对 John 和 Jim 修改论文的反应时,可以说"John, where Jim had had 'had', had had 'had had'; 'had had' had had an unusual effect on the teacher."。数个 that 也可以连在一起,例如:在句子"He said, in speaking of the word 'that', that that 'that' that that student referred to."。

下面给读者介绍一个你可能想跟朋友玩的语法游戏。给站成一排的人每人发张纸,让他们在七个字组成的句子"Woman without her man is a savage"中认为需要的地方点上标点。通常大男子主义者会很快说句子不需要标点,而且他是正确的。在大男子主义中一些空谈者把平衡的逗号放在前置短语之间,"Woman, without her man, is a savage",从语法上,这也是正确的。男女平等主义者,并且偶尔舞弄文墨的人,会在 woman 后加破折号,将逗号置于 her 之后,呈现为"Woman—without her, man is a savage"。

谨慎而言,我们都能理解语言上的性别歧视可以导致 savage 结果。充斥着陈腔滥调的科学论文写作是不科学的。不论何时,在句子无法理解时,通常是由于句法错误。但有时,错误的语法不但有趣而且易于理解,以下例子摘自招聘广告"For sale, fine German Shepherd dog, obedient, well trained, will eat anything, very fond of children(出售,优良的德国牧羊犬,温顺,受过良好训练,不挑吃,很喜欢小孩)"。

第二节　避免术语和官腔

一、避免术语

根据字典,jargon 有三种含义:①混乱的、难以理解的语言;奇怪、怪异、粗俗的语言或土语;②专门术语或某一特殊领域或团体的典型习语;③以冗长累赘为特点、令人费解且经常是矫饰的语言。英文写作时,应尽量避免使用读者不易理解的术语。正如 William Zinsser 指出的那样"Clutter is the disease of American writing. We are a society strangling in unnecessary words, circular constructions, pompous frills and meaningless jargons."。

尤其注意避免符合上述第一和第三种定义的术语,符合第二种定义的术语(专业词汇)在写科技文章时很难避免,但是在定义或解释过之后就可以使用这样的专门术语了。很明显,文章是为了给相关专业的读者看的,只有那些不常用的专业词汇才需要解释。下面就是一个因使用术语而使句子难于理解的例子:

May I suggest that you apply for a POD?

如何修改这个句子呢?

我们建议改为:

May I suggest that you apply for a Personal Overdraft?

以下句子均表述不清:

(1) I suggest that you apply for a PIL.

应改为:I suggest that you apply for a Personal Instalment Loan.

(2) The managers will discuss your proposal in due course.

应改为:The managers will discuss your proposal on Friday.

(3) Please remit the relevant amount as soon as possible.

应改为:Please send your cheque for US$40 by 21 June 200X.

(4) You can deposit cheques at designated ATMs.

应改为:You can deposit cheques at designated Automatic Teller Machines.

(5) One of our CSOs will contact you later.

应改为:One of our Customer Service Officers will contact you within 24 hours.

有些作者追求标新立异,从不用 use——而用 utilize,从不用 do——而用 perform,从不用 start——而用 initiate,从不用 end——而用 finalize(或 terminate),从不用 make——而用 fabricate。他们以 initial 开始,以 ultimate 结束;以 prior to 表示以前,以 subsequent to 表示之后;以 militate against 代表禁止;以 sufficient 表示足够;以 plethora 代表太多。偶尔作者也会疏忽,使用 drug 一词。这都是我们要避免的。

专门术语是一种特殊的语言,只有专门的团体才知道它的含义,而科学是普遍的,因此科学论文就应该以通俗的语言来写。

当然,偶尔使用专业术语也是不可避免的,如果这个领域的从业者和学生能懂得这些术语也不会有问题。如果你的潜在读者没有任何人能认出这些术语,你应该使用更简单的术语或详细地解释你所使用的难解的术语(行话)。

二、避免官腔

Speak in a Bureaucratic tone 几乎是所有科学家的通病,他们常常省略了动词(smothered his verbs),掩盖了主语(camouflaged his subjects),并且将它们隐藏在像灌木丛一样多的修饰语中(hide everything in an undergrowth of modifiers)。一切事情都要说明它的组成要素、可行性、更替性、有效性,都要加以分析说明执行情况、禁忌和附属效应等。术语或官腔是由清晰、简单的词语组成,但是当这些词串联到一起时意思就不那么容易理解了。正如下面一段:

General Injury. No person shall prune, cut, carry away, pull up, dig, fell, bore, chop, saw, chip, pick, move, sever, climb, molest, take, break, deface, destroy, set fire to, burn, scorch, carve, paint, mark, or in any manner interfere with, tamper, mutilate, misuse, disturb or damage any tree, shrub, plant, grass, flower, or part thereof, nor shall any person permit any chemical, whether solid, fluid or gaseous to seep, drip, drain or be emptied, sprayed, dusted or injected upon, about or into any tree, shrub, plant, grass, flower or part thereof except when specifically authorized by competent authority; nor shall any person build fires or station or use any tar kettle, heater, road roller or other engine within an area covered by this part in such a manner that the vapor, fumes or heat therefrom may injure any tree or other vegetation.

（以上这些可以翻译成：不要扰乱生长的万物。）

专门术语并不意味一定要使用专业词汇。当面临两个词语的选择时，行话主义者总是会选择较长的一个。行话主义者确实有自己的癖好，他们会把简短的陈述转换成一长串词语，但通常一长串词语还没简单的词汇表达得清楚。我相信任何人在看到烦琐的 at this point in time（此时此刻）的时候肯定更易理解简单的 now（现在）的含义。if（如果）所表达的意思用 in the event that（在……情况下）替代并不会有什么改善。特殊情况下 case 一词用来代表一箱货物或一例流感患者不难理解。事实上在很多情况下都使用 case。

有一个因为省略它而非使用它所带来麻烦的（某些情况下）词语是 about。作者们似乎不愿意使用能使读者更清晰明白的 about，而是使用冗长模糊的词语，如：approximately，pursuant to，in connection with，rein reference to，reference，in relation to，regarding，in the matter of，relating to，the subject matter of，in the range of，relative to，in the vicinity of，respecting，more or less，within the ballpark of，on the order of，with regard to，on the subject of，with respect to。

总之，在写作医学论文时要时刻牢记避免术语和官腔，运用清楚明了的语言客观地进行陈述。

第三节　缩写词的使用

一、少用缩写词

在自己的著作里，要将缩写控制到最低限度，这样编辑将会更加喜欢你的文章，人们读你的文章时也会感谢你。无论出于美观、简练、节省版面抑或其他考虑，千万别忘了首先要考虑的应该是读者并且只能是读者。如果你使用的缩写成了大多数读者阅读的障碍，那将得不偿失。所以，从道义上来说，作者在进行科学论文写作时应尽量做到运用正确、简单、明了的表达方式对读者传授科学研究的目的、方法、结果、结论和意义，即做到对读者负责。

使用缩写的原则：除了标准的计量单位和在所有杂志上都通用的国际单位制（SI）的缩写，大多数期刊还允许那些没有定义的标准缩写如：etc.，et al.，i.e.，和 e.g.（i.e. 和 e.g. 经常被滥用；i.e. 即 that is，e.g. 即 for example）。因为大多数期刊使用共同的缩写标准，当打算使用缩写词时，首先要把它完整地拼写出来，并在括号内注明缩写。文章的第一句话介绍时应该写"Bacterial plasmids, as autonomously replicating deoxyribonucleic acid（DNA）molecules of modest size, are promising models for studying DNA replication and its control."。

二、使用缩写的准则

（一）文章标题里不能用缩写词

在标题中使用缩写不仅会使读者感到困惑，还会受到检索和摘要服务业的强烈反对。

（二）使用统一的缩写词

在书写医学论文时应使用正规的缩写词形式,需以权威出版社发行的医学专著、正规编辑部出版的医学专业期刊或大专院校的统一教材为准。如果缩写标准不统一,文献检索服务将非常困难。即使缩写是标准的,也会出现索引和其他方面的问题。我们现在使用的一些缩写也许几年前还不被认可。比较不同版本的生物学编辑委员会手册中所列的缩写就会发现这一问题。当术语自身改变时就会出现令人意想不到的变化。今天学生可能会为 DPN（diphosphopyridine nucleotide）这样的缩写而苦恼,因为它的名称变为了 nicotinamide adenine dinucleotide,缩写也相应变为 NAD。

（三）摘要中的缩写

只有在多次运用一个较长的名词时才可以替换为缩写。如果使用缩写,在摘要中第一次出现时必须写出其全称,如乙型病毒性肝炎（以下简称乙肝）、急性心肌梗死（AMI）、完全胃肠外营养（TIN）、人类免疫缺陷病毒（HIV）等,因为摘要将单独出现在文摘杂志中。正文里缩写的使用,目的在于减少篇幅纸张以及降低印刷成本。另外更有意义的是,可以帮助读者了解如何正确使用缩写词。

（四）切忌将口头缩略语写入论文

不同地区的医务工作者在日常工作中都可能存在一些约定俗成的口头语或者缩略语,但一定不要将这些非正式或者不规范、不通用的语言写进医学论文。

三、良好的习惯

要有一个好的习惯,在最初写手稿的时候应该把术语拼写完整,然后反复检查手稿中的长单词或短语是否可以用缩写表示。文中出现很少几次的术语不能使用缩写。如果一个术语经常出现（3~6 次）,而且它有标准缩写,介绍这一术语后便可使用缩写（一些期刊允许有标准缩写的术语不需介绍而可以直接使用缩写）。如果一术语没有标准缩写,不要自己制造。除非这一术语在文中频繁的出现或单词较长迫切需要缩写。通常如果指代明确你可以使用代词（它,它们）来避免缩写,或通过使用替代的表达,如"抑制剂""底物""药物""酶""酸"等。

按惯例,正文中首次出现缩写时应该逐一介绍。另一种方法,可以考虑在引言或材料和方法中单独一段介绍（标题"缩写词表"）。例如将正文中出现的有机化学药品缩写表列于正文前。后一种方法（一些期刊要求）适用于相关的反应试剂的书写。例如：

缩略词	英文名称
IEX-1	immediate early response gene X-1
IEG	immediate early gene
UVB	ultraviolet radiation b
RT-PCR	reverse transcription-polymerase chain reaction
Bp	base pair

缩略词	英文名称
PBS	phosphate buffer solution
DAB	3. 3'-diamino benzidine
FCM	flowcytometry
EGFP	enhanced green fluorescent protein
EB	ethidium bromide
mRNA	messager ribonucleic acid
OD	optical density
GFP	green fluorescent protein
PCR	polymerase chain reaction
PI	picolinium iodide
PS	Phosphatidylserine
DEPC	diethyl pyrocarbonate
EDTA	ethylene diamine tetraacetic acid
Mcl-1	myeloid cell leukemia-1
NF-κB	nuclear factor-κB
SDS	Sodium dodecyl sulfate
SDS-PAGE	sodium dodecyl sulfate polyacrylamide gel electrophoresis
Acr	acrylamide
AP	Ammonium persulphate

四、计量单位

计量单位一般缩写。例如:应该写为"4mg"(单复数用同样的缩写)。当不伴随数值使用时计量单位不用缩写。你可以这样写"Specific activity is expressed as micrograms of adenosine triphosphate incorporated per milligram of protein per hour."。

随便使用斜线会引起误解。这一问题经常在表示浓度时出现。如果说"加入 4mg/ml 硫化钠",是什么意思? 写成"每毫升溶液中加入 4mg 硫化钠"会更容易使人明白。

五、国际单位

科学语言中比较重要的一部分便是国际制度(SI)单位为前缀的缩写词。这一最新的度量系统是所有学生在进行科学研究时都必须要掌握的。《CBE 种类手册》(CBE 写作手册委员会,1983)和 Huth's(1987)的《医学写作与格式》都是获得全面信息的很好来源。

通常来说,基本单位,补充单位和推导单位都属于 SI 单位的经典单元。其还包括七个基本单位,即米、千克、秒、安培、开尔文、摩尔和坎德拉。除此之外,弧度和立体弧度是平面和立体的补充单位。推导单位表示基本单位或补充单位的代数值。一些 SI 推导单位存在特殊的名称和符号（SI 单位 metre 和 litre；美国国家标准与技术研究所，其次是美国化学协会和其他一些出版商，仍在沿用美国传统的拼写，meter 和 liter）。

六、其他情况

关于缩写词用 a 或 an 是一个常见的问题。可以写 a M.S. degree 或 an M.S. degree？按照旧的规则在单词前面用 a 发辅音，单词前用 an 发元音（例如：字母 M）。因为在科学文献里我们只使用常见的缩写，不需要读者费脑子去拼写，缩写前面的冠词应该与缩写的第一个字母而不是与第一个字母的发音相协调。因此，虽然 a Master of Science degree 的书写是正确的，但是 a M.S. degree 是错误的。因为 M.S. 的读音为 em es 所以合适的结构应该是 an M.S. degree。

生物学文献习惯在第一次出现后把有机体的名称省略。第一次使用时，应该全部拼写出来，如 Streptomyces griseus，在以后的使用中，可以省略属名但不能省略种类，应写成 S. griseus。假设一篇文章涉及 Streptomyces（链球菌）和 Staphylococcus（葡萄球菌）两种类型，则需要在下文中反复地拼写出它们的全称。如果使用 "S." 缩写表示，读者会感到迷惑而不知道所指的是哪一个。

此外，还有一个问题是将中英文缩写词夹杂使用，如将血常规写成 "血 Rt"，血钾写成 "血 K"，淋巴细胞写成 "淋巴 C"，肝癌写成 "肝 C"，这些都是应当避免的不规范写法。

第四节　文章中动词时态与语态的应用

一、科学论文写作中的时态

在科技论文中，看起来容易的动词时态在应用中的错误并不少见。原因是存在一些不清楚论文时态与论文内容及论文体裁之间关系的作者和编者。研究前已经做过的工作、研究过程中所做的工作、当时的研究结果及已经存在客观真理，这些都需要作者通过动词时态表达出来，都与论文内容密切相关。同时，也需要通过应用某一特定的时态来体现论文体裁所提供的特定背景。

无论何时在引用已经发表的文章时，要以尊敬的态度对待，引用时要用现在式时态。如："Streptomycin inhibits the growth of M. tuberculosis（链霉素抑制 M 结核球菌的生长）"这样说是对的。无论何时引用或讨论先前已发表的文章时，均应该用现在式时态。因为正在引用的是确定的知识，例如：可以说 "The Earth is round."（If previously published results have been proven false by later experiments, the use of past rather than present tense would be appropriate.）。而提起自己现在的科研工作应该用过去时，因为你的工作直到被发表时，才是确定的知识。如果你确定每种颜色链球菌属最佳的生长温度是 37℃，应该说 "S. everycolor grew best at 37℃（过去时）"；如果你在引用先前的结论，即使这个结论可能是你自己的，正确的表述应该是 "S. everycolor grows best at 37℃"。在标准的文章中，应不停地在过去时和现在时中来回转换。

摘要多用一般现在时。目的、方法、结果及结论部分多用一般现在时，背景介绍常采用一般过去时。一般过去时用于描述论文撰写前作者已做的工作。如果是描述研究的成果、得出的结论,用一般现在时。如果描述具体的研究过程,则用一般过去时。如果描述研究结果对未来的影响,用一般将来时。如果是过去的研究成果,但是对现在得出的结论有影响,用现在完成时。如果是引用已经成为公认的事实,则用一般现在时。如:

Thirty-seven consecutive renal transplant recipients were studied prospectively for joint disease。

(作者)连续对 37 例肾移植患者是否有关节病变做了前瞻性观察。

至于前言以及讨论,大部分应是现在时。因为这些部分常常强调先前已确定的知识。假设你的研究是关于链霉素对每种颜色的链球菌属的效果,时态转换如下。

在摘要中,可能这样写:"The effect of streptomycin on S. everycolor grown in various media was tested. Growth of S. everycolor measured in terms of optical density was inhibited in all media tested. Inhibition was most pronounced at high pH levels."。

在前言中,标准的句子应是:"Streptomycin is an antibiotic produced by Streptomyces griseus (13). This antibiotic inhibits the growth of certain other strains of Streptomyces (7,14,17). The effect of streptomycin on S. everycolor is reported in this paper."。研究目的一般用过去时态。"The purpose of this study was to investigate factors that may participate in the production of innocent ejection murmurs."。本研究旨在调查产生非病理性喷射性杂音的可能因素。

在材料与方法部分,可这样写:"The effect of streptomycin was tested against S. everycolor grown on Trypticase soy agar (BBL) and several other media (Table 1). Various growth temperatures and pH levels were employed. Growth was measured in terms of optical density (Klett units)."。

在结果部分,可这样写:"Growth of S. everycolor was inhibited by streptomycin at all concentrations tested (Table 2) and at all pH levels (Table 3). Maximum inhibition occurred at pH 8.2;inhibition was slight below pH 7."。

在讨论部分,可这样写:"S. everycolor was most susceptible to streptomycin at pH 8.2, whereas S. nocolor is most susceptible at pH 7.6 (13). Various other Streptomyces species are most susceptible to streptomycin at even lower pH levels (6,9,17)."。

简而言之,当提及先前已发表的文章时,应用现在时态,而当提及现在的结果时应该用过去时态。

(一) 何时用现在时

1. 一般现在时通常用来表述论文发表时的情况

About 50 cases of leptospirosis are diagnosed each year in the United Kingdom, with an overall mortality of 5%, renal failure, in association with jaundice, is commonly held responsible for this figure. Over a period of 18 years, 6 cases of leptospirosis complicated by renal failure were treated at the Royal Air Force Renal Unit; there were 4 survivors …

美国每年确诊为螺旋体病约 50 例,总死亡率达 5%。造成这些死亡的原因一般认为是肾衰竭合并黄疸。18 年来,有 6 例合并肾衰竭的患者在皇家空军肾病科进行治疗。有 4 例存活……

2. 一般现在时常用来介绍论文内容　常用动词有:report(报告)、describe(描述)、present(提出,介绍)、discuss(讨论)、review(评述)、emphasize(强调)、stress(强调)等。如:

In this paper, we report the effect of plasma exchange in a patient with this syndrome.

本文报道一例这种综合征患者血浆置换疗法的效果。

A case of a 27 years old man who developed anemia after fracture of sella turcica is reported.

本文报道一例 27 岁患者在蝶鞍骨折后发生贫血。

在介绍本文内容时,还可用系动词 be 代替以上动词。如:"本文是一篇……报道"、"本文是一篇……分析"等句式中的"是"均要用现在时。如:

This study is a description of a patient who exhibited diabetic ketosis associated with an alkalosis rather than acidosis and a review of eight previously reported cases.

本文报道一例有碱中毒而不伴有酸中毒的糖尿病酮症患者,并对既往报道的 8 例做了综述。

在介绍"本文"目的时也需要运用现在时。这一"目的"与前文所提的"研究目的"并不相同,前文所指的是在开始研究前要设立确定的研究目的,其早于研究过程中的一切行为,因此需要运用过去时。而"本文"的目的则是指全文的中心思想,所要运用的不定式动词大多具有"叙述""说"等含义。如:

The purpose of this report is to emphasize the value of radiation therapy.

本文旨在强调放射治疗的价值。

3. 作者结论的表达 在进行各种研究工作时,作者都会得出结论,无论结论是肯定还是否定,都需要以一般现在时来叙述,因为科学的结论通常都具有普遍真理的性质。如:

We conclude that the principles of the test system allow increased safety and accuracy in hospital drug handling.

我们的结论是:这种试验制度的一些原则可以提高医院药物管理的安全性与精确性。

The authors conclude that labetalol when combined with a thiazide diuretic is an important therapeutic advance in the treatment of the difficult hypertensive subject.

我们的结论是:拉贝洛尔与噻嗪类利尿剂合用是治疗难治的高血压症的重要进展。

由上述例句可以看出,通常应该用一般现在时来表达作者的结论,但也存在应用一般过去时的情况。虽然两者在语法上都是正确的,但却表达了作者完全不同的态度。一般现在时体现了作者对于该结论具有普遍真理性质的认识,而过去时则体现了作者对于该结论不具有普遍性的认识,只是把其认作了当时的一个研究结果。如:

This trial showed both drugs to be effective and there was no statistically significant difference between them in their effect.

这一试验表明,两种药物都有效,其效果在统计学上无明显差异。

另一个例外是计算和统计分析的结果应用现在时,尽管陈述的对象是过去时,如:

These values are significantly greater than those of the females of the same age, indicating that the males grew more rapidly.

还有一个例外是一般的陈述或已知的真理。可以说"Water was added and the towels became damp, which proves again that water is wet."。很多时候你需要不断地转换时态,"Significant amounts of type Ⅳ procollagen were isolated. These results indicate that type Ⅳ procollagen is a major constituent of the Schwann cell ECM."。

(二)何时用过去完成时

一般用过去完成时表示在开始研究之前就已经做过的工作或存在的状态。如:

In a 22-year-old male, who had been irradiated 16 years previously for Hodgkin's disease, a radiation-induced thyroid carcinoma developed.

一例 16 年前因患霍金森病接受过放射治疗的 22 岁男患者发生放疗诱发的甲状腺癌。

当有两个前后相连的行为出现在研究过程中时,通常以过去完成时表达先发生的。如:

Two patients with primary spontaneous pneumothorax died despite intensive treatment. In the first the pneumothorax had been present for 10 days, …

两例原发性自发性气胸患者,虽然得到积极治疗,仍然死亡。第一例患者气胸已持续达 10 天之久……

(三) 何时用现在完成时

当出现以下情况时,需要运用现在完成时。一是存在持续到撰写论文时的行为或状态;二是在具有不受时间限制永恒的现在时动词的行为动作之前就已经完成的行为。如:

Three patients have been now free from recurrences for 5 years, 13patients for 4years, 11 patients for 3 years, and 9 patients for 2 years。

迄今为止,无复发者 5 年 3 例,4 年 13 例,3 年 11 例,2 年 9 例。

Radionuclide examinations provide considerable information in evaluating patients who have received renal transplants.

放射性同位素检查对接受过肾移植的患者的评价,能提供重要资料。

另外,过去时间的背景常用现在完成时来表现。通常现在完成时放在开始作为先导,然后后续跟接一般过去时。这样的现在完成时便为过去提供了时间背景。如:

The authors have examined the lungs from five patients who died with the adult respiratory distress syndrome. Pressure volume curves were obtained and bronchoalveolar lavage fluid was studied on a surface balance. The pressure volume curves revealed reduced compared to normal or near normal lungs. A significant loss of volume was also found …

我们检查了 5 例呼吸窘迫综合征成人患者的肺脏,取得了加压容量曲线资料,对支气管肺泡灌洗液的表面平衡做了研究。与正常或接近正常的肺脏相比,加压容量曲线提示顺应性降低,肺活量也显著减少。

(四) 何时用将来时

一般将来时表示将要发生的事情,论文中描述以后要做的工作或预期的结果时使用。如:

As greater clinical correlation is obtained, then use-fulness of thyroglobulin determinations will increase.

随着甲状腺球蛋白测定与临床的相互关系日益密切,其诊断价值也将随之提高。

(五) 论文摘要中几个常用动词不同时态的意义

1. report 与 describe

(1)一般现在时:表示"本文报道"。如:

Three patients with rheumatoid arthritis are reported who appeared to have allergy to prednisolone.

本文报道 5 例男性神经性食欲缺乏患者,其年龄在 13~23 岁。

（2）一般过去时：表示在撰写论文时也已报道过。因此不是"本文报道"，而是已由其他文章报道过。如：

In 1968, studies of infectious hepatitis in volunteers were reported.

对志愿人员进行传染性肝炎的研究，在 1968 年就已有报道。（本句中的 report 根据内容可以看出不是"本文"报道，而是"别的文章"已有报道。）

（3）现在完成时：用现在完成时态即可表示"另文报道"，也可表示"本文报道"。如：

A patient with plasma cell leukemia and Ig G(K) M-component, who developed a hyperviscosity syndrome is reported. To our knowledge, this complication has not yet been reported in plasma cell leukemia.

本文报道一例合并有 IgG（K）M 血症的浆细胞白血病患者出现高黏稠综合征。就我们所知，浆细胞白血病的这一并发症迄今未见报道。（本句中第一次出现的 report 是"本文"报道；第二次出现的现在完成时态的 report 则不是"本文"，而是"别的文章"没有报道过。）

2. present　present 一词用一般现在时与 report 相同，表示"本文报道""本文介绍"。如：

Two cases of haemobilia due to haemorrhagic cholecystitis are presented。

本文报道 2 例出血性胆囊炎引起的胆道出血。

在英美医学杂志中出现的一般过去时态的 present，用"本文报道"或"另文报道"之类含义来解释，往往解释不通。而且，在目前国内出版的英汉辞典中也找不到恰当的解释。在 *Webster's Third New International Dictionary* 中对 present 有一段释文可以用得上："to come forward as a patient"。如：

Three elderly patients presented at one hospital in a 2-week period with acute urinary retention precipitated by the hyperosmotic non-ketotic diabetic state.

在两周内有三名上了年纪的患者因高渗性非酮症糖尿病继发急性尿潴留而来医院就诊。

present 的过去时态与 with 连用时，含有"呈现""表现"之意。如：

A successful pancreatogram was obtained at endoscopic retrograde holangiopancreatography in 53 patients with calculous biliary disease. Twenty-eight patients presented with jaundice and 25 with pain.

我们对 53 例胆道结石患者经内窥镜做逆行胰胆管造影，成功地获得了胰造影图。表现为黄疸的患者 28 例，表现为腹痛的患者 25 例。

present 的过去时态还可能有别的含义，但不太难理解，故从略。

3. review　review 一词在论文摘要中往往因时态应用的不同，而具有不同的意义，而其时态的应用又与该动词宾语的含义有关。

（1）一般现在时：Review 用于一般现在时态时，含有"本文综述""本文评述"的意义。搭配 review 连用的各种词语通常都要叙述一定的内容。如：

The (pertinent) literature is reviewed.

本文综述了有关文献。

Chemotherapy experience is briefly reviewed.

本文扼要地评述了化学治疗的经验。

（2）一般过去时：review 用于一般过去时态时，就不能表示"本文综述"或"本文评述"。因"综述"与"评述"是作者在撰写论文时的行为，所以用现在时。过去时态是表示作者在撰

写论文之前的行为,即是作者所进行的工作仍在研究过程中。此时,它便具有"复查""回顾"的含义。如:

Eighty-seven cases of male breast cancer seen over 30-year period were reviewed.

我们对 30 年来所遇到的 87 例男性乳腺癌患者做了回顾性研究。

我们不少医务工作者已习惯将 review 一词译成"复习",如"复习文献"等。我们认为"复习功课"是汉语的固定搭配用法,而"复习文献"似搭配不当。

二、主动语态和被动语态

现在我们来讨论语态。有学者认为,尽量减少被动语态在英文科学论文中的出现频率。原因是主动语态表达意思较被动语态简明扼要。也有学者认为,在任何形式的写作中,主动语态比被动语态更严密、更精简、更清楚、更有效。在医学论文写作中,人称代词通常决定动词的语态。因此,第三人称的被动语态比第一人称的主动语态更常见。如:We suggest that …(我们建议……)往往写成 It is suggested that …;We conclude that …(我们的结论是……)往往写成 It is concluded that …。

如何使用人称代词在科技论文中分为两派。一派是主张广泛使用被动语态,少用第一、第二人称代词,尤其是单数第一人称代词。例如 I think …,I feel …,I believe … 等这些与科学精神不符的表达。他们认为科技论文不应强调某个作者及其看法,而应强调客观事实,让事实来反映出真理。另一派的看法是,亲切、自然和直截了当也应该在科技论文中体现。如:不应拐弯抹角地说 It was decided that …;而应直率地说 I decided that …(我断定……)。

这派意见认为,研究报告属于个人叙述文章,应以第一、第二人称代词为主。如果以被动语态为主,就会出现文词过长,动词与动作执行者混乱不清的现象。因此美国 *Science* 杂志在"投稿须知"中列出:被动语态少于主动语态,因为被动语法需要词语较多,易将动作与动作执行者混淆。因此选择第一人称,拒绝第三人称。凡能用单数第一人称的地方,就不用复数第一人称……

但是目前第三人称仍在国外医学文摘中占有绝对优势,单数第一人称及第二人称代词少见。在 1980 年底 42 卷《工医学文摘》(*Excerpta Medical*)内科分册中 400 篇文摘的统计中,第三人称 357 篇(89.3%)、we 30 篇(7.5%)、the author(s)代替第一人称 13 篇(3.2%)。在 Medline 检索系统收录的发表于 1996 年至 2003 年 5 月不同生物医学期刊的结构式英文摘要中随机挑选 900 篇,分析其各篇中的时态、语态使用情况时发现,"目的"和"讨论"里主要采用主动语态,而"方法"和"结论"里主要采用被动语态。

在论文摘要中使用 I 是罕见的,这里不讨论习惯用第三人称文摘的写法,而对表达"我"时的四种处理方法进行重点介绍。

1. 复数第一人称 we 的使用。无论单数还是复数的编者、著者第一人称在报道性文章中多用 we。

We still consider, due to the above, that enterolithotomy alone is a sufficient primary rocedure, and that only in cases of new biliary tract complaints can cholecystectomy and closure of an evevntual fistula be considered.

由于上述原因,我们仍然认为最初单纯做肠取石术就已足够了。只有在出现了新的胆道症状时才考虑切除胆囊及封闭可能产生的瘘管。本文作者仅一人,这个 we 实际上是指 I。

2. 不带动作执行者被动语态的使用。可通过论文摘要的语意看出作者本人是动作执行者。

Two cases of angiosarcoma of the heart are described.

我们（本文）报道两例心脏血管肉瘤。

上面例子的谓语 are described 是不带动作执行者的被动语态。从文字内容可以看出动作执行者就是文章作者本人，这种写法还比较常见。

3. 用 the author 代表 I，用 the authors 代表 we。应注意，英语习惯不用 the writer 代表 I。

The author presents the experience with 264 patients with secondary renovascular hypertension.

我们（作者）介绍 264 例继发性肾性高血压的治疗经验。

4. 在科技论文中，第一人称不仅可用 the author 代替，this study，this report，this paper，this article 等也可代替。如：

This study reports our first year's experience of endoscopic sphincterotomy for common bile duct stones.

本文报告作者在第一年经内窥镜切开括约肌治疗胆总管结石的经验。

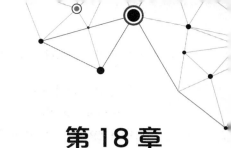

第18章
常用句型及各种数字英文表达

Chapter 18
Commen Sentence Patterns and Number Expressions in English

第一节　常用主题句、描述句和结尾句

正文部分的写作虽然重点不同,但基本结构都大同小异,常由主题句、描述句和结尾句3个部分组成。

一、主题句

主题句扼要说明论文的主题,使论文意旨一目了然。主题句用一般现在时表达,常用句型有:

本文研究了……

This paper reports the result of …

The article describes a study of …

The author presents two typical cases of …

The study deals with the problem of …

To study/identify/examine/explore …

二、描述句

描述句用以概括文章的要点,可包括研究目的、研究方法和过程,以及研究的结果和意义。

1. 表示研究目的的常用句型,用一般过去时表示。

本文的意旨在于……

The purpose of this research was to …

The primary purpose was to …

The object of this research was to …

The study aimed to …

The aim of this study was to …

This study was designed to …

2. 交代研究背景常用的句型,可用过去时或现在完成时,有时也用一般现在时或将来时。

问题的提出是……

This problem advanced …

This problem was brought up …

The problem as such was put forward …

The problem as is outlined now raised (posed) …

3. 说明理论依据常用的句型,可用过去时或者一般现在时。

该理论是……提出来的

The theory of … was created/constructed/developed/formulated/proposed by …

该理论的内容是……

The underlying concept of the theory is as follows …

The fundamental feature of this theory is …

The theory holds/claims that …

根据该理论,可得出……

As can be seen from the theory by …

According to …'s theory, …

In the light of the theory, we have developed a variation method to handle …

Based on the theory, …

应用该理论可以说明……

We can interpret these findings in terms of the above theory.

We can explain these phenomena using the above theory.

The theory can apply to the cases of …

The theory proved to be true for …

4. 提出假设常用的句型,多用一般现在时。

There is an assumption that …

We start from an assumption that …

Our basic assumption is that …

The authors assume that …

We hypothesize that …

We propose the following hypothesis …

5. 描述实验(所用设备)常用的句型,通常用过去时或者现在完成时。

The experiment consisted of three steps …

The test equipment which was used consisted of …

Included in the experiment were …

We have carried out several sets of experiments to test the validity of …

We initiated experiments to prove …

Many studies have been undertaken to verify …

A number of experiments were performed to check …

The present series of experiments have indicated that …

The experiments reported here demonstrated that …

Our experiments failed to prove …

6. 叙述研究过程常用的句型,通常用一般过去时,也可用现在完成时。

研究工作的进行是……

A study was done/made/carried out/performed/undertaken/concluded …

结果的测定……

The effect was measured/determined/examined …

7. 提出研究结果及意义常用的句型,通常使用现在完成时。

我们工作的结果……

This work has given an explanation of/given a clue at/resulted a solution of …

Our work has provided discovery of/facilitated the progress in/contributed to/led to …

The studies we have performed show that …

The investigation carried out by … has revealed that …

These studies have confirmed the opinion that …

Our research has supported the assumption that …

All our preliminary results have shown light on the nature of …

三、结尾句

结尾句是全文的结论或建议,也可提及对未来的展望。用一般现在时,表示普遍真理性。
常用句型:

1. 这项工作可以得出……结论

These studies suggest/believe that …

All these studies lead the authors to/postulate that/conclude …

2. 这些数据使我们得出……结论

These data support us to think/believe/conclude that …

These findings lead us to think/believe/conclude that …

These results assume us to think/believe/conclude that …

From the results we have obtained we can conclude that …

On the basis of our findings it can be concluded that …

3. 现有证据可以表明……

We have at present convicing/compelling/conclusive evidence showing that …

The evidence (obtained from …) favors the current concept of …

Our evidence provided bears out the facts that …

4. 做出评价

Our work involving studies of … proves to be successful/encouraging.

The newly-developed method has certain advantages over the existing ones.

These highly-technical experiments provide evidence for …

5. 对未来的展望

Thus, first extension of the approach could be …

Further studies are needed to determine the importance of …

It also unveil new aspects of the role played by …

It should be an exciting time for researchers seeking to harness this powerful endogenous pathway to treat human disease.

第二节　常用句型

无论是初学者,还是有一定医学英文论文写作经验的人,牢记一些有关医学英语表达的常用句型很有必要。这样做不仅能够提高你的英文水平,保证在写作过程中语言表达的正确性,更能够使你的写作过程变得顺利,缩短写作时间。下面,我们简单介绍一下医学英文写作中比较常用的一些句型。

一、有关 study 的常见句型

study 作名词时表示研究或学习的过程或结果;作动词时表示进行学习或研究的行为;作形容词时表示与学习相关的。名词 study 有单、复数两种形式。

名词 study 与表示"研究方法"的前置定语连用时,一般选用单数形式,如:

A retrospective study 回顾性研究

A prospective study 前瞻性研究

A double-blind,crossover study 双盲交叉研究

A follow-up study 随访研究

A clinical study 临床研究

A randomized controlled study 随机对照研究

名词 study 与表示"研究对象"的前置定语连用时,通常选用复数形式,如:

Macrophage studies 对巨噬细胞的研究

Radioisotope red-cell survival studies 放射性同位素对红细胞存活期所进行的研究

Urodynamic studies 尿动力学的研究

Physical and chemical studies 物理与化学研究

Molecular structural studies 分子结构的研究

Signal mechanism studies 信号机制的研究

常见句型举例

句型(1)

A … study was done in … patients …

A … study was made in … patients …

A … study was carried out in … patients …

A … study was undertaken in … patients …

A … study was performed in … patients …

句型(2)

… studies were conducted in, patients … studies were done in … patients …

(我们)对……患者进行了……研究……

… patients carried out a … study …

… patients performed … studies …

... patients entered a ... study ...

……患者参与了……研究；我们对……患者进行了……研究

句型（3）

In a ... study ... 在一次……研究中

In a study of ... 在对……的研究中

句型（4）

... was (were) studied in ... patients ...

（我们）对……患者进行了……研究

句型（5）

We studied ... patients to ...

... patients were studied to ...

我们对……患者进行研究，以期……

... patients were studied for ...

我们对……患者进行研究，看是否有……

在句型（1）中，study 是名词，用作句子的主语，与之搭配的谓语动词常见的有：do，make，carry out，perform，undertake，conduct 等。在本句型中，这些动词同义，可互换。下面是具体的例子：

例 1 A prospective study was done of PSA levels in 58 patients with prostate cancer.

我们对 58 例前列腺癌患者 PSA 水平作了前瞻性研究。

例 2 Survival studies were carried out in 60 patients with renal cell carcinoma after operation.

我们对 60 例肾癌术后患者进行了生存分析研究。在上述例句中，patient 之前一般都用介词 in，但也见有用 on 的，如：

例 3 Urodynamic studies were performed on 100 consecutive patients with benign prostatic hyperplasia.

我们连续对 100 例前列腺增生患者进行了尿流动力学检查。

在句型（2）中，study 是名词，用做谓语动词的宾语，与之搭配的动词常见的有 undergo（经受）、enter（参加）。这两个动词不同义，一般不可互换。具体例子如下：

例 1 20 patients with benign prostatic hyperplasia underwent urodynamic studies to determine Whether combined with urethral outlet obstruction.

作者对 20 例前列腺增生患者进行尿流动力学研究，以期有无尿道出口梗阻。

例 2 Twenty patients with mild to severe essential hypertension satisfactorily controlled by twice-daily amlodipine therapy entered a double-blind, crossover study comparing the efficacy, tolerability and safety of their usual twice-daily sotalol administration with the same dosage given once daily.

20 例轻度至重度原发性高血压患者经氨氯地平治疗（每天两次）病情稳定后，进行一次双盲交叉研究，比较一天两次与一次用药（剂量相同）的疗效、耐受性与安全性。

在句型（3）中，study 可用于介词 in 的短语中，这也是一种常用的结构。如：

例 1 In an uncontrolled study 45 patients with over active bladder were treated for up to 2 months with solifenacin succinate.

我们对使用琥珀酸索利那新治疗 2 个月的 45 例逼尿肌过度活动患者进行非对照研究

例 2 The effects of sotalol on blood pressure were examined in a prospective and a retrospective study.

我们通过前瞻性和回顾性研究检验了索他洛尔对血压的作用。

例 3 In a study of 250 patients with nocturnal enuresis, ten were found to have recessive spina bifida.

我们检查了 250 例夜遗尿患者,发现 10 例伴有隐性脊柱裂。

例 4 The influence of contrast material on renal venous renin activity was evaluated in a prospective study of 45 hypertensive patients.

我们对 45 例高血压患者作了前瞻性研究,以评定造影剂对肾静脉肾素活性的影响。

在句型(4)中,study 是动词,用做句子的谓语。如:

The characteristics of lymphatic metastasis of lung cancer were studied in 23 patients.

我们对 23 例肺癌患者淋巴转移的特点进行了研究。

句型(5)与句型(4)基本结构相同,只是本句型多包含了一个目的状语。本句型表达"目的"的方式有两种:一是用动词不定式;二是用介词 for+ 名词。如:

例 1 Twenty marrow transplant patients with Lymphoblastic leukemia were studied to determine the usefulness of antibody and antigen detection in the diagnosis of pneumocystis infection.

我们对 20 例患有急性淋巴细胞白血病的骨髓移植患者进行研究,以期确定抗体及抗原测定对该病诊断的价值。

例 2 Thirty-six consecutive marrow transplant recipients were studied prospectively for joint disease.

我们对连续 36 例骨髓移植患者作了前瞻性研究,看是否有关节病变。

例 3 We studied 11 patients with benign prostatic hyperplasia and 10 normal subjects for urodynamic parameters.

我们研究了 11 例前列腺增生患者及 10 名正常人的尿动力学参数。

二、有关各种诊断检查与手术治疗的句型

句型(1)检查名称或手术方式 +was(were)performed(done)+in(on)… patients

句型(2)患者 +underwent+ 检查或手术名称

在句型(1)中,介词 in 与 on 可以互换。请看下列对比例句:

(A) Pre-exploratory choledochectomy was performed in 48 patients with a diagnostic accuracy of 94 percent.

我们对 48 例患者剖腹前作了胆总管镜检查,诊断准确率达 94%。

(B) Four hundred and twenty-five cystoscopes were performed on 380 patients with persistent Frequent urination and urgency complaints.

我们对 402 例持续尿频、尿急症状患者做了 380 次膀胱镜检查。

(A) Thallium-201 myocardial perfusion scintigraphy was performed in 46 patients with coronary artery disease and 12 normal control subjects.

我们对 46 例冠心病患者及 12 名作对照的正常人进行了心肌铊 201 灌注闪烁照相检查。

（B）Biopsy was performed on 42patients with proven cancer of the liver.

作者对 42 例已确诊为肝癌的患者做了穿刺活检。

（A）Two endoscopies were performed with 10-day interval in each subject.

每人各做两次内窥镜检查（间隔时间为 10 天）。

（B）Over a two-year period, 120 Chol cystograms were performed on 80 patients.

两年来，我们对 80 例患者做了 120 次胆囊造影。

（A）In 15 patients with acute pancreatitis caused by biliary disease endoscopic sphincterotomy was performed after diagnostic ERCP (endoscopic retrograde cholangio pancreatography).

在 ERCP（内窥镜逆行性胰胆管造影术）检查确诊后，我们对 15 例胆道疾病引起的急性胰腺炎患者经内窥镜做了括约肌切开术。

（B）Parietal wall vagotomy without drainage was performed on 35 patients.

我们对 35 例患者不用引流施行了壁迷走神经切断术。

句型（2）与句型（1）含义相同，不同的仅是动词的语态。在句型（2）中是主动语态，句中的主语是"患者"。在句型（1）中是被动语态，句中的主语只能是各种检查与手术名称，而"患者"则置于介词短语中。

Fifty patients over a 2-year period underwent bladder resection of bladder Cancer.

2 年的时间里，有 50 例患者因膀胱癌进行了膀胱切开术。

Such patients should undergo coronary angiography for detection of the disease.

这类患者应做冠状血管造影，以对该病做出诊断。

三、表达"测定"的句型

表示测定的动词最常用的是 measure，也可用 determine。能与这类动词搭配的名词可分为三类：

1. 各种化学与生化成分词语，如 antibody（抗体）、antigen（抗原）、potassium（钾）、cholesterol（胆固醇）等。

2. 各种表达含量的词语，如：concentration（浓度）、level（水平）、rate（率）、output（输出量）等。

3. 表示各种功能的名词，如 function（功能）、activity（活性）、change（变化）、affinity（亲和力）、response（反应）、binding（结合力）等。

现举例说明如下：

Serum lipids was measured in 1 680 women attending a screening center.

我们对普查中心的 1 680 名女性做了血脂含量的测定。

Serum high-density-lipoprotein cholesterol was determined in patients with hepatoma, liver cirrhosis and healthy controls.

我们对肝细胞瘤、肝硬化及健康的对照组人员做了血清高密度脂蛋白胆固醇含量的测定。

Levels of serum potassium, sodium and calcium were measured in 58 patients admitted to a coronary unit.

我们对冠心病监护室收治的 58 例患者做了血清钾、钠及钙离子含量测定。

The concentration of cyclic adenosine 3', 5'-mono-phosphate in 16 cerebrospinal fluid samples from eight patients with bacterial meningitis due to several different organisms was determined.

我们对 8 名由几种不同微生物引起的细菌性脑膜炎患者的 16 份脑脊液标本做了 3',5'-单磷酸环腺苷浓度的测定。

The signal transmission function of the dendritic cells was determined.

我们测定了树突状细胞的信号传导功能。

Thyroid-stimulating immunoglobulin activity was measured by radioreceptor assay in sera from patients with Graves' disease, Hashimoto's thyroiditis, and thyroid cancer.

我们用放射受体检查方法对 Graves 氏病、桥本氏甲状腺炎及甲状腺癌患者血清中的甲状腺刺激性免疫球蛋白活性做了测定。

第三节 各种数字英文表达方法

一、大数目中的小数目

要表达"在……例中有……例",可用下列三种结构:①数字 +of+ 数字;②数字 +out of+ 数字;③ among+ 数字 + 数字。这三种表达法意义相同,使用频率以 of 为最高,out of 与 among 次之。要注意:小数目可用作主语,也可不用作主语。不作主语时,往往与介词 in 搭配连用。下面将就具体用法进行介绍:

1. 使用介词 of

Three hundred and forty of 5 145 patients undergoing TURP (transurethral resection of the prostate) required reoperations on this system.

在 5 145 例施行过经尿道前列腺电切手术的患者中,有 340 例需再次做电切手术。

Of 180 previously untreated patients, 20 have died of renal failure.

在过去 180 例未经治疗的患者中,有 20 例死于肾衰竭。

In twenty of the 28 patients, long-term palliation was accomplished.

28 例患者中,20 例患者得到长期症状缓解。

2. 使用介词 out of

Twenty out of 28 patients complained of sleep disorder due to disturbances of microcirculation.

在 28 例患者中,由于微环境紊乱有 20 例睡眠障碍。

Out of four patients with small-cell carcinoma, two showed an objective response to oral treatment.

在 4 例小细胞癌患者中,有 2 例口服药物客观有效。

Death from seminoma occurred in 3 out of 16 patients with nodal metastases <5cm in diameter.

在转移性癌结节直径 <5cm 的 16 例患者中,有 3 例死于精原细胞癌。

3. 使用介词 among

Among 20 patients who underwent pancreatic surgery during the first week of treatment, 5 died.

在胰腺手术的 20 例患者中,第一周内有 5 例死亡。

Among 111 subjects with asymptomatic hyperuricemia followed for 108 months, atherosclerotic heart disease developed in six.

111 例无症状型高尿酸血症患者经过 108 个月随访,有 6 例发生动脉粥样硬化性心脏病。

最后,要提一下数词的书写问题。按正规的写作要求,在句子的开头不可用阿拉伯数字,应用英语数词,但在英美作者的文摘中破格的写法时有所见。在本书中我们对不规范的写法均做了修改。

二、集团数

所谓"集团数"是指以整体形式表现出来的数目,常见的表达法如下:① a total of …;② a series of …;③ a group of …。在英美医学杂志中,这些词组做主语时,其谓语动词既见有单数,也见有复数。如:

A total of 149 patients was followed up for from 1 to 4 years, the average follow-up period being 2.6 years.(谓语 was 为单数)

我们对总数达 149 名患者随访了 1~4 年,随访期平均为 2.6 年。

A total of 134 patients suspected of having pancreatic cancer were given preoperative ultrasonic examinations.(谓语 were 为复数)

(总数达)134 例拟诊为胰腺癌的患者在术前做了超声检查。

A series of 21 patients treated surgically for primary melanoma of the skin of the breast has been studied.(谓语动词为单数 has)

我们对 21 例乳房皮肤原发性黑色素瘤手术治疗的患者进行了研究。

A series of 59 consecutive patients with inoperable carcinoma of the prostate were entered into a national cooperative study.(谓语动词为复数 were)

我们将 59 例不能手术治疗的前列腺癌患者列为全国协作组的研究对象。

A group of 186 patients with transient ischemic attacks of cerebral infarction was found to demonstrate in vivo spontaneous platelet aggregation in 39% of these studied.(谓语动词为单数 was)

在 186 例一过性脑缺血发作引起脑梗的患者中,我们发现 39% 的患者体内发生了自发性血小板凝聚现象。

A group of 86 cirrhotic undergoing therapeutic variceal decompressive procedures were studied.(谓语动词为复数 were)

我们对 86 例施行曲张静脉减压术的肝硬化患者进行了研究。

可是,S. E. Paces 著的 *Common Errors in English*(P.12)却指出:

Wrong: A series of events form history.

Right: A series of events forms history.

这种情形与 a number of 类似。语法家一般都认为 a number of 做主语时其谓语动词应用复数,并指出用单数是错误的,但是事实上仍有用单数的,如 *Advanced Learner's Dictionary of Current English* 中就有一例:

A number of books is missing from the library.

图书馆里有一些书不见了。

不同表达方式的原因与作者写作时的着重点不同有关,如着重从逻辑意义出发,则用复数形式比较合理;如着重把一个前带有单数名词的词组作为一个整体词强调对待时,则选用单数形式,如上例的 A number of books。

上述词组还可用于介词短语中,也即是处于状语地位,这时谓语动词就不受其影响了。

Of a total of 44 episodes of cramps, 26 were treated with hypertonic glucose.

在总数达 44 次的痉挛发作中,有 26 次采用了高渗葡萄糖治疗。

Thirty-two cases of pulmonary contusion were selected on radiological criteria in a series of 250 thoracic traumas.

在 250 例胸外伤中,根据放射影像学诊断标准选出 32 例肺挫裂(作为研究对象)。

Dose-response curves to intravenous salbutamol were constructed after injection of saline or aminophylline in a group of ten asthmatic patients.

一组 10 例哮喘患者在注射盐水或氨茶碱后获得了静脉注射沙丁胺醇的剂量效应曲线。

三、另加数与其余数

"另有多少例"与"其余多少例"的表达方法如下:

(1) another+ 数词 + 名词　其他……;另……;

(2) the other+ 数词 + 名词　其他……;另……;

(3) 数词 +other　另……;

(4) an additional+ 数词 + 名词　另……;

(5) 数词 +additional+ 名词　另……;

(6) a further+ 数词 + 名词　另……;

(7) the remaining+ 数词 + 名词　其余……;

(8) the remainder 其余。

凡有冠词时,数词置于名词之前,如上述结构中的(2)、(4)、(6)、(7)。结构(1)中虽无冠词,但 another 是由 an+other 构成,故仍算有冠词,数词亦置于名词之前。在无冠词时,数词置于形容词或代词之前,如上述结构中的(3)、(5)。结构(8)不与数词连用。现将上述结构按顺序各举一例如下:

Of 20 patients with the zollinger-Ellison syndrome who underwent visceral angiography, only 3 had unequivocally positive studies for primary pancreatic tumors; another 5 patients had equivocal diagnoses based on adequate studies.

在 20 例做了内脏血管造影的 Zollinger-Ellison 综合征患者中,仅 3 例确诊为原发性胰腺肿瘤;另虽有 5 例通过适当的检查,但诊断不能最后确定。

Circulating platelet microthrombi was evaluated during the acute and convalescent phases of illness in 44 patients admitted to the hospital for chest pain … Circulating platelet microthrombi were significantly increased during the acute phase in 22 patients with transmural myocardial infarction compared with values in the other 22 patients without myocardial infarction.

我们检查了 44 例因胸痛住院的患者,对急性期与恢复期间循环血中血小板微血栓进行计数……。22 例透壁性心肌梗死患者与另 22 例无心肌梗死的患者相比,前者在急性期循环血小板微血栓大大增多。

Twelve patients with primary kidney cancer died of renal failure; three others died of multiple metastases.

12 例原发性肾癌患者死于肾衰竭;另外 3 例患者死于多发性转移。

One hundred and fourteen evaluable patients with measurable metastatic breast cancer were treated with a combination chemoimmunotherapy program, an additional 117 patients with the same program with the addition of bacillus Calmette-Guerin by scarification.

我们对 114 例能进行评价的,有可测指标的转移性乳腺癌患者进行了化学免疫联合治疗,而另外 117 例类似的患者除用化学免疫联合治疗外,还加用卡介苗划痕治疗。

The authors used the whole lung section technique to review the macroscopic pathology in 12 patients who died with Legionnaires' disease. None of these patients had been treated with erythromycin.

Abscesses were present in 2 cases and nodular infiltrates in 2 others.

In 5 additional patients, Legionnaires' disease had been treated with erythromycin.

作者用全肺切片技术对 12 例死于军团菌的患者做了肉眼病理学复查。患者无一例接受过红霉素治疗。

有两例见到多处脓疡,另两例有淋巴结浸润。

另有五例患者曾接受过红霉素治疗。

A total of 178 patients were available for follow-up. Of these 2 proved to have carcinomas on immediate follow-up, and a further 2 patients developed cancers in the same breast, one 4 and the other 7 years after aspiration.

可随访的患者共 178 例。在这些患者中,有 2 例一开始随访就确诊有癌症。另 2 例同一乳腺癌症复发,分别见于针吸后 4 年和 7 年。

The remaining 18 of the 67 patients, who lost an average of 17kg experienced a mean increase of 2.1mg/dl in serum uric acid.

67 例患者中其余的 18 例,体重减少 17kg,血清尿酸平均增加 2.1mg/dl。

In 25 of the 111 patients hypertension developed; their mean weight was not significantly higher than that of the remainder.

在 111 例患者中,有 25 例发生高血压;他们的平均体重并不明显超过其余的人。

四、平均数与中位数

"平均数"的常用表达词语有 average 和 mean;表达中位数最常见的为 median 一词。表达法如下:① average 平均为;② average+ 名词,平均;mean+ 名词,平均;median+ 名词,中位;③ an average+ 名词 +of+ 数词,平均为;A mean+ 名词 +of+ 数词,平均为;A median+ 名词 +of+ 数词,中位数为;④ an average of+ 数词,平均为;An mean of+ 数词,平均为;A median of+ 数词,中位数为;⑤ on(the)average,平均。

(1)在第一种结构中,average 是动词。

Survival following splenectomy averaged 25.5 months.

脾切除后存活时间平均为 25.5 个月。

On the twenty-third day following injury, urine volumes averaging from 50 to 100ml per 24 hours were obtained.

受伤后第 23 天,尿量平均为 50~100ml/24h。

（2）在第二种结构中 average、mean 和 median 都是形容词。

The average age of the patients is 50.

这些患者的年龄平均为 50 岁。

The mean age of the sham group was 38.6 years.

假手术组的平均年龄为 38.6 岁。

The median survival for the 12 patients was 25 months.

这 12 例患者的中位生存时间为 25 个月。

（3）在第三种结构中，average、mean 和 median 都是形容词，但在被它们修饰的名词后有 "of+ 数值" 的介词短语。

This leaded to an average reduction of 1.2mg/100ml within 24 hours.

这一情况导致 24 小时内平均减少 1.2mg/100ml。

Out of these patients 12 achieved a partial response with an average duration of more than 6 months.

在这些患者中有 12 例部分有效，持续时间平均在 6 个月以上。

Pruritus has recurred in 15 patients after a mean remission of 3 months.

15 例患者痒疹在平均缓解三个月后又复发。

One hundred and fifty-five men with a mean age of 53 ± 8 years underwent serial exercise testing 3 to 52 weeks after myocardial infarction.

155 例平均年龄为（53 ± 8）岁的男性患者，在心肌梗死后 3~52 个星期进行了一系列的运动试验。

（4）在第四种结构中 average、mean 和 median 都是名词。它们后面要接 "of+ 数值" 的介词短语。

Among 67 patients studied, 49 lost an average of 20kg.

在所观察的 67 例患者中，有 49 例体重平均下降 20kg。

The course of rheumatoid arthritis was analyzed in 50 newly-diagnosed adults followed prospectively for an average of over 5 years.

我们对 50 例新确诊的类风湿性关节炎成人患者作了平均 5 年以上的前瞻性随访，对该病病程作了分析。

They found that serum potassium concentration was lowered from an average of 5.8 to 4.0mmol/L.

他们发现，血清钾浓度从 5.8 降到了 4.0mmol/L。

Sixteen patients were known to remain in remission for a mean of at least 10.6 months after the first or second course of treatment.

在第一或第二个疗程之后，16 名患者症状继续缓解，平均至少为 10.6 个月。

Follow-up information was obtained for a mean of 21 months in all 109 patients.

我们平均用了 21 个月的时间，取得了所有 109 例患者的随访资料。

Patients ranged in age from 10 to 76 years with a median of 48 years.

患者年龄在 10~76 岁之间，中位数为 48 岁。

（5）在表达平均数时，如句中无恰当的名词可与形容词 average 搭配连用，就可用第五种结构 on（the）average。这一结构中 average 是名词，冠词 the 可以省略。如：

The patients were hypertension during 6.5 years on the average.

这些患者高血压的时间平均为 6.5 年。

The onset of claudication had on average been 7.5 months previously.

以往发生跛行时间平均为 7.5 个月。

It is 5cm long on average.

平均长度为 5cm。

五、一般数值表达法

（1）（a+ 名词 +of）+ 数词：“（a+ 名词 +of）+ 数词”是一种常见的表达数值的结构。其中的“名词”一般都是表示“数值”概念的名词或动名词，如：

1) a total of 总数为……

2) a series of 连续数为……

3) a period of 为期……

4) a maximum of 最大量值为……

5) a minimum of 最小量值为……

6) an incidence of 发病率为……

7) a mortality of 死亡率为……

8) an accuracy of 精确率为……

9) a dose of 剂量为……

10) an average of 平均数为……

11) an mean of 平均数为……

12) an average duration of 平均持续时间为……

13) a median follow-up interval of 随访平均间隔时间为……

14) an average reduction of 平均减少……

15) a mean remission of 平均缓解时间为……

现举例如下：

Daily fever persisted with temperatures reaching a maximum of 39.8℃ on the fourth hospital day.

在住院第四天，全天持续发热，最高达 39.8℃。

The patient was initially treated with ampicillin for a period of 10 days.

患者最初用氨苄西林治疗了 10 天。

Nosocomial infection was noted in 5 patients with a mortality of 60%.

有 5 例院内感染，死亡率为 60%。

The first two patients were admitted at night and blood glucose estimations were not done. This led to a delay of 16 and 12 hours respectively before the appropriate therapy was instituted.

前 2 例患者是在夜间住院的，故未做血糖分析，这就使患者分别延迟 16 小时及 12 小时才进行适当的治疗。

Initial laboratory studies included the following; arterial blood gases showed an oxygen tension (PaO$_2$) of 52mmHg, a carbon dioxide tension (PaCO$_2$) of 29mmHg, a PH of 7.48, a hemoglobin level of 12.6g/dl, a white blood count of 8 600/mm^3, a prothrombin time of 15.4 seconds with a control of

12.2 seconds, a serum bilirubin of 3.7mg/dl (total) and 3.0mg/dl (direct).

最初的实验结果如下：经动脉血气分析，氧分压为 52mmHg；二氧化碳分压为 29mmHg；PH 为 7.48；血红蛋白浓度为 12.6g/dl；白细胞计数为 8 600/mm³；凝血酶原时间为 15.4 秒（对照为 12.2 秒）；血清总胆红素为 3.7mg/dl，直接胆红素为 3.0mg/dl。

（2）动词 + 数词：表达数值还可用"动词 + 数词"的句型。常用的动词有 account for（占），represent（占）两词。Account for 可后接任何数词，包括百分数；而 represent 一般后接百分数词。

Primary nocardia infection without known underlying disease accounted for only 4 of 17 infections.

在 17 例患者中，无基础疾病的原发性诺卡氏菌感染仅占 4 例。

Melanomas in this location accounted for 1.8% of a total of 1 140 patients with primary clinical stage I and Stage II melanomas treated during a 28-year period.

在 28 年里，在经过治疗的总数达 1 140 例的原发性临床 I 期及 II 期的黑色素瘤患者中，黑色素瘤发生在这一部位的占 1.8%。

Infections with M (Mycobacterium) intracellular avium represented 27 percent of all mycobacterial infections seen during this period.

在这一时期所发生的全部分枝杆菌感染中，细胞内鸟（型）分枝杆菌感染占 27%。

（3）多个数值的特殊表达法：当有多个名词附有不同数值时，"a+ 名词 +of+ 数词"结构不再适用。这种情况下，可将各数值直接置于该名称之后，数值与名词之间用","隔开，但不是必须适用，可省略。

The relationship of antibody-coated bacteria to clinical syndromes was: asymptomatic acteriuria, 15% (27/178); cystitis, 8% (6/75); acute hemorrhagic cystitis, 67% (4/6); prostatitis, 67% (2/3). and acute pyelonephritis 62%(16/26).

被抗体包裹的细菌与临床综合征的关系是：无症状细菌尿 15%（27/178）；膀胱炎 8%（6/75）；急性出血性膀胱炎 67%（4/6）；前列腺炎 67%（2/3）；急性肾盂肾炎 62%（16/26）。

Liver function test results were bilirubin 0.4mg, serum glutamic oxaloacetic transaminase 65U (normal less than 40U), alkaline phosphatase 260U (normal less than 110U).

肝功能检查结果是：胆红素 0.4mg，血清谷草转氨酶 65 单位（正常值在 40 单位以下），碱性磷酸酶 260 单位（正常值在 110 单位以下）。

六、百分位

百分位可用 percent，当然也可用符号"%"。

在应用百分数时应注意是否需用介词 of。如"5% 的病例"和"5% 的葡萄糖"如何译？前者应译为 5% of the cases，后者应为 5% glucose。为什么前者用 5% of，而后者只用 5%？这是因为 5% of the cases 中的 5% 是 the cases 的一部分，所以要加介词 of。而 5% glucose 中的 5% 只是表示 glucose 的浓度，是说明 glucose 的性质，并不是它的一个部分。再举例如下：

X-rays of the chest, colon, and biliary tract revealed pathology in 30%~40% of the patients.

这些患者中有 30%~40% 经过胸部、结肠及胆道 X 线检查发现有病理变化。

In 30 percent of bacteremias, the site of origin could not be identified with certainty.

30% 的菌血症不能确定感染的原发部位。

Approximately 15 percent of strains of *E. coli* causing bacteremia underwent 99 percent or greater killing by pooled normal human serum.

引起菌血症的大肠杆菌，大约有 15% 的菌株被混合的正常人血清杀灭 99% 或更多一些。

One patient had a 50 percent regression of a large pulmonary metastasis which, upon surgical removal, showed active osteogenic sarcoma.

一例患者的大块肺转移灶缩小了 50%，经手术切除检查，证明是活动性骨肉瘤。

七、数值分别为的表达

在表达三个及以上的人或事物各具不同的数值时，可用 respectively（分别）一词进行表述，例如：将"敏感性为 85%，特异性为 98%，预测准确率为 98%，分类正确率为 91%。"译为 sensitivity was 85%, specificity was 98%, predictive accuracy was 98%, correct classification rate was 91%，就显得句型过于单调。这时，可用 respectively 一次改写为 Sensitivity, specificity, predictive accuracy, and correct classification were 85, 98, 98 and 91% respectively.

respectively 在应用过程中往往放置于句子的末尾，而且在该词之前一般都有逗号，也可不用逗号，该词也可置于句中。现再举几个例子，并请注意可有不同的译法。

The patients were respectively 28 and 36 years old women of good health.

（1）患者分别为 28 及 36 岁健康女性。

（2）两患者均为健康女性，一例 28 岁，一例 36 岁。

Serum alkaline phosphatase and aspartate aminotransferase values were increased in 15 and 18 cases respectively.

（1）血清碱性磷酸酶及天冬氨酸转氨酶升高者分别为 15 例及 18 例。

（2）血清碱性磷酸酶升高者为 15 例，天冬氨酸转氨酶升高者 18 例。

The annual mortality rate in such populations has averaged about 7 and 11% in patients with 2 and 3 vessel disease, respectively.

在这类人群中，两根血管病变与三根血管病变的患者年死亡率平均各为 7% 及 11%。

八、倍数

在英语医学论文中常见的表示"倍"的词是 times 和 -fold。

在英语中"一倍"不说 one time，应说 once；两倍不说 two times，应说 twice；三倍以上才说 three（four, five …）times。但"2~3 倍"可说 two or three times 或写成 2 or 3 times。此外，"一倍半""两倍半"也可写成 1.5times、2.5times。

-fold 是后缀。可与其他的字组成新字，如 twofold, threefold（也可写成 two-fold、three-fold）等。

表达倍数的句型如下：

（1）A is 3 times as deep as B.

1）A 的深度是 B 的三倍。

2）A 比 B 深两倍。

（2）The depth of A is 3 times the depth of B.

The depth of A is 3 times that of B.

1）A 的深度是 B 的三倍。

2）A 比 B 深两倍。

（3）A is 3 times deeper than B.

1）A 的深度是 B 的三倍。

2）A 比 B 深两倍。

（4）A increases 3 times.

1）A 增加了两倍。

2）A 增加到（原有的）三倍。

这四种句型所表示的倍数关系都是相同的,都是 1×3=3,也即:是原来的三倍,或比原来的多两倍。这里要特别提出三种句型,A is 3 times longer than B 对这一句型结构,就是以英语为母语的人也会有两种不同数值的理解,有人理解为:A 比 B 长三倍,即 A 的长度是 B 的三倍。B. Evans 编的 *A Dictionary of Contemporary American Usage* 中有一段说明对我们写作很有帮助,现摘录如下:

The word "times" may be used in comparing a large thing with a small one, as in "it is three times as large:" and "it is three times larger:" The first form is perfectly clear but the second is ambiguous. It means to some people "three times as large" and to others "four times as large". for this reason, it should be avoided. When a small thing is compared with a large one, the word: "times" should not be used. The small thing is "one-third as large as" or "two-third smaller than "the other".

将大的事物与小的事物加以比较时,可用 times 一词,如 "it is three times as large … 及 it is three times larger …,前一种结构表达的概念非常清楚,而后一种结构的含义却模棱两可,有的人认为它表示"三倍",有的人又认为是"四倍",因此应避免使用。将小的事物与大的事物加以比较时,不要用 times 一词,应说:"这一事物是另一事物的 1/3"或"比另一事物小 2/3"。

以上所述是本节第一、第三种句型结构的用法。现在再看第二种句型,在句型（2）中 3 times 本身就是定语成分,所以不要在后面接介词 of,如:

The arterial pressure might rise simultaneously to about 1 times normal.

动脉压可能同时升高到正常的 1 倍。

倍数词后接的名词有定冠词时,倍数词应置于定冠词之前,因此,语法上称这种倍数词为"前置限定词"。如:

The left ventricle has approximately twice the thickness of the right ventricle.

左心室的厚度约为右心室的两倍。

倍数词后接的名词如在前面已经出现过,应用 that（those）来代替,如:

The volume of the systemic circulation is about 7 times that of the pulmonary system.

体循环的容量约为肺循环容量的 7 倍。

Consequently, the sulphonamide levels of sulphadiazine were 2.5 times those of sulphamethoxazole.

因此,磺胺嘧啶的磺胺含量是磺胺甲噁唑的 2.5 倍。

由后缀 -fold 组成的词可用作一般形容词。如后接名词有冠词时,冠词要置于这个词的前面,如:

The hallmark of the inflammatory process is a four to fivefold, or more, elevation of serum transaminase levels.

血清转氨酶浓度升高 4~5 倍以上，是炎症过程的标志。

在句型（4）中，倍数词 times 与后缀 -fold 都可与动词直接搭配连用。如：

Neonatal death increased by more than two and a half time.

新生儿期死亡率增加了 2.5 倍多。

The diameters of these vessels increase only fourfold.

这些血管的直径只能扩大到 4 倍。

除上述四种句型结构外，还有一种"倍数词 +as much as……"句型。在这种结构中，倍数词既可与动词搭配连用，也可与名词搭配连用。如：

The ventricles rest almost twice as much as they work.

心室休息的时间几乎是工作时间的两倍。

Cow's milk contains about twice as much protein as human milk.

牛奶中蛋白质的含量是人奶的两倍。

When burned, fats produce almost two times as much energy as does the same amount of carbohydrates.

脂肪在氧化时所产生的能力是等量碳水化合物的 2 倍。

九、比率

表示 A 与 B 的比例常用的形式有：

ratio of A and B

A：B ratio

A/B ratio

ratio of the two

现将上述结构各举一例如下。

The ratio of total cholesterol to HDI cholesterol fell insignificantly.

总胆固醇与高密度脂蛋白胆固醇的比率下降不大。

Notably more males than females were affected (male to female ratio, 14：4).

男性患者显然多于女性（男女比例为 14：4）。

The male: female ratio was 5：4.

男女比例为 5：4。

A retrospective survey of patients with infective endocarditis at St. Bartholomew's Hospital in the decade 1966~75 showed a male/female ratio of 1.5：1.

对 1966—1975 十年间在 St. Bartholomew's 医院治疗的感染性心内膜炎患者进行的回顾性调查表明男女之间的比例为 1.5：1。

There was no correlation between transport rates and the ratio of the two conversion pathways.

这两种转换途径的比例与输送率之间并无关系。

有时 ratio 一词还可省去不用，如：

The female: male was 2：1 in the left bundle branch block and left anterior hemiblock groups and 1：1 in the group with right bundle branch block.

女性与男性的比例在左束支传导阻滞及左前阻滞组为 2∶1；在右束支传导阻滞组为 1∶1。

ratio 一般总是指两个数值相比，可是，相比的两个数值的后一数值如是 1，如 2∶1、3∶1 等，这后一数值 1 有时可省略不写，这时，ratio 的意思是"比值"，如：

The 5-year age-race adjusted mortality rate for smokers was 24.3 compared to 18.8 for nonsmokers, yielding a 5-year mortality ratio of smokers to nonsmokers of 1.29.

吸烟者的五年年龄及种族调整死亡率为 24.3，而非吸烟者为 18.8，吸烟者与非吸烟者的五年死亡率的比值为 1.29（或：吸烟者与非吸烟者的五年死亡率之比为 1.29∶1）。

The ratio of male and female has been falling steadily, and now stands at about 1.2 for hospitalizations and about 1.5 for deaths.

男女之比已逐步下降，目前男女住院数之比约为 1.2∶1，死亡数之比约为 1.5∶1。

十、数值的范围

数值上下波动的范围一般用 from … to … 或 between … and … 加上另一个表示"幅度变动"的动词来表达，但 from … to … 也可以单独使用。

常见的句型结构如下：

range from … to …　在……之间　range between … and …

with a range of … to …　在……之间

Vary from … to …　在……之间

Vary between … and …

from … to …　从……到……

现按上述结构分别举例如下：

The duration of therapy ranged from six to eighteen months.

治疗时间为 6~18 个月。

Serum potassium concentrations ranged between 3.5 and 5.5mmol/L.

血清水杨酸盐浓度在 3.5~5.5mmol/L。

The patients ranged in age from 33 to 80 years.

患者年龄在 33~80 岁之间。

Their average age was 32.6 ± 1.5 with a range of 12 to 54 years.

他们的年龄在 12~54 岁之间，平均为（32.6 ± 1.5）岁（注意：range 如是名词，后面只能接 of … to … ，不可用 from … to …）。

The fraction of unchanged drug reaching systemic circulation varied between 0 and 38% assuming a liver blood flow rate of 1.53L/min.

假设肝血流量为 1.53L/min，那么进入体循环的未经改变的那部分药物占 0~38%。

The dosage to be used for intravenous infusion varies from 1ug/min to 20μg/min usually ranging between 3 and 10μg/min.

要使用的静脉灌注剂量在 1~20μg/min 之间，而通常则在 3~10μg/min 之间。

要特别注意 from … to … 的用法，这一词组应看成一个整体，相当于一个名词的作用，甚至可做主语，该词组如需要与其他介词连用时，介词要置于 from … to … 整个词组之前，此外 from … to … 中的 from 往往可省略。

Various studies reported asthma to be present in from 2.3 to 4.8 percent of this age group.

据各种研究报告，该年龄组哮喘的发病率为 2.3%~4.8%。

An adult who is up and about, but relatively inactive, needs 20 to 30 percent more calories than required under basal condition. For one engaged in a sedentary occupation, this extra energy requirement rises to from 30 to 40 per cent above basal.

一个成年人如起床走动，但活动量不大，其所需的热量比基础代谢多 20%~30%，一个伏案工作的人所需要的能量要比基础代谢多 30%~40%。

As a rough indication of their size, from 10 to 1 000 bacteria (depending upon the species) could, if lined up, span a pinhead.

10~1 000 个细菌（随菌种而异），如能排列成线，就相当于针头大小，这就是对细菌大小的粗略估计。

十一、约略数的表达法

约略数的表示法为将含有"约略"含义的词或词组与一个确定的数值搭配在一起连用，表示"约略"含义的词或词组较多，且大多为副词性的，只有 approximate 一词是动词。这类词或词组常见的如下：

（1）approximate 大约为

（2）approximately 大约

（3）about 大约

（4）some 大约

（5）or so …… 左右

（6）almost 几乎

（7）nearly 差不多

（8）over 超过……以上

（9）above 超过……以上

（10）more than 超过

（11）greater than 大于

（12）less than 不到

这些词在句中的位置与汉语的习惯有所不同。如汉语可以说"我们大约治疗了 10 名病人"，"大约"置于动词之前。在英语中，这类副词一般都要紧接数词，如：we treated about ten patients。在需要应用介词时，介词也要置于整个"略数词"之前，也即是置于含有"大约"之类含义的副词或词组之前。在上述例词（组）中 or so 是例外，要置于数词之后，请看下面例句：

The loss of water from the skin and respiratory tract approximates 750ml per day.

从皮肤和呼吸道丧失的水分每天约 750ml。

She had radiation-induced hypothyroidism which persisted for approximately 10 years.

她患放疗诱发的甲状腺功能减退已有十年左右。

These patients have an average annual mortality rate of only about 2%.

这些患者的平均年死亡率约 2%。

Figure 3-26 illustrates a situation in which hyperventilation had been present for some 30 hours.

图 3-26 表明,换气过度已有 30 小时左右。

The eye except for the anterior one fifth or so of its circumference, is enclosed in a bony case.

眼球除了前 1/5 部分外,其他均嵌在骨眶内。

One patient had monethyglycylxylidide concentrations almost twice that of lidocaine.

一名患者的单乙甘氨基二甲苯胺化合物的浓度几乎是利多卡因的 2 倍。

The incidence of appendicitis in older patients has risen nearly sevenfold over the last four decades.

40 年来,年龄较大的人的阑尾炎发病率增加了将近 6 倍。

In over 90% of the cases significant chest pain is due to coronary disease.

90% 以上的胸部剧痛与冠心病有关。

The patient weighed above 200 pounds.

该患者体重超过 200 磅。

Of these 26, 12 had an elevated SGPT (serum glutamic oxalacetic transaminase) for greater than 1 year.

这 26 例中,有 12 例血清谷草转氨酶(SGPT)升高已一年以上。

约略数还可用符号"<""">"来表示,如:

Hypothermia, rectal temperature <97.6 ℉, was noted at the onset of bacteremia and prior to shock in 83 patients.

83 例患者在菌血症及休克前发现体温过低,肛门温度在 97.6 ℉以下。

关于约略数值的表达法还应注意一点:表示约意义的副词一般应与确切的数值连用,而不应与约略数值连用。如可以说 about 10,approximately 100 等,而不应说:about more than 10,about less than half,about several 等。About three or four 虽也有人用,但仍以删去 about 为好。

十二、持续时间的常用句型

按英、美医学论文的写作习惯,病例数往往不置于标题中,而是置于摘要正文开头第一句来表达。这时,摘要开头第一句不仅叙述病例数,而且还交代该研究共持续了多少时间。表达这种持续时间的常用词有:during、period、for、within,常用句式结构如下:

during the past 5 years;over the past 5 years 近五年来

during a 10 years period;over a period of 10 years;in a 10 year period 在为期十年中

during the period 1970-1975; during the 1970-1975 period; in the period 1970-1975 在 1970—1975 年期间

in 1970-1975;in the years 1970-1975;for the years 1970-1975 在 1970—1975 年间

between 1 January (,) 1970 and 31 December (,) 1975 在 1970 年 1 月 1 日至 1975 年 12 月 31 日期间

From January (,) 1970 to December (,) 1979; from January 1970 through December 1975

从 1970 年 1 月至 1979 年 12 月

for five years　为期五年

within 12 hours　12 个小时之内

上述各组中,每组的含义基本相同。在第 5 组中,from January through December 是美国说法,意思是"从一月到十二月底"。现举例说明如下:

1. 第一种结构

Over the past 10 years, 23 addicts presented with the nephritic syndrome and/or renal insufficiency.

十年来,有 23 名成瘾者呈现肾病综合征及 / 或肾功能不全。

2. 第二种结构

During a five-year period, 105 patients with intestinal obstruction, secondary to metastatic disease, were seen.

在 5 年中我们诊治了 105 例继发于转移性肿瘤的肠梗阻患者。

3. 第三种结构

Eight patients have been admitted with gallstone ileus to the Heming Central Hospital during the period 1960-1977.

1960—1977 年间,赫明中心医院收治了 8 例回胆结石引起肠梗阻的患者。

4. 第四种结构

In 1970-71, 5 249 Copenhagen men aged 40-59 were screened for hypertension.

1970—1971 年,我们对哥本哈根 5 249 名 40~59 岁的男性做了高血压普查。

5. 第五种结构

Thirty-four suspected primary bone neoplasms were evaluated by needle biopsy between 1976 and 1978.

在 1976—1978 年间,我们用针吸活检对 34 例拟诊为原发性骨肿瘤的患者进行检验。

6. 第六种结构

We investigated 27 patients with colon cancer who underwent surgery and were followed for 5 years.

我们对 27 名接受过手术治疗的结肠癌患者进行了为期 5 年的跟踪调查。

7. 第七种结构

The birth weight of newborns was recorded within 12 hours.

新生儿的体重在出生后 12 小时以内进行了记录。

此外,有时需要表示"在第几天",可以用"on/at day+ 数字"来表示,如:

On day 20 after tumor cell inoculation mice were killed and liver weight and number of liver metasets were determined.

At day 14 of gestation, rats destined for reduced uterine perfusion were clipped as described below.

十三、剂量

叙述剂量时,常用 dose 与 dosage 两词,现先说明一下这两个词含义上的区别。根据

Dorland's Illustrated Medical Dictionary 的释义, dose 是: a quantity to be administered at one time, 也即是说, 是一次用的剂量。dosage 的释义是: the determination and regulation of the size, frequency, and number of doses, 意思是决定和调整各种剂量的大小, 频率与次数, 简言之, 就是 "剂量学"。这两个词在词典上含义很清楚, 可是实际应用时却很复杂。现按实际应用情况分别叙述如下:

（1）表示一次剂量时只能用 dose, 特别要用 a dose of 这结构。

Tamsulosin given in a dose of 0.2mg once a day for two weeks.

使用盐酸坦索罗辛, 每次 0.2mg, 每天一次, 连续 2 周。

Amlodipine was given orally in a dose of 2.5mg 24 hourly.

口服氨氯地平片, 每次 2.5mg, 24 小时一次。

（2）如不是指 "一次量", 而是指 "一天量" 或 "总剂量", 则 dose 与 dosage 往往可通用。如:

Gastrointestinal intolerance restricted dosage to 50mg daily.

由于胃肠道不能耐受, 故剂量限制在每天 50mg。

The patient was treated with penicillin in a dosage of 4g/day.

患者采用氨苄西林治疗, 剂量为每天 4g。

（3）如是泛指性剂量, 则应用 dosage。如:

In determining dosage regimens, it is quite important to know the extent of drug accumulation.

在决定剂量方案时, 必须知道药物在体内蓄积的程度。

（4）dose 与 dosage 还可用复数式, 表示 "各次" 或 "各种" 剂量。

The dosages used were several times higher than those used in earlier studies.

所用的各种剂量比先前所用的剂量大几倍。

（5）叙述剂量时, 也可不用 dose 或 dosage, 而是直接写出用药量, 如:

Azathioprine, 125mg/day, was restarted after recovery from the bone marrow suppression, and prednisone, 10mg/day, was continued.

在骨髓抑制恢复后, 仍继续使用泼尼松, 每天 10mg, 并重新启用硫唑嘌呤, 每天 125mg。

在这种用法时, 剂量数前后往往用逗号隔开, 但有时也可不用逗号。

十四、年龄表达法

年龄在医学文献中经常使用, 表达方法也较多。现将常见的基本结构介绍如下:

a 50-year-old patient

a patient aged 50 years

a patient aged 50

a patient 50 year of age

at the age of 50 years; at the age of 50

除上述四种常用的基本结构外, 表达约略年龄与年龄范围的方法也极多, 常见的如下:

over (the) age (of) 50 (years) over 50 years of age

under (the) age (of) 50 (years)

above (the) age (of) 50 (years)

below (the) age (of) 50 (years)

before (the) age (of) 50 (years)

after (the) age (of) 50 (years)

more than 50 years old

less than 50 years old

older than 50 years

younger than 50 years

aged 50 years and over

50 years of age and under

at 50 years of age or less

in women 50 years or older

between the ages of 30 and 50 years

from 6 to 12 months of age

aged 30 to 50 years

ranging in age from 50 to 80 years

现以基本结构为主,结合约略年龄表达法,举例说明如下:

(1)第一种基本结构的中心词是 old。要注意,在这结构中 year 一般不用复数式,不要写成 a years old patient,而应写成:

Trauma and blood transfusion led to profound, persistent infectious mononucleosis in a 21-year-old man.

一例 21 岁男性患者,因外伤和输血引起重度持续性传染性单核细胞增多症。

在文摘中 old 大多置于名词之前,但也有置于名词之后的。这时,year 就应该用复数式。如:

Age is associated with slightly lower triiodothyronine levels, but only in men 60 years or older or in women 80 years or older.

碘塞罗宁含量偏低与年龄有关,但这种情况仅见于60岁以上的男性及80岁以上的妇女。

(2)第二种基本结构的中心词是 aged。这个词是形容词,不是动词过去式。这一结构中的 years 可以省略,但不可加用 old,不要写成 aged 50 years old,而要写成:

The incidence and prevalence of diabetes mellitus were determined in 3 733 Pima Indians aged 5 years or over by periodic examinations over a 10-year period.

在为期 10 年中,我们对 3 733 名 5 岁以上的比马印第安人进行了定期检查,并确定了糖尿病的发病率与流行病学情况。

(3)在第三种基本结构中 years 不可省略。如:

All patients were black men 18 to 45 years of age.

所有患者均为 18~45 岁的黑人。

(4)在第四种基本结构中,the、of 和 years 都可省略。本结构与第二种结构相同,也不可加用 old。但不可以说:at the age of 50 years old。简言之,有 age 或 aged 时,不可再用 old。year 在 age 之后可省略,在 age 之前不可省略。如:

After age 50 the cause which is most frequently overlooked is calcific aortic stenosis.

50 岁以后最容易疏忽的病因是钙化性主动脉瓣狭窄。

(5)还可用补叙的写法来表达年龄,这时年龄的前后一般要用逗号隔开,但也可不用逗号隔开。如：

Patient B, age 30 years, had complained of primary infertility for two years.

患者（B）（30 岁）患原发性不孕症 2 年。

（6）要注意，在表达年龄范围时要用 ages 的复数式。如：

Esophageal cancer most occur between the ages of 50 and 70 years.

食管癌最常见于 50~70 岁的人。

（7）表示平均年龄可用 a mean age of 或 an average age of 这种结构。如：

155 men with a mean age of 53 ± 8 years underwent serial exercise testing 3 to 52 weeks after myocardial infarction.

155 例男性患者（平均年龄为 53 岁 ± 8 岁）在心肌梗死后 3~52 周进行了一系列的运动实验。

（8）age 与介词 at、in 连用时含义不同。与 at 搭配，是指"在……年龄"；与 in 搭配，是指"在人生中的一段时间内"。如：

It may occur at any age.

这在任何年龄都可以发生。

还要注意，在 in old age、in middle age 中，不用冠词 the；"青年"这一概念不用 young age，应用 youth 来表达。

十五、表示时间概念的前置定语

表示时间概念的词组，即："数词 + 时间性名词"，往往可用作定语置于另一名词之前。这种时间概念的前置定语有如下几种结构：

（1）a+ 数词 + 时间名称单数 + 名词

（2）a+ 时间名称单数所有格 + 名词

（3）数词 + 时间名称复数 + 名词

（4）数词 + 时间名称复数所有格 + 名词

（5）数词 + 时间名称 +of+ 名词

在医学文献中，上述（1）、（4）、（5）三种结构使用最频繁，第三种结构极罕见。

A 27-year-old English house wife was admitted on 1 March, 1977 with a 10-day history of fever.（第一种结构）

一名 27 岁的英国家庭主妇因发热 10 天于 1977 年 5 月 1 日住院。

In less than an hour's time the patient will go to sleep, and when he wakes up he won't feel any pain.（第二种结构）

不要一个小时病人就可入睡，等他醒后就一点不痛了。

On pretreatment menstrual cycle in Subject A and another cycle studied after two months therapy with dexamethasone, 0.25mg given orally twice a day, are compared in Figure 4（第三种结构）。

我们将患者 A 治疗前的一次月经周期与用地塞米松治疗 2 月后（0.25mg 每天口服两次）的另一次月经周期加以比较（图 4）。

A 38-year-old drug addict was admitted to the hospital with chest pain of four days' duration（第四种结构）。

一例 38 岁的药物成瘾者因胸痛 4 天住院。

During 1 year of maintenance therapy with 800mg cimetidine daily，3 of 19 patients relapsed（第五种结构）。

用甲腈咪胺每天 800mg 维持治疗一年期间，19 例患者中有 3 例复发。

十六、"治疗后一周"与"治疗一周后"

one week after treatment

after one week of treatment

第一句是"治疗后一周"，这个一周是指治疗以后经过一周时间，这一周时间并未再进行治疗。

第二句是"治疗一周后"，这个一周是指治疗持续的时间。

在 one week after treatment 的结构之前，还可以使用其他介词，如：

In one week after treatment=One week after treatment

Within one week after treatment

在治疗后一周之内的某一时间

For one week after treatment

在治疗后整个一周的时间段里

现将两种结构的用法举例如下：

（1）第一种结构：表示"×× 后多少时间"。

Three days after admission the patient became febrile.

入院后 3 天患者发热。

（2）第二种结构：表示"×× 多少时间以后"。

After 1 year of medical treatment 69 stones of the 3 major coronary branches showed no significant change.

内科治疗 1 年以后，3 根主要冠状动脉分支的 69 个结石无明显改变。

十七、统计学意义常用的句型

There was/is（no）significant difference in ...　（不）存在显著差异

The difference in ... was/is significant　差异显著

No significant difference was found/observed in ... 没有发现显著差异

... and ... differ significantly in ... 差异显著

十八、一些常见的英文文章语言技巧

如何指出当前研究的不足以及有目的地引导出自己的研究的重要性：通常在叙述了前人成果之后，用 however 来引导不足，比如：

However, little information ...

　　　　little attention ...

little work …

little data …

little research …

or few studies …

few investigations …

few researchers …

few attempts …

or no

none of these studies

has (have) been less

done on

focused on

attempted to

conducted

investigated

studied

(with respect to)

Previous research (studies, records) has (have)

failed to consider

ignored

misinterpreted

neglected to

overestimated, underestimated

misled

thus, these previus results are

inconclusive, misleading, unsatisfactory, questionable, controversial …

Uncertainties (discrepancies) still exist …

这种引导一般提出一种新方法,或者一种新方向。如果研究的方法以及方向和前人一样,可以通过下面的方式强调自己工作的作用:

However, data is still scarce

rare

less accurate

there is still dearth of

We need to

aim to

have to

provide more documents

data

records

studies

increase the dataset

Further studies are still necessary …

essential …

为了强调自己研究的重要性,一般还要在 however 之前介绍自己研究问题的反方面,另一方面等等。比如:

(1) 时间问题:如果你研究的问题时间上比较新,你就可以大量提及对时间较老的问题的研究及重要性,然后说(however),对时间尺度比较新的问题研究不足。

(2) 物性及研究手段问题:如果你要应用一种新手段或者研究方向,你可以提出当前比较流行的方法以及物质性质,然后说对你所研究的方向和方法,研究甚少。

(3) 研究区域问题:首先总结相邻区域或者其他区域的研究,然后强调这一区域研究不足。

(4) 不确定性:虽然前人对这一问题研究很多,但是目前有两种或者更多种的观点,这种 uncertainties,ambiguities,值得进一步澄清。

(5) 提出自己的假设来验证:如果自己的研究完全是新的,没有前人的工作进行对比,在这种情况下,可以自信地说,根据提出的过程,存在这种可能的结果,本文就是要证实这种结果。

We aim to test the feasibility (reliability) of the …

It is hoped that the question will be resolved (fall away) with our proposed method (approach).

(a) 提出自己的观点

we aim to

this paper reports on

provides results

extends the method

focus on

he purpose of this paper is to

furthermore, moreover, in addition, we will also discuss …

(b) 圈定自己的研究范围

前言的另外一个作用就是告诉读者包括评审者你的文章主要研究内容。如果处理不好,评审者会提出严厉的建议,比如你没有考虑某种可能性,某种研究手段等等。为了减少这种争论,在前言的结尾你就要明确提出本文研究的范围:

时间尺度问题:如果你的问题涉及比较长的时序,你可以明确地提出本文只关心这一时间范围的问题。

We preliminarily focus on the older (younger).

或者有两种时间尺度的问题(long-term and short-term),你可以说两者都重要,但是本文只涉及其中一种。

研究区域的问题:和时间问题一样,明确提出你只关心这一地区。

(c) 最后的圆场

最后,还可以总结性地提出,这一研究对其他研究的帮助。或者说,further studies on … will be summarized in our next study(or elsewhere)。

总之,其目的就是让读者把思路集中到你要讨论的问题上来,减少争论(arguments)。正确清楚地表达自己的研究成果和观点是写好英文科研论文的基本要求。否则,无论研究结果多么重要,科研论文都会被审稿人拒之门外。句型的选择和应用贯穿于英文文章写作的始终,恰当的句型和地道的英语表达方法不仅会给审稿人留下较好的印象,提高稿件录用的概率,同时也显示自己卓越的表达能力,使读者在轻松阅读中了解你的科研成果。

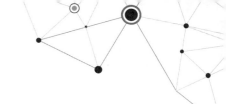

第19章
医学论文的伦理、权益及版权

Chapter 19
Medical Ethics, Rights and Copyright

第一节　医学研究的伦理

　　医学伦理学（medical ethics）是评价人类的医疗行为和医学研究是否符合道德的学科，其内容涉及生物学、医学、环境学、教育、科学研究、经济学、人类学等，属于伦理学的一个分支学科，是一门研究医疗卫生实践和医学科学发展中人类、医学团体与社会之间道德关系的科学。

一、医学伦理的必要性

　　近年来，国内外一些重大的学术不端行为在学术界引起轩然大波。韩国首尔大学黄禹锡教授在胚胎干细胞研究中的弄虚作假行为，使得人们对生物医学研究中的伦理问题越来越关注。此次事件中所涉及的论文造假行为给医学工作者提出警示：医学论文中的伦理学问题必须引起重视，对伦理学问题的认识能力必须提高。尤其是以患者或者正常人为研究对象时，由于活体会暴露于各种危险因素中，此时伦理要求就更为重要。美国国家卫生研究院（National Institutes of Health，NIH）解释了医学伦理的必要性："The objective of clinical research is to develop generalizable knowledge to improve health and/or increase understanding of human biology. This objective requires human subjects who could be at risk of harm even as they are contributing to scientific knowledge. Human subjects are a necessary means to the end of greater knowledge. Consequently，because people can be used as a means，clinical research has potential for the exploitation of human subjects. Ethical guidelines are the main mechanism used to minimize the chances of exploitation of research participants."。

二、医学伦理国际准则

　　随着社会的发展，各界对生物医学研究和临床试验的伦理学问题的关注日益增加。一些国际指南对人体进行生物医学研究的伦理和科学标准做了明确规定。其中具有代表性的有《纽伦堡法典》《赫尔辛基宣言》《贝尔蒙报告》《涉及人的生物医学研究的国际伦理准则》等，主要包括：

Nuremberg Code-Nuremberg Military Tribunal, 1947

Declaration of Helsinki-World Medical Association, 1964, '75, '83, '89, '96, 2000

Belmont Report-National Commission for the Protection of Human Subjects of Biomedical and Behavioral Research, 1979

45 CFR 46-DHHS, 1981, '91

Guidelines for Good Clinical Practice for Trials on Pharmaceutical Products-WHO, 1995

Good Clinical Practice: Consolidated Guidance-International Conference on Harmonisation-Technical Requirements for Registration of Pharmaceuticals for Human Use

Convention of Human Rights and Biomedicine-Council of Europe, 1997

Guidelines and Recommendations for European Ethics Committees-European Forum for Good Clinical Practice, 1997

Medical Research Council Guidelines for Good Clinical Practice in Clinical Trials (pdf)-Medical Research Council, United Kingdom, 1998

Guidelines for the Conduct of Human Research Involving Human Subjects in Uganda-Uganda National Council for Science and Technology, 1998

Ethical Conduct for Research Involving Humans-Tri-Council Working Group, Canada, 1998

National Statement on Ethical Conduct in Research Involving Humans-National Health and Medical Research Council, Australia, 1999

这其中,最为著名的是《纽伦堡法典》和《赫尔辛基宣言》。《纽伦堡法典》是一套人体试验准则,来源于第二次世界大战之后的纽伦堡审判的结果。

The Declaration of Helsinki was developed by the World Medical Association (WMA), as a set of ethical principles for the medical community regarding human experimentation, and is widely regarded as the cornerstone document of human research ethics. (WMA 2000, Bošnjak 2001, Tyebkhan 2003)。

《赫尔辛基宣言》制定了涉及以人体为对象进行医学研究的道德原则,包括以人作为受试对象的生物医学研究的伦理原则和限制条件,也是关于人体试验的第二个国际文件,比《纽伦堡法典》更加全面、具体和完善。以下摘录部分《赫尔辛基宣言》的主要内容:

Basic principles

The fundamental principle is respect for the individual, their right to self determination and the right to make informed decisions regarding participation in research, both initially and during the course of the research. The investigator's duty is solely to the patient or volunteer, and while there is always a need for research, the subject's welfare must always take precedence over the interests of science and society, and ethical considerations must always take precedence over laws and regulations. The recognition of the increased vulnerability of individuals and groups calls for special vigilance. It is recognised that when the research participant is incompetent, physically or mentally incapable of giving consent, or is a minor, then allowance should be considered for surrogate consent by an individual acting in the subject's best interest. In which case their assent should still be obtained if at all possible.

Operational principles

Research should be based on a thorough knowledge of the scientific background, a careful assessment of risks and benefits, have a reasonable likelihood of benefit to the population studied and be conducted by suitably trained investigators using approved protocols, subject to independent ethical review and oversight by a properly convened committee. The protocol should address the ethical issues and indicate that it is in compliance with the Declaration. Studies should be discontinued if the available information indicates that the original considerations are no longer satisfied. Information regarding the study should be publicly available. Ethical publications extend to publication of the results and consideration of any potential conflict of interest. Experimental investigations should always be compared against the best methods, but under certain circumstances a placebo or no treatment group may be utilised. The interests of the subject after the study is completed should be part of the overall ethical assessment, including assuring their access to the best proven care. Wherever possible unproven methods should be tested in the context of research where there is reasonable belief of possible benefit.

《赫尔辛基宣言》在医学研究的基本原则中,有一条关于医学论文写作和发表的伦理原则:作者、编辑和出版者在发表研究结果的时候都应遵守伦理义务。作者有义务将涉及伦理问题的研究结果(无论是阴性还是阳性结果)公开,并对报告结果的完整性和准确性负责。医学研究者应该坚持合乎伦理的报告原则。同时,其中的资金来源、所属单位和利益冲突都应该在发表的时候说明。不符合本宣言原则的研究报告不应该被接受和发表。医学论文的伦理问题会在后文具体阐述。

医学研究中伦理原则主要包括以下几个方面:

1. **知情同意**　是指使受试者充分了解研究目的、过程、可发生的风险、收益及方式并自主决定是否参与研究。《赫尔辛基宣言》第 24 条指出:"合格的涉及人类受试者的医学研究,每位潜在受试者必须得到足够的有关研究目的方法、资金来源、任何可能的利益冲突、研究人员的组织隶属、研究期望的好处和潜在危险、研究可能造成的不适,以及任何其他相关方面的信息","在确保潜在研究受试者理解了信息后,医生或另一位有资格的人必须获得潜在研究受试者自由表达的知情同意,最好为书面形式。如果同意的意见不能用书面表达,非书面同意意见应被正式记录并有目击证人"。这是因为医学科研与临床医疗的目的不同。医学科研的根本目的是发现研究新的疾病诊疗方法和某种药物的有效性,而临床医疗的目的在于解决患者健康问题。因此医学研究活动并不一定对受试者有益。所以在实施有一定风险的临床干预措施之前,受试者必须对研究目的、意义、方法、预期利益和潜在的伤害充分知情,自愿参加研究工作,并在知情同意书上签字。

2. **科学性和合理性**　医学研究的科学性是指研究项目的设计必须符合科学原理和方法,必须立足于科学文献、必须以充分的实验室工作和动物实验为基础,才能产生可信有效的数据。合理性是指必须符合医学伦理学的基本原则要求,必须依从严谨的方法学。

3. **研究对象选择的公正性**　是指公正的选择受试对象,以确保弱势群体免受危险性研究的伤害和避免特权机构及人群从中非法获益。

4. **遵从对照原则**　在研究设计中要设立对照组,并按照完全随机的原则把受试者分配到各研究组中。在试验结束之前,研究者和受试者都不知道受试者所接受的究竟是哪一种干预措施(双盲)。《赫尔辛基宣言》第 32 条指出:"一种新干预措施的益处、危险、负担、有效性等,必须与当前被证明最佳干预措施进行对照试验"。

5. **保密原则**　临床医学科研中的保密原则是指:不泄露与受试者有关的任何信息;为使医学研究结果真实可靠,对受试者采取的某些无害措施对受试者保密。《赫尔辛基宣言》第 23 条指出:"必须采取一切措施保护研究受试者的隐私和为个人信息保密,并使研究最低限度对他们的身体精神和社会地位造成影响"。

第二节　医学论文的伦理道德问题

一、原创性

任何形式的出版物都应考虑各种法律和伦理原则。论文写作要遵守国家法律法规,遵循科学道德和医学道德的要求。如果要将别人或者自己的著作再版,为了避免被指控剽窃或侵犯版权,必须获得许可。

以《新英格兰医学杂志》(NEJM)为例,其投稿须知的第一段话就明确要求稿件必须原创。

Manuscripts containing original material are accepted for consideration if neither the article nor any part of its essential substance, tables, or figures has been or will be published or submitted elsewhere before appearing in the *Journal*. This restriction does not apply to abstracts or press reports published in connection with scientific meetings. Copies of any closely related manuscripts must be submitted along with the manuscript that is to be considered by the *Journal*. The *Journal* discourages the submission of more than one article dealing with related aspects of the same study.

同样,《柳叶刀》杂志也对投稿稿件的原创性作出了明确的说明,且规定不能一稿多投。

Manuscripts must be solely the work of the author(s) stated, must not have been previously published elsewhere, and must not be under consideration by another journal.

原创性要求所揭示事物的现象、属性、特点及所遵循的规律应是前人没有做过或没有发表过的,即首创或部分首创,要有所发现、有所发明、有所创造、有所前进,而不是对前人工作简单的重复、复述、模仿和解释。通常向杂志投稿(综述除外),就意味着它是未出版过的原创性研究成果或一些新的观点,绝对不能考虑一稿两投,并且投稿一旦被接受就将不能以相同的形式发表在其他杂志上,如果没有编辑的许可也不允许以英语或其他语言再次发表。以短篇论文为例,它可以再版许多次而不违反道德原则,而一篇原创的研究性论文则只能在最初的杂志上发表一次,即使再版获得了版权许可但人们也普遍认为这违反科学伦理。无论国内还是国外的不同杂志,重复发表相同资料和观点的论文,可能使一些人只考虑自我宣传而不顾医学伦理。

如果作者想在另一出版物重新发表全部或大部分以前发表过的内容,无论什么缘故,都不会获得编辑部任何许可,只有其中的表格和插图,可以被引用在综述中再次发表。如果出版物的原创性低,整篇论文都可以再次发表,例如,某些特殊的机构经常允许重新出版一些卷册的论文集,一些特定主题的研究论文集或特定学科的论文汇编。在这些情况下,考虑到道德和法律的要求,都应该争取获得再发表的许可。

二、医学论文署名的伦理学要求

作品署名问题在现代科学研究中突现是有原因的。在 19 世纪以前,作品署名是不存在争议的。一百多年前的科学家几乎都是"个体户",科学家步入科学殿堂,纯粹是出于好奇心和兴趣。这样,在作品署名上除了表明该作品是他的之外,无任何其他实际意义。由于当时科学与社会联系并不紧密,使得个人研究成为可能,科学作品的个人署名成为必然。19 世纪以后科学研究蓬勃发展,从事研究的人也急剧增加,这就导致了竞争,而竞争的基础通常是发表的论文数量,这就使得一部分科研人员为追求论文数量而越轨在作品上署名。这是作品错误署名的来源。进入 20 世纪,科研项目呈现出高度综合性,科学研究也从个人模式进入团队合作模式,靠一个人的力量是很难再维系下去了。由于这个原因,每篇论文的作者也就明显增多了。美国的一项调查显示:国际医学年鉴和新英国医学杂志每篇论文作者的数量平均从 1925 年的 1 位增加到 1985 年的 6 位。合作研究的兴起,导致多人署名现象的出现,客观上也就为一些越轨署名提供了可能性。

科研论文中所列作者的名字要符合科学伦理的要求,每个作者都要对这篇文章负责任。当文章被发现造假时,某些署名的作者会声称不知情而逃避责任。经典的语句是"我真的不知道我的合作者做了什么"。但是这不能成为推卸责任的借口。文章的每一名作者必须对文章的科学性、真实性和原创性负责。但是在现代科学研究中,并不是每个作者都能达到该要求。为了某些利益在论文上挂名或是在论文上造假的情况时有发生,这就违背了作品署名的原则,即作者必须已参加过足够多的研究工作并能对作品的内容承担责任而且能保证它的合法性。一些杂志已经采取了更具体的指导方针,即署名作者必须参与下列一种或几种:①实验的设想和系统性的设计;②具体操作了实验并收集和保存了重要的资料;③分析和解释过原始资料;④参与了手稿的准备和修改。

同样以《新英格兰医学杂志》(NEJM)为例,其投稿须知中规定只有以下情况才可以作为文章的作者。

(a) the conception and design or analysis and interpretation of the data …

(b) the drafting of the article or critical revision for important intellectual content.

(c) final approval of the version to be published.

Each author must sign a statement attesting that he or she fulfills the authorship criteria of the Uniform Requirements. At least one person's name must accompany a group name (e.g., Thelma J. Smith, for the Boston Porphyria Group). As part of the submission process, authors must indicate whether any writing assistance other than copy editing was provided.

1991 年 10 月,我国 14 名学部委员曾在联名发表的《再论科学道德》一文中指出:"只有对一篇论文从选题、设计、具体实验到得出必要结论的全过程都有了解和参与,并确实对其中一个或几个具体环节做出贡献的,才能当之无愧地在论文上署名。如只具备后者,可由作者在文末道谢,但不宜作为作者之一,因为他无法对论文负责。"如美国医学杂志指出作者署名的价值:①为了表明文责自负;②记录作者的劳动成果;③便于读者与作者的联系及文献检索(作者索引)。

三、医学论文的版权

医学论文的版权即医学论文著作权,是指该作者对其作品享有的权利(包括财产权、人身权)。版权的获得有两种方式:自动取得和登记取得。在中国,著作权法规定,作品完成就自动有版权,这即版权的自动取得。登记取得是指在作品完成后到相关部门登记获得。根据性质不同,版权可以分为著作权及邻接权,简单来说,著作权是指作者本人对其作品的所有权;邻接权的概念,是指作品在发行和传播过程中有关产业的参加者的所有权,比如出版权等等。

一般情况都是出版者拥有版权,这样他们将有法律依据,以自己的利益并代表在其期刊上发表论文作者的利益,阻止未经授权的再次出版。这样,出版社和作者就可以共同防止被剽窃、盗用已发表数据,防止为了广告或其他目的进行未经授权的重新出版,和其他潜在的滥用。

每个期刊都有版权,论文的法定所有权属于版权所有者。重新发表他人的著作时要得到许可,从法律的角度讲是因为它涉及版权法。因此,如果你想要重新出版受版权保护的论文,你必须获得版权所有人的同意,否则将会有被起诉侵权的风险。

同样以《新英格兰医学杂志》(NEJM)为例,其投稿须知中对稿件版权的说明:

The Massachusetts Medical Society is the owner of all copyright to any work published by the Society. Authors agree to execute copyright transfer forms as requested with respect to their contributions accepted by the Society. The Society and its licensees have the right to use, reproduce, transmit, derive works from, publish, and distribute the contribution, in the Journal or otherwise, in any form or medium. Authors may not use or authorize the use of the contribution without the Society's written consent, except as may be allowed by U.S. fair-use law.

在美国,根据1909年的版权转让法,向期刊提交手稿的行为被假定为作者的所有权转移给了出版社。在出版的时候,有版权证明并填写了版权转让书和交付了著作权登记所需的必要的费用,文章的所有权便由作者移交给出版社。

美国1976年的版权法要求从此不再自动转让版权而必须有书面形式的转让。缺少书面的版权转让证明时,出版商可推定为已经获得在其期刊刊登文章唯一的特权;出版商将具备再版,影印和拍摄缩微胶卷或授权他人这样做(或从法律上防止其他人这样做)的权力。同样,版权法指出版权保护开始于"当笔离开论文时",由此可认识到作者的知识产权和出版的过程是分离的。因此,现在大多数出版商要求每个作者在投稿时或者在接受发表时把版权转让给出版商。转让生效后,出版商给每位作者一份"版权转让"证明。

新版权法的另一个新特点是涉及了作者的影印本。一方面,作者都希望看到他们的论文被广泛接受。另一方面,出版商不希望牺牲期刊的利益实现这一目标。因此,新版权法通过定义"合理使用"来解决这些冲突,允许某些类型的图书馆和用于教育的复印(也就是说,可以不经许可也不付版费而复印),同时也保护出版商反对未经许可的复制。

为了使授权影印系统更简便地使用期刊论文并免除付给出版商的版税,版权结算中心(Copyright Clearance Center)应运而生。许多出版社都已经加入了这一中心。这一交易清算中心使用户可以不必得到先前出版社的许可而随意拷贝,用户只需要把版税交给中心就可以了。

由于科学伦理和著作权法都是重要的基本法则,所以每个科学家都必须对它们十分敏感。基本上,如果你未获得版权所有者的许可,就意味着你不能重新出版表、数字和文字。即使这样,标明再版来源非常重要,通常要用一句重要的话来表明"再版(期刊或书)许可;版权(年)和版权所有者"。

根据《中华人民共和国民法通则》和《中华人民共和国合同法》侵犯版权的行为包括以下几点:

(1)未经著作权人许可,发表其作品的;

（2）未经合作作者许可,将与他人合作创作的作品当作自己单独创作的作品发表的;

（3）没有参加创作,为谋取个人名利,在他人作品上署名的;

（4）歪曲、篡改他人作品的;

（5）剽窃他人作品的;

（6）未经著作权人许可,以展览、摄制电影和以类似摄制电影的方法使用作品,或者以改编、翻译、注释等方式使用作品的,本法另有规定的除外;

（7）使用他人作品,应当支付报酬而未支付的;

（8）未经电影作品和以类似摄影电影的方法创作的作品、计算机软件、录音录像制品的著作权人或者与著作权有关的权利人许可,出租其作品或者录音录像制品的,本法另有规定的除外;

（9）未经出版者许可,使用其出版的图书、期刊的版式设计的;

（10）未经表演者许可,从现场直播或者公开传送其现场表演,或者录制其表演的;

（11）其他侵犯著作权以及与著作权有关的权益的行为;

（12）未经著作权人许可,复制、发行、表演、放映、广播、汇编、通过信息网络向公众传播其作品的,本法另有规定的除外;

（13）出版他人享有专有出版权的图书的;

（14）未经表演者许可,复制、发行录有其表演的录音录像制品,或者通过信息网络向公众传播其表演的,著作权法另有规定的除外;

（15）未经录音录像制作者许可,复制、发行、通过信息网络向公众传播其制作的录音录像制品的,著作权法另有规定的除外;

（16）未经许可,播放或者复制广播、电视的,著作权法另有规定的除外;

（17）未经著作权人或者与著作权有关的权利人许可,故意避开或者破坏权利人为其作品、录音录像制品等采取的保护著作权或者与著作权有关的权利的技术措施的,法律、行政法规另有规定的除外;

（18）未经著作权人或者与著作权有关的权利人许可,故意删除或者改变作品、录音录像品等的权利管理电子信息的,法律、行政法规另有规定的除外;

（19）制作、出售假冒他人署名的作品的。

以上第（1）至第（11）项行为,侵权人应当根据情况承担停止侵害、消除影响、赔礼道歉、赔偿损失等民事责任。第（12）项至第（19）项行为,侵权人除了承担上述民事责任外,同时损害公共利益的,可以由著作权行政管理部门责令停止侵权行为,没收违法所得,没收、销毁侵权复制品,并可处以罚款;情节严重的,著作权行政管理部门还可以没收主要用于制作侵权复制品的材料、工具、设备等;构成犯罪的,依法追究刑事责任。

另外,在著作权许可使用或转让等合同中,当事人不履行合同义务或者履行合同义务不符合约定条件的,应当依照《中华人民共和国民法通则》和《中华人民共和国合同法》等有关法律法规承担民事责任。

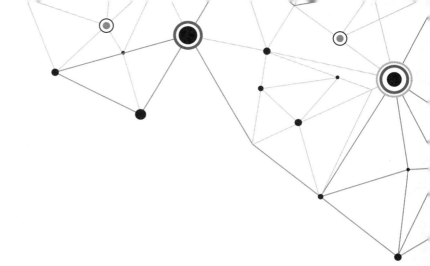

第二部分

国际知名专家介绍如何撰写医学英文科研论文

Part 2

Tips and Experiences of How to Write
Medical Research Papers in English From
Renowned Experts Internationally

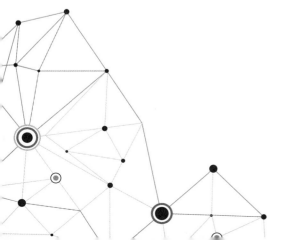

第 20 章
怎样开始临床研究：态度、诚实、知识与规则

Chapter 20
How to Start Clinical Research: Attitude, Introspection, Knowledge and Discipline

Stephen Shei-Dei Yang

Many clinicians have difficulty in initiating clinical research. As a clinician, I have published more than 100 peer reviewed articles (mostly SCI articles) in 100% clinical topics. My personal stories may be helpful to someone who wishes to start clinical research. Attitude, introspection (self-examination), knowledge and disciplines are the four principles that open the door for clinical researches.

A. Attitude

What do you want to be, an ordinary doctor or an expert? Your attitude decides your achievements.

If you decide to be an ordinary doctor, then you can stop reading now. If you want to be an expert in a small field, or even make a great contribution to human, then you can start to change your mindset and take the following advices to become an expert. The process to become an expert or a physician scientist can be painful, time consuming and lonely. However, the fruits of your efforts are rich and sweet. You will have joy in finding something new in knowledge and improving health of people.

I finished resident training in one of the best medical centers in Taiwan in June, 1991. Since then I have left medical center till now. I was appointed as Chief of Urology in a public regional hospital in January 1993. Though the regional hospital had few facility and support for academic activity, I enjoyed doing operations. One year later, I felt bored because my medical life was fully occupied by hernia repair, ureteroscopic lithotripsy (URSL) and transurethral resection of prostate. I tried to make some efforts that few urologists would try at that time: applying URSL in cases with upper ureteral stones. Three years later, I found that my surgical outcomes were superior to most doctors in Taiwan and around the world. This experience became my first SCI article in 1996 [1]. I overcame the low self-confidence in academic performance.

B. Introspection (Self-examination)

Look at your clinical outcomes honestly and compare them to the published results.

This is the fundamental approach to improve personal medical quality and to start the investigation of clinical science. Through review of personal clinical outcomes, one can recognize the strength and weakness of one's medical practice. If personal outcomes are superior to the published results, it is a good chance to be reported to the world in a good SCI journal. If personal outcomes are worse than the published results, one should improve his/her techniques as the experts' suggestions. If you have done everything you know to improve your techniques, but the clinical outcomes are still worse than the published ones, there should be something unknown in this field. Find out the causes and do not be afraid to report it.

When I studied abroad in 1995, I learned about the high incidence (10-30%) of contralateral hernia after unilateral inguinal hernia repair in children. Inserting an endoscope through the opened hernia sac to check the contralateral side was emerging to prevent the occurrence of metachronous contralateral hernia. Coming back to Taiwan in 1996, I started to follow this trend in the world. In the mean time, I review our cases to see if our surgical outcome were similar to the published reports. After the review, we had a 10% contralateral occurrence of hernia after repairs of unilateral hernia in children and adolescents. Since this is nothing new, it was published in a local, non-SCI journal [2]. We recognized that we have the same clinical problem as the world and this article serves as the fundamental data for later comparison of new surgical technology.

In 2003, we had already done 43 cases of examination of contralateral hernia sac in children with unilateral hernia. We prophylactically repaired the contralateral side of ingeuinum in 4 cases when a patent processus vaginalis was detected. However, we still had 4 (11.3%) cases of contralateral hernia at one year followup. We stopped inserting endoscope into the opened hernia sac in 2004. We were afraid of reporting our poor results because of low confidence in this field. After the Western experts reported the unsatisfied results of transinquinal endoscopy in the prevention of contralateral hernia, we published our outcomes in a local journal in 2008 [3]. If we dare to report it in 2004, this will be breaking news at time and might be published in a high impact SCI journal.

C. Knowledge

1 Learn new idea through studying abroad as a tutor of a well-known expert, being a copycat of a new technique or new drug, attending important conferences. Developing a new technique or a new concept is the fruit of these hard works.

1.1 **Studying abroad is a short cut to become an expert.** I studied in Brown University, USA in 1995. My mentor, Anthony A. Caldamone, inspired me greatly. He opened the door of pediatric urology to me. The dramatic operation: tubularized incised plate (TIP) urethroplasty just appeared in the world. Fortunately, he is one of the 6 pioneers in this new operation. I learned it there, and practiced it in Taiwan, just like a copycat. Since most hypospadias surgeries in Taiwan are proximal type, we, together with my local mentor (Prof. Shyh-Chan Chen) in Taiwan, had to start TIP urethroplasty in proximal hypospadias. We were lucky to achieve excellent results and published them in 2000 [4]. In two years, we published 6 related articles in hypospadias repair.

Piet Hoebeke is the key person who inspired me the field of pediatric urology. I attended an educational course regarding pediatric lower urinary tract dysfunction in Gent in 2000. This course opened me a new research field which I devoted myself till now. One should study abroad for a short, medium or long time as long as he or she is eager to learn something new.

1.2 **Attending important conferences.** In 2002, I and my senior resident, Yao-Chou, Tsai, attended the Asia Pacific Association of Pediatric Urology in Hong Kong in 2002. We learned the laparoscopic technique of careful dissection and knot-tying in the treatment of varicocele and single port laparoscopic hernia repair. We were not satisfied with transinguinal laparoscope examination of contralateral hernia sac, and did not agree with the concept of ligating hernia sac without dissection. We did something different when we went home.

　　1.3　Develop a new technique. We developed a new technique by laparoscopic dissection of hernia sac with intra-corporeal suture ligation of the peritoneum. The new mini-laparoscopic procedure completely follows the principle of open surgical treatment of hernia. The results were published in 2007 [5]. The recurrence rate of the same site was 2%, and the contralateral occurrence of new hernia was 1%. We successfully reduce the second operation. Since we do not manipulate spermatic cord and vas deference, we believe that our technique should be good for fertility and be the new standard of pediatric hernia repair. Tsai YC won the Young Investigator Award in the 2008 World Congress of Endoscopic Surgery. Up to April, 2014, we have published more than 10 articles related to inguinal hernia.

　　2　What is normal?

　　In the era of functional medicine, the norm of a specific function may not be well defined. Actually, most definitions are based on expert opinion with very low level of evidence. In my interested field of lower urinary tract symptoms/dysfunction (LUTS, LUTD), I started to establish normal references of uroflowmetry and post void residual urine (PVR) in Taiwanese children in 2003. I was confused that about 20% of Taiwanese children did not have a "normal bell-shaped" uroflowmetry. On the contrary, most published rates of abnormal uroflow pattern from Caucasians were around 3-10%. I was surprised that the rate of abnormal flow pattern in children from Hong Kong was also around 30%. What's wrong with the ethnic Chinese children? Through a large scale investigation on 1 128 children, we concluded that most (98%) Taiwanese children could have a normal bell-shaped uroflowmetry curve if they did it twice [6-7]. The high rate of abnormal uroflow pattern is due to bladder over distention, not cultural/social problem. Based on the large data and the assistance of Dr. Shang-Jen Chang, we published a series of papers regarding the normal reference values for PVR, Qmax, and optimal bladder capacity (Table 20-1). International Children Continence Society adopted these normal reference values as new standardization in 2014. The argument of the physiological meaning of expected bladder pushes us to develop the concept of "optimal bladder capacity". Under our definition of optimal bladder capacity, the reproducibility of normal flow pattern, Qmax, and PVR were 94.4%, 95.8% and 89.0%, respectively.

Table 20-1　Summary of "normal" reference values of lower urinary tract function in children [8]

Parameters		
Age in years	4-6	7-12
PVR in% of BC	<10%	<6%
PVR in ml	<20	<10
Flow pattern	Bell-shaped	Bell-shaped
Qmax in ml/s	≥11.5	≥15.0
Optimal BC	Between 80ml and (age in years*37ml) for children aged 3-8 years.	

PVR=postvoid residual urine, Qmax=peak uroflow rate, BC=bladder capacity,

3　Find out the evidence.

In the era of evidence based medicine, the scientific world welcome new evidence to update "old" concept. Randomized controlled study to prove or against a common practice is highly welcome and usually published in a high impact SCI journal. Conducting a RCT is not easy, but usually results in great achievement.

In 2001, we started to look at the necessity of internal ureteral stenting (double-J stent) after an uncomplicated ureteroscopic lithotripsy. Just before the accomplishment of the study, similar RCT was reported. We were a little frustrated. However, our paper was quickly accepted by Journal of Urology [9]. Indeed, a solid concept requires several good RCTs directing to the same conclusions. The second or third RCT on the same topic is still welcome. If RCTs direct to different outcomes, then further RCTs are highly interested in major journals. In the urological fields, many articles arguing about the treatment options of localized prostate cancer in elder men and the use of prophylactic antibiotics in the prevention of recurrent UTI in children. Many of these debates are published in the most respected journal: New England Journal of Medicine.

D.　Discipline

One has to comply with the aforementioned principles day by day. It is impossible to get results very quickly. A good study usually takes for more than one year. Collecting the data to establish normal bladder function of children took me 5.5 years. I have a tutor who is a neurosurgeon. Dr Hsien-Ta Hsu asked me to guide him to start writing of his first paper at the age of 46 years. We worked together for 2 years to get the first paper published [10]. In these 2 years, he learned how to think and write logically. Now, he becomes an independent clinician scientist and published several SCI papers. The sign to convince me to continue the teaching is that he read English newspaper every day. He has a good discipline in improving language skill, so does his academic skill.

Sometimes, one may go to the wrong directions and get no conclusion after heavy works. However, carefully examine on what you have done, you can still get new insights for the next research topic. Never give up if you ran in the wrong road. Check out what's wrong. Restart and you will find the correct way to success.

Conclusions

There is no magic way to find a topic to start with and no simple way to get achievements. Change your attitude. Examine your clinical outcomes. Learn new knowledge. Follow good discipline. Success will come to you!

References and Mile stones in Yang's clinical research

1. Chen SC, Yang SS, Chen YT, Hsieh CH. Tubularized Incised Plate (TIP) Urethroplasty on Proximal Hypospadias. BJU Int, 2000, 86, 1050-1053. (Corresponding author)【Though I am a copycat of TIP urethroplasty, I am among first few doctors to extend its indication to proximal hypospadias. This article has been cited for more than 50 times.】

2. Chang SJ, Yang SS. The Inter-observer and Intra-observer Agreement on the Interpretation of Uroflowmetry Curves of Kindergarten Children. J Ped Urol, 2008, 4:422-7. (corresponding author)【This fundamental work opened the gate to the study of normal lower urinary tract dysfunction in children.】

3. Chen YT, Chen J, Yang SS, Hsieh CH. Is ureteral stenting necessary after uncomplicated ureteroscopic lithotripsy? A prospective, randomized controlled trial. JUrol, 2002, 167:1977-80. (Corresponding

author)【This is our first RCT. After this painful beginning, we have no difficulty in conducting new RCTs.】

4. Hsu HT, Chang SJ, Yang SS, Chai CL. Learning Curve of Full-Endoscopic Lumbar Discectomy. Eur Spine Journal, 2013, 22:727-733. (corresponding author)【This is my first paper outside of urology. Guide a freshman into in scientific world is not easy. However, it is possible as long as he is eager to become an expert.】

5. Tsai YC. Wu CC. Yang SS. Minilaparoscopic herniorrhaphy with herniasac transection in children and youngadults, a preliminary report. Surgical Endoscopy, 2007, 21 (9): 1623-5. (corresponding author)【This is our new approach to hernia and we believe it should be the new standard for herniorraphy in children.】

6. Tsai YC, Wu CC, Yang SS. Posterior Wall Enhancement is Not Necessary in Patients ≤18 Years Old with a Primary Inguinal Hernia. Journal of Taiwan Urological Association, 2007, 18:151-153. (corresponding author)【This is the first clinical review of personal outcomes in hernia repair. It became the corner stone of the future studies.】

7. Tsai YC, Wu CC, Yang SS. Transinguinal Laparoscopy for a Pediatric Inguinal Hernia: the Inability to Predict the Occurrence of a Contralateral Metachronous Inguinal Hernia. JTUA, 2008, 19:94-97. (corresponding author)【Because of low confidence in this field, we did not report our outcomes in time. Otherwise, such an important finding should be accepted in a high impact SCI journal.】

8. Yang SS and Hong JH. Electrohydraulic Lithotripsy of Upper Ureteral Calculi with Semirigid Ureteroscope. J Endourol, 1996, 10:27-30.【This is my first SCI paper when I served in a public regional hospital.】

9. Yang SS, Chang SJ. The Effects of Urinary Bladder Over distention on the Voiding Function of Kindergarten Children. J Urol, 2008, 180:2177-2182.【This new finding extend our view to new researches in children and adults.】

10. Yang SS, Shih S, Chang SJ. Tzu Chi Nomograms for pediatric lower urinary tract function. Tzu Chi Med J, 2014, 26:10-14.【Summary of our research on normal LUT function in children.】

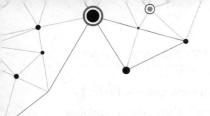

第 21 章
如何做动物实验

Chapter 21
Animal Experimentation — What to Do

Jens Chr. Djurhuus

Introduction

Diagnostic and treatment dilemmas in clinics occur every day which is a strong incentive to be curious and take the pains to acquire more knowledge in order to answer the questions with the ambition of improving diagnostics and treatment for the benefit of the patients.

When an attempt to solve the problem and answer the questions in the clinical setting by investigating patients has proven futile, the next step will be experimentation. There may be a choice between *computer simulation or tissue sample analyses* or, if that is not sufficient, *animal experimentation*. Usually it ends up being a combination of all three, where the animal experimentation led to new knowledge which can be further elucidated by way of cell and computer technique.

To perform

Animal experimentation is a complex process. Many considerations have to be taken before the actual study, and permissions have to be acquired. Not least in the European Union there is an increase in the requirements to perform animal experimentation[1][2]. There is a trend towards making them universal and a basic requirement for publishing. We will return to that later in this chapter.

Planning phase

In the planning phase it is important to realise which questions should be addressed, and consequently what kind of models should be used and usually also developed. It is preferable that the study is going to take place in an institution where conditions for animal experimentation are present and thereby one is able to choose from the whole spectre of animals from c. elegans and zebrafish, across rodents to large animals, especially pigs, animals which all can be genetically modified. State of the art anaesthesia equipment and laboratory test facilities should be available. It is also important that state of the art investigational methods are available. This includes access to electrophysiological measurements, including telemetry and high-tech state of the art imaging facilities, such as ultrasound with multiple frequency probes, x-ray, gamma camera facilities for isotope organ function studies, MR and PET and perhaps MEG.

---

① Animal research: A balancing act: Editorial,Nature Medicine, 19, 1191, 2013

② Directive 2010/63/EUDirective 2010/63/EU

An experimental technical staff trained in working with different kinds of animals and veterinary assistance is also fundamental to ensure high quality animal experimentation based research.

Besides monitoring the physiological manifestations which are to be investigated, it is also essential to ensure homeostasis during the experimental procedure. Aside from monitoring blood pressure and blood gases together with electrolytes it may be advisable to monitor urine production ratetoo.

All of these parameters are only obtainable in animals which allow for sampling of these parameters predominantly in large animals.

Albeit there might be theoretical risks of transfection it is also preferable that clinically oriented animal experimentation takes place in the absolute vicinity of a hospital clinical setting. Thereby it is possible for clinicians to ping-pong between clinical work and experimentation, with mutual benefits for the clinicians to participate and for the research to profit from the clinical knowledge and the technical skills.

Concerning housing of the animals there is an increase in demands to the quality of facilities inside the European Union. To be acquainted with the current demands one should consult the European Directives on animal experimentation, where how much space each animal should have are specified, what kind of environmental enrichment should be available to the animals, how many air shifts there should be in the facility per time unit, temperature, humidity, what kind of, and how much, straw and other material should be on the floor, and also finally specifications concerning food[1]. These requirements may appear somewhat harsh, but in general they ensure the quality of the research, and it also makes it easier to comply with later, and specify how the animals have been kept by simply stating that it complies with international regulations.

Prerogatives

Before any experimentation is undertaken, it is important that the education and license needed for the study are obtained. In Denmark, special surgical skills from clinicians are required for the experiment, one can work with animals only if they have a specific education with a course in animal experimentation. And one cannot apply for permission to perform a study unless these qualifications are fulfilled. On the EU level there is a non-binding Education and Training Framework issued in February 2014[2].

The large amount of researchers, especially PhD students, who want to do animal experimentation ensures that the frequency and the quality of courses clearly fulfil the demands. In Denmark it is organised as formal courses in universities to ensure that the capacity, timeframe and frequency of these courses are sufficient to cover the demands so that the educational demands do not hamper the progress of the research.

The courses ensure that researchers have obtained knowledge about the legislation and theory about handling laboratory animals, and how to conduct a study with clear reference to the *three*

---

① EU Directives, Directive 2010/63/EU

② FELASA Working Group: Standardisation of Enrichment

Rs(Replacement, Reduction and Refinement), which are described later. The courses also include how to premedicate and anaesthetise and pain cover different laboratory animals, and finally they include basic operative procedures, both in rodents and in larger animals such as intubation, access to vessels and procedures in the thorax and abdomen.

Choosing the model

Having obtained the permission to perform animal experimentation, it is time to make considerations as to what kind of model should be used to answer the specific questions. In our lab priority is on the analogy level, because the lab is tuned in to answer clinical questions as sufficiently as possible, not least due the demand for clinical relevance, but that has to be seen in the light of that we have access to an abundance of animal models, as previously mentioned, from c. elegans, zebrafish, genetically manipulated rodents to large animals with the exception of non-human primates which are specialised in comparative anatomy, physiology and pathophysiology.

Parallel to the decision about analogy level, and thereby choice of animal, considerations about the *three Rs* have to take place.

Most of the achievements in this avenue have been gained from previous experimentation.

Replacement requires that previous findings have eliminated the need for animal experimentation and that it is substantiated scientifically that the "lower level" animal models or even cell cultures or simulation can be used in the future.

Refinement is crucial and closely related to *reduction*. The prerogatives to refinement or reduction are that you are doing your research in an advanced and reputed setting.

Techniques

Telemetric monitoring is getting widespread use. It can be used both in small and large animals. One can measure pressure flow, EMG, EEG, there is practically any physiological manifestation using telemetry. The advantage of using telemetric investigations is that you can measure in the unrestrained animal and for a prolonged period of time, both within the specific procedure but also on a long term basis.

Implants include osmotic pumps which can be used for continuous or interrupted administration of agents for time period up to a month. We have used it in many experiments especially in orthopaedics (ALZET Osmotic Pumps).

We used a pioneering prototype telemetry system more than 25 years ago to monitor the peristaltic activity of the upper urinary tract measuring pressure in the renal pelvis on both sides. It was established that there is a basic peristaltic frequency particular to each side, which means that it is not the same on the two sides. There can be transient deviations from the frequency but it always goes back to the original, even with continued stimulation, and the specific basic frequency of peristalsis was shown to be constant for up to nine months. These results became part of the evidence to show that pressure-perfusion study response used to identify upper urinary tract obstruction clinically depended on this basic peristaltic rhythm more than on the so-called obstruction. The higher the peristaltic rate was, the more pronounced was the pressure response.

The drawback of telemetric measurements is that the amount of information obtained is immense. Therefore, advanced signal analysis equipment is warranted.

Species aspects

It is also a challenge to what hitherto has been found from a lot of animal studies. Rodents are night animals and most of the investigations done hitherto are done during daytime due to investigator convenience. With the information, for example on the circadian rhythm of blood pressure it becomes evident that future studies in night animals should be done according to their physiology and not the physiology of the researcher.

Characteristics of measurements and physiological manifestations

In signal processing it has to be taken into consideration that working with rodents is working with highly active animals. A mouse can easily have a heart rate of up to 400/minute. This is a challenge, both to basic sampling but especially if one wants to monitor derivatives of the blood pressure, for example the rate of change, the dp/dt. Therefore one has to be aware of the basics of working with sampling of signals.

First, one has to substantiate the characteristics of one's measuring system. If fluid-filled catheters are used connecting the organ, which is measured to a transducer, it has to be established what kind of dynamic properties the system has. Usually such systems are damped which means that they have a limitation to what frequency they can transmit pressures. They may also have uneven characteristics, damping some frequencies and amplifying others, and therefore it is crucial that they are tested before insertion for frequency characteristics. Even solid state transducers may have limitations, but here it is mainly the sampling system which is the limitation.

If one uses solid state transducers one has to bear in mind that they are "looking" in only one direction. It means that if they are inserted into a non-captive organ they would not measure the true changes in pressure during, for example, a peristaltic event. We examined the peristaltic activity of the gut using a six point system each measuring its share of the circumference. None of the pressure measurements showed the same, and therefore it is crucial to be aware of that you might depict activity, but it would be difficult to quantitate. Even in a captive system solid state transducers may show different results depending on orientation. This is of course not animal experimentation specific but is also relevant in measurements in humans.

The actual study

Pilot studies

When it has been decided upon which animal model, which type of anaesthesia and what monitoring equipment should be used, it is time to the final adjustment before the study is to commence. It is very important to realise that pilot studies are a crucial part of the process. It is through the pilot studies that one can realise what can be done, what the possible influence of anaesthesia might be, how the animals should be treated during operation, and when it is time for the final adjustment with regards to preparation of the animal in the day or the days ahead of the procedure: How long should the animal fast before operation? How should the fluid regimen be before? Should they be pre-treated and what kind of drugs should be used?

These pilot studies are probably the most important part of the whole process. Therefore relevant time should be used and a log book should be designed.

During the planning and after the pilot studies it is mandatory that everything else but the intervention, which should elucidate the questions posed, should be made as simple, consistent and clear as possible.

Animal studies are, unlike most clinical studies, studies where there should be a non-negotiable focus on consistency, as clear cut answers to the questions posed should be aimed for.

This does not mean that unforeseen results, both during the pilot studies but also in the real study, should be discarded. Most of the original observations which have been made, and practically all fundamental achievements in science, have been the result of researchers not discarding their unforeseen results or outliers. In short unforeseen results are not failures until clearly proven.

When procedures have been established, calculations are to be made to ensure that the number of experiments is sufficient, and not more, to provide the result(s) warranted.

The experiment

One of the cornerstones in animal experimentation is that it allows for controls in terms of sham procedures. The sham procedures have to be planned preferably after the pilot studies in order to decide exactly what the experimental procedure and what the sham procedure is. The sham procedures have to be exactly as the experimental procedures, except for the intervention which is done to elucidate the question posed. It means that operation time has to be the same and also the surgical procedure should be identical.

A fixed procedure has been established, and it is time to adhere to it throughout the experiment. It is fundamental that all experiments are treated as if they were clinical cases, which means that meticulous records should be kept, and in a separate log book records should be kept as to when the measuring system is calibrated and with which procedures.

After having finalized the pilot studies, one can then decide on the number of animals which should be used strictly adhering to the procedure which has been decided upon.

Analyses and publication

Animal experimentation should be treated in the same manner a clinically based research. It should be considered unethical if a study is not published. If not, the risk is that others may repeat the study in a situation where repetition is not necessary.

The research group should, even from the beginning, make a time schedule as to when the analyses have been finalized, a so-called *frozen file,* followed by a time limit for the finalization of the manuscript.

Conclusion

Without animal experimentation advances in our knowledge, new diagnostics and new treatment would be impossible. But animal experimentation is a discipline requiring the highest skills and a comprehensive knowledge about means available.

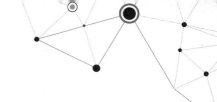

第 22 章
现代科学的挑战:行为规范和作者的责任

Chapter 22
Challenges in Modern Science with Special Reference to Code of Conduct and the Responsibility of Authors

Jørgen Frøkiær, Jens Chr. Djurhuus

1 Setting the scene

Challenges Research nowadays is increasingly an interaction between many disciplines. This may be in the form of multidisciplinarity where identifiable scientific disciplines participate in a project, but where it is evident from the final result what the contribution has been from each of the disciplines. The scientific work may also be transdisciplinary where the scientific work in one major discipline benefits from the interaction from another discipline. Finally, it may be interdisciplinary where the different disciplines merge into a new scientific concept. Regardless of the number of disciplines contributing to a research project science is today characterized by a collaborative effort and this interaction challenges the overall responsibility for the end product.

Collectively these new challenges together with an increase in trends towards multi-authorships even within one discipline calls for considerations as to what is an author, and do all authors have the same responsibilities or might there be one, the corresponding and/or the senior author, who has special responsibilities as to the quality of the work. Other challenges are the change in scientific paradigms from the long-term findings and thorough study to the short-term finding and the pressure of fast publications preferable in so-called high impact journals. Also the restrictions to format and limitations in manuscript lengths by the publishers tend to push researchers to make clean statements and to fractionalise their work.

2 Research integrity

The consequences of complex collaborations are that the patch work consists of multiple contributions of results based on various methods which are not necessarily familiar to every collaborator. One fundamental issue is therefore that research collaborators can have confidence in each other's faculties (expertise) as researchers.

In the Singapore Statement on Research Integrity four fundamental capabilities have been outlined:

- Honesty in all that concerns research
- Responsibility in research work
- Professional code of conduct and fairness in cooperation with other researchers

- Good stewardship of research on behalf of others[1]

3 When are you an author?

ICMJE, The International Committee of Medical Journal Editors, which is an organisation, composed of multiple scientific journals, amongst others Chinese Medical Journal, has produced recommendations for conduct, reporting, editing and publication of scholarly work in medical journals. The ICMJE has set up criteria for being an author. The criteria are fairly strict and consist of a description of an author who has contributed substantially to all aspect of the process, including the conception or design of the work, or a person who has substantially contributed to the acquisition, analysis and interpretation of data together with being a person who has participated in drafting the work and revising it critically; and has been part of the final approval of the version for publication; and has agreed to be accountable for all aspects of the work, ensuring that questions related to the accuracy and integrity of any part "work" is an appropriate investigator.

4 The role of the senior author

The senior author's role and responsibilities are subjected to an intense dispute, and rightfully so, because the nature of how knowledge is generated has changed dramatically over the last decades. The question is what a senior author should be responsible for. In the medical and life sciences fields, a senior author is often a person who is placed at the last position in the row of authors, and there is anticipation that this person is the guarantee of the work which has been performed. This is of course an immense task in multicentre clinical trials and in genetics, but even more so when different fields of research are incorporated in a scientific work. The ICMJE has not offered a clear attitude as to the senior author responsibility. And many journals do not specifically detail what they anticipate. However, there is a trend, and an increasing trend, towards that the senior author should have more responsibility than the rest of the authors.

5 Responsibilities of senior team members on multi-group collaborations

The editors at the Nature journals assume that at least one member of each collaboration, usually the most senior member of each submitting group or team, has accepted responsibility for the contributions to the manuscript from that team. This responsibility includes, but is not limited to: (1) ensuring that original data upon which the submission is based is preserved and retrievable for reanalysis; (2) approving data presentation as representative of the original data; and (3) foreseeing and minimizing obstacles to the sharing of data, materials, algorithms or reagents described in the work[2].

According to this statement there can be no doubt that the senior author has the full responsibility of the quality and the content of a scientific paper, not only from the point of view of the ethics and the permissions but also with regard to honesty and dishonesty.

The Dutch cardiologist Don Poldermans has together with co-authors produced high impact papers with recommendation-consequences concerning the use of anti-arrhythmics in relation to cardiovascular surgery. In the ground breaking papers it turned out that some of the patient material

---

[1] Singapore Statement on Research Integrity, September 2010

[2] Nature's website, Scientific Reports, Editorial and publishing policies http://www.nature.com/srep/policies/index.html

seemed constructed involving a junior author. As a consequence of this finding Poldermans had to step down from his post at the Dutch university where he was employed. There are numerous examples of scientists who came into similar situations and where the key question is whether or not they had knowledge about falsification of data prior to submission of data and publication.

In Denmark the dispute has been about a similar responsibility for a very prominent senior author. The Danish Committee on Research Dishonesty analysed work performed by a young researcher who had committed dishonesty together with the senior author. It was claimed that the senior author should have discovered reuse and manipulation of images. A large proportion of researchers in the Danish research community has objected fiercely to that, and claims that an author can only be responsible for one's own contribution but not others. This has been brought even further in the debate by researchers questioning if other authors, in particular a senior author, can be responsible for fractions of a work they do not understand. And that can certainly be the case when, example given, quantitative research in an article is combined with qualitative and when social science is combined with hard-core medical and molecular science. The question then is if a combined article is the right format? There is no doubt that a comprehensive strategy in translational research requires input from more than one discipline and as such make the project complex. However, one could dream of an alternative approach where the work was presented in chapters where it was obvious which kind of research approach had been used. This can of course only be relevant in multidisciplinary research. If interdisciplinary and transdisciplinary research is the case, there can be no doubt that all of the work should be understood by all the authors and especially the senior author.

6　How do we ensure research integrity in Denmark?

The Danish Committee on Scientific Dishonesty (DCSD) handles scientific misconduct or suspicion of it on the national level

For many years we in Denmark have had a committee system to deal with scientific dishonesty. It was pioneered in medicine but has spread to other scientific fields so that we today have three committees:

(1) one for scientific dishonesty for health and medical sciences.

(2) one for scientific dishonesty for natural, technical and production sciences.

(3) one for scientific dishonesty for cultural social sciences.

The three committees each have a chairman and six members. The members must be recognised scientists who are appointed by the Danish Minister of Higher Education and Science. That happens after consultation with the Council for Independent Research. The chairmanship is held by a judge of the Danish Supreme Court appointed by the minister.

The Danish Parliament has defined scientific dishonesty as falsification, fabrication, plagiarism and other serious violations of good scientific practice.

The process in DCSD

The process is that a person, or maybe a group, in open or anonymously put forward allegations on research misconduct to the committees. In order for the committees to investigate an allegation, the matter must fall within the mandate of the committees, which means that the allegation must relate to a scientific product, an article, a thesis or similar. It must be of importance to Danish research and it must concern scientific dishonesty, in case of disagreements on the quality of research this falls outside the mandate of the committees. Finally the respondent must be scientifically trained within the field of scientific product in question.

If these criteria are met the respondent receives a copy of the complaint, and the respondent is requested to submit a response within an appropriate time frame. The comments, when they are sent, are forwarded to the complainant and thereafter the complainant is requested to submit a response within an appropriate time frame. This is again sent to the respondent, and the respondent is requested to submit a response within appropriate time. Then again the complainant is informed and finally the committee is making a conclusion. The decisions made by the committees are made public on a yearly basis. In later years, more prominent cases have been a matter of public debate as with senior author responsibilities referred to later.

This ping pong process should ensure that both the complainant and the respondent have a fair process.

This committee system is a national committee system, but also at research institutions such as the Danish universities, especially the multi-faculty, which amounts to five, there is a local committee consisting of local university peers.

7 The institutional level at Danish universities

Especially at the multi-faculty universities there is a process going on renewing and formatting standards for responsible research activity. Again, the pioneers here are in health sciences where the challenges seem to be even more eminent due to the nature of the research work which can have severe consequences for patients and society, and where multi-author research is performed both within the institution but more so in many institutions. Danish health sciences research is 40% international with institutions all over the world each having their standards for responsible research activity.

At Aarhus University there has for long been a committee with representatives from all the faculties. However, this committee has more or less had a niche role with limited impact, which has made it more the trend to go directly to the national level instead of the institutional level.

Both from the point of view of having a clear statement from the institution about responsible research practice which can be presented to and adhered to when the institution's researchers are working trans-institutional and in order to a construction which can deal with the current trends in code of conduct and research integrity, the Danish research institutions, in particular Aarhus University has a process ongoing to renew tools to handle responsible research practice.

The Faculty of Health at Aarhus University has developed new standards and guidelines guiding researcher through the process of developing the project including preparation of the protocol, specifying what the protocol should contain. But before anything is done it is required that all participants in the project specify their functions and responsibilities. It is also required to pinpoint the leader of the project and what function and competence this leader should have. Moreover, it is recommended to specify which functions and responsibilities the potential external collaborators should have. A specific issue in Denmark since 1st January 2000 is immaterial rights which also have to be dealt with in the preparation of the project. It is furthermore the attitude of Aarhus University to comply with the guidelines set forward by ICMJE. Finally, since most of the research today is externally funded it is mandatory to pinpoint who has the responsibility for financing and for providing the funding.

8　Experimental studies

In experimental studies, which include animal experimentation, it is required that permission is applied for and obtained from the Danish Committee on Animal Experimentation. It is also obligatory that all involved in animal experimentation should have a special course in performing studies based on animal material.

In clinical studies it is unequivocal that the Helsinki Declaration with the revision in 2008 is adhered to, and that the studies are applied for and accepted by the local committee on scientific ethics, respectively in special cases the national committee. This ethical committee is composed of laymen and scientific personnel in equal numbers. It is the responsibility of the researchers and also of the scientific committee members to explain the studies to the laymen in a format which offers full understanding.

After the ethical committee an application is sent via one of Denmark's five regions to the National Board of Data Security. Also, if the research project involves drugs or utensils the Danish National Board of Health has to approve.

As a consequence of the ICH Directive research initiated in drugs as well as utensils has to comply with Good Clinical Practice (GCP) and will be monitored by the official Good Clinical Practice Committee, of which Denmark has three. Moreover, all clinical studies have to be made public in international database, example given clinical trials.gov.

Clinical studies involving laboratory tests have to be performed in a laboratory complying with Good Laboratory Practice (GLP).

Denmark has a long tradition in using registries for analysis of diseases, their prevalence and for analysis of the effect of treatment. Therefore, specific guidelines have been elaborated as to how to handle that type of data. The specific issue is tissue samples. Here it is mandatory to ensure that the patient/person has not specifically forbidden that the material can be used for research.

Concerning publication and authorship it is the declaration from Aarhus University that all results of concluded studies should be published. That is regardless of whether they have negative or inconclusive results. This should be done as soon as possible, and concerning authorship the ICMJE rules should be adhered to.

It is stated that a decline of authorship, if the person is entitled to according to ICMJE rules, ghost-writing, gift-authorships, guest-authorships all are violations of responsible research practice. It is recommended that a senior author should take responsibility for all content of the article.

9　Conflicts of interest

Here referral should be made to ICMJE Form for Disclosure of Potential Conflicts of Interest. Aarhus University adhere to these guidelines.

In order to enforce the guidelines, and to cope with multi-, inter-and transdisciplinary activities, Aarhus University is appointing a committee with representatives from all faculties. The committee is supposed to handle most of the questions concerning responsible research practice. In order to facilitate good research practice each faculty will have a so-called "ombudsman". An ombudsman is an old Nordic institution who can evaluate and guide in issues concerning inter-person conflicts, but also conflicts between persons and authorities. The institution in Denmark is dating back to the mid-20th century when a state ombudsman institution was established by the Danish parliament. It is crucial and fundamental that the person is totally independent and can make his or her recommendations or judgements according to what the person thinks is just right. This institution has spread to many other countries, and now it is established within the scientific community where an ombudsman is available for persons who may suspect misconduct and needs advice about what has to be done about it. Through the interaction between the complainant and the ombudsman it is decided by the complainant what should be done if it is something which can be handled between the researchers, if it is something which needs to be carried further on, and there the university committee comes into play. The complainant can also go to the Danish national committee on scientific dishonesty, but it is recommended, also from the point of view of use of resources, that most of the activities are done locally, but also openly, so that both the scientific society and the community on national and international level know that the institution can take proper care of issues concerning conduct and misconduct in science.

As mentioned in the introduction the conditions for scientific publishing has changed over the years. When a doctoral thesis of up to 100 pages in the mid-1980's could be published in full internationally journals, it was because at that time the scientific community and the publishers believed that extensive state of the art surveys were of fundamental importance.

Since then the conditions have changed. The state of the art review incorporated in a PhD thesis today is usually published in a limited number of copies, and the journals have increased their demands that articles are succinct, compressed and with a limited number of tables, figures and even references. Therefore, there is a tendency towards splitting up the scientific work in small slices, called "salamisation". That is on the expense of an overview of what the author and his/her group has produced over a period of years. One loses the general overview. Also due to the demand for compression and the limitation in the number of references, reference to other parts of the published material in other papers are neglected which may hamper the possibility for other researchers to perform their own analysis possibly combining findings in several papers. This "salamisation" may be a restriction to bringing our knowledge forward. Fortunately, in the process of having Open Access, not only to publications, there is a trend in the European Union towards that the raw data should be made available to the research community. This may counteract the effect of "salamisation".

第 23 章
如何发挥新生物医学技术在大学医院的作用

Chapter 23
A New Bio-Medical Technique in an University Hospital Environment

Hans Stødkilde-Jørgensen

Along the advances in modern bio-medical technology, patients build up expectations about more precise diagnostics and therapeutic interventions subsequently. This requirement is justified by the large budgets which most countries allocate to bio-medical research and development and to the health sector in general, regardless if this is public or private. Sometimes, the expectations are ahead of the stage of instrumental maturation and the clinical implementation of new technologies. Indeed, the expectations among patients are often boosted by researchers and developers themselves in unification with investors and companies. However, it is often forgotten, that translation of new technologies from the basic research communities into relevant clinical diagnostics or therapeutic entities is a long process-stretching from implementation of early ideas about new techniques in the laboratory to the pre-clinical methodological maturation and finally ending with clinical testing.

Quality control in a broad sense is crucial throughout this process. Staff members should be trained in evaluating the technological stage, reproducibility and true quality of the data forming evidence for introduction of new methods in practical clinics. Especially for new diagnostic technology and methods, parameters like sensitivity and specificity are fundamental. To this could be added that well documented procedures and follow-up studies are necessary in the practical therapy. All these factors are the building stones that allow further advancements in patient treatment through a continued methodological development. Even when a new instrument or treatment principle has passed the different testing stages, the general clinical cost/benefit has to be taken into consideration. If the clinical value is not convincing or the costs in a broad sense cannot be justified, it might never reach such a high priority that it should be employed in clinical use. Introduction of new bio-medical research or clinical technology relies on a number of technical and organizational factors and is unfortunately often burdened by high financial expenses for equipment, installation facilities and system application. Indeed, purchase costs and installation budgets can most often be foreseen, but running costs in the following years might be more difficult to estimate as they depend on factors like available personal expertise, utility costs, technical servicing and of course how frequently this equipment is used in general.

1　Translation of basic research results to clinical use-the important pre-clinical step

New scientific results from chemistry, physics and molecular biology often form the developmental beginning of clinical diagnostics and therapy, for example in the form of new scanner technologies or therapeutic agents. Indeed, areas like nanotechnology and genetic engineering have in the recent years demonstrated the importance of strong developments coming from the fields of natural sciences. The translation process of the results into a clinical environment requires a number of pre-clinical steps, where technology is enhanced and matured for daily use demanding a high level of patient security, stability etc. The pre-clinical developmental stage often includes animal-based research. Finally, new technology must be followed by a cluster of substantial data regarding diagnostic or therapeutic value, functional stability and in-depth evaluated data on the technology outcome. Another important building block is the scientific documentation and publication which allows sites around the world to compare results and reproduction and hereby push the development forward. These factors secure that new technologies do not only rely on concept data proof, but are based on comprehensive data securing solid evidence forming the fundament for clinical introduction.

2　A new scanning technique translated from research environments to clinical sites

Design, implementation and verification of pre-clinical scanning technology, meant for introduction to clinical use, is of course very much dependent on the scanning type, and there might, furthermore, be a relatively large difference from brand to brand although there are many principal similarities. To illustrate aspects of new diagnostic method introduction a good example is an upcoming magnetic resonance scanner technology which right now is entering clinical use. The technique is called MR-hyperpolarization and has its scientific origin in quantum physical phenomena's. Having been refined in the physicist's and chemist laboratories for the last 10-15 years this methods' pre-clinical stage refinement is now being completed and has recently been used to study patients in California [1].

Very briefly described MR-hyperpolarization or Dynamic Nuclear Polarization (DNP) is a new MR-scanning technology for in-vivo quantification of metabolic processes with an extremely high sensitivity [2, 3, 4]. The DNP technology allows a rapid and highly-sensitive in vivo detection of pre-polarized 13C compounds (bio-probes) with a signal enhancement of more than 10.000 (Figure 23-1) [5]. This substantially increases the detection limit for quantitative measurements of specific metabolic fluxes involved in processing important intermediates in lipid, sugar and amino acid metabolism [2].

A solution (few ml) of a bio-active molecule (bio-probe), where one of the ^{12}C atoms is exchanged with a ^{13}C atom, is hyperpolarized in the polarizator. The solution is injected into the patient a few seconds after finishing the polarization process. The MR-spectroscopic scanning process runs through the next few minutes with a time resolution of about 1 sec. Up to four different bio-probes can be polarized simultaneously.

Bio-probes are molecules designed to trace specific metabolic fluxes in living tissue by exchanging selected ^{12}C atoms with ^{13}C atoms that can be hyperpolarized (Figure 23-2). Injection of a bio-probe will result in a very strong MR-signal from the main molecule and its breakdown products, thus being quantitated with extremely high sensitivity. Even though [1-^{13}C]pyruvate is the only bio-probe used in humans until now, a number of bio-probe molecules for tracing various metabolic processes in animals are already available [3]. [1, 4-13C] fumarate might be the next bio-

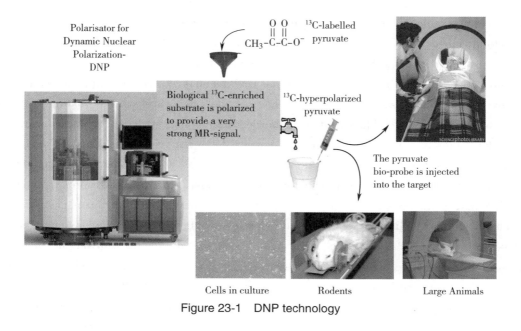

Figure 23-1　DNP technology

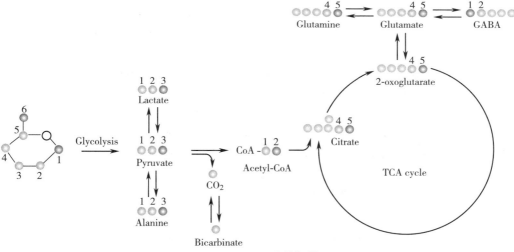

Figure 23-2　生物探针

probe introduced for human use, because of its large potential in quantification of metabolic effects in tumors due to therapy. Other examples of experimental bio-probes are lactate, acetate, leucine and glutamine, but the range of theoretically available bio-probe designs is long.

Different ^{12}C atoms in e.g. glucose or in pyruvate can be exchanged with ^{13}C for hyperpolarization and traced through the various steps of the glycolysis. The colouring of individual carbon atoms allows tracing them through the individual glycolytic steps in the figure. ^{13}C exchange on specific carbon positions allows for quantification of both intermediary and end product when injected into a living organism. Other steps in the TCA flux can be traced as well.

Examples of research fields and clinical applications connected with DNP technology

Metabolic changes detected by DNP have, in experimental tumors, been shown to correlate with response to chemotherapy [6]. Therefore, the DNP technology is expected to provide an enhanced prediction of therapeutic effects in pancreatic cancer in correlation with its potential to detect possible metabolic markers of response or resistance in patients.

Another oncological application area of the DNP technology is the combination with hadron therapy. Commercially available proton accelerators allow deposit of particle (hadron) radiation energy very locally in a solid tumour thus minimizes radiation damage to healthy tissue nearby and additionally minimizes the risks of secondary cancers following years later. The DNP technology can identify areas in e.g. the prostate gland that present the most abnormal metabolism and thus the highest malignity and as a result DNP might hereby be used for guidance of the hadron radiation.

The DNP methodology can also be used for in vivo quantification of fluxes of lipid, sugar and amino acid metabolism in lifestyle related diseases. It allows possible acquisition changes in metabolic fluxes in liver and muscles following a dietary shift to proteins with varying amino acid composition and load (e.g. low glycine) in nutrients. Another example is branched-chain amino acids (Leucine, Isoleusine and Valine) dietary programs. A final example is DNP application in studies of enzymatic controlled metabolic fluxes with studies of the metabolic inflexibility in diabetic or obese persons switching (metabolic flexibility) between utilization of carbohydrates and lipid derivatives. This includes ketone bodies as fuel substrates and preventive interventions like exercise, high glucose diet, high fat diet or anti-inflammatory treatment affecting the dys-metabolic state of obese subjects, with or without diabetes or metabolic syndrome.

Metabolic and pharmacological studies in cells cultured in MR-compatible bio-reactors are future applications of DNP due to the high sensitivity of this technology. For surface adherent cells a substantial concentration of cells can be achieved in a reactor. An example is endothelial progenitor cells which are believed to be influential on tissue regeneration by enhancing the formation of new blood vessels in ischemic tissue. Other relevant cell types are various cancer cell lines. A design example of an MR-compatible bio-reactor is shown in Figure 23-3 below. The bio-reactor is located deeply in the system circumvented by the MR-electronics (RF-coils) and connected to various fluid lines.

Upper: a vertical MR-compatible bio-reactor prepared for ^{13}C DNP metabolic measurements in cells grown on a scaffold located inside the reactor. Lower: microscopy of progenitor cells. They adhere to hydrophilic surfaces of 3D printed scaffold with predefined spaces between fibres. Adherent cells on the fibres (stained for nuclei) are shown to the right. With the cells in position inside the bio-reactor, this is submerged into the RF circuitry and pushed forward to the iso-centre of a high-field horizontal magnet.

3　The organizing and practical implementation

The committee given the mandate to organize planning and practical DNP implementation has to consider whether sufficient budgets are available to complete the installation and cover the running costs as well as secure that the human expert resources are available, as DNP requires presence of experts with different educational backgrounds. Many managers experience that operating new technologies in medicine often calls for educated expertise from physicists, engineers or pharmacologists.

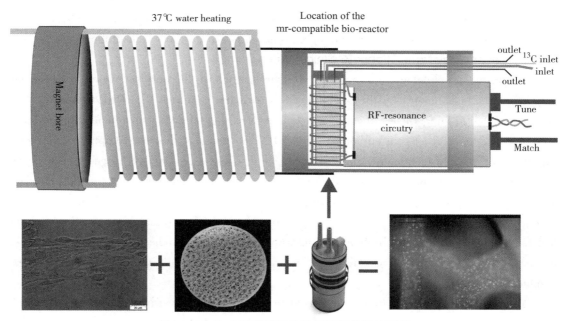

Figure 23-3　MR 兼容性生物反应器的设计举例

A training capacity must be available from the vendor and is also required at the location where the equipment is installed. Furthermore there is a need of local partnerships with educational institutions in order to secure accession of early stage researches. When entering the operating phase a set of training programs for both researchers and technical personnel should always be established to secure continued operation.

Methods developed in the research laboratories often have to go through different steps of product maturing before they can enter daily clinical practical use. The technology must be stable in terms of nearly 100% up-times and in case this is not fulfilled the system must be monitored with service assistance with very short response times. Normally the uptime should be described in the purchase contract. Nevertheless, when initiating research with a system like the DNP, a system only recently released on the market and with one main contractor, it is still composed by an assembly of products from various subcontractors, and therefore requires that both vendor and buyer accept that special technical and educational attention is needed for a long time after operation start.

In order to secure that operation remains user-friendly for the technical and clinical personnel, effort must be made to develop a user interface that is logical and easily understandable.

Questions about licensing and IP rights arise when developing new technology. With the DNP technology this is especially complicated and both a purchase contract and a so-called sterile-use license agreement are needed at purchase. While the purchase contract, as they often do, describes hardware items, delivery dates, uptime etc., the second contract binds the purchasers' possibility of teaming up with third parties and addresses the ownership of new technical and chemical developments intended to be operated on the DNP system. As mentioned above the DNP system relays on ^{13}C enriched substrates, of which many have already been developed for experimental purposes [3] and only a few of these will enter clinical use. In that case there will be a large commercial value for the selling company. Therefore, the DNP purchaser will, via the sterile license contract, be urged to cede ownership on bio-probes developed at the buyers' institution.

4　Technology translation into clinical use

Maturating a technology in a pre-clinical environment with the purpose of preparing use for patients normally commences within a group of relatively few countries. The DNP technology now being up-scaled to human usage is at present time in less than ten locations around the world and only three sites are at present authorized to use DNP in humans. In order to optimize and gain experience of this new technique various international discussion and data exchange platforms have been established. In Europe it has been agreed that one well-recognized university centre (Cambridge) will produce the necessary bio-probe packing's for others. This will secure a stable quality of the product. The DNP technology requires materials that do with stand submersion into fluid helium with temperatures close to the absolute zero and within seconds later are heated to room temperature. In such hostile environments fragments might be torn off and could result in embolism when injected into the blood stream.

An additional effect of sharing toxicology data openly is that it can be used by sites in all the other countries. The production process for bio-probes does include addition of substances that are potentially dangerous for an organism if there are traces of leftover in the bio-probe sample.

Countries do have diverging rules regarding the commencement of patient examinations with a new technology, which until then has been applied only pre-clinically. Indeed, even in EU-countries there are different regulations, but the discrepancy is most often not invalidating for the exchange of pre-clinical experience from for instance animal based studies. Translating the DNP technology into human applications is already initiated in California and will soon be done at both Oxford and Cambridge University in Great Britain. For patients at Aarhus University Hospital in Denmark the introduction of DNP will be offered for diagnostics early 2015. The first group to be included will presumably be patients suffering from pancreatic cancer.

5　Reporting scientific results from developmental pre-clinical studies

In many countries most of the practical research is carried out by early stage researchers who do have a righteous expectation of being able to publish according to the effort they add to the ongoing development of the project. It must, though, never conflict with license contracts or violate patents issues. In many cases the first publications will be a mixture between technical proof of concept data and results achieved from biological application studies.

By its very nature the first publishable data on technologies applied on new fields are often accepted relatively easy by the relevant journals. It is though very important that the publications are precise – especially when presenting new technologies where many details are enclosed allowing others to redo the experiments exactly the same way [1]. Published studies were the DNP has been applied is now increasing in number. Just in the first half of 2014, 162 publications appear in PubMed searching with the keyword "hyperpolarized 13C". Until now some of these have been based on limited materials, whereas others have been preliminary reports. Yet, it is evident that the publication activity has been increasing since the introduction of DNP technology a few years ago.

Key references

1. Nelson SJ, Kurhanewicz J, Vigneron DB, et al. Metabolic imaging of patients with prostate cancer using hyperpolarized [1-^{13}C]pyruvate. Sarah J. Nelson. Sci Transl Med, 2013, 5:198ra108.

2. Schroeder MA, Clarke K, Neubauer S, et al. Hyperpolarized magnetic resonance: a novel technique for the in vivo assessment of cardiovascular disease. Circulation. 2011.4; 124:1580-94.

3. Kurhanewicz J, Vigneron DB, Brindle K, et al. Analysis of cancer metabolism by imaging hyperpolarized nuclei: prospects for translation to clinical research. Neoplasia. 2011; 13:81-97.

4. Hurd RE, Yen YF, Chen A, et al. Hyperpolarized 13C metabolic imaging using dissolution dynamic nuclear polarization. J Magn Reson Imaging. 2012; 36 (6): 1314-28.

5. Ardenkjær-Larsen JH1, Golman K, Gram A, et al. Increase of signal-to-noise of more than 10,000 times in liquid state NMR. Discov Med. 2003; 3:37-9.

第 24 章
科研文章摘要和论文的撰写:欧洲经验

Chapter 24
Writing a Scientific Abstract and Paper: European Experience

Fawzy Farag, John Heesakkers

1 Introduction

Are you finished with collecting the data of your research? You must have exerted great efforts to conduct a well-structured research with a clear research question and good methodology! Did it take you so long to analyze the data and get the results? You must be impressed with what you did! But how can you be sure that colleagues and other people interested in your scientific field will be impressed with it too? How can you be sure that you can communicate your message to them?

In fact, the most important part of scientific work is the way you describe it in writing and get it published in a journal or to get it presented in a conference. There, you get comments, fruitful discussions and feedback of your colleagues. This shades the light on new aspects of your research, stimulates more spots on grey matter of your brain to explore your topic in more depth and to get more out of it!

The general advises of developing your skills in writing a scientific paper were outlined by Peter Hall [1] in 10 golden lessons:

(1) "Develop your skills by reading"

(2) "Have something to say"

(3) "Understand the structure of a scientific article"

(4) "Understand the simple rules of writing"

(5) "How to decide where to send your paper"

(6) "Instructions to authors and the need to worry about details"

(7) "Understand the steps after manuscript submission"

(8) "Understand what editors like"

(9) "Be aware of what editors do not like! "

(10) "Do not give up and understand the peer review process"

The detailed recommendations and guidelines to improve your skills in writing a scientific paper are addressed elsewhere in this book. In this chapter, we will guide you to learn how to write a well structured abstract for urological conference and how to write a scientific paper and get it published in top ranked urological journals.

2　How to write an abstract for a urological conference?

What we mean by the word abstract is a condensed summary of a full text article describing the methodology and results of a scientific experiment [2]. An abstract for a scientific meeting must be concise due to the limited number of words and figures. However, your abstract must give enough information about the methodology followed in conducting the study and the outcome of it. This is of paramount importance to get accepted at a urological conference.

The most important advice to have a good abstract is to have enough time to write it! David Pearson [2] stressed this point by paraphrasing a golden statement of his mentor "if you want a 10 minutes summary, I can have it for you a week from today; if you want it to be 30 minutes, I can do it tomorrow; if you want a whole hour, I am ready now".

An abstract in general consists of the following items [3]: title, list of authors, introduction, materials and methods, results, discussion. However, some urological conferences have their own modified formats. An example is the International Continence Society (ICS): http://www.ics.org/publications/abstracts which recommends the following format: list of authors, title, hypothesis/aim of study, study design, materials and methods, results, interpretation of results, table/figures, concluding message.

We will go through the individual components of the abstract step by step now. We will use an abstract of our research group that has been presented at the annual meeting of the European Association of Urology (EAU) in 2011, for example: http://www.uroweb.org/events/abstracts-online/

Near infrared spectroscopy: A novel non-invasive diagnostic method for detrusor overactivity in patients with overactive bladder symptoms. A preliminary and experimental study

Farag, F.[1], Martens, F.[2], D'Hauwers, K.[2], Feitz, W.[2], Heesakkers, J.P.[2]

[1]St RadboudUniversityNijmegen Medical Centre and Sohag University Egypt, Dept. of Urology, Nijmegen, Netherlands, The, [2]St RadboudUniversityNijmegen Medical Centre, Dept. of Urology, Nijmegen, Netherlands, The

Introduction & Objectives

Near infrared spectroscopy (NIRS) is an optical technology. It detects the hemodynamic changes in biological tissues via non-invasive measurement of changes in the concentration of tissue chromophores such as oxyhemoglobin (O_2Hb) and deoxyhemoglobin (HHb).

Objective: To address the accuracy and reproducibility of NIRS to detect the hemodynamic effects of Detrusor Overactivity (DO).

Material & Methods

Forty one patients with overactive bladder (OAB) symptoms underwent one or more filling cystometries with simultaneous, transcutaneous NIRS of the bladder (Figure 24-1). The separated graphs representing both tests were presented to 3 urodynamicists with 3 weeks between the first and second presentation. The graphs showed curves with and without DO episodes with the bladder sensations marked. The urodynamicists marked pressure changes suggestive of DO in the cystometry curves. For NIRS curves they marked definite deviations from baseline. Analysis was done to

---

determine the sensitivity and specificity of NIRS for DO. Fleiss and Cohen's Kappa statistics were used to estimate the inter-and intra-observer agreements respectively.

Results

The sensitivity and specificity of Hbsum (O_2Hb+HHb) curves for DO were 62-97% and 62-79% respectively (AUC 0.80-0.82; p<0.001). O_2Hb curves had 79-85% sensitivity and 82-91% specificity for DO (AUC 0.80-0.85; p<0.001). The sensitivity and specificity of HHb curves were 71-82% & 77-82%, respectively (AUC 0.73-0.84; p<0.001). The inter-and intra-observer agreements to trace the effect of DO on NIRS curves were substantial (Kappa >0.6).

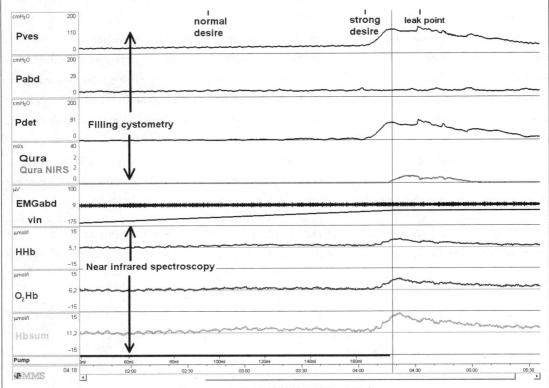

图 24-1　HHb 曲线的敏感度和特异度

Conclusions

NIRS is a potential non-invasive diagnostic method to detect DO. Its value to study the pathophysiology and treatment results in OAB syndrome will be tested.

(1) Title

A title should be catchy, determined, clear, simple, and not of highly technical character so that the readers of your abstract will not give up early before they read it to the end! And preferably, avoid abbreviations unless they are accepted internationally [3].

The number of words of a title should be about 10-12 words [4]. Perhaps you have already noticed that we used an affirmative format on writing the title of our abstract "*Near infrared spectroscopy: A novel non-invasive diagnostic method for detrusor overactivity in patients with overactive bladder symptoms. A preliminary and experimental study*". Classically, you can follow one of 3 ways to write a title for your abstract; a descriptive way that describes the main information of the abstract, an interrogative way where you can raise a question to stimulate the reader's mind to think about what is coming in the context of your abstract, or an affirmative way where you just summarize the results of your study [3].

(2) List of authors and their affiliations

It is expected that the first place of the authors' list is preserved for the researcher who was most involved in the research. The last author is, most of time, the most senior researcher [4].

(3) Introduction

The research topic of this abstract goes over the use of a relatively new technology for urologists. Therefore, we had to explain its nature briefly to the readers first, to be able to communicate further components of the abstract to them successfully: "*Near infrared spectroscopy (NIRS) is an optical technology. It detects the hemodynamic changes in biological tissues via non-invasive measurement of changes in the concentration of tissue chromophores such as oxyhemoglobin ($O_{2+}Hb$) and deoxyhemoglobin (HHb).*

(4) Objectives

The objectives of an abstract are measurable behaviors that you expect a reader of your abstract to be able to perform, after reading it [4]. In the example, you see that the behavior was to address/approach a particular scientific method through which we were able to investigate the accuracy and reproducibility of NIRS to detect the potential hemodynamic effects associated the event of involuntary detrusor contractions of the urinary bladder in patients with overactive bladder syndrome: "*To address the accuracy and reproducibility of NIRS to detect the hemodynamic effects of Detrusor Overactivity (DO)*".

(5) Materials and Methods

When you read the methods section of an abstract, you learn how the study was designed, its population and how they were sampled, the primary and secondary outcome(s) and measurements done to assess them. [4].

The primary study outcome was the sensitivity and specificity of the new noninvasive diagnostic technique, NIRS of the urinary bladder, to detect the events of DO compared to conventional filling cystometry. To address the primary outcome, certain measurements were done. First, the basic measurement was to perform conventional filling cystometry simultaneous with the noninvasive NIRS of the urinary bladder: "*one or more filling cystometries with simultaneous, transcutaneous NIRS of the bladder*". Then, to measure the number of DO events detected or missed by the NIRS compared the conventional cystometry: "*The separated graphs representing both tests were presented to 3 urodynamicists* "*For NIRS curves they marked definite deviations from baseline*", "*Analysis was done to determine the sensitivity and specificity of NIRS for DO*". The secondary outcome was to determine the reproducibility of this new technology in detecting the hemodynamic effect of DO. To measure this secondary outcome, the following measurement was performed: "*The separated graphs representing both tests were presented to 3 urodynamicists with 3 weeks between the first and second presentation. The graphs showed curves with and without DO episodes with the bladder sensations marked.*", "*Fleiss and Cohen's Kappa statistics were used to estimate the inter-and intra-observer agreements respectively.*"

(6) Results

You may present only the most relevant data, start with the key primary and secondary outcome(s) and the related statistics/significance level [4].

In the example the primary outcome was presented as follows: "*The sensitivity and specificity of Hbsum ($O_2Hb+HHb$) curves for DO were 62-97% and 62-79% respectively (AUC 0.80-0.82; p<0.001). O_2Hb curves had 79-85% sensitivity and 82-91% specificity for DO (AUC 0.80-0.85; p<0.001). The sensitivity and specificity of HHb curves were 71-82% & 77-82%, respectively (AUC 0.73-0.84; p<0.001).*"

The secondary outcome was presented as follows: "*The inter-and intra-observer agreements to trace the effect of DO on NIRS curves were substantial (Kappa >0.6).*"

(7) Conclusions

On writing the conclusion of your study, you should briefly describe the main outcome of it. Pay attention to presenting robust conclusions supported by the results obtained from your current study [4].

Please have a look at the conclusion we made of our study in the example abstract: "*NIRS is a potential non-invasive diagnostic method to detect DO. Its value to study the pathophysiology and treatment results in OAB syndrome will be tested*". You will see that we concluded that the NIRS of the bladder could be a diagnostic method for DO in patients with OAB, but we were very determined when we used the words "*potential*" *and* "*will be studied*". Moreover, in the title of the example abstract we wrote "A preliminary and experimental study". All these extra words make the core message of our abstract very clear to readers that we are developing a novel diagnostic technique for DO in patients with OAB syndrome but this technique is still under development and needs further investigations before we can use it in daily clinical practice.

(8) General remarks

Perhaps you already noticed that we used only 250 words to describe all components of the study from the introduction through the objectives, methods, results, till the conclusions. This seems to be too small number of words to describe such a big study! You have to know that all international conferences make strict guidelines to authors who are willing to submit their abstracts to the reviewers committee of these conferences. This in part could be ascribed to the large number of abstracts submitted to a specific conference and hence, the big number of abstracts assigned to each single reviewer that sometimes reaches up to 400 abstracts!

Therefore, you need to read carefully instructions to the authors offered by every conference committee before you start writing your abstract. Most conferences allow between 250 and 300 words. You can check the exact number of words used in your abstract through the word writing program you are using. Most conferences use special online submission systems that allow only the named number of words to be submitted [5]. In all cases, this restricted number of words will exclude the title and authors list and affiliation. Please bear in mind that the 250-300 include the tables and figures in your abstract. In other words, a single table or figure counts as 250 words!

(9) Tips

Complete sentences on writing an abstract are not always needed [5]. You may need to rewrite your abstract many times before you reach a concise format, use an active voice, use more generic terms, describe abbreviations early in the abstract then use the abbreviations only through the abstract, avoid empty phrases like "*studies show*"[4].

3　How to write a scientific paper?

In the previous part of this chapter, we presented the way we followed in writing an abstract summarizing the research work we did on NIRS for the diagnosis of DO. We showed you how we followed the instructions to authors available on the EAU website to make it in an acceptable format by the reviewers till it was accepted for presentation in a poster session during the annual meeting of the EAU 2011.

In this part of the chapter we will guide you to learn how to write a scientific paper of a clinical study. We will use our publication [6] in European Urology as an example: *Near-infrared spectroscopy: a novel, noninvasive, diagnostic method for detrusor overactivity in patients with overactive bladder symptoms-a preliminary and experimental study*". This publication is the extended format of the same study we presented as an abstract in the previous part of this chapter.

(1) Title

"*Near-infrared spectroscopy: a novel, noninvasive, diagnostic method for detrusor overactivity in patients with overactive bladder symptoms-a preliminary and experimental study*"

As we have shown before, we intended to make it a catchy, determined, and clear title. We avoided using highly technical terms and abbreviations. Again, we used an affirmative format on writing the title. Other formats you can use on writing a title could be descriptive or interrogative formats.

(2) List of authors and their affiliations

As we learned in writing an abstract, the first place of the authors' list is preserved for the researcher who was involved the most in the research. The last author is in most of time the most senior researcher or project leader [4].

(3) Abstract

Writing an abstract at the beginning of a scientific paper is somehow different from writing an abstract to present at a congress.

In general, an abstract should contain the following items: Background, Materials and Methods, Results, and Conclusions. These items briefly represent the main sections of any scientific paper: Introduction, Materials and Methods, Results, and Discussion. Each item of the abstract should contain 1-3 sentences. In the background, you need to present a statement of the hypothesis. In the Materials and Methods section you need to briefly present the design, experimental and statistical aspects of your study. Finally, on concluding your abstract, you need to summarize your impression about the results and make it clear whether the results were supportive to your original hypothesis or not [7].

European Urology journal regularly updates the guidelines to authors on its website http://www.europeanurology.com/resources-for-authors/submission-guidelines#35-original-articles. The latest abstract format in 2014 restricts the number of words to 300. You may find the following proposal of a well structured abstract on the website of the European Urology:

"*Background: The abstract should begin with a sentence or two explaining the clinical (or other) importance of the study question.*

Objective: State the precise objective or study question addressed in the manuscript (e.g., ''To determine whether …''). If more than one objective is addressed, the main objective should be indicated and only key secondary objectives stated.

Design, Setting, and Participants: Describe the basic design of the study. State the years of the study and the duration of follow-up. Describe the study setting to assist readers to determine the applicability of the report to other circumstances, for example, general community, a primary care or referral center, private or institutional practice, or ambulatory or hospitalized care. State the clinical disorders, important eligibility criteria, and key sociodemographic features of patients. The numbers of participants and how they were selected should be provided. In follow-up studies, the proportion of participants who completed the study must be indicated. In intervention studies, the number of patients withdrawn because of adverse effects should be given. For selection procedures, these terms should be used, if appropriate: random sample (where random refers to a formal, randomized selection in which all eligible individuals have a fixed and usually equal chance of selection); population-based sample; referred sample; consecutive sample; volunteer sample; convenience sample.

Intervention(s): The essential features of any interventions (surgical or medical) should be described. The nonproprietary drug or device names should be used unless the specific trade name is essential to the study.

Outcome Measurements and Statistical Analysis: Indicate the primary and secondary study outcome measurement(s) and the main statistical analysis.

Results and Limitations: The main outcomes of the study should be reported and quantified. Complications or sequelae of the interventions used must be detailed. Particular attention must be paid to estimates of treatment effect and confidence intervals and not just to p-values. All randomized controlled trials should include the results of intention-to-treat analysis, and all surveys should include response rates. Limitations of the study should be acknowledged.

Conclusions: Provide only conclusions of the study directly supported by the results, along with implications for clinical practice, avoiding speculation and overgeneralization. Indicate whether additional studies are required before the results should be used in usual clinical settings. Give equal emphasis to positive and negative findings of equal scientific merit."

Please have a look at the abstract of our example:

"*Background: Near-infrared spectroscopy (NIRS) is an optical technology. It detects the hemodynamic changes in tissues via noninvasive measurement of changes in the concentration of tissue chromophores such as oxyhemoglobin (O2Hb) and deoxyhemoglobin (HHb). Involuntary bladder contractions may cause changes detectable by NIRS.*

Objective: To address the accuracy and reproducibility of NIRS to detect the hemodynamic effects of detrusor overactivity (DO)."

Design, setting, and participants: A prospective cohort study was carried out on 41 patients with overactive bladder symptoms.

Measurements: Forty-one patients underwent one or more filling cystometries with simultaneous NIRS of the bladder. The separated graphs representing both tests were presented to three urodynamicists on two occasions, 3 wk apart. The graphs showed curves with and without DO episodes with the bladder sensations marked. Thirteen of 47 graphs (28%) with DO and 16 of 58 graphs (28%) without DO were excluded due to motion artifacts. The urodynamicists marked pressure changes suggestive of DO on the cystometry curves. For NIRS curves they marked definite deviations from baseline. The sensitivity and specificity of NIRS for DO were determined. The inter-and intraobserver agreements were determined.

Results and limitations: Valid data from 33 of 41 patients (80%) were included in the analysis. The interobserver agreement to trace the effect of DO on NIRS curves was "substantial" (kf > 0.6). The sensitivity of the Hbsum (O2Hb+HHb) curves for DO was 62-97% with a specificity of 62-79% (area under the curve [AUC]: 0.80-0.82; p<0.001). O2Hb curves had 79-85% sensitivity and 82-91% specificity for DO (AUC: 0.80-0.85; p<0.001). The sensitivity and specificity of the HHb curves for DO were 71-82% and 77-82%, respectively (AUC: 0.73-0.84; p<0.001). These values represent the performance of NIRS in the data sample that is not contaminated with motion artifacts; they are not representative of a general clinical setting.

Conclusion: NIRS is a potential noninvasive, reproducible, diagnostic method to detect DO."

To what extent does it comply with the proposed format by European Urology?

(4) Background and Objectives

The Background or Introduction section of a scientific paper goes over the research question. Therefore, it needs to give an insight into the available knowledge in literature that is related to the current research question which should be relatively new! The Objectives of the study then follows. Finally, a reader of your paper is expected to build a clear overview of your research question and the objectives of your study. Please make this section concise, the Introduction or Background of should not be a "literature review" therefore only key publications of relevance should be cited [8]. Please have a look at the Background of our example article:

"Overactive bladder (OAB) syndrome is highly prevalent in Western culture [1]. It negatively affects the patient's quality of life [2]. Filling cystometry is the standard urodynamic test to detect detrusor overactivity (DO) [3]; however, it is invasive and may cause patient's discomfort and urinary tract infections (UTI) [4]. Therefore, a noninvasive diagnostic tool that can replace conventional cystometry is recommended, especially for patients who undergo regular urodynamic evaluation.

Doppler ultrasound studies have revealed significant variations in blood flow of the bladder wall during the voiding cycle [5, 6] and bladder contractions in animal models [7]. DO is assumed to cause substantial variations in oxygen supply and consumption of the bladder wall during involuntary muscle contraction. Near-infrared spectroscopy (NIRS) as an imaging technology can

> *monitor the hemodynamic changes during bladder filling and voiding. Light in the near-infrared area is capable of penetrating the skin to the underlying tissues and is absorbed by naturally occurring chromophores such as oxyhemoglobin (O2Hb) and deoxyhemoglobin (HHb). NIRS enables detection of oxygen-dependent hemodynamic changes in biologic tissues by measurement of the relevant changes in the concentration of tissue chromophores relative to baseline. Total hemoglobin (Hbsum) is an indicator of total blood perfusion that can be derived from the sum of O2Hb and HHb[8].*
>
> *Urologic applications of NIRS cover various urologic disorders [9]. NIRS was previously reported to be an independent predictor of bladder outlet obstruction (BOO) with a good correlation between NIRS and pressure flow parameters [10]. Previously, we showed that transcutaneous NIRS of the bladder is feasible to detect DO episodes as the involuntary detrusor contractions have characteristic imprints on NIRS signals [11]. The objective of this study was to determine the accuracy and reproducibility of NIRS during cystometry in detecting DO episodes. Therefore, the sensitivity and specificity of NIRS changes compared to cystometry were investigated after exclusion of NIRS data contaminated with motion artifacts. Moreover, the inter- and intraobserver agreements of DO diagnosis in NIRS curves were determined.*"

Using 323 words only, we were able to communicate to readers the basic information about the new technology we applied in our research and its previous applications in medical field and in particular, in urology field. Therefore, the reader was prepared to receive the research question of our study "*to determine the accuracy and reproducibility of NIRS during cystometry in detecting DO episode*".

(5) Patients and Methods

In this section of your paper, you need to describe the actual steps you followed in order to find answer(s) to your research question. The Methods section is the most important section of your research because in one way or another, a reader of your paper must be able to repeat your methodology! You need to mention the ethical approval of the study and the institute in charge besides the availability of a signed informed consent by human subjects included in your study. You may arrange your Methods section in consequent headings, e.g., Participants, Ethical approval, Measurements, Statistical method. Or another setup according to the content of your paper [8].

The major items to be clearly detailed in the Methods section are the basic study design, the location where it was performed, participants (their basic characteristics and character of interest for which they were included). You also need to state the inclusion and exclusion criteria of your study. For randomized controlled trials, you need to state the way you did that.

> "*Patients*
>
> *The study group consisted of 41 consecutive adult patients referred to Radboud University Nijmegen Medical Centre, The Netherlands, for urodynamics between 20 August 2009 and 28 December 2009. Inclusion criteria were men or women >18 yr old with urgency with or without incontinence, frequency, and nocturia. Exclusion criteria were abdominal scars, hematuria, and*

> *a history of mixed incontinence. One patient was diabetic and one was treated for hypertension. Antimuscarinics were stopped >3 d before urodynamics. This study was approved by the local ethics committee."*

The Measurements or Intervention whether they were diagnostic, drug therapy, or surgical, need to be explained as detailed as possible, with clear mentioning of the study endpoint.

> *"Procedure*
>
> *Patients completed a 24-h voiding diary. Patients with clinical benign prostatic hyperplasia (BPH) and voiding symptoms suggestive of BOO completed an International Prostate Symptom Score (IPSS) questionnaire. Urinalysis was performed to exclude UTI and hematuria. All patients underwent cystometry (Solar, Medical Measurement Systems, Enschede, The Netherlands). A gas-filled urethral catheter (6 Fr/Ch) was inserted to monitor intravesical pressure (Pves), while abdominal pressure (Pabd) was monitored using a rectal balloon. Water was infused at room temperature with filling rates of 10-50ml/min as requested by the patient's physician. The same rate was used when several cystometries were performed in the same patient. Transcutaneous, noninvasive bladder monitoring with NIRS (URONIRS, Urodynamix Technologies Ltd, Vancouver, Canada) was performed simultaneous with cystometry. An emitter and a sensor were connected to a rubbery self-adhesive patch, 4cm apart. The patch was placed on the abdomen 2cm above the pubic symphysis across the midline [12]. Baseline NIRS reading for 30 s was followed by testing the effect of cough and Valsalva maneuver on NIRS signals. Patient movements, straining, and urine withholding were restricted. Surface Electromyogram (EMG) monitoring of the abdominal wall muscles (EMGabd) was used to rule out motion artifacts. Bladder sensations and events were recorded.*
>
> *The cystometries were diagnosed by a urodynamicist according to the International Continence Society guidelines to identify patients with and without DO. NIRS data were imported and automatically synchronized in the urodynamics database. Graphs contaminated with motion artifacts were excluded (Fig. 1). For rating purposes, the cystometry graphs and NIRS graphs were separated and coded. Graphs with DO were used as cases (Fig. 2) and graphs without DO as controls.*
>
> *Inter-and intraobserver variability*
>
> *The cystometry graphs consisted of three curves representing Pves, Pabd, and detrusor pressure (Pdet). NIRS graphs consisted of three curves representing HHb, O2Hb, and Hbsum. Flowmetry and EMGabd curves wereadded to the cystometry and the NIRS graphs. Rating was done by three experienced urodynamicists on two occasions 3 wk apart. The cystometry graphs and the NIRS graphs were presented separately and randomly to the raters. The raters did not know which NIRS graph belonged to which cystometry graph. The urodynamicists had to look for pressure changes suggestive of DO for the cystometry graphs and definite deviations from baseline in each NIRS curve (O2Hb, HHb, and Hbsum)."*

The statistical methods need to be clearly stated including the power calculation, setting of level of significance (p value) and the statistical tests and software used in the study.

"*Statistical methods*

The inter- and intraobserver agreements were analyzed using Cohen's kappa (kc) and Fleiss' kappa (kf) statistics [13]. Kappa values were interpreted based on the convention by Landis and Koch:<0, no agreement; 0-0.20, slight agreement; 0.21-0.40, fair agreement; 0.41-0.60, moderate agreement; 0.61-0.80, substantial agreement; and 0.81-1.0, almost perfect agreement [14]. Receiver operating characteristic curves were used to determine the diagnostic value of NIRS in predicting DO. The Mann Whitney U test was used for differences between groups."

(6) Results

On reporting the results, you need to follow the same order you followed in describing the data in the Methods section. Report final number of subjects included in final analysis and how many dropouts and reason for these dropouts. Describe the demographics of your patients. Start with the primary outcome followed by the secondary outcome(s). Avoid double reporting of data in tables and text! Stick to one way of reporting measurements. Finally, save your comment on the results to the Discussion section! data of study subjects [8].

This study included 34 men and 7 women (mean age: 62 14 yr) with overactive bladder (OAB) symptoms. The mean body mass index was $26kg/m^2$ (range: 20-33). Seventeen patients had neurogenic disorders, 21 men had BPH, and 3 had idiopathic OAB. The mean frequency was 12 3 voids per day (range: 6-17). The mean IPSS was 17 (5-33) for patients with BPH.

Fifty-two cystometry sessions with simultaneous NIRS were performed. The cystometries identified 23 patients with DO who underwent 34 cystometry sessions. Forty-seven DO episodes were identified. To get optimal NIRS graphs, only 34 of 47 DO graphs were selected for the final analysis based on the stability of Pabd and EMGabd curves. Each DO episode was considered an individual case. The median bladder filling at start of DO episodes was 137ml (range: 12-492ml). The median Pdet change at DO was $42cm\ H_2O$ (range: $6\text{-}215cm\ H_2O$). Cystometry identified 18 patients (one cystometry each) without DO. Their data were used for control purposes. Each control cystometry session was divided into equal parts, which included sensation marks. A total of 58 control graphs were obtained of which 16 (28%) were excluded based on the stability of Pabd and EMGabd. Thirty-four of the remaining 42 graphs were randomly selected as individual control cases using SPSS (SPSS Inc, Chicago, IL, USA).

Table 1 shows the results of the two rating sessions. The overall diagnostic agreement for the three observers was 92% for cystometry graphs (kf=0.84). For the NIRS, the observers agreed on 81% of the HHb curves (kf=0.63), 84% of the O2Hb curves (kf=0.69), and 81% of the Hbsum curves (kf=0.61). The AUC value ranges for the diagnostic performance of NIRS for the three observers were 0.73-0.84 for HHb; 0.80-0.85 for O2Hb, and 0.80-0.82 for Hbsum (p<0.001). The intraobserver agreement for cystometry was kc=0.85-0.97; for NIRS, kc=0.53-0.79 for HHb, 0.65-0.76 for O2Hb, and 0.67-0.75for Hbsum. The sensitivity of NIRS For DO as an average of the three observers was 92% for Hbsum, 82% for O2Hb, and 77% for HHb. The specificity was 86% for O2Hb, 80% for HHb, and 72% for Hbsum. However, it should be mentioned that these high values do not represent *the actual sensitivity and specificity in the general clinical setting, but only in an optimal study sample (72%) not contaminated with motion artifacts. The performance of NIRS would have been lower if analysis of the whole group, including motion artifacts, was done. To rate false-positive and false-negative DO diagnoses in NIRS graphs, only graphs with at least two curves marked with a deviation were counted as positive. Although 16 of 58 control graphs (28%) were excluded for motion artifacts, the NIRS graphs were rated falsely positive in 6 of 34 (18%) controls. The NIRS curves showed no deviation in 5 of 34 (15%) DO episodes. The median change in Pdet at DO was significantly lower in these false-negative cases as compared to the true-positive cases (20 vs 47cm H_2O; p<0.005) (Table 2). Twenty of 29 true-positive cases had DO at a filling volume <100ml, while 1 in 5 false-negative cases had DO at a volume <100ml. No adverse events related to NIRS occurred.*

Readers prefer to read tables and see figures, it helps them to understand the results and get an overview of the entire outcome of your study. Pay attention to the clarity of numbers and symbols used in your tables. Always make them clear. You may explain any symbol or abbreviation used in the table in the legend of this table. Your tables must have informative titles and preferably indicate the statistical test if any significance level is reported in the table.

Table 1　Results of the two rating sessions[*]

Patients, n=34		Session I				Session II			
		Cy. %	HHb %	$O_2Hb\%$	Hb_{sum} %	Cy. %	HHb %	O_2Hb %	Hb_{sum} %
Observer 1	Cases	100	82	85	97	100	82	88	97
	Controls	9	18	18	38	9	23	21	53
Observer 2	Cases	100	71	79	88	97	68	65	73
	Controls	21	23	9	26	9	26	9	38
Observer 3	Cases	100	79	82	91	97	62	62	65
	Controls	0	18	15	21	0	18	18	21

Cy=Cystometry; HHb=deoxyhemoglobin; O_2Hb=oxyhemoglobin; Hb_{sum}=total hemoglobin

* The ratio of the graphs rated with the answer 'yes' to the total number of detrusor overactivity graphs in the upper row (true positives) and the ratio of the graphs rated with the answer 'yes' to the total number of control graphs in the upper row (false positives) are shown for each observer. The columns in the table represent the results of rating the cystometry and the individual near-infrared spectroscopy curves, respectively, during the two rating sessions.

Table 2　A comparison of some relevant demographic and urodynamic parameters between the true-positive and false-negative cases based on near-infrared spectroscopy diagnosis.

	Cases, n=17, 34 DO episodes		
	True positives n=14 patients, 29 graphs	False negatives n=3 patients, 5 graphs	p value*
Mean BMI ± SD (range)	$25.8 \pm 3 kg/m^2 (20.5\text{-}31)$	$25.4 \pm 4 kg/m^2 (20.8\text{-}28.4)$	0.63
Median filling volume at DO, ml (range)	131 (12-492)	149 (59-171)	0.51
Median peak pressure at DO, cm H_2O (range)	47 (11-215)	20 (6-24)	0.004

DO=Detrusor Overactivity; BMI=Body Mass Index; SD=standard deviation.

* Mann Whitney U test.

(7) Discussion

You should focus on discussing the answers you found for the research question and the meaning and implication of the primary outcome. You need to discuss the interpretation of your findings in light of existing knowledge and compared to other publications on the same topic. Report the limitations of your study in an honest way, because reviewers and readers will find it anyway! Finally, your conclusions must be based on the actual findings of the study [8].

This is the first clinical study that tests the application of NIRS during the filling phase of the voiding cycle. Our objective was to determine the accuracy and reproducibility of NIRS in detecting DO episodes during cystometry.

Cystometry detects the mechanical effect of DO. NIRS is used to measure the changes in concentration of bladder wall chromophores relative to baseline in response to bladder events. The assumption is that changes in activity and consequent oxygen consumption cause chromophore changes. This real-time feature of NIRS is unique in comparison to other non-invasive diagnostic techniques that are examined for DO [15, 16].

There are three possible reasons that can explain the characteristic imprint of DO on NIRS signals. The first possibility is an auto-regulatory hemodynamic mechanism in the bladder. The second possibility is the mechanical compressive effect of DO on the bladder wall vasculature. The third possibility is the effect of bladder wall movements during DO, leading to momentary changes in blood volume lying within the NIRS imaging scale.

High inter-and intraobserver agreements are mandatory for assessment of the clinical applicability of any new diagnostic test. Agreement among the urodynamicists was 'almost perfect' for cystometry, while it was 'substantial' for NIRS (K_f=0.84, 0.61, 0.69, and 0.63 for cystometry, Hb_{sum}, O_2Hb, and HHb curves, respectively). This might be explained by the familiarity of the urodynamicists with the classic setup of the conventional cystometry.

NIRS curves had a good diagnostic performance as predictors of DO, giving a range of AUC values of 0.80-0.85 for O_2Hb curves, 0.73-0.84 for HHb curves and 0.80-0.82 for Hb_{sum} curves, as calculated for the three observers. NIRS was highly sensitive to detect DO episodes: 92% for Hb_{sum},

82% for O_2Hb and 78% for HHb. Hb_{sum}, curve being the sum of O_2Hb and HHb, can explain its higher sensitivity for DO.

NIRS is susceptible to motion artifacts[17]. In order to have NIRS applied reliably, artifacts should be avoided. Figure 3 shows the imprint of cough and Valsalva's maneuver on NIRS. Therefore, 28% of the graphs were excluded from analysis. The overall specificity of NIRS parameters for DO was 86% for O_2Hb, 80% for HHb and 72% for Hb_{sum}. There were six false-positive cases out of the 34 control graphs. This implies that observers still see some deviations in NIRS curves in absence of DO. One explanation could be a DO episode that was not detected by cystometry. Radley et al. found that conventional cystometry classified only 32 of 106 women with OAB symptoms as having DO, while ambulatory urodynamics classified 70 women as having DO[18]. Another explanation could be the wash-out effect of accumulated vasodilator substances as part of the regulatory mechanisms to maintain blood perfusion to the bladder wall during filling[19]. A third possibility would be a misinterpretation of the physiologic, systemic, hemodynamic fluctuations of respiratory signals or cardiac pulsations[17]. This is unlikely because normally these fluctuations are regular, rhythmic and of low amplitude.

NIRS failed to identify 5 of 34 cases with DO as compared to urodynamics. Explanations could be a bladder contraction with low amplitude or the bladder lying out of reach of the NIRS imaging scale due to a small bladder volume or a thick abdominal wall. Twenty of 29 true-positives had DO at filling volumes <100ml, while only 1 in 5 false-negative cases had DO at <100ml. Only the difference in P_{det} was significant between the false-negative and true-positive cases. Therefore, a bladder contraction with a low P_{det} seems to be the main reason for the false negativity.

Our study has some limitations. More men were included than women, while generally OAB symptoms are more prevalent in women. This can be explained by the high inclusion number of men with BPH. We excluded 28% of the graphs due to motion artifacts. It was mandatory in our methodology to have non-contaminated data in order to evaluate the scientific value of NIRS in the diagnosis of DO. We believe that the sensitivity and specificity were high in our series because they were tested only within a selected data sample. However, the situation should be different when the clinical applicability of NIRS will be addressed. Recently, algorithms were developed for cancellation of motion artifacts[21]. This could be applied to improve future study set-ups.

No laboratory screening was done to exclude systemic vasculopathies.

(8) Conclusions

The conclusions should be real conclusions from the study you did, the results that you obtained, the critical appraisal from the findings based on the existing literature and the balance between your findings and flaws and the literature to date. Try to be concrete and not repetitive with respect to the abstract.

In the current study, we showed that NIRS is non-invasive and reproducible with high sensitivity for detecting DO. Its value for clinical trials evaluating treatments for DO remains to be determined. NIRS curves correlate well with DO episodes detected by conventional urodynamics. NIRS seems to detect the hemodynamic changes caused by detrusor contractions. This implies that

> *NIRS can be used to study the regulatory mechanisms of blood perfusion to the bladder during filling as well as the hemodynamic phenomena accompanying DO. NIRS is a potential non-invasive diagnostic tool for DO in patients with OAB symptoms.*

(9) General remarks on the setup of the manuscript

Urological journals recommend various formats to be used on writing a manuscript. These formats obligate authors to use certain number of words, specific writing font and size and line spaces. They also ask for specific reference style. Some journals ask even for more information about the role of each author and his or her exact contribution to the manuscript. We present here an example of the manuscript setup as recommended by the official website of the European Urology: http://www.europeanurology.com/resources-for-authors/submission-guidelines.

"For submission and review, acceptable manuscript file formats include Word, Word Perfect, EPS, and Text, Postscript, or RTF format. Use 12-point font size, double-space text, and leave right margins unjustified with margins of at least 2.5cm. Each page should be numbered in the upper right corner, beginning on p. 2. Add continuous line numbering.

Title Page

The title page should include a word count for the text and abstract separately. Authors' full names, highest academic degrees, and affiliations should also be included (see list below). If an author's affiliation has changed since the work was done, the new affiliation also should be listed. For indexing purposes, 3 10 key words should be supplied in alphabetical order (see example below)

Title

Authors (first name and initials followed by surname, e.g., Juan X. Alvarez)

Affiliations (if multiple affiliations are listed, indicate with lowercase letter footnotes following the respective authors names)

Contact information for corresponding author, including full mailing address, telephone number, fax number, and e-mail address

For indexing purposes, 3-10 keywords should be supplied in alphabetical order. Headings

Units of Measurement

Units of measurements must conform to the Systeme International (SI): year(s), yr; month(s), mo; days, d; hours, h; minutes, min; seconds, s; grams, g; liters, l; meters, m; sample size, n; degrees of freedom, df; standard error of the mean, SE; standard deviation, SD; probability, p.

Numerals and Abbreviations.

Use numerals for all values greater than ten and those followed by a unit; otherwise, spell out (e.g., 18 patients, 0.8 g/ml, 47%, 37 8C, six cases). Spell out numbers at the beginning of a sentence. Abbreviations must be defined at first use in each of the following: text, tables, and figure legends."

References

1. Bliss DZ. Writing a successful research abstract. J Wound Ostomy Continence Nurs, 2012, 39:244.

2. D Andrew, MT David, FE Babl. Review article: A primer for clinical researchers in the emergency department: Part III: How to write a scientific paper. Emergency Medicine Australasia

Ema, 2012, 24 (4): 357-362.

3. FF Farag, FM Martens, KW D'Hauwers, et al. Near-infrared spectroscopy: a novel, noninvasive, diagnostic method for detrusor overactivity in patients with overactive bladder symptoms-a preliminary and experimental study. EurUrol, 2011, 185 (4Suppl): e870-e871.

4. Hall PA. Getting your paper published: an editor's perspective. Ann Saudi Med, 2011, 31 (1): 72-76.

5. Pierson DJ. How to write an abstract that will be accepted for presentation at a national meeting. Respir Care, 2004, 49 (10): 1206-1212.

6. Taboulet P. Advice on writing an abstract for a scientific meeting and on the evaluation of abstracts by selection committees. European Journal of Emergency Medicine, 2000, 7 (1): 67-72.

7. GJ Wood, RS Morrison. Writing abstracts and developing posters for national meetings. J Palliat Med, 2011, 14 (3): 353-359.

8. Van Way CW 3rd. Writing a scientific paper. Nutr Clin Pract, 2007, 22:636-40.

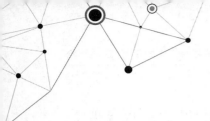

第 25 章
如何写好科研论文

Chapter 25
How to Write Good Scientific Text

Yrjö T. Konttinen, Ahmed Al-Samadi

Summary

Writing a good scientific paper starts when the project is initiated. Writing is but one of the last phases of the process of publishing. Although it is possible to produce an original article or review all alone, in biomedical science one usually works in a good group and team of coworkers. Production of experimental data requires good financing, facilities and reagents. This does not necessarily mean that all the money has to be in a research account when the work starts but it should be possible and realistic and likely that funding can be raised as work proceeds. Research team and funding form the material platform on which the knowledge, insight, working hypotheses and work process can be built. Even though the most "perfect" research leaders cannot always be 100% right, group leaders anyway have substantial knowledge and experience, which usually provides the framework of and direction to the research. Old and in particular new group members need to study hard to read themselves into the current research topic. Dialogues and discussions with team members make this fun and improve the learning curve. New ideas, interesting research questions, a testable working hypothesis, aims and other parts of the research plan should be carefully prepared-well planned is half done. Often already now the introduction and materials and methods are taking shape and many of the key references can be added. Some pilot experiments with negative and positive controls might be extremely useful. Experiments and hypotheses probably form multiple cycles in a closed loop control system. It is often a good idea to verify the central findings by using several methods with different premises, e.g. to study the phenomenon of interest at protein, mRNA and functional level using cell culture, experimental animal model and patient samples. Experimental data may make it necessary to modify the original working hypothesis because facts change theory and hypothesis, not *vice versa*. Senior and junior members of the team usually execute most of the practical research. Be open-minded and work hard but relaxed. Ask for advice. It is good to frequently report to the team leader but also in larger group meetings for feedback and ideas for the paper. At the end, one may notice that one is at the road's end-but that is not the road one was planning to take. Do not worry, expected findings often too predictable and boring, unexpected may be more interesting. To to prepare the results section: try to illustrate all main results in form of simple figures, microphotographs, drawings, flow charts and tables. Try to make them self-explanatory. This mill finally produced the solid good stuff, which can now be formulated to a paper. Clearly thought will be clearly written. Formulate the story line, which is clear and logic. Shortness and clarity are virtues. The story should be progressive and evolving and may contain some surprise moments. Selecting a proper target journal helps to produce text according to Author Instructions and a good match between the quality of your work and the scope, ranking and impact factor of the target journal may speed up the publication process. It helps to prepare already before first submission a flow chart: if the work is not accepted to the target journal, where to submit it 2nd, 3rd, 4th etc. time. Good work published in a very modest journal may get hundreds of citations, whereas publishing in a top journal does not guarantee anything and may not be cited at all. It is the substance of the work, not the publication platform, which is important here.

Introduction

These reflections are based on scientific experience of the lead author, an internist, now Professor of Medicine, based on Hirsch index 61; 45 supervised PhD theses; work as a post-doc with Professors Nathan J. Zvaifler and Harry G. Bluestein at UCSD; Professor Robert J. Winchester at NYU; Professor Paul Davis and Anthony S. Russell at UEA and Professor Pierre Meunier at Université Claude-Bernard; hosting later in my own group post-docs from 32 different countries; peer reviews done for over 150 different international journals; and handling of 50-100 papers a year as a Co-Editor of Acta Orthopaedica during their peer review process. It was also much affected by learning from Professor Julia M. Polak at the Royal Postgraduate Medical School in London, now part of the Imperial College School of Medicine.

Like any competitive and challenging task, writing an article does not start by just positioning the starting line, in this case a blank computer screen. It takes a lot of exercise and doing to get there, to have something to write about. At the point of writing, the scientific work is often already rather well formulated or "written" in the mind of the lead scientist, even before the final article writing starts.

A short summary on the foundations of and roadmap to a good paper is presented in Figure 1. Select a team with adequate financing and output. Study the substance of your project. You will find many good references to be used later on. This work, communication and creative thinking will form the basis of the central process, which is creation of an idea formulated to a testable hypothesis, invention of the wheel. That process is important for later writing the introduction of your paper. The wheel is the driving force in the subsequent work cycles consisting of shuttling between experimental testing of the hypothesis and reformulation and adjustments of the working hypothesis. When planning the design of your experiments and what methods you will be using you are already being prepared to write the Materials and Methods section of your final article. During experimentations, results are gradually produced. This practical and intellectual exercise does not happen in a vacuum, but inspires to thinking, discussions and presentations. Much is dependent on your attitude. Be open-minded, relaxed and enjoy your work. See challenges instead of problems, opportunities instead of work pressure. Depending on the level of ambition and the practical circumstances, when it feels that the work is finally done, it is time to start to formulate the discussion section, to develop the final story line.

Team

Selection of the team is often dependent on one's future plans, e.g. what medical specialty one after graduation would like to select. In some universities research is very dominated by strong leaders so one has often in practice to select the group led by the Department or Institution Head, to be able to do research first and later continue to specialize to the clinical area of interest or even do both at the same time. It is therefore good if research also at the local level can be organized so that there are real options and sound competition. In practice, this often happens so that in one larger group there are several smaller teams, led by team leaders, who in practice guide, teach and on daily basis support younger researchers.

For people in basic sciences and in particular for post-docs going to sabbaticals abroad, it is possible to select a group among many different alternatives. One can then check the direction, quality and output of the work of different potential host groups and then make a personalized choice corresponding to one's needs. If possible, it is useful during lunch and tea time or using e-mail, mobile and skype to clarify how the group members experience their research work: do they find their work exciting and is it stimulating and fun to work in the group? Is the team spirit good? How much do they get support from the group leader and at the bench? After finishing in the group, do the researchers maintain contact with it, also afterwards? That a group is located at a top university does not need to mean that also the group is at a top level, it can only be its address. Or even if the group is at a top level, it might base on the phenomenon in which "researchers are thrown to the water to find out which of them can swim." If there are many candidates to such a group, this type of "natural" selection, survival of the fittest, is naturally one way to go, but it might not necessarily be your first choice. A less known university with a top-level group might be a much better choice, but then the selection process then becomes more important and needs to be more specific. It might be a good idea to meet your future host in person in some international meeting. Do not buy a pig in poke!

It is difficult to do good research as a military exercise and hard work, without enjoying it. Doing research should be like playing and doing sports: fun and motivating. This gives much better results than just trying to make progress by force. At last, it is good to remember, according to the slogan from the USA army: "Do not only ask what your team can do for you, but also ask what you can do for your team." When you are a team member, also you contribute to the team spirit and to the success of the group.

Financing

As they sing, money makes the world go round … a mark, a yen, a buck or a pound. Adequate financing, facilities, equipment and reagents are necessary for biomedical research. There is a harsh competition of financing. Few groups have permanent, institution-based or otherwise secured financing. Most struggle for external funding which can sometimes be lavish, but is often short-term and uncertain. It is wise to check the history of the group and how it is going now for the group. Are they getting results? If so that is assuring. This is often the best predictor of the future: they are using money and producing results, according to the "publish or perish" rule. Funding is however also affected by external circumstances, such as the general economic situation which varies in group, university, local, state, national and worldwide scale.

Often researchers can together with the supervisor or host seek personal funding for the researchers. This is often neglected. Many younger researchers are too passive and waiting to get their share of the group's funding-although a much better strategy to make them attractive could be to seek personal funding from domestic, foreign or international sources and be self-financing. This will definitely improve one's chances to be able to select the group of choice as described above. Such grants can provide continuity for the PhD work or post-doc sabbatical. Do not just trust on good luck, seek opportunities and be active yourself!

Studying

Study the topic of your research by using textbooks, PubMed, patents, pdf-reprints and other data sources, including naturally work of the host group on the current topic. Try first to clarify the concept, understand the processes and build a framework, where to place more detailed information. Discuss the topic with the group members and meetings and take regular and web-courses whenever it seems that this will significantly improve your readiness. Do not just passively study, take time to try to comprehend the data and landscape more deeply, try to build your own theoretical framework or mind map and try even to challenge the current points of view. If not else, it is good exercise and will help to solidify old and create new engrams. You are anyway hoping to find a new path. This studying provides the theoretical basis used to do the work and then write the paper. Studying is naturally a continuous and life-long learning process for a scientist. Never miss a good chance to learn something new.

It is a good idea to go back to the basics, in particular always after one gets experimental results. It is very common that a properly performed and controlled pilot experiment does not fall out as expected. This might have trivial reasons, which always need to be considered, but it is also possible that the expectations were wrong and that "the thing" works differently from what one was thinking. Many good experiments are wasted because too little time is used for contemplation. This should not be a moment of frustration but a challenge and opportunity to restructure one's own thinking. For an eager scientist, experimental results are like food for the hungry, food for thought. So after "cooking" in the laboratory, enjoy-and think. What were you trying to do and what did you get? Data cannot be changed to fit your theory, but theory and the content of your future paper must be prepared so that it fits the facts you found.

Basics and our state-of-the-art are often not at all as solid as they look like. There are countless uncovered molecules, interaction, phenomena and processes just waiting to be discovered under the surface and beyond the horizon and I think that nobody seriously predicts that one day in the distant future, everything will be uncovered and understood. Because we cannot learn everything by studying books and other already existing documents, let us get practical and combine theory and practice into a productive cycle.

Research idea and hypothesis

Team (class), funding (financing), knowledge and skills might perhaps be enough for a pupil but, but for reasons mentioned above, not for a scientist. Scientist needs to be creative to design a good approach to solve technical and theoretical problems at the frontier of science and knowledge. Because research is a continuing or usually at least a long-term process, ideas which form the basis of future research have already been inspired by and more or less formulated based on earlier published work and unpublished own experiments. Experimental results challenge all the time the creative scientific process. The Golden Book of Nature does not easily give away its secrets but it takes a lot of work and thinking to understand better how it works.

A theoretical framework and a working hypothesis will help forward. A working hypothesis should be based on current knowledge on how things work and clear understanding what we now know about it, but also vision beyond that, what happens or actually could below the surface, where we cannot see clearly yet. Can we learn to understand or predict things better than before, by using our hypothesis as a tool? Hypothesis should be formulated so that both "yes, it is true" and "no, it is false" answers to it, proving or disapproving it, are interesting. In randomized clinical trials but also in experimental research one should have a rough idea what are the risks for false positive and false negative results. Doing an experiment many times with the same cell line or mouse strain may give statistically significant but misleading results. Also observational and high through-put discovery data needs to be repeated and tested adequately.

Sometimes the work is stuck so that clear and reproducible results are obtained and validated, but do not fit into the frame or current thinking. One should then try to create a firework of ideas. A real brain storming session or sessions together with the group members could be a good idea. One should not be afraid of coming with silly ideas or solutions because that prevents the creative process and free associations. On the contrary, in a good brainstorming session scientists should almost compete about who can come with the most imaginative idea. It can be a lot of fun! These ideas should be recorded so that they can later be more critically evaluated.

Without accurate knowledge of the state-of-the-art, a theoretical framework to place old data and new findings, without research questions, driving hypothesis and direction, one can easily drown in the sea of information, the level of which is rapidly rising.

Theory-practice cycles

A theoretical framework and a working hypothesis help to find a good research path-and to make a good research plan. This already shapes the future paper quite far. A good research hypothesis is a bit like trying to solve a detective story: one can, based on the history (published literature) and findings (experimental results), make an educated guess (a hypothesis) but this should be rigorously tested. In a simple setting this testing refers to that we study the dose and time effect of an input variable on a measurable out-put variable at the same time when all the other confounding variables (factors) are standardized. In a murder case, if one suspect (a solution) can be excluded, then a new hypothesis could be done before going back to the field work to test it (design and execution of new experiments). Because the first solution at least for the time being was excluded, one has to come one step further in finding new ways to tackle with the problem to find out if the working hypothesis is true or not. If the hypothesis is truly interesting, proving it wrong might be a most interesting finding. There is some publication bias, however, based on a tendency to only publish positive findings. On the other hand, finding the hypothesis to be true might be considered to be boring, too predictable.

In research, theory (framework, hypothesis, interpretations, understanding) and practice (experiments and analysis) go hand in hand, in productive cycles. What makes your ideas, your research questions and working hypothesis fresh and original? Dare to think differently, try to see the same data but to understand it in a new way, formulate a new hypothesis. If your laboratory does not have extremely good funding, I mean in the worldwide scale, you are not likely to be able to beat the top teams consisting of professional, hardworking, professional and well-funded scientists, not by brute force at least. Maybe you can develop a new idea-and let them to study it in detail.

Thinking and discussing

To prepare a good paper, it is good if one can use time for thinking about the basics, state-of-the-art and visions of the future. What did we know and what did we learn?

One does not need to work alone. One good way is to develop new ideas and angle of views together with group members. Use them to test your interpretation of your findings. The ideas and the story line of the future paper were already once scrutinized when the research plan was prepared. Now it might be a good time to participate in a national or international meeting to present the preliminary data in form of an oral presentation or a poster. This means that one will have to produce *ad interim* progress report about the current state of the project. This is useful exercise. Often a poster presentation in a well-organized congress with poster sessions and poster presenters being there at their posters available is the best way to get feedback from other scientists. Usually the best discussions in the scientific meetings occur in front of posters, not in front of a large audience in the keynote or plenary lecture hall. Establish cross-scientific and international networks. Such lectures and short oral presentations have another type of function. Good social skills and networking are often more important than a high IQ.

What would today's world be without internet, software and hardware (computers). Ask the wizard. Use tools like STRING (Search Tool for the Retrieval of Interacting Genes/Proteins) and GO (The Gene Ontology) to get an idea of the protein-protein interactions (pathways) and gene product properties and their attributes involved. Once you have results these programs can give hints which would be very difficult and time demanding to search from PubMed and study as described above.

Often it goes so that one already thinks that now I have it, now I know how it works. Suddenly lots of data, information and experimental results fall together. However, when more papers are published and more experiments done to produce new data, the picture will become diffuse again, until a new order again starts to rule.

Attitude

Try to be relaxed when thinking and working. You do not need to come to the answer right away. Lacking the anxious waiting and reflection and-finally-the excitement at the moment of discovery and understanding would make a scientist's life mentally poor. It is impossible to understand all at once, because the very task is to reveal new data and to create new order in chaos (as harmony probably looks to us due to lack of knowledge), which is not there yet.

Try to be relaxed and enjoy, like you would when playing a mahjong or tangram. If one would have ready models how to place tans to form different shapes, one could rapidly come to many different solutions. But would it be any fun-to play it that way? Instead, it is really fun to struggle and plan the pilot "experiments", to exercise error and trial and finally get the pieces to fall together so that a new silhouette is formed. Scientist should not be or become anxiou (in a negative meaning of the word) because one does not have an immediate and final answer at hand. Trial and error approach, working hypothesis and experimental results are needed to get closer to new data and understanding. If the results do not fit with the hypothesis, hypothesis has to be reformulated and the tans have to put together in a new way. One is getting further away from everyday dogma, against some new solutions.

It is good to start to think, how things really work, not just to read, memorize, repeat and verify what most of the other have already reported. Enjoy creative thinking because in the virtual world, in the human brain, different scenarios and different solutions to them can be rapidly created at a low cost.

Sometimes it really helps just to take time off, to relax and forget everything: a mind put into motion will work even at the unconscious level and maybe upon returning back from a real holiday to laboratory, the right solution is there, in front of your nose-this is my own experience. In retrospect the solution often feels much more simple than expected. One is hoping to be able to develop in such a direction that the path from the question to an answer would be relatively straight. On the other hand, if the solution is all too simple and easy, it might be trivial, and not anything important-although it might, sometimes ingenious solutions are simple.

Story line

A scientific article should not be just a pile of data without a story and coherence although different omics and data bases deposited in the net can be a veritable source of information for a skillful scientist. Just reporting data without understanding is too descriptive and not hypothesis driven. Members of the group, which planned the work, designed experiments and collected data, become now coauthors writing the final paper.

As is understood from above, work done when writing the research plan and giving presentations of the preliminary results make the team well-prepared for this work. It is easy to see the story line, the red thread running through the whole article.

Try to use clear logic, and simple and exact language. Avoid unnecessary abbreviations because they do not make the text more scientific and can make reading more difficult.

All parts of the text should be systematically organized to the same sequential order. If for example immunostaining was mentioned as the first method in the Abstract, it should be described first also in the Materials and methods, it should be reported first in the Results and, depending on, the interpretation of the staining results should be first discussed in the Discussion. This inherent coherence will in part contribute to easy reading of your text, which feels well-structured.

It might be good to first write the summary (abstract) or to improve the one which perhaps was already submitted or even published in Abstract Book of an international meeting; notice that some journals do not allow pre-publication abstracts. Writing the abstract helps to crystallize the work because of the often very low number of words (e.g. 200) or characters and spaces allowed in the abstract.

Then write the introduction: why was it important to do this work? Introduction should be written so that it is easy to understand, even for somebody who is not working in your narrow and specialized research area. Its main function is to introduce the topic but in particular to wake interest in the readers. It should not be too detailed and it should not be a new summary of the work in the introduction format. It is not not a mini-review of the subject. It is good to finish the introduction with a well formulated working hypothesis which drives the work through.

Materials and methods were already written earlier in the research plan. Their final description might require some slight changes if it perhaps during experiments was noticed that some of the circumstances had to be slight modified from the original protocol, first written down to the research plan. Materials and Methods should be written like to peers, who are at a professional level. This means that you can use exact "engineering" language and expect that the people reading this part of the article are experts and can follow the method description. This section should anyway be written in such a detail that the experiments can be reproduced by others, following the same methodology.

In the Results, describe the most important data preferably with clear figures, photos, drawings, flow charts and tables. It is often good to plan the figures first. The text and the figure legends are then easy to write. Data should not be repeated in the text, in the figure and in the figure legend. Sometimes data is in addition provided in the table. This is too much. Data should be mentioned only once. Mark your figures so that an intelligent reader does not even need to read the figure legend to basically very rapidly understand what you did and what you found.

Discussion should be for and against, pro and con. Develop first and follow then the story line. Let the story flow and progress logically rather than paining lavishly with full color palette loose and non-coherent colourful pieces of descriptive data. Figures are to attract the eyes, text of the discussion is to stimulate the brain and thinking. Do not break the story line in the middle, by jumping to some irrelevant side-track. However, do not tell all at once. It is probably possible to write the text in the same way as it was presented it in an international meeting, so that you move quite naturally from your starting point via the experiments and results to their interpretation, in a logical chain. It is good if you can make your audience to listen to you or read your paper so that they cannot stop, for example to rapidly reply to an e-mail. It helps here if you come up with something unexpected when still following you logical story line. Although it is a totally different genre, discussion of a good scientific article has some similarities with a good detective story, like Sherlock Holmes. It makes you wake up too late at night, simply because the story is too fascinating for you to stop reading. Clearly thought is clearly written. Via the research question and working hypothesis your article helps to reach a new level of understanding.

As is seen above, at this late stage, writing the draft article, the good basic work done studying literature to start with and always when planning experiments pays off. Most of your references have been probably already collected when planning and performing the work, preparing the research plan and the presentations. One can at each and every step describe what the premises (current state of the knowledge) were, what the research question was, how it was solved and how the results are interpreted. It is always good if one can point out what exactly is new in the paper submitted for publication.

Final refining

After the first draft is ready, go it through a couple of times alone. After you have finished the first draft, it is a good idea to discuss this work individually with your coworkers. You can with them, hopefully a handful at least, go through the story line. Is the thinking correct? Does the story line run smoothly? Is everything presented in different sections of the paper in the same and logic order? Is the language clear and simple? Are the figures and tables self-explanatory? Is the most relevant literature cited?

It does often take only perhaps half an hour to two hours to discuss the paper with a coworker or friend: a lot can be accomplished in a short time. At that stage it is not necessary yet to systematically check the text for writing mistakes and spelling errors using software which automatically corrects writing mistakes and checks the language and grammar for eventual mistakes. If you are not a native English speaker and have not yet had an opportunity to reach a good level of English writing, it is good if you have such a coworker.

The final test might be to ask some other scientist in another field to read the paper first once and then ask him/her to tell what was written. If the story line was running nicely, they will be able to summarize the content of the paper, otherwise they might only be able to recollect some detail of it.

第 26 章
同行评审期刊中发表学术文章的流程

Chapter 26
A Flow Chart for a Novice Researcher to Publish a Scholarly Article in a Peer-Reviewed Journal

Tian-Fang Li, Jonathan D. Holz, Hui-Wu Li

Overview

This chapter of the book will discuss our own experiences in manuscript preparation which includes more than 50 papers published in prestigious internationally-circulated, peer-reviewed journals of medical research, and more specifically, in musculoskeletal research journals. Most of this advice is derived from our own experience, but some useful skills summarized by other scientists are also cited here.

A well-written paper clearly conveys your thoughts and shares your findings with others. A successful protocol for publication implements the following steps: experimental design, experimentation, documentation, data collection and analysis, and finally publication. The major components of a manuscript include: the primary question or questions you want your research to answer, a description of the experiments done to address these questions, the most significant and novel findings arising from these experiments, the implications and impact your findings will have in your field, and the future directions your research will take based on these findings. Before designing any experiments or planning your study, you should thoroughly read the relevant background literature in your field. Also you should completely disclose all of the rationale behind your study as well as your experimental plan to your mentors, your colleagues, and your friends who are working in different fields. Their feedback will be important for you in organizing your thoughts on experimental design and methodology, as well as writing. The opinions from both experts and non-experts are important in helping you conduct well-designed experiments to cover topics of interest in your field and to ensure universal appeal and clarity, respectively. Start writing as early in the process as possible; and be aware that you will probably need to revise your manuscript a minimum of ten times. Use simple words to clearly present your findings. Remember that it is the quality of your science, not the artistic beauty of your writing, which helps you publish in a good journal. However, scientific writing is a form of storytelling: it does require that you make your story vivid and catchy. For a novice writer, it is of pivotal importance to avoid flowery language and verbosity, as they will convolute the importance of your findings and conceal your ideas from readers. Of note, a common mistake when writing your first paper is the use of unnecessary intensifiers such as fairly, greatly, very etc. These intensifiers will increase the readers' emotion, but at the same time reduce their objectivity towards your manuscript. Try not to use "there is/there are" sentences. For example, a wordy sentence "there are a group of mice that exhibit characteristic features of arthritis …" can be replaced by a simpler one "these mice exhibit characteristic features of arthritis …" Remember, clarity, conciseness and logic are the key elements of a good paper. An important step in becoming a highly skilled writer is to keep practicing. Read research papers as many as possible in the top journals of the field and try to absorb and digest the contents of the papers. During these processes, you will get a sense about how to write a paper and will get some very constructive criticisms from your peers/friends. No matter how harsh the reviewers' critiques are do not get desperate and do not take these negative comments as personal. It happens to anybody. Although it is still intimidating even for a well-established scientist with hundreds of publications, one can gain the confidence gradually through a constantly-improvement of writing skills. In all situations, try your best to avoid any scientific misconduct.

Why publish

Publishing a high-quality paper in your field's leading journals is important for many reasons. It serves as a passport to your scientific community. You claim priority in your field through publishing papers. The accomplishment of writing a manuscript demonstrates in-depth understanding of your project, and indicates that you have been working in this area for years. Additionally, the scientific merits of a discovery will naturally be attributed to the first researcher who reports it in a journal. More practically, research papers will advance your academic career and help you continue to obtain research funds to support your future studies. In most cases, promotions are dependent on the papers you published and the subsequent grants you were successfully awarded. If you don't publish, no one will know what you and your colleagues have been doing, and the assumption will be that you have done nothing. Personal communications and unpublished data will leave your research work largely unnoticed. For these reasons, it is often true that scientists without publications can no longer conduct any elegant research.

Important tips

- Carefully design experiments and identify your audience
- Read the instruction for authors carefully and follow all rules of a specific journal
- Be organized, and start writing early
- Use simple and short sentences, instead of long and difficult ones
- Use the active voice in most sections except for the Methods section
- Make your ideas flow and present your study logically
- Control your urge to edit at the beginning of manuscript preparation
- Perform multiple revisions based on the comments of both experts and non-experts
- Avoid wordiness and unnecessary intensifiers
- Use strong verbs and avoid unnecessary nominalizations
- Pay particular attention to self-plagiarism, e.g. when you are citing your own work, don't simply copy and paste.
- Never submit your manuscript simultaneously to more than one journal.

Experimental designs

The importance of a well formulated experimental design cannot be over-emphasized. Carefully designing your experiments sets the end-points necessary to confirm or reject your hypotheses, and lends credibility to your findings and conclusions. Both of which are prerequisite to successful publication in a good journal. At the outset of your project make sure that your ideas are original and innovative, by scouring previous literatures and speaking with experts. You must have deep enthusiasm for your own ideas. You should also ask around to confirm that your peers and friends are likewise excited by your new insights. A good research project should be question-driven, e.g. you need to first ask a question and propose experiments to answer that question. However the experiments you propose to answer your question must meet the following criteria: Are your proposed experiments feasible and operational? Do you and your colleagues have the necessary skills and experience to complete these experiments? Do you and your mentor have the relevant instruments and equipments in your department or university? Are your experimental approaches reproducible? Are the outcomes measureable and able to be evaluated? Are there any technical difficulties in performing the proposed experiments? Will your findings raise new questions for future studies? When designing an experiment, never forget to include the appropriate controls: they are critical in ensuring the reliability of your results and are essential for a good publication. It is common for a new researcher to become too ambitious with their designs. Remember that it is impossible to solve all problems at one time, and you must be able to get things done within a certain time-frame.

Start writing a manuscript

Search all relevant literature sources to make sure that your questions are new (innovative) and important (significant). Remember that novelty and significance are the most important factors for successful publication in a top journal. When writing, try to understand what the reviewers want in your paper. The most important step in publication is to persuade the editors, reviewers, and your future readers that your study has merits, so you want your final draft to be as good as possible. Remember that it is your science, not your English writing, which matters the most. No one can get everything right when writing a first draft of a manuscript, so simply let your ideas flow and don't be distracted by your writing skills. Control your desire to edit until writing is complete. During this time, you share your draft with your colleagues, fellow students, mentors and friends, and expect many harsh, but helpful, criticisms from them. However, don't get discouraged and never take these criticisms personally. Constructive criticisms will help you to remove many flaws prior to submission and in the end will save you a lot of time. Your first manuscript must be written and rewritten at the very least a few times. It is wise to take a break after finishing the first draft and then read it again a few days later. Revise your manuscript as soon as you receive new comments or criticisms.

Every author has his or her own habits of writing. I usually start writing the Introduction section immediately after the initiation of my experiments. By doing so, I will gain an in-depth understanding of my project. The experimental designs may need to be adjusted if different or additional experiments need to be performed. Upon completion of all the experiments, I will start organizing the figures and preparing the figure legends. The Results section will then be expanded based on the results and legends. After that, I will finish the Materials and Method section and finalize the Introduction section. The Discussion and Conclusion will be written after all these sections are written satisfactorily. It is at this time that I fully realize the novelty and significance of my project, the limitations of my experimental approaches, and the direction of future studies.

Authorship

All authors must contribute in a significant way to different aspects of manuscript preparation including concepts, ideas, designs, data analysis, results interpretation, etc. The first author listed on the publication should be the person who plays the major role in designing and performing the experiments, as well as in data collection and analysis. The first author must also be responsible for coordination of the experiments, presentation, and publication of the manuscript under the supervision of the senior author. The senior or corresponding author is usually a principal investigator on a research team, a mentor of students and postdoctoral fellows, and a recipient of research funding. This author is not necessarily involved in every detail of conducting experiments, but provides critical input on experimental design and data interpretation. The corresponding author reads the instructions from the International Committee of Medical Journal Editors. A corresponding author should also take responsibility for potential scientific misconducts.

Title

A good title should contain the fewest possible words that adequately describe the content of a paper. The title must be attractive and interesting. Potential readers usually scan hundreds of titles in their field, and may skip to other papers if the title of your paper cannot catch their eyes. Without compromising the sufficiency of experimental information, a title should be as concise and clear as possible. At the same time, it must accurately reflect the conclusions you made at the end of your manuscript. However, one must be very cautious to avoid any possible overstatements and inappropriate interpretation of the novelty of your findings. A good title will lead to increased citation of your article by attracting more readers. Number of times your paper is cited is a good indicator of your contribution to your field.

Abstract

An Abstract is a summarized version of the entire manuscript. Similar to the Title, an abstract (of about 250 words) should briefly describe your objectives, most important findings, and provide interpretation and conclusions based on your results. The vast majority of readers only spend a short time browsing a large number of abstracts in their research fields, and only a small portion of the dedicated readers with very specific interests in certain topics will finish reading the whole paper. Thus, it is critical for authors to write an appealing and convincing abstract in a concise and precise way. The Abstract should also be interesting and engaging to a broader readership.

I often start writing an abstract after finishing the other sections of the manuscript so that I have a good overview of the entire study. The Abstract should start with a brief introduction comprised of background information and the important questions that have yet to be answered. Strong rationale should be provided as to why the questions are being asked and why it is important to answer such questions. The Methods section in the Abstract will tell the readers what experiments were conducted to explore the central hypothesis. The Results section, the heart of an Abstract, demonstrates the novel and important findings. The Conclusions should summarize your results in a very accurate way and emphasize the importance of your study so that the readers may easily grasp the take-home messages. However, the Results must be interpreted with great caution to avoid overstatements. At the end of the Abstract, I often briefly describe the implications of the study and potential follow-up studies. Try to avoid writing an overly enthusiastic abstract because such an abstract will present a biased picture and can mislead general readers.

Keywords

Carefully select keywords that will help readers find your paper. In addition, the reviewers may be selected based on your keywords. I often read the entire manuscript a few times before selecting representative words that are neither too general nor too specific.

Introduction

An Introduction conveys your thoughts to your potential readers. You should immediately get to the point at the beginning of this section and tell readers that your current study will serve as a bridge between your new findings and previous findings made by other groups. In addition, you have to convince your readers that you are exploring the most important unanswered questions. The first few sentences must be appealing and straightforward to keep your readers' attention. Emphasis should be put on the specificity, novelty, and general relevance to the broader scientific community. Each paragraph of the Introduction section should contain an opening sentence that conveys its main idea and should conclude with a sentence that transitions naturally into the next paragraph. The readers will rapidly lose their patience if you keep them searching for the main idea of a paragraph. It is also important to confirm that your experimental approaches are well validated and very reasonable. The reliability of your results should be concisely discussed. To make your manuscript as interesting as possible, you should discuss only the most important predicted findings.

Materials and Methods

This section should provide succinct but detailed descriptions of the experimental approaches utilized in your study. The detailed information will help the researchers in other groups to reproduce your results. Incomplete or incorrect descriptions may invite criticisms from both editors and reviewers, potentially leading to rejection. However, previously published methods, especially those from your own group, can be omitted and referenced. It is unnecessary to comment on or discuss your approaches here, as that should be done in the Discussion section. This section is the only one in which passive voice, instead of active, is predominantly used. Critical information regarding the validation and rationales of experimental approaches should be explained clearly in this section. Detailed information should be provided about the preparation and application of the materials that were used in the study. A brief research protocol describing the measurements and calculations used in this study should also be included. It is advisable to consult statisticians to make sure your analyses are correct and appropriately represented. To make this section more clear and logical, it is preferable to use subtitles. The description of preparations, measurements, and the protocol should be organized chronologically. When your study involves human subjects or laboratory animals, you must follow the ethical guidelines listed in the most updated version of the Helsinki Declaration.

The approval from your own institute should be mentioned. However, the editor will be the most important person in judging if your experiments were carried out in an ethically acceptable manner.

Results

This section is the central part of the manuscript summarizing years of your hard-work. As in other sections, cohesion and flow are crucial for the presentation of Results. Clarity and objectiveness are also important considerations. With simple and short sentences, this section should guide the audience through the observations you made. If your findings are not consistent with your primary hypotheses; a plausible explanation of such a contradiction can be offered in the Conclusions. It is absolutely unethical to willfully distort your original data to comply with your proposed hypothesis. At the end of each paragraph, a few sentences are needed to explain the transition to the next set of experiments. I usually don't include much, if any, interpretation in the Results, just let them speak for themselves.

Discussion

This section also must be well-organized. Many revisions are needed before the Discussion can be finalized. Generally speaking, the present tense, instead of past tense, should be used in this section. Often times, an outline is needed to organize your thoughts in a logical way. Typically, A Discussion will start with a reiteration of your working hypotheses and a summarization of the supporting results. The discussion should focus on your findings and should not cover side issues without significant relevance to your research topic. However, all findings, including those without statistical significance, should be discussed and you should explain why your Conclusions are appropriate. After providing the answers to the questions raised in the Introduction, the analysis and interpretation of the major findings should be provided. This section should conclude with a few sentences focusing on the implications and potential impact of these observations. While this section must be very specific, you can expand your implications to cover broader areas. While exaggeration and overstatement of your results should be carefully avoided, it is often reasonable to make extrapolations from your data. Continuous practice will help you get a sense for the extent to which you may speculate without affecting the objectivity of your findings. A structured and well-outlined Discussion will be useful for a beginner to prevent speculations from going too far. A thorough discussion about the conflicting and unexpected observations should be provided and alternative explanations should be discussed. All limitations and weaknesses with regards to the methods and the results will be discussed with a focus on their potential effects on validity. If your research has clinical significance, explain how your findings will impact clinical outcomes, the contributions to your specific research field, and how it serves to improve the overall understanding of the mechanisms of disease. Collect all observations, both from your own and other groups, to defend your conclusions. As it is impossible to get all things done in one study, you can propose future experiments to follow up your current study. However, it is advisable that you don't propose too many experiments or experiments that are too complicated for you to accomplish. It is also likely that the editors/reviewers will ask: why did not you do these experiments in the current study?

Conclusions

Some readers approach your paper by a glancing at the Abstract at the beginning and the Conclusions at the end of the manuscript. Then, they will decide if they will read the entire paper. The Conclusions briefly summarize the whole manuscript and provide support for the validity of your studies. The function of this section is to positively affect the audience as they complete your manuscript. The Conclusions must convince your readers of the importance of your study. Bear in mind that the function of Conclusions is not to reiterate or summarize all previous sections of your manuscript; that is covered in the Abstract. While the Conclusions are also likely to touch on potential broader impacts or even mention new research topics for future study, it is not appropriate to overstate the impact of your findings.

Figures and tables

Well-organized figures are the most effective way to present research findings and the driving force behind a decent publication. Good figures should speak for themselves. Don't put too much information into any one figure. Figures containing too many panels will be too formidable for your readers and cause them to stop reading. Because of publishing costs, use color figures only when they are necessary to convey additional information. Figure legends should provide sufficient details so that your readers do not need to move back and front to the Materials/Method and Results Sections to find the rationales and contexts. However, make sure that you are not repeating the text that has been fully described in the Results section. Simplicity and clarity are equally important for Tables and Figures, avoid using long and boring Tables. Never try to manipulate or alter your pictures, the editorial board has many tools to detect manipulations.

References

Relevant references will spare you a lot of time in repeating previously-conducted laboratory work. Citing the work from other groups is a way to show your respect to them. However, your space is valuable, so only cite references wherever they are absolutely necessary. Personally, I prefer to cite original articles, instead of review articles. If possible cite the most recent findings rather than an older manuscript. However, if there are many similar papers, it is fine to cite the review papers written by scientific leaders of your fields. Cite references that directly agree or disagree with you. If you are familiar with your research field, you will notice any progress made in the field. You will also become familiar with the prominent scientists who have made significant contributions to the current understanding of the topics you are working on. Remember to cite papers from these scientists or they will feel offended. Remember they may be potential reviewers of your manuscript. You must convince the reviewers that you read and understand the work you cited or they will think that you lack expertise in your field. Try not to cite personal communications and unpublished data. Don't cite articles published in languages other than English.

Editing and polishing

You have to be fully aware that major structural changes will likely be needed for your manuscript. At the beginning phase of writing, don't waste your time on editing sentence structure and grammar. Let your ideas flow onto the page and make sure your construction is logical. When putting separate sections together you must have a bird's-eye-view of the entire paper. It is at this time you may ask yourself: are major structural changes needed? Are my ideas well-organized? You may need to rearrange sections of the manuscript and the order of the contents. Repeated editing is needed to find unnecessary words, mistakenly written phrases, or misconstructions. Trivial changes should be made and these include wording, the structure of sentences, grammar, spelling, punctuation, etc. Try to avoid there is/there are sentences.

Cover letter

It is worthwhile to spend some time writing a well-polished cover letter. A good cover letter should be as fervent and convincing as if you were applying for a job. It is your opportunity to speak directly to the editors about the important findings you made in your study and present the reasons why you chose to submit your manuscript to this specific journal. You should clearly and concisely demonstrate the importance, novelty, and potential ramifications of your study; in this phase it is important not to understate any of these qualities. If you realize a conflict of interest, you can write to the editor to exclude certain reviewers.

Waiting for the decision letter

After submission and while you are waiting for a reply, imagine that you are an editor of the journal and think about what kind of questions you would ask when you read a manuscript. You may ask whether the findings in the manuscript are novel and interesting. Are they significant or just incremental? Are conclusions correctly drawn based on the results?

It is rare that your manuscript is accepted without any questions or request for additional experiments. In most cases, the letter from the editorial board will ask you to make some revisions following the suggestions from the reviewers. These can be either minor or major revisions. If major revision is needed, you may be asked to significantly change your text or to perform a number of new experiments. A minor revision request indicates that your manuscript is close to the publishing standard set by the editorial board of this journal, but it does not guarantee an acceptance, so you still need to be careful when responding to their critiques. You may need to make small changes to your text or references and some simple but important experiments may be needed before submitting your responses to their comments.

A rejection letter from the editors is always disappointing, but don't panic. It can happen to anybody, either a young researcher or a well-established scientist. No matter how reluctant you are, you have to read the comments word by word to understand why your manuscript has been rejected. Sometimes you may feel that the critiques raised by the reviewers are not fair, or even stupid. Control your anger. Don't be anxious or emotional; don't feel this is an unfair process. Leave it alone and wait for a few days. When you next open your documents, you may already have a clear strategy about how to respond to these difficult questions. Remember that the same group of people may serve as reviewers for other journals, so never just copy and paste to the new format of a new journal. Take full advantage of this opportunity to improve the quality of your manuscript and try to address all comments that led to the rejection.

Resubmission

When submitting the revised version of your manuscript, write a letter that will win the heart of the editors and reviewers. As you have spent years on the experiments and manuscript preparation, it would be absurd to send a careless response letter, even if you think the reviewers did not understand your studies. If the editors feel that you are not very serious in addressing the issues, you are taking an unnecessary risk of being rejected. However, you must show them that you believe strongly in your research and that you really cherish the findings you made in your studies. Never show any disrespect for your own work just to make the reviewers happy. If you don't trust your results, who else will? So be respectful and confident at the same time.

第 27 章
如何构思一篇医学英文文章

Chapter 27
How to Profile an English Medical Article

Jianying Zhang

近些年,SCI 收录文章对于中国学者日趋重要,越来越多的高校和科研机构对于 SCI 收录文章的要求也逐渐提高,尤其是医学科研院校。很多高校已经将 SCI 收录文章作为博士毕业的硬性条件,因此,越来越多的医学科研工作者开始或已经将撰写英文文章作为总结自己科研工作的方式。但也有很多初次接触英文文章者,不知如何下手,如何动笔。笔者认为,在写英文文章时,构思很重要,有了构思就有了框架,就容易开始。本章就我们多年撰写和发表英文文章的经验,以我们刚刚发表的一篇英文文章为例,探讨如何构思一篇医学英文文章。

一、开始写文章之前应该做些什么?

1. 回顾所作的研究,从以下几个方面考虑:
(1)你所作的研究具有创新性和实际意义吗?
(2)你是否检索了该领域最新的研究成果?
(3)该研究的发现是否经过正确的分析方法进行了验证?
(4)实验方法是否有效和可靠?
(5)你的发现可以告诉读者一个很好的故事还是一个不完整的故事?
(6)这个研究和目前的研究热点有直接的关系吗?
(7)这个研究能否为一些研究难题提供解决方案?
如果所有的答案是"yes",那么你就可以开始着手写文章了。

以我们发表在 *Clinical Immunology* 杂志上的一篇题为"Using immunomics approach to enhance tumor-associated autoantibody detection in diagnosis of hepatocellular carcinoma(运用免疫组学手段提高肿瘤相关抗体在肝癌诊断中的价值)"的文章为例。该研究实际上并没有运用非常先进和新颖的技术,只是应用了肿瘤免疫学方面最经典的几种研究方法,例如酶联免疫吸附试验(ELISA)、蛋白免疫杂交(Western blotting)等对肝癌患者血清和对照血清的 14 种肿瘤相关抗原的抗体进行检测并分析。但是我们在构思文章时,将创新性侧重于对新概念的应用,即"免疫组学(immunomics)"。免疫组学新兴的研究热点,是研究免疫相关的全套分子、它们的作用靶分子及其功能,免疫组学包括了免疫基因组学(Immunogenomics)、免疫蛋白质组学(Immunoproteomics)和免疫信息学(Immunoinformatics)三方面的研究。经过查阅最新文献,未见类似的研究题目,而且该研究题目涉及了目前较为热门的研究领域,抓人眼球,容易被杂志编辑部的主编所接受和受到读者的青睐。

2. 仔细考虑你的目标

(1) 这是一篇什么类型的文章? 通常有以下几种:

1) Full-length methodology research(original articles):全文论著;

2) letters/rapid communications/short communications:来信 / 快讯 / 短讯;

3) case studies/case reports:病例研究 / 病例报道;

4) review papers:综述。

在其他章节已有关于这几种文章类型的详细描述和解释,此处不再赘述。

(2) 你的目标读者是谁? 这篇文章发表出来后是想让哪些读者看? 是该领域专家,或者多学科的研究人员,还是普通的读者? 针对不同的阅读对象,需要调整文章内的相关信息和写作风格。再小学科的杂志也有其不同背景的阅读人群,而且每个杂志都有自己的独特风格,在撰写文章之前要多看一些杂志的文章,了解其风格,从而确定本次的文章适合投向哪类杂志。另外还要考虑读者群,文章是面向全世界读者还是当地读者。

(3) 投哪个杂志合适? 要考虑发稿范畴(查阅相关杂志的网址和最近发表的文章)、文章类型、读者群和最近的研究热题(快速浏览最近的文章摘要)。

考虑到我们的这篇文章主要侧重于肿瘤免疫学方面的研究,因此,首先将杂志范围确定在 Immunology 方面,然后根据以往发文章的经验,将影响因子(impact factor)规定在 4 分左右,又查阅了最近几年该研究方向发表文章的杂志分布情况,将目标定在了影响因子 3.77 分的 *Clinical Immunology* 杂志。

二、怎样构思一篇英文文章?

在撰写文章之前,首先要了解文章的结构,大致分为 title page、main text(including introduction, methods, results and discussion/conclusion)、acknowledgements、references 和 supplementary materials。对于每部分的详细功能和要求在其他章节已有描述,在此不再赘述。关键问题是,在撰写文章时以什么顺序写呢? 大多数的研究人员喜欢按照上述顺序一一撰写,但我们多年来是按照另外一种特殊的顺序撰写的。以下详细介绍撰写顺序,并以我们发表的文章为例进行解释和说明。

1. **结果部分**　在结果部分,要注意尽量用图和表概括结果,但不要在文字叙述中重复图表的数据内容。

(1) 在撰写文字之前,先准备好高质量的表格和图片:图和表是一篇文章的精髓,大多数的编辑和读者在拿到一篇文章时,首先要看的就是图和表,了解这篇文章的主要研究内容以及研究结果,从而决定是否继续阅读全文。很多情况下,如果一篇文章的图表制作粗糙,表达结果不清晰,让人很难一目了然,在投稿时,首先主编的那一关就过不了,连同行评议的机会都没有了。因此,图表一定要做得清晰易懂,要让作者在不阅读全文的基础上就能明白你做了什么,结果是什么。

我们的文章在准备图表时费尽了心思。由于对 6 组个体研究对象血清,以及一组系列血清的 14 种肿瘤相关抗原(tumor associated antigens,TAAs)的抗体进行了 ELISA 检测和 Western blotting 的验证,数据繁多,结果繁杂,要想把这些结果用有限的图和表来表达清楚确实不是一件容易的事。我们首先通过 Table 1（The properties of 14 TAAs）对 14 种 TAAs 进行了简单的介绍，并附上最新的相关文献，以便读者查找和了解这些 TAAs 的情况（注：本章提及的所有图表可以参考我们已经发表的文章：Liping Dai et al. Using immunomic approach to enhance tumor-associated autoantibody detection in diagnosis of hepatocellular carcinoma. Clinical Immunology, 2014 Mar 22; 152(1-2): 127-139。Table 2（Frequency of 14 anti-TAAs in the different conditions）显示了 14 种 TAAs 抗体在六组研究对象中的表达阳性率，并通过"*（$P<0.05$）"和"*（$P<0.01$）"标识出统计学卡方检验的结果，让读者对这次研究的总体结果一目了然。Table 3（Sequential addition of antigens to the panel of 14 TAAs）显示了 14 种 TAA 抗体的结果——累加时，肝癌组（HCC）、肝硬化组（LC）、慢性肝炎组（CH）和正常对照组（NHS）的抗体阳性率。而 Table 4（Evaluation of the panel of 14 TAAs in the diagnosis of HCC）则着重展示 14 种 TAA 抗体累加时，各组合在肝癌诊断时的流行病学评价指标，说明联合检测的重要性。Table 5（Antibodies to 14 TAAs of serial sera from 16 HCC patients in different time point）是利用一批肝癌患者的系列血清（从诊断前一年左右至诊断时）在诊断前一年内的 14 种 TAA 抗体变化的情况，提示这些抗体可以用于肝癌早期诊断。最后，表 6（Sensitivity of combined use of both AFP and 14 anti-TAAs in HCC detection）显示了 14 种 TAA 抗体与甲胎蛋白（AFP）联合检测可以提高诊断价值，这是临床工作者关注的话题。

Figure 1（The range of antibody titers to different tumor associated antigens is expressed as absorbance units obtained from enzyme immunoassays）利用散点图呈现了各组 14 种 TAA 抗体的 ELISA 结果（OD 值）及平均值，与 Table 1 相辅相成，使读者对结果有了更清晰地了解。Figure 2（Some representative sera show immunoreactivity to 14 TAAs, which were verified by Western blotting）则是对上述结果的进一步的验证。Figure 3（Analysis to determine the presence or absence of co-expression of antibodies to any combination of two of the 14 TAAs）利用彩色条图显示了 14 种 TAA 抗体两两组合的阳性率在各组中的分布情况。Figure 4（The expression of autoantibodies for the representative HCC patients with serial bleeding serum samples）是两个代表性肝癌病例系列血清的 14 种 TAA 抗体 Western blotting 结果，显示了在诊断前一年左右 TAA 抗体在患者血清中已经呈现高表达，提示可作为肝癌早期诊断的生物指标。

以上的图和表不仅从广度上，也从深度上显示了 14 种 TAA 抗体在肝癌早期诊断中的作用和意义。由于在设计文章时，我们对图表的设计进行了优化，专家审稿后，几乎未对这些图表进行任何修改，直接用于发表。

（2）撰写结果文字部分。图表准备完毕后，接下来就是根据图表撰写结果文字部分。

结果第一部分，我们介绍了 14 种 TAA 抗体在肝癌及其他对照组的频率与滴度（Frequency and titers of autoantibodies in HCC against a mini-array of 14 TAAs）。该部分由 Table 1、Table 2、Figure 1 和 Figure 2 的结果组成。首先简单介绍了 Table 1 的内容，由于表中给出了参考文献，读者可以自行查阅感兴趣的相关文献，所以在结果中不再赘述。〔原文：As shown in Table 1, a panel of 14 TAAs was carefully selected and included in the present study, including ten oncoproteins such as three IMP proteins (IMP1, IMP2/p62, IMP3/Koc), CIP2A/p90, RalA, c-Myc, survivin, cyclin B1, 14-3-3 ζ, MDM2, and four tumor suppressors such as p53, CAPERα/HCC1.4, p16 and NPM1. Of these 14 TAAs, 10 TAAs were used in the previous studies except CAPERα/HCC1.4, MDM2, NPM1 and 14-3-3 ζ.〕

接下来介绍 Table 2 里提供的数据信息。首先对 Table 2 里所包含的研究对象信息做了简单描述（原文：Table 2 shows the frequency of autoantibodies to the panel of 14 TAAs. The sera examined in this study include sera from 76 patients with HCC, 30 patients with CH, 30 patients with LC and 89 normal human sera as well as controls representing non-cancer autoimmune diseases including 51 patients with SLE, and 94 with PSS. A positive result for antibody in ELISA was taken as an absorbance reading above the mean+3SD of the 89 normal human sera.）。由于表里已经详细列出每种抗体在各组中的频率数值，接下来对 14 种抗体检测结果在各组中的分布做一概括，就没必要重复表里的结果 [原文：Higher frequency of antibodies against individual TAA in HCC was found with TAAs such as survivin, CAPERα, RalA, p62, Koc, MDM2, cyclin B1, p53 and 14-3-3 ζ, compared to normal human sera（p<0.01）. In chronic hepatitis, antibody frequency to any individual TAA ranged from 0 to 6.7%, and in liver cirrhosis, it ranged from 0 to 13.3%. The reactivity of anti-TAA antibodies in normal human sera was very low, ranging from 0 to 3.4% to any individual TAA. Sera from patients with autoimmune disorders also showed very low frequency of 14 anti-TAAs with no more than 5.9% and established that antibody reactivities observed were cancer specific and not attributable to nonspecific immunoreactivity.]。

由于 Table 2 只显示了 14 种抗体在各组中的频率，我们又通过 Figure 1 显示了这些抗体在各组中滴度的差异，使读者对各组间抗体的差异有了更深入地了解。因此在这一段，我们对 Figure 1 提供的信息进行了简单描述，并说明通过 Figure 2 的 Western blotting 结果验证了 Figure 1 的结果。[The titers of 14 anti-TAA antibodies in different conditions are shown in Fig. 1. The high titer in many HCC sera and distinct difference between HCC and other conditions such as chronic hepatitis, liver cirrhosis and normal individuals were also demonstrated in this figure. Many HCC sera showed absorbance readings several-fold above the cut off（mean of 89 NHS+3SD）, indicating that antibody responses in some HCC patients were quite robust and not just mildly elevated. All of the sera with positive results in ELISA were verified by Western blotting with purified recombinant proteins. Fig. 2 shows that some representative patients with HCC produced multiple autoantibodies, whereas normal individuals rarely showed multiple autoantibodies to the 14-TAA panel.]

结果第二部分介绍 14 种抗体逐渐累加时可以增加肝癌的检出率（Stepwise increase in the rate of anti-TAA positivity with successive addition of antigens）。我们选择阳性率从高到低的顺序——累加 14 种抗体，结果肝癌的检出率从 21.1% 增加至 69.7%，明显高于肝炎、肝硬化和正常组。[原文：As shown in Table 3, antibody frequency to any individual TAA in HCC was variable from 5.3% to 21.1%. When we added the antigens to the panel starting with CAPERα-TAA which had the highest occurrence of autoantibody in HCC to successive TAAs with lower occurrence, there was a stepwise increase of positive antibody reactions up to 69.7%, which was significantly higher than the frequency of antibodies in chronic hepatitis（30.0%）, liver cirrhosis（36.7%）and normal individuals（17.0%）.]

流行病学中诊断实验的评价指标往往被用来评价一种或几种生物标志在临床诊断中的意义。本文也用到了相关知识，包括灵敏度、特异度、阳性预测值和阴性预测值等。[原文：Subsequently, we evaluated the accuracy of these 14 TAA panel as the diagnostic biomarker platform for HCC（Table 4）. The sensitivity in diagnosing HCC compared to normal individuals was from 21.1% for one TAA(CAPERα) to 69.7% when we added the TAAs stepwise to 14 TAAs, while the specificity decreased from 100% to 83%. The positive predictive value(PPV) and negative predictive value(NPV) for this 14 TAA array were 77.9% and 76.3%, respectively.]

似然比(Likelihood ratios,LR)也是评价诊断实验的指标,但文献中并不常用,考虑到本文的读者人群主要为临床和免疫学专业人员,故对似然比做了较为详细的介绍,以及其在诊断中的意义如何判断。[原文:Likelihood ratios(LR) are the preferred diagnostic measures when the prevalence of disease is higher or lower than 50%. The range of LR+is 1(neutral) to infinity(very positive). The higher the LR+for a diagnostic test, the greater the confidence we estimate a person as a true patient. The range of LR− is 0(extremely negative) to 1(neutral). The lower the LR−, the greater the confidence we judge a person who does not truly have a health problem. The LR+and LR− of 14 TAAs panel were 4.10 and 0.37, respectively, and the interpretation is that it is likely that a positive test comes from a person with HCC, and that a negative test is insufficient to rule out HCC.]

第三部分分析了 14 种抗体两两组合在几组研究对象中的阳性率(Preferential reactivity of HCC sera with certain antigens),结果发现肝癌组血清中两种抗体同时阳性的频率明显高于其他几组。[原文:Most of the normal human sera showed the absence of coexpression of antibodies to any combination of two of the 14 TAAs. Similar results were observed in chronic hepatitis and liver cirrhosis sera. There appeared to be an increase in frequency of coexpressed antibodies survivin and CAPERα in HCC(5.3%), however, which did not reach statistical significance. Nevertheless, the frequency of HCC sera coexpressing antibodies to survivin and RalA was highest(10.5%) among all the combinations and statistically significantly higher than NHS. Some other combinations of any two antibodies in HCC, such as anti-survivin with anti-Koc, anti-p53, anti-MDM2 or anti-RalA; anti-CAPERα with anti-RalA, anti-p62, anti-MDM2 or anti-1 433 ζ, anti-RalA with anti-Koc or anti-p62, also showed the statistically significant increases compared to normal sera(Fig.3).]

本文除了以上对 14 种 TAA 抗体在肝癌患者血清以及慢性肝病和正常人血清中的阳性率进行分析以外,还对 16 例肝癌患者诊断前一年内的系列血清进行了 14 种抗体的检测,结果发现多种抗体在诊断前几个月,甚至诊断前 1 年就可以检测出来。14 种抗体联合检测时,阳性率高达 87.5%。[原文:Seventy-nine serial serum samples from 16 HCC patients were also available in the current study for the detection of autoantibodies against 14 TAAs. All these patients had been previously diagnosed as liver cirrhosis or chronic hepatitis and serum samples had been collected every three months before they were diagnosed as HCC. At least two to four samples before diagnosis were available for each patient. These are very valuable serial serum samples which are likely to represent early stage of HCC patients and the presence of autoantibodies in these samples might be biomarkers for early stage of HCC. The frequency of 14 anti-TAA antibodies at the diagnostic time point ranged from 12.5%(Koc) to 50%(survivin and CAPERα), and most of these antibodies could be detected in 3 to 12 months before the diagnosis of HCC(Table 5). The interesting result was that the positive rate of autoantibodies was as high as 87.5% at the time point of one year before diagnosis when the panel of 14 TAAs was taken as the marker for detecting HCC.]

最后一部分介绍了 14 中 TAA 抗体与甲胎蛋白（AFP）联合检测在肝癌诊断中的价值（Simultaneous use of both AFP and mini-array of 14 TAAs as markers in HCC detection），结果发现 14 种抗体联合 AFP 检测肝癌的阳性率高达 79.1%，更有意义的是 14 种抗体的检测能发现 43.8% 的 AFP 阴性的肝癌患者。〔原文：In the present study, 43 to 76 HCC sera were available for studies to determine the relationship of AFP to anti-TAA responses（Table 6）. Twenty-seven of 43（62.8%）HCC sera had abnormal serum AFP level（≥100 ng/ml）. The sensitivity of AFP alone as marker in HCC detection was consistent with the previous report. Of interest was that 7 of 16（43.8%）HCC sera with normal AFP level（<100 ng/ml）were autoantibody positive to the 14 TAA array. If both 14 anti-TAAs and AFP were simultaneously used as diagnostic markers, 34（13+14+7）of 43（79.1%）HCC patients could be correctly identified. Elevated AFP and anti-TAA appear to be independent but supplementary serological markers for the diagnosis of HCC.〕

2. 讨论　讨论是一篇文章中最重要的部分，大多数被杂志编辑部拒稿的稿件就是因为讨论部分太薄弱。讨论部分应该主要描述：你的结果意味着什么？所用的方法是否可靠可信？你的发现和其他研究有什么联系？研究有什么局限性？

在撰写讨论部分时，有以下几个注意事项。

（1）要和结果部分相对应地进行讨论，但不要重复结果；

（2）要和前言部分前后呼应，不能各说各的，或前后矛盾；

（3）不要介绍一些在文章前些部分没有提到过的术语；

（4）避免一些不确切的表达方式，例如，"higher temperature" 或 "at a lower rate"，应该用量化的语言进行描述；

（5）可以在合理的解释下进行推测，但是这种推测必须建立在事实的基础上，而不是想象；

（6）将自己的结果和其他人已发表的文章进行比较，但不能回避和自己结果不一致的情况。

对于这种情况应该直视它，并且说服读者，让读者相信你的结果是对的。

本文在设计讨论部分时，也费了不少心思。由于 TAA 抗体作为血清标志物在肿瘤检测中的临床意义评价方面的文章，我们实验室已经发表了多篇文章，每篇文章在设计和撰写时都要有独特之处，才能引起编辑和读者的兴趣。本文主要侧重于新概念的应用，即 immunomics（免疫组学），因此，这篇文章讨论的亮点就是 immunomics 理念的应用。

讨论一开始，我们先介绍了目前 TAA 抗体在肿瘤诊断应用中存在的主要问题，即灵敏度低的问题，并指出这种弊端可以通过联合一系列的 TAAs array 以增加检测的灵敏度和特异度，而这种策略正是 immunomics 理念的体现。这和前言部分做到了前呼后应。（原文：Many investigators have been interested in the use of autoantibodies as serological markers for cancer immunodiagnosis, especially because of the general absence or a significantly lower frequency of these autoantibodies in normal individuals and in non-cancer conditions. The drawback for this approach is the low sensitivity when a single or individual TAA is used to determine the presence or absence of an autoimmune response in cancer. This drawback can be overcome by using a panel of carefully selected TAAs to increase the sensitivity and specificity, which deals with the concept of "cancer immunomics".）

紧接着我们介绍了 immunomics 方法中的两种策略，并指出本研究应用的是其中的

"hypothesis-driven immunomics"，并通过两个例子说明此策略目前在肿瘤 TAAs 抗体检测中研究先例和成果。[原文：In terms of "immunomics", there are two strategies based on the aims: either to discover new putative biomarkers (autoantigens and autoantibodies) called "discovery-driven immunomics" or the aim is to assess the relevance of putative markers already described as "hypothesis-driven immunomics". The latter one can potentially use two main approaches: immunotests (from classical ELISA to protein biochips) and research of autoantigens using a peptide signature. Wang et al. developed a phage-display library derived from prostate cancer tissue, and a phage protein microarray, to analyze autoantibodies in serum samples from patients with prostate cancer and controls. In this study, a 22-phage-peptide detector was constructed for prostate cancer screening, with 81.6% sensitivity and 88.2% specificity. Similar to our study, a decision tree was constructed to classify prostate cancer by a five-TAA-panel using ELISA, with 79% sensitivity and 86% specificity. The findings of Wang et al. as well as our panel of TAAs are not fully optimal with respect to sensitivity for adoption in a screening program, and could be improved by the inclusion of additional tumor antigens.]

本研究共选择了 14 种 TAAs，其中有六种是首次应用在肝癌检测的 TAA array 中。并简单介绍了这六种 TAA 的情况，其他八种 TAAs，由于在以前的研究中已有介绍，故在本文不再赘述。[原文：In the present study, a total of 14 TAAs were selected to comprise a mini-array approach to detect anti-TAA autoantibodies in 76 patients with HCC. Six of these 14 TAAs, including RalA, CIP2A/p90, CAPERα, MDM2, NPM1 and 14-3-3ζ were newly added to this TAA array, and the other eight TAAs were the same ones as used in our previous study. RalA, CIP2A/p90 and CAPERα were identified and evaluated as TAAs in previous studies. Mouse double minute 2 homolog protein（MDM2）, also known as E3 ubiquitin-protein ligase, is an important negative regulator of p53 tumor suppressor. Nucleophosmin 1（NPM1）, known as nucleolar phosphoprotein B23 or numatrin, a multifunctional nucleolar protein, has emerged as a p14ARF binding protein and regulator of p53.14-3-3 ζbelongs to the 14-3-3 family of proteinswhich mediates signal transduction by binding to phosphoserine-containing proteins and acts as a suppressor of apoptosis and has a central role in tumor genesis and progression. The results have shown that all these six TAAs can induce relatively higher antibody responses ranging from 10.5% to 21.1% in HCC than that in normal individuals.]

下面一段介绍本研究的主要结果以及临床意义。14 种 TAAs 联合检测可以使灵敏度提高至 69.7%，而且，由于有些 TAAs 在诊断前 1 年即可检测到，因此可以用于肝癌的早期诊断。另外，14 种 TAAs array 还可以作为临床中 AFP 检测的互补方法。[原文：The frequency of autoantibodies against 14 TAAs in autoimmune diseases such as SLE and PSS were as low as that in NHS, and it was significantly lower than that in HCC sera. The frequency of autoantibodies to 14 TAAs in HCC sera ranged from 5.6% to 21.1%, and the cumulative frequency was 69.7% while using a combination of the 14 TAAs. Of interest is that some of these anti-TAA autoantibodies can be detected at least one year before the diagnosis of HCC. This indicates that the panel of 14 TAAs as targets for detection of autoantibodies might be used as valuable biomarkers for the early diagnosis of HCC. In our previous study, we have investigated another group of HCC patients, and found that 7 of 8 HCC patients with autoantibodies against multiple TAAs had normal range of serum AFP levels. Six of these 8 HCC patients with anti-TAA antibodies were also confirmed to have well to moderately differentiated HCC with comparatively small nodules of HCC（<30mm）. In the present study, 43.8% of HCC sera with normal AFP level had anti-TAA autoantibodies. The results have further supported our previous hypothesis that anti-TAA antibodies may be used as supplementary serological markers for the diagnosis of HCC, especially for the AFP-negative cases.］

最后,对本研究做了总结,提出合理地选择 TAA 加入 TAAs array 可以增加肝癌的检出率,但真正要想应用于临床,还需进行临床可靠性检验。因此,全面地分析和评价不同的 TAAs 组合将有利于寻找针对不同肿瘤的特异性的 TAAs 抗体,并最终应用于临床诊断。［原文:In summary, this study further demonstrates that malignant transition in HCC can be associated with autoantibody responses to certain cellular proteins which might have some roles in tumorigenesis, and suggests that a mini-array of multiple carefully selected TAAs can enhance antibody detection for immunodiagnosis of HCC. As noted in this study, our efforts were aimed at increasing both the sensitivity and specificity of antibodies as markers in HCC detection to include antigens which might be more selectively associated with HCC and not with others. We conclude that multiple anti-TAA antibody detections improve predictive accuracy even if further work would be necessary to validate the detection of anti-TAA autoantibodies as a clinically reliable approach. A comprehensive analysis and evaluation of various combinations of selected antibody-antigen systems will be useful for the development of autoantibody profiles involving different panels or arrays of TAAs in the future, and the results could be useful for diagnosis of specific types of cancers.］

3. **材料与方法** 将文章最重要的两部分结果和讨论完成后,接下来就是材料和方法部分。这部分的要求是做到准确可靠,并具有可重复性。也就是说,读者在看了这篇文章后,可以用相同的或类似的方法重复出来。但这并不是说,就一定要把实验的每个细节面面俱到,对于已有文献报道的方法可以用参考文献的形式发表出来,作者可以参考原始文献。对于生物标志物在临床诊断中应用的文章,方法里应该介绍细致的检测试验的质控方法。另外,研究对象的临床信息尽量详细,包括性别、年龄、临床分期、病理组织类型等等。

本研究在进行 TAA 抗体在肝癌诊断中的应用评价时,由于选择的研究对象有多组,每组在研究中起到的作用不同,因此,在材料方法里利用较大篇幅对研究对象的样本进行了介绍,包括类别、数量、来源。其中包括 76 例肝癌血清,30 例慢性肝炎和 30 例肝硬化血清,89 例体检人群的正常对照血清,并对其中 76 例肝癌血清的临床资料进行了详细描述,实际上,此处也可以表格形式展现,但由于本文已有足够多的表格,因此利用文字进行描述。［原文:Sera from 76 patients with HCC, 30 patients with chronic hepatitis（CH）and 30 patients with liver cirrhosis（LC）were obtained from the serum bank of the Cancer Autoimmunity Research Laboratory at University of Texas（El Paso, Texas, USA）. Eighty-nine normal human sera（NHS）were originally obtained from the serum bank in the AutoimmuneDiseaseCenter at the Scripps Research Institute（La Jolla, CA, USA）. Of the 76 HCC patients, 71（93.4%）were histologically confirmed, 50（65.8%）were male, and 26（34.2%）were female. Mean age was 57.0 ± 11.2 years（range, 23-77 years）. Fifty-two（68.4%）patients were positive for HBV, 6（7.9%）patients for HCV, and 4（5.3%）for both HBV and HCV. Forty-eight（63.2%）had previous history for chronic hepatitis, 13（17.1%）patients had liver cirrhosis, and 9（11.8%）patients had no previous history of either chronic hepatitis or liver cirrhosis. Based on the Chinese general diagnostic guidelines for liver cancer, 23（30.3%）patients were in clinical stage I, 14（18.4%）in stage II, 24（31.6%）in stage III, 8（10.3%）in stage IV, respectively, and 5（6.7%）patients had no available data as to clinical stages. In the present study, 43 sera were available for AFP testing. The AFP test kit was provided by GenWay Biotech（San Diego, CA）. The results showed that 62.8%（27/43）sera had abnormal AFP levels（N100 ng/ml）whereas 16（37.2%）had normal levels（b100 ng/ml）. All cancer patients were diagnosed according to established criteria；their serum samples were collected at the time of initial cancer diagnosis, when the patients had not received any treatment such as hemotherapy or radiation therapy.］

本文还包括 79 份来自 16 位肝癌患者的系列血清,这些血清均来自肝癌患者诊断前一年内,每三个月采样一次,对于这些血清的检测,可以反应自身抗体在肝癌发生过程中的变化,是一组非常难得和有价值的血清。（原文：Seventy-nine serial serum samples from 16 HCC patients were from Shinshu University School of Medicine Affiliated Hospitals in Matsumoto, Japan. The serum samples included at least two to four samples obtained several months prior to clinical detection of liver malignancy. All of the patients had previous history of chronic hepatitis or liver cirrhosis.）

另外,本研究还检测了 51 例系统性红斑狼疮（systemic lupus erythematosus, SLE）患者血清和 94 例进行性系统性硬皮病（progressive systemic sclerosis, PSS）患者血清,目的是验证 14 种 TAA 抗体的肿瘤特异性。［原文：In addition, as representative of patientswith know immune reactivity to other autologous cellular antigens, sera from 51 patients with systemic lupus erythematosus（SLE）and 94 patients with progressive systemic sclerosis（PSS）were available from serum bank of the Autoimmune Disease Center（Scripps）and were evaluated with the same immunoassays for their response to the 14 TAA panel.］

接下来介绍主要的实验方法,包括 14 种 TAA 的表达纯化,以及免疫学常用的 ELISA 和 Western blotting,这些都是大家熟悉的方法,在此不再赘述。

最后,别忘了陈述该研究的研究对象知情同意和伦理学证明。这在撰写医学科技论文中,尤其是涉及患者的时候,必不可少。（原文：This study was approved by the Institutional Review Board of the University of Texas at El Paso and Collaborating Institutions, and informed consents from all human subjects were obtained for experimentation.）

4. 前言　前言部分往往在文章中起到承接的作用,并说服读者为什么你的工作将可以推进这一研究领域的进步。前言应该言简意赅,过长的前言会让读者感到不耐烦,因此切记前言不可长篇大论,更不能写成综述;尽量引用一些最新的相关文献,但不宜过多;不要忽略或回避那些和你研究结果相反的研究;一些非标准的缩略词,在这部分应该给予定义。

我们在撰写前言时,主要从以下几个方面进行陈述。

（1）你想解决的最根本的问题是什么? 本研究所关注的问题是:肝癌患者往往在诊断后 1 年内死亡,这主要归因于缺乏敏感的早期诊断方法。［原文：Hepatocellular carcinoma（HCC）is the third most common cause of cancer-related deaths worldwide. The majority of people with HCC will die within one year of diagnosis. The high fatality rate of HCC can partly be attributed to a lack of sensitive detection methods for early diagnosis.］

（2）在这个问题上,目前有一些解决的办法吗? 最好的办法是什么? 这种方法的局限性是什么? 迄今为止,AFP 是在肝癌诊断中应用最广的血清标志物,但是,特异度不够高,而且灵敏度也是和肿瘤的大小相关的。因此,AFP 在肝癌诊断中的应用并不是最优的,急需开发另外的标志物。[原文:Up to now, alpha-fetoprotein(AFP)is the most widely used serological marker used in HCC diagnosis. However, it is well documented that its specificity is not high enough, especially in the context of chronic liver diseases and cirrhosis, and its sensitivity is related very much to the size of the tumor. Therefore, the efficacy of AFP in the screening for HCC is not optimal and additional biomarkers are urgently needed.]

（3）你的研究将怎样解决这个问题？许多研究表明,人类的免疫系统可以识别癌细胞中的抗原变化,从而诱导机体产生相应的自身抗体,这些抗原叫"肿瘤相关抗原"。这些肿瘤相关抗体被称为机体发生癌变的"报告者"。利用血清学筛选实验以确定肿瘤相关抗原的分子特征,这种方法也称为"cancer immunomics（肿瘤免疫组学）"。[原文:There are many studies demonstrating that the immune system can recognize antigenic changes in cancer cells, leading to development of autoantibodies against these antigens which have been called tumor-associated antigens(TAAs). Therefore, these autoantibodies have been called "reporters" from the immune system which identify antigenic changes in cellular proteins involved in the malignant transformation process. Determining the molecular identity of targets of such autoantibodies (autoantibody signatures) would be relevant for serological screening tests for malignancies, an approach which has been called "cancer immunomics".]

我们以往的研究利用八种 TAAs 对肝癌血清进行自身抗体检测,单项指标的灵敏度都不高,但将八种抗原联合进行检测时,灵敏度增加到 59.8%。由此,我们提出利用 TAAs mini-array 进行肝癌检测的理念。但是,目前这种方法仍然需要不断地增加新的抗原来完善,这也正和"cancer immunomics"的理念契合。在该研究中,我们又精心设计了 14 种 TAAs 的 mini-array 进行肝癌的检测。（原文:In our previous study, we screened sera from 142 patients with HCC for autoantibodies using a target panel of eight selected TAAs comprising IMP1, IMP2/p62, IMP3/Koc, p53, c-Myc, cyclin B1, survivin and p16/INK4a, and demonstrated that no individual TAA was sensitive or specific enough for HCC detection. Autoantibody to any individual TAA in this panel ranged from 9.9% to 21.8%, but reached 59.8% to the panel of eight TAAs. This study demonstrated the importance of developing multiple or a mini-array of TAAs as an approach in immunodetection of cancer. It also addressed an important issue that highlights a promising way for the development of biomarkers in cancer, dealing with the concept of "cancer immunomics" and promoting a global analysis of the autoantibodies in cancer. Importantly, implementation of such an approach requires the careful selection of target TAAs since it appears likely that there might be selective TAA panels for different cancers. In the present study, we explored this hypothesis using a panel of 14 TAAs for detection of autoantibodies in HCC to determine the possibility and usefulness of such a panel of TAAs in HCC immunodiagnosis. ）

5. 摘要　当以上所有部分都完成后,才开始撰写摘要。在投稿之前一定要看清楚杂志要求的是哪种类型的摘要。主要有以下三种类型的摘要:

（1）陈述式（或描述式）摘要:列出所要讨论的题目,以便让读者决定是否要看全文,这种摘要一般用于综述文章或会议报告。

（2）信息式摘要:根据文章的结构进行总结,提出问题、所用方法、案例研究以及结论,但是不需要每部分的题目。

（3）结构式摘要：按照目的、方法、结果和结论四部分总结文章,这种模式常见于医学杂志。

一个好的摘要应该能深深地吸引住读者,让读者感兴趣,从而希望继续看到全文。一篇好的摘要应该是精确和诚实的,能够单独成立的,简洁和独特的,要尽量少用缩略词。简单地说,就是用摘要去推销你的文章。

我们在撰写摘要时,查阅了 clinical immunology 杂志的要求,摘要少于 150 字。而我们文章的内容非常丰富,这就要求我们在写摘要的时候,尽量选择最重要的结果进行阐述。考虑到文章的题目提到了 "cancer immunomics" 这个名词,我们主要选择了 14 个 TAAs mini-array 检测肝癌血清的结果,以及与 AFP 联合检测的结果。［原文:To explore the possibility of using a mini-array of multiple tumor-associated antigens（TAAs）as an approach to the diagnosis of hepatocellular carcinoma（HCC）,14 TAAs were selected to examine autoantibodies in sera from patients with chronic hepatitis,liver cirrhosis and HCC by immunoassays. Antibody frequency to any individual TAA in HCC varied from 6.6% to 21.1%. With the successive addition of TAAs to the panel of TAAs,there was a stepwise increase of positive antibody reactions. The sensitivity and specificity of 14 TAAs for immunodiagnosis of HCC was 69.7% and 83.0%,respectively. This TAA mini-array also identified 43.8% of HCC patients who had normal alpha-fetoprotein（AFP）levels in serum. In summary,this study further supports the hypothesis that a customized TAA array used for detecting anti-TAA autoantibodies can constitute a promising and powerful tool for immunodiagnosis of HCC and may be especially useful in patients with normal AFP levels. ］

以上几部分是文章的主干部分,其他的部分,例如题目、作者、致谢、参考文献等部分,在其他章节已有详细的介绍,本章仅就我们在撰写文章的过程中的一些经验进行探讨,供大家参考。

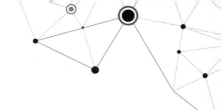

第 28 章
如何撰写科研书籍和文章

Chapter 28
How to Write Scientific Book Chapters and Articles

Jacques Corcos

During my career, I had the good fortune to edit seven books, including four textbooks. To do so, I invited more than a hundred authors to participate in these publications. In the meantime and thanks to my students, colleagues and collaborators, my name has appeared on more than 200 peer-reviewed scientific articles. The following chapter is a brief summary of lessons learned from my long-standing experience with editing book chapters and writing or reviewing scientific articles.

1 WRITING SCIENTIFIC BOOK CHAPTERS

As editor, first of all, I learned that choosing an author has to go beyond friendship and acquaintances. A good author is before anything else an expert in the field. Almost anybody can do a good literature review and summarize trends in specific domains of medicine, but much more is required for book chapters. Personal experience, allowing for critical literature review and introducing some personal data and ideas, is definitively a plus.

It is a challenge for authors to write good chapters. As experts in the field and usually having a strong opinion on the topic based on personal experience, it is essential to stay objective and balanced. There is no unanimity in anything in medicine. Even in human anatomy, an observational topic *par excellence*, opinions and descriptions differ. In physiology, huge differences of opinion are based on experimental results in animals and human beings. As soon as we reach the level of pathophysiology and disease description with symptoms and treatments, the truth and its contrary can be found in the literature. Well-balancing a review becomes a major goal for authors.

Three important items of information have to be considered by authors before designing their chapters:

- what is the place/pertinence of their chapter in the book?
- what is the table of contents and who are the other contributors?
- For whom is this book being produced?

Let's take an example to illustrate these three points: Imagine a chapter for a book on overactive bladder. Considering the topic, it is clear that a chapter on the functional anatomy of the lower urinary tract or on surgical treatments will be less relevant than a chapter on pathophysiology or pharmacological management. It doesn't mean that less attention will have to be put in writing such a chapter; it could be relatively short and more general with fewer details than if it was published, in a surgical technique book, for instance.

The position of the chapter among other chapters and who is writing the other chapters are pertinent to avoid duplications and contradictions. If an author who is cited as reference in a specific domain writes a chapter, it is probably easier to refer to him or her when writing our own chapter than to repeat or even worse to contradict him/her.

Finally, it is obviously essential to know to whom the book is being directed. The book could be a pocket book, a practical book for medical students, or a textbook for residents and established specialists. Thus, clearly the way to write, present and/or illustrate each chapter will be different. We will be more general in a book for students, trying to stay as close as possible to generally accepted ideas and managements than in a specialist textbook where, in contrast, all-important controversies have to be covered.

According to another general rule, writing a book chapter should be as didactic as possible. This means that the reader easily understands the text and that there are clear introductions, summary tables and illustrations after each sub-chapter.

A good chapter begins with an introduction explaining, in brief, why the topic is essential in this book. Authors' experience and their publications in the field can also be presented in the Introduction. Then, the plan of the entire chapter should be exposed. Each chapter or group of chapters must have its own introduction exposing the problem and its own conclusion, summarizing what has already been depicted in a visual way (tables with points, figures, algorithms, etc.). The body of each chapter must reflect the author's opinion and/or experience but obviously also review existing literature in an unbiased way. Finally, the chapter must have its own conclusion, summarizing the entire chapter and suggesting future research or work to be done in the domain.

Illustrations have to be abundant, whenever possible. More illustrations and tables reduce the number of words and usually make a chapter easier to read. When allowed, colors are also an appreciated addition to illustrations. A clear legend is mandatory with all illustrations, making sure that all abbreviations are defined/clarified.

Language is extremely relevant in writing scientific literature. Nowadays, invited authors are from all over the world, and many of them are not native English speakers. Editing by a native English-speaking individual, ideally a professional editor, is highly recommended to ensure that the text and tables are easy to read and without contradictions.

In conclusion, writing a scientific English book chapter follows relatively rigid rules that, unfortunately, most authors are not following. Too often scientific book chapters are long litanies of existing studies without interruption or summaries. It is often difficult to understand the link between these studies and determine which are more important than others.

2　WRITING SCIENTIFIC PAPERS

A scientific paper is very different from a book chapter. Most of the time, it will be an original article reporting research. Occasionally, it will be a review. There are different types of possible reviews so I won't go too much into detail with these options and will give advice on scientific papers in general.

The **Title** must be clear, concise and present a good idea of what the research is about. It may sometimes also include methodology type used (pilot, randomized, randomized controlled, etc.). Finally, it may mention type of research: clinical or basic.

The **List of Authors** has to follow the rule of "who did the research and wrote the paper". Usually, the order of authors has to be discussed by the team, with the most senior author named last. People who did not contribute directly to the publication should not be included among the authors, but their contributions, if considered relevant, should be acknowledged at the end of the manuscript.

Another irritant or controversial issue arises when the research is done by or for a pharmaceutical company. Employees of the company, at any level, should not appear among the authors because they are paid employees and have a significant conflict of interest. This issue draws many opinions and statements from different ethics committees, which are not usually followed by industry. Authors' affiliations must follow journal recommendations.

Article structure is usually the same throughout and includes six sections plus references: the Abstract is a summary of the work in a nutshell; the Introduction explains the problem that the research is aiming to solve; the Materials and Methods section shows what has been done to solve that problem; the Results explain what has been found; the Discussion places the results in the context of what is known and unknown about the problem; the Conclusion summarizes the observations made; and the Reference list is comprised of articles cited throughout the text. Most journals are using this structure, but variations are possible, depending on the type of article or journal recommendations to authors. It is always strongly suggested to have a good look at a few articles in the targeted journal and to carefully read the "Instructions to Authors" before starting to write an article.

The **Abstract** is what readers are going to read first, before eventually perusing the article. It must be clear, concise and to the point. The Abstract has to be written last, once the paper is finished, because then we have a much better idea of the pertinent elements of the article. It needs to have the same structure as the article, with five other sections: Introduction, Materials and Methods, Results, Discussion, and Conclusion.

The **Introduction** sets out the problem that the reported research tries to solve. It explains the rationale for such research in the context of existing literature (with references) and states the working hypothesis and how that research will enhance knowledge on a specific topic.

The **Materials and Methods** section is of paramount importance because it explains in extreme detail how the experiment has been conducted. The studied organism(s) (animals, plants, humans, etc.) and what has been done to them are detailed every step of the way: Where was the study conducted? When? Which equipment was deployed? (and the name the suppliers). What were product quantities? etc.

Statistical analysis has to conclude the section. It has to relate which probability was postulated to decide significance, which software was used, how the data were reported (mean, percent, etc.) and measures of variability (SD, SEM, CI, etc.). Finally, what statistical tests were used and, eventually, why (asymmetrical groups or type of randomization for example)?

The **Results** present key data in the text and illustrations. If data are displayed in a table or graph, for instance, they don't have to be repeated in the text but have to be cited to ensure better understanding of logical research flow. Statistical analysis of data presented in graphic manner can be explained in the text or in a footnote below the illustration. Each illustration must be self-understandable; meaning that reading it must be enough to understand what it shows without having to go back to the text. Table legends appear above tables, whereas figure legends go below figures.

The Discussion aims to interpret results in the context of what is already known about the topic. It has to start by referring to the study hypothesis mentioned and to the reference(s) cited in preceding sections. A concise but complete literature review is mandatory, showing how others have contributed to better knowledge of the topic. Then, describe the results and how they further advance (or not, if they are negative) knowledge of the topic. Always discuss limitations of the reported study and, if possible, explain them. Propose new steps for future studies.

The Conclusion outlines what is new and important in the reported study and at what degree the working hypothesis described in the introduction has been demonstrated.

Acknowledgements, when necessary, close out the manuscript, mentioning the name(s) of people who have helped in the study, without having been actively involved in the research: for example, a statistician, a nursing team, a pathologist, etc.

References are cited according to journal specifications in terms of number and set-up (format).

In conclusion, writing an article is a journey, often a complicated one, following rules that authors must carefully respect to avoid the disappointment of rejection related to poor presentation. This simplified guide to writing articles gives broad strokes to follow for successful submission.

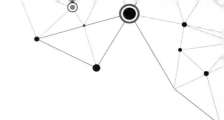

第 29 章
如何修改准备出版的手稿

Chapter 29
How to Revise Manuscripts for Publication

Tze-Woei Tan, Wayne W. Zhang

Introduction

Writing scientific article is one of the most important elements to become a successful academic physician. It is however regarded by many as difficult task, especially when the manuscript is prepared in one's non-native language. Publication is the best way to report one's ideas and outcomes, and is the cornerstone for the advancement in medical science. It is also the most important measure used for academic promotion and career advancement.

Topics on how to prepare and write a manuscript for successful publication are covered extensively in this book and elsewhere (Holmes Circ 2009, Liumbruno Blood 2013, Success in academic surgery). A good manuscript can only come from a well-designed study and appropriately collected clinical data. For submission to English journals, the manuscript ideally should be prepared in English. If the manuscript was written in Mandarin and later translated, it should be done based on idea and not word by word translation. It is always helpful to get the manuscript reviewed by native English speakers or professional translators prior to submission. It is important to choose the journal that you would like to submit and publish in. The articles need to be appealing to the readers of the particular journal. Ideally it should be done prior to writing so that the manuscript is prepared in the appropriate format and requirement. Read the "Instruction to Authors" carefully and it is usually different among journals. Try to minimize grammatical and spelling errors, and submit in appropriate format because the first impression of editors and reviewers about your manuscript are extremely important. Submission to associated journal after presentation at a national meeting can also increase the chance of getting the manuscript accepted (Kaifi JSR 2013), and is usually required especially for the plenary session.

The manuscript undergoes peer-review after submission. This chapter is going to concentrate on how to revise a manuscript after peer-review process, with the goal for resubmission and successful publication.

Peer-Review Process

This process usually takes 2 to 3 months depending on specific journal. The editorial office can return the manuscript to authors for revision if it is not submitted in the required format or does not meet specific requirements. After the manuscript is received, it is usually assigned to 2 to 4 reviewers by the editor. The assigned reviewers are usually experts with adequate knowledge of the field, and have volunteered their times to review articles for the journal. The reviewers have appropriate times to respond and decide whether to review the assigned articles. Occasionally the assignment was refused, and the manuscript reassigned to others. Some journals will ask authors to suggest reviewers and these are taken into consideration during assignment of reviewers.

The reviewers have specific time period in keeping with protocols to review the specific assignment. Suggestion to accept or reject the manuscript for publication will be provided to editorial office with associated comments. Two different categories are provided by each reviewer: one for the authors and is the same one provided in letter reply to authors; while the other one specific for editors and is blinded to authors. Decision is usually made by the editor in keeping with reviewers' comments. In the event of disagreement among reviewers, final decision is made by the editors. Four different types of decisions are made: Accept, minor revision, major revision and reject. The decision is sent back to authors in mail or email.

Decision from Journal

"Accept" and "minor revision" are the two best possible decisions for the submitted manuscript. For accepted manuscript, a proof will be sent to authors for revision and correction. The revision should be minimal at this point, and do not attempt to pursue major revision for the accepted manuscript. One important thing to check is whether authors contact information and afflictions are accurate. The returned corrected proof will be in line for journal publication. It might take up to 6 months from acceptance to publication depending on the waiting list for the journal. It is a nice gesture to send a "thank you" email or letter to the editors for reviewing and accepting the manuscript.

All of us should be happy if the decision turned out to be "minor revision". This implies that the editorial office is interested in publishing the manuscript pending minor correction. Review the reviewers' comments carefully, try to revise the manuscript and resubmit it as soon as possible. The revised manuscript is usually accepted for publication provided all the reviewers' comments are addressed appropriately.

When the manuscript is interesting but requires major improvement, the decision will be "Major revision". All the reviewers' comments will be sent to authors in the decision letter. The reviewers' comments are usually made from the readers' point of views, and the aim is to make suggestions to improve the manuscript for acceptance and publication. Do not withdraw the manuscript. The editorial office is interested in the manuscript, or else the decision will be "Reject". The manuscript should be revised appropriately and resubmitted. The ways to reply to reviewers' comments will be addressed in the next section.

The manuscript can be rejected with comments or without comment. For rejection with comments, possible statements from the editor are: "We cannot accept your manuscript in the current form. It needs to be rewritten completely for possible reconsideration"; "Members of our editorial board have reviewed your manuscript. I regret to inform you that they have decided not to accept it for publication. The reviewers' comments are attached at the bottom of this letter". This manuscript needs to undergo major revisions for resubmission to the same journal, or should be submitted to other journal altogether. A lot of reviewers' comments are relevant even for rejected manuscript and can be used for revision.

When the manuscript is rejected without comments from the reviewers, the statements used by the editor are: "We regret to inform you that your manuscript does not meet criteria for publication in our journal"; "Similar studies or cases have been reported previously. We do not think this article adds more to the existing literatures"; "Thank you for submitting your interesting manuscript, but we believe this topic is beyond the scope of our journal. In order to reach appropriate audiences, we recommend you to submit your work to other journal". The rejected manuscript should be submitted to other journals. Appeal by writing to editor politely to promote your article or request to change reviewers can be done but is rarely successful.

Responding to reviewers' comments

It is important to address every single question and comment in the reviewers' comments. Please be respectful to reviewers and reply politely as the revision is likely to be sent back to the original reviewers. Responding to reviewers should be written logically and serially. If agree with the reviewers, author's answers should be done appropriately and listed after each reviewer's comments. Corresponding changes made in the manuscript should be listed next along with page and line. If disagreed, reply politely and provide evidences. Examples for respond are listed below. Three different documents are required for resubmission: respond to reviewers' comments, manuscript with changes in red (track-change version) as well as manuscript with all accepted changes (clean version). The revised manuscript should be resubmitted within the provided time line.

Comment 1. Please clarify whether your cohorts receiving vaso-active agents included those receiving only intraoperative vasoactive agents administered by the anesthesiologist.

Respond: Thank you for pointing this out. Patients receiving only intraoperative vasoactive medications were not included in our cohorts. This was clarified in the manuscript.

"We defined clinically significant postoperative hypertension or hypotension as the need for the administration of IVMED such as phenylephrine, dopamine, nitroglycerine, or nitroprusside either as intermittent administration or continuous infusion in the postoperative period following CEA. Patients who received only intraoperative vasoactive agents were not included." was added to page 4, line 22-23, page 5 line 1-4.

Comment 2. It is of concern that 2 patients in the observation group required an amputation. This suggests either a delay in diagnosis or treatment. It is hard to postulate what circumstances would lead to an amputation. I presume that this information was not available to the authors.

Respond: Thank you for pointing this important point out. We do not have the specific information for the two patients in the observation group that required an amputation due to limitation of the dataset.

Comment 3. Without data concerning the findings on completion imaging and what procedures were done if any to remedy abnormalities found the last sentence of the conclusions on page 12 line 20-23 cannot be validated.

Respond: Thank you for the comment. We have changed our conclusion to "Our study suggests that CIM does not improve short term and one-year bypass graft patency in both autogenous and prosthetic infrainguinal LEB. Surgeon strategy of routine and selective CIM, especially in patients with end stage renal disease, LEB with autogenous conduit, popliteal artery inflow and distal target are as effective for infrainguinal LEB."

See redline manuscript conclusion (page 13, line 5-10): "Our study suggests that CIM does not improve short term and one-year bypass graft patency in both autogenous and prosthetic infrainguinal LEB. Surgeon strategy of routine and selective CIM, especially in patients with end stage renal disease, LEB with autogenous conduit, popliteal artery inflow and distal target are as effective for infrainguinal LEB".

References

1. Holmes D R, Hodgson P K, Nishimura R A, et al. Manuscript Preparation and Publication[J]. Circulation, 2009, 120 (10): 906-913.

2. Kaifi J T, Kibbe M R, LeMaire S A, et al. Scientific impact of Association for Academic Surgery and Society of University Surgeons plenary session abstracts increases in the era of the Academic Surgical Congress from 2006 to 2010. Journal of Surgical Research, 2013, 182 (1): 6-10.

3. Liumbruno G M, Velati C, Pasqualetti P, et al. How to write a scientific manuscript for publication[J]. Blood Transfusion, 2013, 11 (2): 217.

Selected readings

1. Kibbe MR. How to write and revise a manuscript for peer-review publication. In: Chen H, Kao LS, editor. Success in academic surgery, part 1. Springer-Verlag London, 2012. P. 147-166.

2. Holmes D R, Hodgson P K, Nishimura R A, et al. Manuscript Preparation and Publication[J]. Circulation, 2009, 120 (10): 906-913.

3. Provenzale J M. Revising a manuscript: ten principles to guide success for publication[J]. American Journal of Roentgenology, 2010, 195 (6): W382-W387.

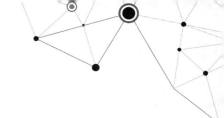

第 30 章
发表英文论文注意事项

Chapter 30
Some Important Points to Publish an English Paper

Ruixia Huang, Jahn M. Nesland, Zhenhe Suo

In this chapter, we present our experiences and suggestions on how to achieve a high quality paper to address prestigious international journals.

1 Be familiar with the addressed journals

Before you start to write your paper manuscript, it's crucial to determine which journals you aim at addressing, i.e., submit your manuscript to a proper journal since various journals have their expected topics and accept papers with different requirements. Based on our experiences, there may exist two means for determining a proper journal with respect to our manuscript. The first way is to perform a systematic review on the existing journals based on the contribution of our work, for instance, approximately estimating to which extent of contribution our work can fall into, e.g., outstanding achievements or incremental work based on the previous work. The second way is to discuss with experts around us (e.g., research scientists, postdocs and PhD) for useful advice since they usually gain sufficient experiences for specific journals if they have tried them before.

Moreover, it is always helpful to carefully read a set of published papers on the specific journals that we plan to address beforehand. The objective of such behavior is to acquire a basic knowledge about the relevant journals such as the topics that the journals are interested in and the required extent for contributions. Meanwhile, through such pre-reading, we can easily determine the feasibility of submission, i.e., whether it is worth to submit our manuscript. Another advantage of doing so is due to the long time for reviewing, which is common for most of journals. In other words, reviewing journal papers usually requires several months for the first round and further takes another several weeks or months for revising the paper (no matter major revision or minor revision) before final decision (rejection or acceptance). Therefore, it would waste plenty of time if the paper that we are working on is out of the scope of the corresponding journals or the quality is much higher or lower than the expectation of the related journals.

2 Keep the manuscript well organized

When the contribution is considered as clear (e.g., splendiferous results have already been obtained by certain conducted experiments), it is time to start to write the manuscript, which holds the contribution we have already achieved. As the first step, the structure of the manuscript should be made as clear as possible. Based on our experience, one good journal can usually be organized in the following structure, e.g., introduction, materials and methods, results, discussion and conclusion. More specifically, 1) *Introduction* should briefly introduce the underlying knowledge that is related with our study which aims at strengthening better understanding for both reviewers and future authors on the problem identification, i.e., why the problem is proposed and its difficulty to solve, i.e., what are the significant challenges? 2) *Materials and methods* refer to the detail information about the materials and the complete method or techniques we used to address the existing problems or challenges. Notice that the designed experiments should be complete and replicable in order for readers to repeat. Based on our experience, this part is always the most important section of the manuscript that should be written as explicitly as possible; 3) *Results* will mainly put the emphasis on the findings we have obtained based on the materials and methods. All the results should be presented in the order of our experiment design in a logical way. The results for the experiments can provide sufficient evidences for the research questions that are tackled. Typical figures and tables with specific information should be presented as needed; 4) *Discussion* should compare our work with most of the excellent existing works in terms of presenting the similarities and differences between them. The purpose of this part is to demonstrate the advantages of our contribution as compared with the current works in the literature. 5) *Conclusion* concludes the whole manuscript such as the problem that is dealt with, the methodology we invented or adapted and the findings extracted from the experiments. Notice that this part is usually used to emphasize the main contribution of the whole paper and additionally presents a list of future work plans.

3　Be careful with the journal requirements

In addition, it is also of paramount importance to make everything satisfy the journal's requirements, e.g. figures, tables and the form of citing references as we may have discussed in other chapters in this book.

To meet the requirements of the journal you want to submit your paper to, first of all, you need to read "Author Guidelines" carefully word by word. It is like the data sheet to a new product you want to use or the detail rules of the game you want to play. It may be called different names in some journals, e.g. "Publication Criteria" and "Manuscript Guidelines". If you do not read the data sheet carefully before you use the new product, you may destroy it. If you do not know the game rules well before you play the game, you may lose it. "Author Guidelines" can guide you whether the theme of your paper is ok for the journal, and avoid some tiny issues that may delay your publications.

You should especially pay more attention to the requirements of figures and tables. You may notice that most of the journals require the resolution, file size and some others of the figures. However, if you don't read the requirements carefully, you may neglect that some journals need you to delete alpha channels in the figure for publication, which we already experienced before, and that did delay the proceeding time of the manuscript from production part to reviewers.

Here we would like to share some experiences regarding answering reviewers' questions about some small mistakes on the manuscript preparation:

Dear ***,

Thank you for your efforts to help us format your manuscript for publication. There are just a few more issues to resolve before we can proceed:

- Funding information should not appear in the Acknowledgments section or other areas of your text, but must be entered into the online Editorial Manager in the Financial Disclosure field. Please remove this text from the manuscript and let us know if you require any changes to the Financial Disclosure that currently reads: This study was funded by grants from Inger and John Fredriksen Foundation and Radium Hospital Research Foundation and The Norwegian Cancer Society. The funders had no role in study design, data collection and analysis, decision to publish, or preparation of the manuscript.

Note: To update this information in Editorial Manager please reply to this e-mail and have PLOS staff make the change.

- Within tables, there should be no returns or tabs within the cells and no complicated merged/ split cells. Tables that do not conform to these requirements may give unintended results when published. Problems may include movement of data or loss of spacing. If you replace hard returns with a single space, the data will remain in the same cell; if you intend to start a new line, please create a new table row. For best results, please ensure your tables are in a uniform grid. For more information, please see our Guidelines for Table Preparation: http://www.plosone.org/static/figureGuidelines. action#tables.

[Please unmerge the vertically merged cells in Table 1 (columns 1, 2, 6). To start a new line, create a new table row.]

4　Deal with revised comments in a good manner

It is also of great importance to deal with the comments and answer the reviewers in a proper way. Sometimes you can save a relatively not so hopeful manuscript if you pay more attention with the writing attitude and choose proper words. Sometimes it may cause disaster if the answers are terrible. You should have your own opinion, which can be accordance or different with the reviewers. You can be confident with your own opinion, but never be too aggressive and deny the reviewers' suggestion too directly unless you have well prepared to be rejected.

4.1　When the comment is luminous

If the comment is unquestionably scientific and reasonable, or if we are advised to do some more reasonable experiments, we always agree with the reviewers and be grateful to the useful suggestion in the answer, and do the corresponding revision in the paper.

It is also very common that there is some confusion in the text especially when the authors are not from English native speaking country. It is very important to be humble and try to make the expression clearly to authors.

4.2　When you made an obviously silly mistake

Sometimes even when you have checked a number of times before you submit your manuscript, the reviewers can find some unexpected and totally silly mistakes, like inconsistent number, etc. In this case, the paper can be rejected due to this reason. If you are pretty lucky, you will be asked to explain it. Then it is very essential to explain clearly why this silly problem can happen, and don't forget to express honestly sorry about that.

Reviewer's question: Regarding the inconsistency with the numbers in the manuscript and table 1.

Our answer: We really appreciate the discovery of the mistakes. This study was performed in a manner of double-blind. The pathologists were responsible for performing and scoring the immunohistochemistry (IHC) work, and clinicians were responsible for collecting and summarizing the clinical data of the patients. And then both pathologists and clinicians provided their data to a statistician for additional statistical analyses. However, there were two cases not qualified by the pathologists, but somehow their IHC scores were still kept in the database of the clinical doctors, which created problem for the final results shown in the Table 1.

4.3　When the comment is debatable

If it is OK for you to either change it to satisfy the reviewer or not, we suggest you to show some respect to the reviewer. State your opinion respectively. And you need to try the reviewer's suggestion and show the results. Explain the difference in two different ways and tell the reviewer you and coauthors decide to choose which one. Do some corresponding change in your paper if in need.

4.4　When you don't agree with the reviewer in some point

If you don't completely agree with the reviewer in some points, it is sometimes very difficult to answer. You can state your opinion humbly but not deny the reviewer's question point-blank. For example in our experience:

Reviewer's question: The data are broken down to categories that are not always making clinical sense. For example, the age grouping is not clinically relevant: the prognosis or even physical status of the group 40-50 years of age is not necessarily different from the group 50-60 years of age. The authors can decide in broader categories i.e.<50, >=50 or <65, >=65yrs, that may add more strength in their data. Same for histology and FIGO staging, it may be more interesting I/II vs. III/IV or I/II vs. IIIA/B vs. IIIC vs IV, although admittedly the FIGO grouping is authors' preference.

Our answer: We are grateful for the comments and suggestions about these. Firstly about the age grouping, we were not certain what the best way to group age was. Therefore, we decided to divide the patients between 40 to 70 years of age by 10 year age difference, and the others were either younger than 39 or older than 70. The suggestion to divide the patients into two groups is fine for us. Therefore, we have regrouped the patients and modified the table accordingly. Concerning the FIGO stage statistical analysis, we discovered that there are only 6 cases with IIIA and IIIB, and others are IIIC. Therefore, it is not ideal to have a very small group with only IIIA and IIIB. After several times discussions within the coauthors, we decided to divide the patients into FIGO stage I+II, stage III and stage IV, based on the suggestion of the reviewer.

第 31 章
医学研究和发表论文技巧

Chapter 31
Tips for Medical Research and Publication

Wei Cheng

1 Research approach

1.1 Learn from experience

I would like to share my experience as an academic surgeon, with the new generation of doctors in China. I moved through the ranks of lecturer (University of Hong Kong), associate professor (Chinese University of Hong Kong) and chair professor (Monash University, Australia) in the last 30 years. The lessons I share come from my experience as a reviewer for journals, editorial board member of magazines, supervisor of PhD students as well as author and presenter of manuscripts.

1.2 Why publish?

First, one may ask, why do we publish? The fact is that without publication, one cannot be recognized for one's discovery. I met Donald Nuss at a meeting. He is the guy who pioneered Nuss operation. He has been practicing Nuss operation for 10 years before he presented his technique at a meeting in US. Suddenly, the whole world adopted his approach. This has change the practice of managing pectus excavatum. In reality, both in China and in the Western countries, institutions prefer academic surgeons to head a teaching hospital department. Publication does not only advance one's career, required for promotion, it actually make you a better surgeon. When we write, we, like writers, become thinkers. Those who think about his work would constantly improve his work and set a higher standard.

1.3 Ask a good question

How do we do research. The key factor, in my opinion, is to ask a good question, a question of which you don't know the answer. A while ago, some researchers noticed that mice lick their wounds and wonder why. They created some wounds of the same size over the ventral and dorsal aspects of the mice and found that the ventral wound where the mice could lick healed faster than the dorsal wounds where the mice couldn't like. The result was the Epithelial Growth Factor (EGF) in the saliva. Today, EGF is being used to facilitate wound healing in burn's patients. In a word, curiosity is the most important thing. Albert Einstein said: "imagination is more important than knowledge". In addition, "If we knew what it was we were doing, it would not be called research, would it? ".

It follows that, before we spend money and energy doing one piece of research, it is worthwhile to search in the literature and the web thoroughly to make sure that nobody has done similar study before. When I was doing my PhD in Toronto, my subject was the role of *Sonic hedgehog* gene on anorectal malformation. While studying the hindgut, I noticed that the bladder development was abnormal. This was something entirely new. I finished the major part of my PhD thesis on p63 gene, a job offer of associate professor at the Chinese University of Hong Kong came up. So I rushed back to Hong Kong. Once I started clinical work, my laboratory research slowed down. A Japanese group published what I found first, in *Development*, with impact factor of 9.6. By the time I published the same finding a year later, being the 3rd in the world, in *Urology*, the impact factor has dropped to 3.9. From this lesson, one learns two things, your work needs to be novel and you need to be the first one to publish it.

1.4　How to be creative?

How do you become innovative and creative? Of course, you don't make something out of nothing. You need to learn from others. John Hutson is a professor of pediatric urology from Melbourne. He spent 30 years researching undescended testis. Before he started, he told me, he read everything ever published on the subject, about 200 papers. Only then can you be sure that what you do will be new. Inspiration may also come from being well informed. Yves Heloury is also a professor in pediatric urology in Melbourne. Although he is a French and English is not his first tongue, he spends about half an hour each day scanning through all the pediatric surgical journals for new and interesting articles. He always knows whenever I publish a paper and sends me interesting papers now and then.

Talking to your fellow researchers are also important. At university of Toronto and Monash University research institutions, retreats were organized whereby each research student share their research work. This is very important, as these studies often use the newest techniques on the "hottest" topics. Informal exchange is also important. When I was in Great Ormond Street Hospital, the week often ended with a visit to the pubs at the corner. With a pint of beer in hand, I would ask my fellow researchers if I could "borrow" some of their antibodies etc. My original PhD research topic at University of Toronto was on *Shh* (Sonic hedgehog) gene. My supervisor Peter Kim is a pediatric surgeon. While having a group meeting with a developmental biologist working on p63 in brain development, he noticed that the p63 knock-out mice have abnormal lower trunk. I was asked to study it. It turned out to be an important discovery, showing that p63 gene is responsible for bladder development. Hence, exchange of ideas is very important. I am writing this paragraph while attending the APSA, i.e. American Pediatric Surgeon Association conference in Phoenix. Attending the meetings, in many ways, is as important as reading the journals yourself. Many research ideas come from these conferences.

To create a platform or an environment of exchange of ideas, Mr. Perutz, the head of Cavendish physics laboratory Cambridge University, in the 1950s, organized a tea room for the researchers. His wife would bring home made cakes to "lubricate" the exchange of ideas each week. In that period, the laboratory produced 5 Nobel Prize winners.

I met Dr. Tom Krummel many years ago in Hong Kong. Dr. Krummel is currently the President of American Pediatric Surgeons Association and the head of surgery at Stanford University. His has created many innovation. In the last 15 years as the leader, they have created 34 start-up companies and many new technologies. His philosophy is 1) gather people of different disciplines together, 2) see the global trends, 3) allow people to fail but learn from the failures. The reason is simple. Innovation is to "figure out what works, you have to figure out what doesn't work". That makes sense. Krummel quoted Sammuel Becket on innovation: "Ever Tried, Ever failed. No matter. Tried again, failed again. Failed better."

1.5　Practical suggestions of where to start your research

During my years working at Queen Mary Hospital, Hong Kong University, I witnessed many excellent surgeons who have gained world recognition. There were Prof. John Wong for his esophageal cancer work, Prof. William Wei for his nasopharyngeal carcinoma resections and Prof. S.T. Fan for his liver surgeries. What they had in common was that they worked on Asian diseases, i.e. esophageal, liver and nasopharyngeal carcinomas are rare in the West. By doing so, they easily became international experts. Prof. Li Long in Beijing similarly focused on choledochal cysts, an Asian congenital anomaly, which made him known throughout the world.

To be effective, one needs to assemble a multi-discipline team. You need your team of pathologists, radiologists and pediatricians to write a manuscript. In Sick Kids Hospital, Toronto, the new pediatric surgeons have additional training in epidemiology and statistics (pediatric surgeons Paul Wells did a Master of Statistics and Epidemiology in Edinburgh and Priscilla Chu did a PhD in molecular biology before joining the faculty). These are the in-house experts in research and publication. Of course, you may forge multi-centre or multi-national collaborations.

Writing a manuscript is like doing operations, start with something easier, i.e. case report, case series, retrospective study. More persuasive papers are prospective randomized trial, clinical pathological studies or combined cell biology, molecular biology, animal studies, clinical studies.

2　Publications

2.1　背景研究

请先到 PubMed 上查清楚。别人发表过的,再写就没什么意思了。至少要从另一个角度去分析您的数据。发表的唯一的价值是新。

2.2　标题

标题十分重要。因为读者是否看你的文章是基于你的题目在 PudMed 中能否吸引读者的注意力。请看以下三个标题:

（1）Operation A is better than operation B for disease X

（2）What is the best operation for disease X?

（3）Comparison of operations for disease X

标题（1）是个结论。标题（2）是个问题。标题（3）是研究的类别。基础科研的文章和北美的习惯通常喜欢用标题（1）,即让读者一目了然。其他两个标题,读者看了之后还不知其结论。读者在检索文献时,如果看到您以结论做出的标题,一定会下载这篇文章。

2.3　思路

一般的杂志通常是很公式话的要求作者遵循 IMRAD 的次序写文章, 即 Introduction（引言）,Method（方法）,Results（结果）and Discussion（讨论）。我在多伦多大学读研时,上了一堂写论文的课。

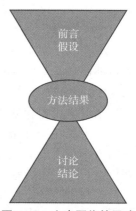

图 31-1　文章写作的思路

其中记忆最深的是这个钥匙孔形的写作方式。

2.4　引言

引言的功能从广到窄的一个过程。以下是我自己的公式,仅供大家参考。

(1)介绍所研究的疾病。这疾病对社会造成的负担,给患者带来的痛苦。言下之意,本研究之重要。

(2)文献中有什么是已知的。

(3)什么是未知的。什么是有争议性的。

(4)我们想做的研究:我们的假设。

(5)目的:例如,To test our hypothesis,we have carried out a prospective randomized trial to compare treatment A and treatment B,specifically the outcomes of mortality,and morbidities …(一句话)。

2.5　方法与结果

方法中一定要提及:①伦理委员会的批准;②家长同意书;③ inclusion and exclusion criteria;④统计学方法。

结果:最好用附标题,结果的先后次序,应显示出思想的逻辑性。譬如:①两组的年龄,性别,和病情没用分别;②治疗方面,唯一的分别是药物 A,或术式 A 等;③ A 组比 B 组的成活率高 X%。

2.6　讨论

讨论是从小到大的一个解释过程。如果您不知道如何着手,您不妨参考我的公式:

(1)总结研究的独特性。例如:本研究有史以来第一次证明了手术 A 比传统手术的优越性。

(2)文献中对您对支持。A 君也做过三例相似的手术,均成功。或在大鼠的实验中,A 手术可以降低门静脉血压。

(3)文献中的不同意见一定要一一解释。X 君的结果和我们的相反,可能是病人的年龄段和我们不同,或病情的等级也许不同,也许所用的方法有所不同。

(4)drawback:本研究的不足之处是:①这是一个回顾性的研究,需要个前瞻性的研究;②病例数量仍太少,所以不能达到统计学的意义。

(5)结论(take home message)。十组数据,十个研究,得到一个结论,这是篇好文章。一组数据,有十个结论,那是不科学的。最忌讳的是没用数据便做结论,譬如:X 病应尽早手术,但结果中没有做早期和晚期手术的对照。

2.7　摘要

摘要的文字不要重复论文中的文字。应用最精简的语句阐明研究最重要的结果。审稿人对那些和文章中一模一样的摘要会反感。

2.8　细节

争取他人的意见非常重要。所有的作者都应该参与论文的修改。

如果您在国际杂志上发表,一定要找那些英文是母语的人修饰文章。那些自称是英语好的人不算。同时也要请教统计学专家。如果英文不是您的母语,切勿用复杂的句型。最好化整为零。用一些很简单的句子。出错的机会便会减少。

一些生物的专业用语要特别小心。例如斜体字,*SHH* 是指人类基因,*Shh* 是指小鼠同源基因,*hh* 是指果蝇同源基因。正体字 SHH 是指蛋白。Shh–/– 是指小鼠基因敲除,SHH+/–

则是指人类杂合子基因突变。这些细节,审稿者会留意到。基础研究的文章最好在投稿前,最好让基础科学家看看稿子。

2.9　大忌

(1)浮夸。审稿人一眼就能看穿这浮夸的语句。

(2)懒惰。如果不用 spell check,连英文拼写,格式要求都做不到的话。审稿者不免觉得你对投稿不认真,对他不尊敬。第一关恐怕也过不了。

(3)人身攻击。你可以不同意某些作者的说法,但一定不可以攻击他。原因是在科学领域中,很难说谁错谁对。说不定你攻击的正是审稿者。那你的文章就不用发表了。

2.10　投稿

论文重写是一个学习的过程。我自己的博士论文,重写了十六次。每次修改,都有错误。如果您的文章被一本杂志退回来,不要泄气。好好总结评委的意见。修改文章。再投其他杂志。如果您解释了您的缺点,下一次成功的机会自然会高一些。

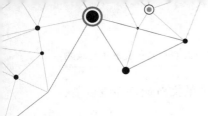

第 32 章
编辑想要的是什么

Chapter 32
What Editors Want

Alan D. L. Sihoe, Jennifer D. Y. Sihoe

1　Introduction

The ultimate goal when a clinician engages in medical writing is-in the majority of instances-to have the writing published in a peer-reviewed scientific journal. In this regard, the single most important factor determining whether or not that goal is achieved is the decision of the editor. One can have the well-written paper on the most perfectly designed study, and it can be given the most glowing comments by the reviewers, but if the editor is not completely satisfied with the submission then it will not get published.

A respectable medical journal nowadays aims to accept 20-30% of papers received, and that figure could drop even further for the more 'prestigious' journals. Journals have a lot of pressure to maintain their status, quality and of course their Impact Factor at the highest levels. They can only do this by tasking their editors to be highly selective and choose only the best papers for publication. As a journal's reputation grows, it attracts even more submissions, and it can afford to accept an even smaller percentage of submitted papers for publication. Therefore, in this environment, it becomes vitally important that clinicians not only research and write well, but also satisfy what the editors want when selecting papers for publication.

This chapter does not teach the reader how to write a scientific paper. That is well covered by the other chapters in this book. Instead, this chapter will assume the reader has already drafted a paper and is preparing to submit to a journal. This chapter will aim to share some of the authors' insights into what journal editors want (or do not want) to see in submitted papers, based on the authors' own years of experience as editors and reviewers. The authors do not make any assurances of success if these insights are heeded, but it certainly does no harm to its chances to gently adapt a paper to satisfy editors' preferences.

2　The Editor's Responsibilities

As noted above, the editor's role in whether a paper can be published is pivotal. The editor has not only the power to select reviewers, but also the power to over-rule the recommendations of reviewers. Once a decision is made, the authors of a paper also have no realistic chance of appealing against the decision. This is not a democratic process, but an essentially autocratic one.

However, as the saying goes, with great power comes great responsibility. The editor's absolute power in determining acceptance is bestowed in return for the observation of four hugely important areas of responsibilities.

2.1　To the Readers

The most commonly used yardstick to judge whether a paper should be accepted is: will this paper be of interest to readers. To make a journal (scientific or otherwise) attractive, it must have contents or articles that of interest to its readers. In turn, to be interesting to readers, an article must have: originality; good writing; reliable content; a subject of relevance to the readership; and-crucially-a message to share with the readers directly. If an article lacks these qualities, it will be boring and it will not be read. This will lead in turn to reduced readership and ultimately a failed journal. Therefore, like a commercial magazine, for a scientific journal the customer (the reader) is all-important. If the author of a paper must submit to the demands of the editor, then the editor must submit to the wants of the reader. A good editor must be in tune with what the readership of his/her journal likes. This means understanding the specialty and where the gaps in the knowledge of the specialty are, realizing what the clinical and/or research trends are within the specialty, what the balance between clinical and basic science interest is amongst readers, and what areas have been over-or under-reported in the recent literature. Before submitting to a journal, a browse through the past issues of that journal over the last 12-24 months is often a good indicator of the direction that the editor perceives the readers wish to take.

2.2　To the Journal

Besides maintaining readers' interests, the editor hopes to maintain a journal's status by carefully guarding its scientific status and reputation. Right or wrongly, this is most often measured by the journal's Impact Factor. The Impact Factor is determined by the Thomson Reuters agency, and it is simply the total number of citations received by a journal over the past year for articles it published in the *preceding* 2 years divided by the total number of "citable items" published by that journal in the same preceding 2 year period. "Citable items" are usually articles (including case reports), reviews, proceedings, or notes; not editorials or letters to the editor. A journal can raise its Impact Factor by publishing very good articles that generate many citations (increase the numerator), or by reducing the overall number of articles it publishes (reducing the denominator). The importance of the Impact Factor cannot be underestimated (even though it is a far from ideal means for judging scientific merit). Authors naturally want to publish in a 'prestigious' journal and that means one with a high Impact Factor. A high Impact Factor will therefore attract more articles, allowing the editors to select only the best-which in turn will increase citations and future Impact Factor. However, if a journal is not selective about what papers it publishes, the lower quality papers fail to interest readers, and in turn, readers uninterested by a paper will not cite it in their own writings. For the journal, the reduced citations will lead to a reduced Impact Factor, and reduced numbers of submissions in future. This is a downward spiral that editors have a great responsibility to avoid. For authors wishing to submit to a high-quality journal, the message is that they must consider how 'citable' their submission is.

2.3　To the Scientific Community

Once a paper is published in any journal, it becomes a permanent part of our collective history and knowledge in science. If someone publishes a paper that says chopping off your right arm can cure asthma, for example, then there is no way from preventing somebody somewhere from believing it to be true and harming someone when that 'message' is followed. Editors and reviewers therefore have a crucial responsibility as gate-keepers preventing mis-guided or even harmful papers from reaching the literature. To a large extent, the strict critical appraisal by the reviewers of a paper according to its scientific quality, ethical content, and potential conflicts of interest will achieve this. However, on top of this, the editor must sometimes intervene to pre-empt the emergence of damaging trends in science. One example is the emergence of a new minimally invasive surgical technique in recent years. In a rush to publish case reports and case series using this technique, one paper was submitted that saying the authors used a wound a few millimeters shorter than that reported by others. Although this paper received positive reviews, the editor rejected the paper. Besides the negligible (and dubious) difference made by a few millimeters, the rejection was made to prevent an anticipated run of copy-cat papers where authors try to publish by simply shrinking their wounds by another millimeter, and unleashing a childish game of 'one-up-manship' in the literature.

2.4 *To the Author*

The editor of a medical journal is almost always a clinician him/herself. So just as he assumes a responsibility for each patient submitting to his/her care, the editor also almost invariably assumes a personal responsibility to every author that submits a paper to his/her journal. It may sound strange to many authors, but it is absolutely true that almost all editors are by nature sympathetic to their fellow clinicians submitting papers and will do everything in his/her power to help. This includes an appreciation that authors would like a speedy decision, so editors do tend to handle submissions as quickly as possible, or as permitted by the editor's own clinical duties. Reviewers are protected by anonymity, but editors are not. And hence editors often work as arbitrators between hostile, scathing reviewers and the authors-a fact often not appreciated by authors. Even with rejections, a good editor will take time to explain the reasons why a paper was rejected, in the hope that the authors can improve their writings in the future. This is a very important task, because if the authors can improve as a result, then there is a better chance that their future writings can benefit more readers (clinicians) in future. If the rejected author feels that he/she has learned something from the submission process and has been treated with respect, then maybe he/she will resubmit future writings to this journal again. In the end, all parties can win even when there is a rejection. Authors facing rejection should bear this in mind of bearing a grudge.

3 The Editor's Workflow

The pathway followed by a paper after it is submitted to a journal has been covered elsewhere in this book. Let us now take a look at the process from the editor's point of view.

Once a paper is received by a journal, the editorial office passes it on to the editor-in-chief. In the case of a larger journal, there are a number of associate editors, each responsible for a particular sub-specialty within that journal's field. The editor-in-chief allocates the paper to the appropriate associate editor who is most knowledgeable in that field. Every journal has a large list of known experts in its field who are known to be capable of giving dependable, objective, scientifically sound appraisals of submitted papers-and the journal often retains these experts as assistant editors, Editorial board members, or reviewer team members. The editor-in-chief or associate editor chooses 2-3 reviewers from these experts (or other clinicians he/she personally knows to be knowledgeable in the field) to appraise each paper submitted. This allocation takes no more than a few days after a paper is received. In a medium-sized specialty journal, an associate editor can typically receive up to a 10-20 submissions a week. Depending on how 'good' a reviewer is, each reviewer may be called upon to review papers from 0 to around 20-30 papers a year on average.

The editorial office keeps track of how long it takes the reviewers to return their reviews. If there is no response or an excessive delay, the associate editor can request other reviewers to do the job. Return of reviews from reviewers is the usual reason for long wait for decisions on a submitted paper-and can take a number of weeks. Nowadays, journals tolerate only a limited delay before seeking alternate reviewers. This is good news for authors, but it means more work for editors in selecting reviewers.

Once the reviews are gathered, the associate editor makes a judgment based on a combination of the reviewers' recommendations and on the criteria listed below in this chapter. Editors do not blindly follow the recommendations of the reviewers, and they usually do personally read and review each paper submitted. A typical editor will do this within a few days of receiving all reviewer's reports for each paper. In addition to the decision, the editor will write to tell the authors what their appraisal found and why a decision was made, and to give comments or instructions to help the authors in addition to what the reviewers have already written. Given the number of papers received each week, an associate editor often ends up writing more words per week than contained in some of the papers received! Editors nowadays also grade the reviewers confidentially. Those who give good reviews will be highlighted for more responsibilities in future, while consistently poor reviewers will also be tagged or not used in future. This is part of the editor's responsibilities to protect authors and ensure they all receive a fair deal.

The editor-in-chief reviews the decisions of the associate editors before sending the decision letter to the authors. For papers requiring revision, it is usually the associate editor who judges whether the revisions re-submitted have adequately addressed and have made an unacceptable paper now acceptable. This is most often done without the help of the reviewers, and is actually a further piece of workload for the associate editor. Authors can improve their chances of acceptance by making thorough revisions that help the associate editor see the improvements made, rather than by making confrontational or argumentative rebuttals of the editor's and reviewers' well-intentioned comments. When the revised papers are received, the associate editor also always aims to return a decision within a few days.

The above summary of the typical editor's workflow is intended to give authors a glimpse into the workload he/she faces every week. Remember, these editors are usually full time clinicians and researchers just like the authors submitting papers to them. Editors receive no pay generally, and must spend literally hours of their own time each week to fulfill their editorial duties. Although they enjoy the job and do not complain, Editors are human after all and under this sort of workload, it is appreciated by editors if submitted papers are made 'easier' to review. A well prepared paper is always appreciated by editors and reviewers, and paying attention to the criteria below will help better preparing the paper for submission.

4　What Editors Want

Other chapters in this book already describe how to write a good paper. However, even when the same criteria for appraising a paper are used, authors and Editors may have slightly different views or place slightly different emphases on each of these criteria.

4.1　Originality

Probably the most commonly used phrase to reject papers in all of medical literature is that a paper "does not add anything new to our current knowledge". This highlights that originality is very important. Obviously, if a paper is the first in the world to describe something new, then it will always be of some educational value to the readers and to the whole world of medicine/science. But if a disease, finding, treatment or opinion has already been published before, what is the point of publishing it again? If one group has already described a certain treatment of disease X in 12 patients, and another group has described the same thing in 34 patients, then a paper describing the same thing in 4 patients is hardly likely to make any clinical impact, interest readers or generate citations. This is an easy 'reject' decision for editors to make.

But that is not to say that the treatment in the example above is never going to be publishable again. To get published, it needs to find something new to report that has not been mentioned in the previous reports of 12 patients and 34 patients. It can be a new way to deliver the technique, a new subgroup of patients it can be given to, a new indication for giving it, a new outcome discovered (good or bad), and so on. To look for this new finding, the authors must thoroughly read the previous literature on this subject and see what their own results show that previous reports have not. They must then highlight that new feature prominently in the title, the abstract, and in the main text of the paper. Preferably, it should be illustrated. The authors must not simply repeat the same kind of results and outcome measures used in the previous papers, and then slip in the new finding as simply an extra sentence at the end of the results section. If the new, original finding is not properly highlighted or 'advertised' prominently, it will be missed by the busy reviewer or editor-and the paper will get rejected.

4.2　Message

Many editors and reviewers regard this as the most important criterion of all: what does this paper have to say to readers. A paper must always deliver a clear, sound and relevant message.

Many novice authors will report that they 'treated 500 patients with disease X', and hope that their extensive experience with a nice large cohort will make their paper publishable. It will not. The reason for rejecting such papers is that they fail the "so what? " test. The editor (and readers) will read such a paper and say "so what? " because the only message is that the authors boast of their own experience. Even saying that their experience "shows this treatment can be safely and effectively done" is boring unless it truly is original (see above). Instead, in the above example the authors must use their experience with 500 patients to deliver a message about how the disease can be treated better in future. Can the authors use their experience to say something useful about patient presentation, selection for treatment, methods of treatment, outcomes of treatment, ways of measuring outcome, and so on? Instead of saying "we treated 500 patients with disease X", Editors would prefer authors that can soundly say "based on our experience with treating 500 patients with disease X, we can recommend that patients with characteristic Y should be treated with method Z". This will turn the results from a boast into a useful educational message for readers.

Part of delivering a good message concerns originality as discussed above. In addition, the message could be useful to readers even if not entirely original if it is still clinically relevant and timely. For example, do the findings in the authors' study or clinical experience provide a timely reminder of a neglected medical principle, a novel insight into an old clinical problem, needed corroborative data to confirm or refute a controversial viewpoint, and so on?

All authors should carefully re-read their own papers before submitting and ask themselves "so what? " If they find that their paper really has no message to give that will change even their own practices in future, then it is safe bet that other readers will not change theirs. If that is the case, it should be asked whether that paper is even worth submitting and publishing.

4.3 Quality of the Science

If the authors do have a message, then the editor must decide whether they have provided enough data to support the message. In other words, is the quality of the science good enough? It is no good giving the message that "a rabbit lives on the moon" if the only evidence supporting it is that "the shadow on it looks vaguely like a rabbit if you squint a bit".

The first step is to check on the hypothesis, or the clinical question that has been framed in the Introduction. What is the clinical scenario being addressed? Is it really a problem that readers recognize in daily practice? If not, is this study even worth conducting in the first place?

Once that is understood, the next step is to see if the method is designed and patients selected to answer that question. For example, a paper was once rejected because it aimed to look at the efficacy of an operation X, but the whole study ended up comparing 2 sub-groups of completely different patients who received operation X for very different reasons. Not only was the comparison invalid (non-comparable groups), but the whole comparative study design failed to answer the posed question about the efficacy of operation X itself (which would have required a control group who did not receive X). As part of the consideration of the study design, the selection of patients is also vitally important. Editors often pay close attention to see if the selection of patients are too loose (heterogeneous cohorts introducing too many confounding variables) or too tight (highly selected cohort with inherent selection bias). Authors submitting papers should provide details and justifications for how they select patients very carefully. The authors must also be careful when selecting and describing outcome measures. Ideally, outcome measures should be validated by previous studies (with references provided), and should be objective and quantifiable. For example, instead of patient self-reporting, could pain be also assessed by analgesic requirements? Outcome measures should be clearly defined. It is not acceptable to just say "large" and "small" to describe two categories of tumor, and instead ">3cm" and "<3cm" may be considered instead.

When giving results in a clinical study. The follow-up is very important. Authors need to reassure editors exactly what means were used to follow-up patients, and exactly how many patients were lost to follow-up. A certain degree of 'loss' of patients to follow-up is often expected, and claims of "100% follow-up" should be expected to be met with skepticism by reviewers. Investigations and schedule of investigations used on follow-up of patients must also be provided. Without clear accounting of these, any claims of survival or disease-free intervals by the authors will again be regarded with suspicion by editors and reviewers. In the results, editors will also be looking for adequate analysis of the data. As already mentioned earlier, it is boring to simply say "we treated 500 patients with disease X". If the authors have really treated so many patients, then why not look for trends and differences amongst the cohort? Editors will be thinking: "if I was a reader and I had 500 patients with disease X, this is what I would have liked to know". For example, if the authors had a Ferrari, it is not good enough to say they owned it. Others would want to ask: how much does it cost, how fast can it go, what is the acceleration, what is the gas consumption, and so on. Authors should anticipate what readers (who are just clinicians like themselves) would have liked to know and try to satisfy such natural curiosity by providing a thorough data analysis.

In the discussion, the editor will be looking for the authors to demonstrate an appreciation of the context of their current study and of its implications. The context means that authors need to tell readers what has already been discovered in this field, and therefore what the current study has added or changed regarding current knowledge. In other words, the authors should try to tell readers what the findings mean. In Watson and Crick's famous (and famously concise) paper on the discovery of the structure of DNA, they wrote in their Discussion: "The previously published X-ray data on deoxyribose nucleic acid are insufficient for a rigorous test of our structure. So far as we can tell, it is roughly compatible with the experimental data, but it must be regarded as unproved until it has been checked against more exact results … We were not aware of the details of the results presented there when we devised our structure, which rests mainly though not entirely on published experimental data and stereochemical arguments." This clearly demonstrates that they were aware of previous similar studies at the time, but they highlighted where their own study was different (and better). Watson and Crick then wrote: "It has not escaped our notice that the specific pairing we have postulated immediately suggests a possible copying mechanism for the genetic material." In this single remarkable sentence, they informed readers of the wider implications of their discovery-far beyond the simple elucidation of a molecular structure, and creating a revolution in the entire world of biomedicine.

Besides discussing context and implications to buttress the scientific quality of the paper, the discussion should also list the limitations of the study. No study is perfect, and reviewers always love to point out faults in someone else's research. This always leaves a bad impression on the editor who would then think: "were the authors trying to hide these faults or were they too careless to even realize? " It is always therefore better for the authors themselves identify their own faults first, acknowledge the faults in the discussion, and then discuss the possible impact those faults may have had on the paper. This will also help reassure the editor that if the paper gets published, the journal is unlikely to receive a nasty 'Letter to the Editor' from a zealous reader pointing out a very embarrassing error that was missed.

Last but not least, the conclusion sentences in both the abstract and main text are always carefully scrutinized by the editors. First of all, the conclusion *must* directly address the clinical question or hypothesis posed in the objective or Introduction. The question is the reason the study was done, so if the final conclusion does not address it, something has gone astray-and the editor will be very wary about accepting. Secondly, the editor always looks to see if the conclusion is directly supported by the results displayed. For example, if the results only show that treatment X was safely performed in a series of 20 patients, but the authors try to claim that X is better than treatment Y, then this is an automatic contra-indication to acceptance.

4.4 Quality of the Writing

The quality of the *science* is not the same as the quality of the *paper*. The authors can perform the most meticulous research yielding the most significant results, but if they cannot write a clear, readable paper to report it then that research becomes useless for readers.

It all starts with the title. The simplest and safest way to write a title for beginners is to simply say what the study was and what was found. For example, "Pre-operative Quality of Life predicts Survival Following Pulmonary Resection in Stage I Lung Cancer: an observational analysis of 131 consecutive patients" is a very good title. It is rather long, but it very clearly tells the reader: who is being studied; what parameter(s) are being studied; what kind of study this is; and the result. Editors love this because they know exactly what they are reviewing at a glance, and they know that once accepted readers will also know exactly what that paper is about. A clear title encourages readers to read the paper, and this in turn will increase the chance of citations by readers. The wrong way to write the title for the same study would be: "Survival after Lung Cancer Surgery". This tells the reader (and the editor) absolutely nothing-and in fact it is highly likely to mislead readers into thinking it is exploring many aspects of survival, when it actually only focuses on one aspect. Authors are encouraged to use detailed, descriptive titles until they have enough experience to know when to try more adventurous titles (such as provocations and questions in the title-which sometimes work, but sometimes backfire horribly).

The abstract is always said to be the most read part of the paper after the title. Editors must assume that many readers will only read the Abstract (or only have access to the Abstract online) and will not read the whole paper. The editor therefore would like the Abstract to tell readers all the pertinent details. Like the title, the Abstract needs to tell readers: what the objective of the study was; who was being studied; how was the study done; what were the findings; what do the findings mean and tell us about the objective. In particular, in terms of 'what the findings were', it is appreciated if actual numerical data are given. It is useless to say, for example, that "treatment X reduced blood loss (p<0.05) and length of stay (p<0.05)" because readers will want to know the size of the effect. Editors want to see "treatment X reduced blood loss compared to Y (300ml ± 50ml versus 480 ± 40ml, p=0.03) and length of stay compared to Y (3 ± 1.2days versus 5 ± 1.4days, p=0.01)". Abstracts are usually limited in terms of word count. It is better to provide more relevant data, and instead reduce words describing background in excessive details. One thing that must be avoided in the abstract is speculative discussion. There is no discussion section in the abstract: only a conclusion that should only be one or two sentences saying what the objective findings in the results say about the objective question. Anything more that speculates about how great treatment X is tends to be treated very harshly by reviewers and editors.

In the introduction and discussion, a very common mistake by the beginner is to spend too many words talking about basic 'textbook' information about the disease or treatment. For example, when writing to a respirology journal regarding a novel treatment of pneumothorax, it is completely pointless writing that: "Pneumothorax is air in the pleural space. It comes in primary and secondary types. Primary pneumothorax affects tall, thin, young men and has an incidence of … ." Authors should be aware that the readership of a specialty journal they are submitting to is more than fully aware of this basic, student-level information. Repeating it here is needless, insults their intelligence, and distracts from the more important messages that the authors need to convey to readers. Other common mistakes include: duplicating what is already said in the introduction by repeating the same information in the discussion; adding a separate 'Conclusion' paragraph (usually unnecessary as the information has already been said somewhere in the discussion); and use of pointless clichés (such as "this warrants further study in future").

In the results section, editors definitely do not like lots of data written in a huge paragraph in the main text. Consider this block of text:

"Surgical procedures included 22 thoracotomies: three for pneumothorax, five for empyema, five for lobectomy, four for wedge resection, four for rib resection and one for pseudoinflammatory tumor removal. We performed 69 thoracoscopies: in 46 cases for pneumothorax, in seven cases for empyema, in eight cases for palmar hyperhidrosis, in four cases for benign disease and in four cases for malignant tumor. Tracheal interventions consisted in five tracheal resection-reconstructions, six tracheotomies and four Montgomery T-tube replacements. We also performed two mediastinoscopies and two mediastinotomies."

Yes, the information is all there, but can the reader easily and quickly assimilate the data and tell what has been done to whom? Wouldn't it be much easier to digest if the authors had used tables or charts? If the reviewers and editors find it tedious to sift through results like this, then it is probably the same forthe ordinary reader. A frustrated editor not only becomes more inclined to reject, but may miss important details in the confusion and end up rejecting even if he/she wasn't irritated enough to do so initially. Authors should take every opportunity to use tables and charts to simplify and clarify their results display, and also to make the paper more physically attractive.

The above advice regarding tables and charts applies equally to figures (including drawings, photos, and increasingly videos). When describing any new device, technique or technological innovation, it is almost essential that the novel item or procedure be well illustrated. In many cases, such items can never be adequately described in words, and there is no substitute for a good photo. Some editors have occasionally made acceptance of a paper conditional on the authors providing appropriate illustration. However, there are two issues to bear in mind whenever including figures. First, it is the authors' responsibility to ensure copyright is obtained when a figure is duplicated from elsewhere. Second, sometimes excessive use of figures can backfire. In a series of 500 patients receiving surgery for liver cancer, is it really necessary to include a histology slide of hepatocellular carcinoma, or to include CT scans of the liver before and after the operation?

The reference section also deserves some attention. First, the references must be formatted exactly according to the journal's exact specifications. This is because increasingly many journals use software that automatically extracts the references into a separate section for the reviewers and editors to see, complete with a hyperlink which they can click to immediately see the reference. If the authors fail to format the reference correctly, the software fails and the editor and reviewers must manually search the Internet to find the reference. Admittedly, not all reviewers look at the references, but some do-and if the reviewer has a hard time doing so, then he/she may naturally have a more negative disposition towards the paper. The second reason that references deserve attention is that in the cases where the reviewer or editor looks up the reference, it is an unforgivable sin if they find that: the reference does not say what the authors say it said; the authors copied whole parts of the reference word-for-word in this paper; the authors' current paper is a duplicate of one of their previous papers quoted as a reference; the reference was written in a language that the authors couldn't have possibly been able to read. All of these examples have occurred before and resulted in rejection of the papers submitted.

In terms of overall writing style, many points have been covered by other chapters in this book. We will give a few tips here. First, editors tend to look for language accessible to all. That means, they prefer writings that are not too flowery and not too colloquial or full of jargon. Nobody expects 'good' English like one would find in a novel. Simple, direct English in short sentences is always the best. Second, the text must be broken into paragraphs and/or sub-sections with separate sub-headings if necessary. Look at this section beginning with "What Editors Want". Imagine if we had not broken it up with sub-headings ("1. Originality"; "2. Message"; and so on), and then if each sub-section had not been broken up into paragraphs. It would have been virtually unreadable, and the strain on the eyes would have been almost painful. It is the same with writing any paper. If the author does not provide 'resting areas' for the reader in-between paragraphs (each with one cohesive theme), then editors and reviewers will also find it hard to read-and end up missing details or rejecting out of sheer irritation.

4.5 Language

One issue that most definitely does *not* have any influence on an editor accepting or rejecting a paper is the standard of English. English is still the second language for most clinicians and scientists worldwide, and hence it provides the most convenient language platform when sharing biomedical knowledge around the world. However, most medical papers around the world in English-language journals are now being written by authors whose native language is not English. Good medical writing is coming from all over the world: Asia, Europe, Africa, Latin America. It is reassuring to know that many editors themselves often do not speak English as the first language. Journals are therefore generally very sympathetic to non-English speakers, and it is never acceptable to reject on the basis of the English alone.

However, having said all that, it is certainly the responsibility of the authors to ensure that their paper is submitted with as good a standard of English as is possible for them. This is for the simple reason that if the reviewers and editors cannot understand a paper, they cannot accept it. Many a times, an editor is forced to reject simply because it is impossible to appreciate what the authors are trying to say.

Journals are not staffed or equipped to dealing with extensive language editing. The publisher (different from the editorial office) may have a limited number of staff helping to proof-read and make minor adjustments to papers that have already been accepted by the editors. However, neither the editorial nor publishing staff have the means to edit the English of every paper that is submitted. Authors must therefore solve the problem of the English by themselves prior to submission. The language editing might be done by a friendly colleague who speaks English as the first language, somebody in the English department of the authors' university, or even by some commercial companies that specially provide such a language-editing service for a fee.

4.6 Legal, Political and Ethical Issues

In the world of academic science, one of the greatest sins is duplicate submission. Once a paper is found to have been submitted after publication (or partial publication) elsewhere, it not only results in automatic rejection but also almost certainly further serious consequences. These range from banning of future publication in the same journal to reporting of the authors to their institute or other relevant agencies-resulting effectively in the end of their academic careers. Detection of duplicate submissions is surprisingly easy. Most editorial offices and publishers have software that can easily scan the internet for similar publications by the authors. The world of medical specialties is also quite small-so there is a very good chance that the editor or reviewer for a given paper will be aware of the authors and/or their previous work. In short, it is not difficult for cheaters to be caught-and many are year after year. Readers of this chapter are strongly warned not to tempt fate by attempting duplicate submissions.

Plagiarism is another sin that is easily detected. As mentioned above, internet-based referencing tools make it very easy for editors to look for similar papers at the click of a button. Whole passages copied from another paper into the authors' current submission are often very easy to spot. Even without the use of such referencing tools, the experienced editor can easily spot when the writing style changes suddenly within a paper-a quite reliable hint that the passage just before or after the change has been written by someone else.

Authors need to fully declare conflicts of Interest. One of the easiest ways to publish a paper is to report the use of a new device, instrument, drug or technology system. However, such papers are often so biased in favor of the novelty they report that they resemble advertisements for the novelty item. Editors are very loathe to turn their beloved journal into an advertising vehicle for industry. Besides being especially strict with assessing the scientific merit of such papers (see above), Editors will be very cautious to detect potential conflict of interest, especially undeclared conflicts. It has been witnessed on many occasions that a paper has been rejected when an editor found that one or more authors had received undeclared support for the item studied, or that one or more authors were even employed by the industry making or selling the item. To reassure editors, authors should not only declare all conflicts, they should also try to avoid using trade names for the items studied. Where possible, generic pharmacological names for any drug and descriptive names for any surgical device should be used in the paper instead.

Ethical concerns are a sensitive issue for many journals and editors. Authors must pay particular attention to the stipulations of each journal's instructions to the authors regarding human trials and animal studies. All the necessary ethical committee approvals and declarations must be included in the paper before submission. If this is not done from the outset, then it looks extremely suspicious when a reviewer points out the omission and the authors subsequently write that "institutional review board approval was obtained". Editors cannot be blamed for being very skeptical in such scenarios, prompting some to find any excuse to reject rather than publish a paper with dubious ethical credentials.

Political correctness is an often ridiculed and lampooned concept. Nonetheless, it remains a serious topic in scientific literature. Racial references with any hint of a derogatory or discriminatory element are absolutely not tolerated. References to gender also must be treated with due respect and caution. In these regards, the authors must always defer to the expectations of the editor and/or the country of the journal. It is not acceptable as an excuse for the authors to say that a certain sex-related reference is acceptable in their own country, for example, if it would cause offence to the readership of the journal. A more specific example is a paper in which the authors remarked that their surgical technique would be "more suitable for young pretty women because they are more likely to be concerned about the cosmetic result". This may well be true in the authors' own country, but this remark would be regarded as deeply offensive to women and inappropriately flippant by the readership of the journal based in the USA. Needless to say, that paper was rejected.

4.7　Suitability for the Journal

Even if all the above considerations are satisfied, the editor may still reject a well-written paper on the grounds that it is inappropriate to the editor's journal. For example, a respirology journal may choose to reject a good paper on a rare disease because it focused entirely on the radiological findings rather than on the clinical presentation and therapy. A surgical journal may also reject a paper on a series of patients receiving a type of operation because it focused on the histology of the resected specimens rather than on the details of the operation. Editors of these journals may respectively advise the authors to re-submit to a radiological and a pathology journal instead.

Authors are therefore advised to consider two points. First, and most obviously, they should always carefully consider which journal they are submitting to and whether their paper is really interesting to the readership of that journal. This has been covered in other chapters in this book, but it is always worth reiterating that authors should browse through the contents of recent issues of a target journal before submitting to see if their paper is potentially relevant to its readers. Second, if the authors do want to submit to that journal, they must adapt their paper to suit that journal's readership. Using the above example of submission to a surgical journal, if the authors want to get the paper accepted, they could inject more details about the operation, provide results that show how the surgery is influenced by the histology (or vice-versa), or how specifically the findings should guide multi-disciplinary care for these patients. If the authors themselves are not surgeons, then they could consider including one of their surgeon colleagues to be a co-author and contribute the relevant sections in the paper.

4.8　Impact on the Literature

It has already been mentioned that one of the editor's responsibilities is to the scientific community as a whole. The editor acts as a gatekeeper, rejecting papers with poor scientific standards or unacceptable legal and ethical issues. The editor also spots trends that may be unhealthy to the specialty and may act to stop them (such as the example of the one-upmanship with the small surgical wounds).

But besides being a blocker of bad influences, the editor also plays a key role as the enabler of good ones. Receiving and handling so many papers week-in and week-out, it is easy for the editor to identify emerging trends in the specialty. The editor may choose to encourage development of a promising clinical direction by selecting good papers studying it for publication together in a special issue, fast-tracking the better ones, or even giving more personal advice on papers on this direction that reviewers have requested revisions of. Authors can pay attention to the directions favored by certain journals when deciding whether to submit to them. The flip-side of this coin, however, is that a journal never wants to be only associated with one topic alone. If there are too many similar papers on a certain topic, conversely a journal may wish to sometimes 'take a break' from that topic because the papers have started to become repetitive and there are fewer new findings emerging.

5　What Editors do *not* really Care about

We have already mentioned that the standard of English is not really a make-or-break issue for editors. However, there are other myths amongst authors about what an editor does or does not look for when accepting a paper. These myths should be exposed now.

5.1　*Friends and Enemies*

An editor does not automatically accept papers submitted by friends, or automatically reject papers submitted by 'enemies'. Inevitably, everybody (whether a clinician, scientist, or anyone) has friends and enemies. But editors are clinicians themselves who treat patients regardless of personal prejudices, and by their own nature as a professional it is not difficult for editors to deal with every submission in a similarly objective manner. In fact, each editor is aware that there may be extra scrutiny when handling submissions by so-called 'friends' and 'enemies', and may subconsciously work even harder to erase any doubts of bias. Authors therefore should never fear submitting to a journal because of personal friction with an editor, nor should they feel entitled to any special treatment if the editor is a 'friend'.

5.2　*Countries and Institutes*

In the same way as dealing with 'friends and enemies', editors also do not hold biases for or against authors from certain countries or institutes. Having said that, an editor may consider the authors' country or institute in two ways. First, editors tend to be wary if a paper advertises its origin from a certain country or institute too loudly. The reason is that if a study is very obviously about a population of country X, then readers will always wonder how relevant that study is to populations in other countries. Studies have shown that papers with a country name in the title tend to generate fewer citations, probably as a result of such reader skepticism. Second, editors are usually aware of rivalries between countries or between institutes within a country. The editor will therefore sometimes choose reviewers carefully to avoid rivalries potentially biasing decisions on a paper. Although an editor can feel confident that he/she will remain unbiased, it is not always possible to say the same for each of the many reviewers. Authors should therefore rest assured that a good editor will always try to look after them even when it comes to finding impartial reviewers.

5.3　Personal opinions on a topic

As mentioned above, an editor may sometimes use his/her position to help a clinical direction develop. However, the reverse is rarely the case. Just because an editor does not perform a certain procedure or agree with a certain clinical direction, that editor should not allow him/herself to block papers studying those things. Most-if not all-editors have risen through the ranks as reviewers themselves. Journals and previous editors become familiar with the personal preferences and dislikes of certain reviewers, and those with very overt, prejudiced stances tend not to rise to become senior editorial staff members. Moreover, recommendations from reviewers that say nothing except "reject-because I don't like or agree with the authors" are usually treated with indifference by a good editor, or even sometimes ignored if the paper otherwise satisfies criteria for acceptance. Once again, authors should rest assured that if their paper is rejected it will not be because of an editor's or a reviewer's personal bias but because of the paper's other failings.

6　Specific Article Types

The above have largely focused on the original article submission to a scientific journal, and these tend to be papers reporting an original research study. However, there are many other types of papers that are submitted to journals. The following considers some of these types.

6.1　Review articles

It used to be said to trainee clinicians that writing a review article was good practice at medical writing in preparation for future authoring of original articles. The truth is, review articles are neither easy to write well nor are they easy to get published nowadays. The reason is that by definition, reviews are not original and hence one of the very tenets of acceptability of a paper is gone. In this age of easy online access to information, few clinicians, scientists or patients rely on a hard copy of a review article in a journal to get a digest of the literature on a medical topic. Online reviews are plentiful and can link easily to the original articles from which the information is taken, and that in turn means review articles do not gain citations like they used to. Editors and journals are also aware, and hence acceptance of review articles is becoming rarer. The exception of course are the very large systematic reviews and meta-analyses. Certain journals also sometimes invite prominent experts in a field to give a summary review of their specialty. But for a simple review article to be submitted to a journal and be accepted nowadays, it needs to be exceptional. One way to catch an editor's attention is to not attempt a bland overview of a topic, but to zoom in on a very specific area of interest within a topic. That is, an author may wish to use a stimulating message to make up for what is lacking in terms of originality. For example, instead of a bland review on pneumothorax, one may wish to focus on the evidence for laser therapy of emphysematous blebs in patients with a first episode primary pneumothorax. A super-specialized focus may be clinically relevant yet unexplored enough that a review article specifically on it may interest editors and readers.

6.2　Case Reports

Editors generally hate case reports. End of story. Scientifically, they have nothing to offer readers. The clinical experience gained from the management of just one or two or even three patients is virtually never sufficient to generate reliable conclusions about how to manage patients or shift current paradigms. Academically, case reports are well known to be almost never cited-and hence they are a sure-fire way to lower a journal's Impact Factor. Many editors of the more established journals are known to automatically and categorically reject any case report submitted. Authors who wish to submit case reports must therefore ask themselves: does this case actually tell readers anything that is completely ground-breaking, novel and important enough that it will change how our peers manage patients? This answer is 'no' in 99% of cases, and if this is so then that case report should not even be submitted. The usual argument that the authors found a 'rare' disease is interesting only to the authors themselves. To any other reader, any case report where 'rarity' is the only feature badly fails the "so what? " test. So what if this is only the 14th case of XYZ syndrome reported in the world? Does it affect how clinicians investigate or manage patients with similar presentations? No-because nobody changes management based on so rare a syndrome. This case report might raise an eyebrow or two, but to a typical editor it has limited real-world value, and near-zero citation potential. The outlet for those who insist on having their case reports published may be some of the newfangled open access journals. However, the pros and cons of this modality of publication are beyond the scope of this chapter.

6.3　Technique papers

In surgery, it used to be thought that describing a new surgical technique would be a useful thing to publish. However, in more recent times, such articles have proven to generate fewer citations that previously thought. Editors of some journals are therefore moving away from accepting these. It may be worthwhile in some cases for authors wishing to publish a technique to accumulate enough of a patient series to publish a proper original article rather than a 'How-to-do-it' type of paper.

6.4　Other types of articles

Besides the classic types of articles already described, some journals offer other categories of articles. These can include: brief communications, new ideas, negative results, proposals for a bailout procedure, best evidence topic papers, Images of the month, and so on. If authors find that their work may not be publishable in traditional journal categories, it may be well worth exploring the many journals in existence today that offer these special article categories. A paper rejected as a classic original article elsewhere may prove interesting and educational for readers if published in these special categories. Again, authors are urged to browse through recent issues of these journals before deciding if their article is suitable for such submissions.

7　Decisions and Revisions

There are only three decisions made by the editor for the vast majority of papers submitted: acceptance, rejection or revision.

Exceedingly few papers are ever accepted outright. If this happens, it is nothing short of a minor miracle. Papers that are accepted need no further discussion here.

Much more likely is the decision of rejection outright. As mentioned already, this will happen to most papers (and nearly all case reports) submitted to any reputable peer-reviewed journal. Therefore, an author should never feel too depressed about being rejected, and he/she should certainly never take the rejection personally. Once the initial anger and sadness subsides, the author should carefully read the editor's decision letter and all the reviewers' comments. In most cases, these contain valuable hints on where the paper failed and could be improved. The author should use this rejection as a learning opportunity to understand how to improve his/her medical writing. It is not unheard of for the author to have a paper rejected by one journal but then accepted by another even more 'prestigious' journal instead. But the key in such success stories is that the author does not instantly resubmit the same paper to another journal. Instead, all the reviewer and editor's comments must be fully responded to and the revised paper is then submitted. It should be remembered that the reviewers of the second journal could well be the same as for the first journal. The world of a medical specialty is not that large, and the number of 'experts' qualified to review a certain article may form quite a small pool indeed. If a reviewer recognizes a paper he/she had previously reviewed for another journal, it is safe to assume that that reviewer will look to see if his/her previous comments had been addressed. If they have not, then that paper is virtually certain to be rejected once again.

For the paper that the editor decides needs revision, the author needs to scrutinize the editor comments very, very carefully. This is because there are often two subtypes of the 'revision' decision. One is the 'accept after revision' decision. In this, the editor has already decided privately that he/she likes the paper, but there are some issues that still need to be improved before it is of an acceptable standard for publication. The author will notice that the editor's comments are generally favorable or neutral, and that the revisions requested are relatively minor (e.g. clearer explanations of some details, improved writing style in some areas, better illustrations, etc). However, the author must never be complacent in such a situation. Disrespectful or dismissive responses to the editor's and reviewers' comments can cause offense and reversal of the editor's support for a paper. Authors should bear in mind that editors and journals are under no pressure at all to accept (and are generally under pressure to reject more papers instead), and all comments made to the authors are made with the genuine intent of helping the authors improve the paper so that the readers can get the most benefit from reading the paper. Off hand dismissal of reviewer comments can be viewed by editors ultimately as disrespect for the journal and its readers.

The other subtype of 'revision' decision is the 'reject unless reworked' decision. Here, the editor basically does not think the paper is acceptable based on all the criteria listed above. However, the editor thinks the paper is salvageable if the authors can make a very determined effort to completely revise the manuscript. In essence, the editor is giving the authors 'one last chance'. Unless the authors do a very impressive job, this paper will get rejected. With this type of decision, the author will notice much more demanding requests from the editor (e.g. demands to rewrite or add whole sections of the text; perform more or different analyses; include more patients; delete unacceptable conclusions; and so on). If the authors read the editor's comments more closely, they should even find the pivotal conditions for not rejecting. These might be flagged by the editor saying that a certain change "must" be made, or that "it is essential" that the authors do something specific. In this sort of situation, failing to respond very thoroughly and sincerely (especially to the pivotal conditions) may signal to the editor that the authors have given up on this submission, and that paper will be rejected.

How authors can respond to the comments of editors and reviewers have already been covered by other chapters in this book. However, we would nevertheless like to share a few more insights regarding what editors would like to see in responses to these comments:

Ⅰ. Do not take any comments or criticisms personally. The editor only makes criticisms because it is felt that a paper has a flaw that can be improved. If the editor dislikes a paper too much, it would have been easier to simply reject outright. The authors should remember that a 'revision' decision is always a sign that the editor is willing to help the authors improve the paper. The authors should therefore respond positively and view the editors and reviewers are blunt but friendly partners in this endeavor.

Ⅱ. Always respond by making changes to the paper, not by replying to the reviewers only. The commonest mistake by novice authors is to think that the reviewers' comments were questions asked because the reviewers themselves were ignorant and didn't know the answers. The authors therefore write personal replies to the reviewers in their 'response to the reviewers' to 'educate' the reviewers, but make no changes at all to the paper itself. This is wrong and disrespectful to the reviewers-who are usually experienced experts in the specialty in their own right and selected specifically to review this paper. The reviewers generally only made their comments or asked their questions not because they wanted to know the answers for themselves, but because they felt that readers would want to know the answers and the authors had not explained them well enough in the paper. The correct response by the authors should always be to tell themselves: "The reviewer only made this comment because we have not made ourselves clear enough in the paper, and therefore we should improve the paper so that it will not remain unclear to either the reviewers or the *readers*". The authors should make the necessary changes in the paper.

Ⅲ. Do not ignore advice to improve the English. As said above, poor English is never a reason on its own to reject a paper. However, when the editor asks the authors to improve the English it usually means that: (ⅰ) the English is so poor that the reviewers and the editor cannot fully understand what the authors want to say; and/or (ⅱ) the degree of language-editing is beyond what the publishers will be capable of coping with. If the authors do not improve the English, then the editor may simply decide (correctly) that readers cannot possibly benefit from reading this paper and reject.

8　The Bottom Line

Ultimately, a paper is accepted or rejected by an editor if he/she feels that by doing so, the editor's responsibilities to the readers, the journal, the scientific community and the authors are fulfilled. In turn, to determine this, an editor assess each submission based on the criteria listed above and assisted by the reviewers' recommendations.

For the authors, what this all translates into is this: if the authors can check and modify their paper so that all the key criteria looked for by the editor are satisfied, then that will help the editor decide that acceptance best serves his/her editorial responsibilities. If the authors help the editor get what he/she wants, then the authors may get what they want too.

References

1. Watson J D, Crick F H C. A structure for deoxyribose nucleic acid. Nature, 1953, 421 (6921): 397-398.

2. Jacques T S, Sebire N J. The impact of article titles on citation hits: an analysis of general and specialist medical journals. JRSM short reports, 2010, 1 (1): 2.

3. Cho B K, Turina M I, Karp R B, et al. Joint statement on redundant (duplicate) publication by the editors of the undersigned cardiothoracic journals. Ann ThoracSurg, 1999, 68:1.

4. Dunning J. How to complete a review for the European Journal of Cardio-Thoracic Surgery and the journal Interactive CardioVascular and Thoracic Surgery[J]. European Journal of Cardio-Thoracic Surgery, 2012, 41 (2): 242-247.

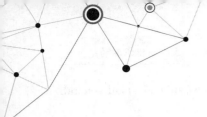

第 33 章
什么样的会议摘要容易被录用

Chapter 33
What Conference Abstract Reviewers Want

Alan D. L. Sihoe, Jennifer D. Y. Sihoe

1 Introduction

In the chapter entitled "What editors want" in this book, we explored the responsibilities of an editor of a peer-reviewed scientific journal and the considerations that the editor must undertake when assessing each paper submitted to that journal. If one understands what the editor is looking for to do his/her job and fulfill his/her responsibilities, then a submission can be tailored for a better chance of acceptance.

However, publication in a scientific journal is not the only way that good clinical works or medical researches can be presented to the world. The best established alternative-or rather adjunct-to journal publication is for the work to be presented at a scientific conference. Such conferences can range from small symposia in a single meeting room to truly massive conventions held at national exhibition centers with thousands of participants. They can range from local institutional workshops, through national and regional congresses, and up to international mega-conferences. In all of these events, the aims are the same: to share one's experiences with the professional community and also to learn from the experiences of others so that patients everywhere will ultimately benefit.

The peculiar thing is, though, that although the same clinical experiences or research study can be delivered both as a journal paper and as a conference presentation, the way that work is assessed for acceptance can be quite different. The criteria used to accept or reject an abstract submitted to a conference can be completely different to those used to assess a paper submitted to a journal. The conference abstracts reviewer will also have different considerations and responsibilities than a journal editor. Therefore, acceptance of a paper by a journal does not guarantee acceptance of the corresponding abstract for a conference, and vice-versa.

This chapter aims to share the authors' experience as abstract reviewers for a good number of medical conferences over the years. This chapter does *not* teach how to write a research abstract (that has been covered elsewhere in this book). Instead, this chapter highlights the key considerations that the abstract reviewer has when selecting abstracts to be presented at a conference. We make no promises that the points made here will ensure abstract acceptance, but delivering what the abstract reviewer is looking for can certainly do the chances of acceptance no harm. We recommend that this chapter be read in conjunction with our other chapter on "What editors want" to best appreciate the differences in the processes.

2　The Relationship between Conferences and Journals

Medical conferences are typically organized and run by professional medical societies or associations. They serve as a focal point for the exchange of clinical knowledge and academic insights between members of these societies and associations, and are hence a vital platform for the educational process in most medical specialties. In addition, they provide a nexus for the meeting of clinicians and scientists of that specialty, promoting the inter-personal networking that is absolutely indispensable in the way clinical and research medicine is advanced today. When an abstract is presented in the context of such a conference, it serves multiple purposes, including:

a. to share the presenters' own experiences and insights;

b. to stimulate interest and debate in the subject among peers;

c. to gather feedback and comments from delegates which may help the presenters' own work in future;

d. to arouse interest in possible future collaborations between presenters and delegates.

Medical and scientific journals are also usually affiliated with one or more professional medical societies or associations. Journals act not only as a medium for the dissemination of clinical and scientific knowledge, but also as a permanent repository of the collective wisdom in the specialty from around the world. Journal archives are the reference library for that specialty. The difference between a published paper and a presented abstract is that the former becomes a permanent record and has a lasting influence on the medical community, while most presented abstracts tend to soon be forgotten after the conference (unless they are then published). However, any presented abstract has the unique advantage of being dynamic and interactive as implied above. The presentation itself allows a two-way interaction between presenter and delegates, whereas a published paper is generally a one-way flow from author to reader (Letters to the editor from readers notwithstanding).

For the professional medical societies or associations associated with both the conferences and the journals, it would be desirable to take advantages of both papers for journals and abstracts for conferences. To this end, some societies request that authors presenting at their conferences must also submit the corresponding paper to the same society's affiliated journal. This is not always the case for most societies and conferences. Nonetheless, it has contributed to the false belief held by some clinicians that presentation is linked somehow to publication. It is essential to correct this misconception now: presentation of an abstract at a conference is most certainly *not* any guarantee that the corresponding paper will be published by the journal of that conference's parent society. The reasons for this are quite simple:

a. from a short abstract it is impossible to judge if the resulting paper is any good;

b. the conference abstract reviewers can be completely different people from the journal editor and reviewers;

c. the criteria for selecting abstracts are very different from those for assessing papers because the two things serve different purposes as above.

Having said that, it is still worthwhile for the paper of a presented abstract to be submitted to the journal affiliated with the conference. Even though the reviewers for the two processes can be different, the general membership of the conference's society is going to be the same as the readership of that same society's journal. If the conference delegates are interested in the abstract, then it is likely they will be interested by the paper. So it is generally still a good idea to submit to the journal of the conference-but just don't expect automatic acceptance just because the abstract got presented.

3　The Conference Abstract Reviewer's Responsibilities

The categories of the responsibilities for a conference abstract reviewer overlap with those of a journal editor or reviewer to some degree (see our chapter on "What editors want"). The difference lies in the priorities and considerations within each responsibility.

3.1　To the Delegates

The abstract reviewer wants most of all to ensure that the scientific program of the conference is interesting for delegates attending it-just as editors of a journal want to ensure that the articles published will interest readers. Only if delegates are satisfied with the program will the conference be successful, and will the delegates attend again next year. But what makes a scientific program interesting for delegates? Readers of this chapter can decide for themselves what they wish to see in a program, but in general most people will want a combination of these factors: novel topics; new techniques or technologies; good basic science research; large well-conducted clinical trials; variety of subjects; interesting clinical cases that are not often seen; and an element of surprise. The difference from reviewing for a journal is that these factors do not just call for educational value but some degree of 'entertainment' value as well. While a journal focuses on publishing articles of quality, a conference needs to keep its delegates intrigued, stimulated and awake as well as educated.

3.2　To the Society organizing the Conference

At the same time as keeping delegates interested, the abstract reviewer must also satisfy the professional society which is organizing the meeting. In most instances, the requirements of the society are the same as the desires of the delegates: good science that also regales and stimulates. However, sometimes the society expects a little more. A society usually sets a theme for a particular conference, and it almost always has a list of different sessions within the conference dedicated to particular fields of interest within the society's specialty. For example, a Thoracic Surgery society may decide that this year's theme is 'minimally invasive surgery', and it may wish to hold sessions within the meeting dedicated to lung surgery, pleural surgery, mediastinal surgery, new technologies, peri-operative oncologic management, and so on. While assessing abstracts, therefore, the reviewer must also ensure that the selection provided for presentations that will fill all these sessions and also match the conference theme. Those hoping to have their abstracts accepted may wish to adapt their submissions to fit the theme and session topics of the conference to increase their chances. It should also be noted that some sessions tend to attract more submissions than others, and hence have lower rates of acceptance. This fact can also be used when deciding the submission strategy.

3.3　To the Scientific Community

The abstract reviewer's obligation to the scientific community is that while giving delegates an interesting assortment of presentations, maintaining the quality of the abstracts must not be compromised. When a journal reviewer has an entire paper to read, it is easy (though time-consuming) to perform a good critical analysis. The conference abstract reviewer only read a short abstract, but must deduce from what little it says whether the science behind it is sound and reliable. This task is not necessarily easy to get right, but this responsibility is important. That is the quality of the selected abstracts often only becomes fully apparent when it is finally presented at the conference. If many abstracts are found to be poor, not only will the reputation of this conference and this professional society suffer and future attendances drop, but it is possible that confidence in the value of attending similar conferences will take a hit. The difference between dedicated scientists learning and sharing experiences at a professional congregation and lazy clinicians taking a holiday together at a resort can be a fine one indeed in the eyes of the lay public. Unless the integrity of the science and professionalism can be maintained at a high level, the important role of conferences in the development of modern medicine can be seriously attacked and eroded.

3.4 To the Abstract Submitter

Unlike with submissions to journals, there are only two possible decisions when submitting abstracts to conferences: accept or reject. The abstract reviewer does not usually give any feedback to the submitters, even if the decision is to reject. There is certainly no option of a 'revision' decision with which the reviewer is obliged to point out where the submission can be improved. However, despite all this, the abstract reviewer does have a responsibility to each person submitting an abstract: fairness. The reviewer and the society organizing the conference have an interest in providing equal opportunities for everyone hoping to present. The abstract reviewer will usually seek (or be advised to seek) abstracts coming from a larger range of different institutes and different countries, rather than accepting multiple abstracts from a small number of 'famous' institutes only. On an altruistic level, this ensures a greater variety of presenters and presentations-which is interesting for delegates and good for scientific exchange. On a more cynical level, attracting more presentations from different institutes ensures greater attendance at the conference. This is a convenient fact for submitters to know because it means that coming from a small institute or country is never a disadvantage when submitting to an international conference. In many cases, it can be an advantage. Indeed, some mega-conferences even hold sessions specifically for presentations by 'international' (overseas) attendees.

4 The Abstract Submission Process

The Scientific Program Committee of a conference is assembled and begins meeting for next year's conference often even before this year's conference is held. Initial meetings will establish the theme and sessions. Usually, there are few changes from year to year, with only detail modifications according to feedback from delegates of previous meetings. A panel of abstract reviewers is then drawn up, and these mostly come from experts within the society or friends of the society.

The call for abstracts goes out typically around 6-9 months before the conference. There is a deadline for abstract submission, but for smaller conferences which receive fewer submissions, the deadline is often extended to the last minute to attract more submissions. For larger, more established conferences, the deadline is very strict indeed and submissions missing the deadline by mere minutes will not be accepted.

Almost all abstract submissions nowadays are done online. The submitter selects which category or session in the meeting is the best fit for his/her abstract. This is very important because the abstracts of a particular category are automatically gathered together for review. Abstract reviewers are also invited to specify which category/session they are most qualified to assess. The conference organizers will then ensure that abstracts of each category/session are allocated to the corresponding abstract reviewers.

Abstracts usually go through at least two rounds of selections. The first round is usually done online with each abstract reviewer given access to abstracts submitted in his/her chosen category, and set a deadline by which all the allocated abstracts are to be assessed. This round is usually done within a month or two of the deadline for submission deadline. Depending on the size of the conference and the number and nature of the categories, each abstract reviewer may typically review from 10 to over 100 abstracts in the first round. Each abstract is also reviewed by at least 2 (and more often 4 or more) abstract reviewers. In this first round, abstracts are usually kept anonymous to maintain review objectivity. Because of the sheer large number of abstracts being handled (hundreds or more for larger meetings), all reviews tend to yield scores-not descriptive comments or even simple accept/reject recommendations. Very often, a standardized scoring system or form is used for all reviews. Details of a typical scoring scheme are given below. The total scores received by the abstracts are used to rank them from best to worst in each category/session.

The second round of abstract selection takes place shortly after the first round, and is not done online but at a meeting in person. Usually, not all the abstract reviewers will be invited to or attend the meeting. Instead, the second round is typically performed by the members of the Scientific Program Committee, perhaps with some invited expert reviewers as well. Second round reviewers will also divide themselves up to handle certain categories/sessions when reviewing. Taking into account the responsibilities and considerations already described above, the reviewers will decide if each abstract should be accepted or not. In the interests of fulfilling the abstract reviewer responsibilities (e.g. maintaining variety, ensuring a diversity of presenters, and so on), abstracts are usually *not* kept anonymous in the second round. However, the objective scores obtained for anonymized abstracts from the first round are used to line up the abstracts in each category, and reviewing starts from the abstract with the best score, moving down the list towards the worst. When enough abstracts are selected for a session, there is no need to continue down to the end of the list. It can be seen that in such a reviewing process, the basis of selection is an objective scoring system, but an element of subjectivity is used in the final selection to allow for fine-tuning and balancing the program.

The very best abstracts may be shortlisted for prizes awarded by the conference, and presentation of these top abstracts may be set at special sessions within the meeting. The next best abstracts tend to be allocated for oral presentation. The best of the remaining abstracts are then allocated for poster presentation-with the final number accepted dependent on the available poster display area. Once all this is done, submitters will be notified of the final decision of acceptance or rejection. This takes place therefore around 3-6 months before the meeting. After the authors of the accepted abstracts confirm that they will attend the conference, the conference organizers will then prepare the final program.

It should be remembered that conferences want to accept as many abstracts as possible to ensure variety and also to attract more attendance. A presenter is automatically also a delegate at the meeting, after all. This more or less is in contrast to scientific journals-where the preference is to accept as few papers as possible to maintain quality and a high Impact Factor. Nonetheless, for most meetings, less than half of all abstracts end up accepted owing to a combination of maintaining high scientific standards and limited sessions for oral presentation and display space for posters. There is no need to feel too dejected if one's abstract is rejected because one will always be in good company.

The above process describes the workflow through a typical international medical conference, and is described for reference only. Obviously, great variations exist between conferences. Some meetings, for example, have abstract reviewers rotate between abstracts laid out all around a room or hall, with the abstract reviewer writing down scores for each abstract he/she arrives at. Nevertheless, regardless of the detail differences between conferences, the basic principles of multiple selections rounds, anonymized scoring by abstract reviewers, and Scientific Committee final selection are common to most major international medical conferences.

5　How are Abstracts scored?

For obvious reasons, we cannot divulge details of the actual marking scheme used by any conference. However, the key elements of any marking scheme are quite self-evident and hardly secret. These are some of the things that abstract reviewers may typically be asked to score.

5.1　Originality

Delegates don't want to hear about similar studies on the same topics at conferences year after year. Originality is vital to stimulate interest and discussion. Even if the same topic is discussed, submitters should try to find a novel approach or insight to the clinical problem that may stimulate abstract reviewers and delegates. For example, nobody wants to hear another case series about laparoscopic colectomy, but what about a new outcome measure or a new indication for this surgery that has never been reported before?

5.2　Impact

A very well written abstract about a very well conducted study will not get accepted unless it has some impact on common clinical practice. It is hard to get excited about therapy X if it only works on left-handed, albino, vegans between the ages of 13 to 16 years. Abstract marking schemes for medical conferences tend to place much emphasis on clinical applicability of the knowledge shared in the abstract. To a large degree, the impact of a research abstract also depends on what the actual results found were. For example, the largest study conducted with the most flawless methodology regarding treatment X will have little impact if the results show it only improves survival by a few days in 2% of treated patients.

5.3　Study Quality

This is perhaps the single element of the marking scheme on which the most points are gained or lost. The quality of a study is judged based on a combination of study design, rigorousness of the methodology, and thoroughness of the data analysis. In terms of study design, the order in terms of increasing number of points scored would be: case report; case series (non-comparative);

comparative study; randomized trial. Extra points may be scored for evidence of good methodology, such as: large sample size; risk-adjustments; blinded studies; and so on. Demonstration of good analysis of the measured data also scores points, including: sample size estimations; meticulous statistical analyses; thorough consideration of all possible correlations between study variables; and so on. If the submitter has done all of these in the study, it is very important that these elements are specifically mentioned in the abstract's methods section, or even in the Title.

5.4　Conclusion

A reasonable conclusion must be drawn. This is the message that the submitters wish to convey to the delegates at the meeting. To gain points, this conclusion must: (i) correspond exactly with the objective and/or title of the abstract; (ii) be directly supported by the data presented in the results of this study; and (iii) avoid speculation.

5.5　Intangibles

Most marking schemes recognize that scoring according to a checklist of features that the abstract may or may not have is not ideal. An abstract that contains all the above features may gain a lot of points, but could still be a dull, unstimulating presentation at the meeting-while a low-scoring abstract could actually provide a very thought-provoking and exciting presentation. Therefore, marking schemes often allow abstract reviewers some extra marks that they are free to give or withhold based on subjective impressions or features not covered by the other scoring elements. These can, for example, be points given for: good writing; how 'fashionable' a topic currently is; or simply how entertaining or well-received the reviewer expects the presentation to be at the meeting.

It can be appreciated from the above considerations that some of the scored elements in an abstract can be modified by the authors before submitting, but many of them cannot. The authors can try to write the abstract in a more attractive way, add more detailed analyses of the data, or compose a more fitting and reasonable conclusion in order to try to gain more points. However, once a study has been completed, no amount of re-writing can change the basic originality, impact, study design or results. For these elements, the best that the submitting authors can do is to try to highlight all the good things they have done in the abstract. For example, if theirs was truly the first study on a topic, and the study itself was a randomized, blinded study on a cohort whose necessary size was already estimated from the outset, then all of these point-scoring elements must be clearly stated in the abstract itself.

6　Tips for Writing the Abstract

As stated previously, this chapter is not aimed at teaching how to write a good abstract. That is dealt with in other chapters of this book. Instead, basing on our own experiences as abstract reviewers and conference Scientific Program Committee members, we can share some tips on how to modify an abstract to best suit what an abstract reviewer wants.

6.1　Title

It is crucial that the Title (the first thing that the abstract reviewer reads) gives a good first impression to capture the attention from among the large volume of abstracts that each abstract reviewer must read. A good title for an abstract does not necessarily mean a flashy or clever one. Instead, the best title is often one that can summarize the whole abstract in one sentence. That means it should contain as many of these as possible: what patients were studied; type of study; factor studied; outcome measured; result. For example: "Drug X improves 5-year overall survival among adult patients with inoperable small cell lung cancer: a case-match study". This Title captures all the necessary elements, and clearly informs the abstract reviewer (and hence conference delegate) exactly what the presentation will be about. If the premise of the study as stated in the Title sounds promising enough, the abstract reviewer may already be predisposed to accept even before he reads further into the abstract. A fancy Title like "Is Drug X the panacea for lung cancer? " may sound catchy, but it tells the reviewer absolutely nothing about the study. It makes the abstract reviewer work harder to find out what the study is about, and that is not appreciated when reviewing over a hundred submissions.

6.2　Proportions of each section

The introductions/objectives, methods, results and conclusions are the 4 sections necessary in virtually all abstracts, but the relative length of each section can be varied to suit the study. It is essential to score points in the above marking scheme by using these sections appropriately because the word count limit for conference abstracts is usually very tight. If the originality or impact of the study is not immediately obvious, it may be worthwhile using a slightly longer Introduction to explain why the study is actually original or significant. If the authors used a clever study design, they may wish to highlight this by expanding the methods section. However, unless these issues do require the extra words to explain, our personal preference is to keep the Introduction, methods and conclusion slightly shorter and spend more words on the results section. This is because a typical oral presentation at a conference is between 6-10 minutes long. It is extremely disappointing if the abstract is accepted, and then it is only found at the time of presentation that the authors only had one result to show the delegates. That would be a very poor presentation indeed. By putting slightly more data into the abstract's results section, the authors can reassure the abstract reviewer that they will actually be able to produce a decent presentation at the time of the conference, complete with results that the delegates can appreciate.

6.3　Tables and Figures

The word count limit-as said-is very tight for conference abstracts. It is not easy explaining a major study and showing all the important results in an abstract limited to between 200-300 words. The submitter should therefore look very carefully at the conference's policy on Tables and Figures. If a Table is allowed for abstracts, then the submitter should definitely try to take advantage and include a Table because Tables are usually not included in the word count limit. The data-which take up a lot of words in the abstract-can be transferred as much as possible from the results section to the Table. Instead, the submitter can use the saved word count to explain very briefly the key findings in words in the results section, or expand a little in the other sections of the abstract. Similarly, if a figure is allowed, this must also be taken advantage of. A photo to show a technique will not only save many words in the methods section, but will also look more attractive to a reviewer. A complex methodology may be explained more clearly (and using less words) if a flowchart was included as a Figure.

6.4　Don't make empty statements

One thing that reviewers hate-but which submitters often do-is to say something in the abstract that is not backed up by showing the data or results. For example, submitting authors sometimes write in the results "we found that A was better than B ($p<0.05$)", or that "we will show in our presentation that X is superior to Y". If A is 'better' than B, then the abstract must say what parameter was used to judge this and what the actual difference was? Just saying "$p<0.05$" without these is completely meaningless. Making a promise that some data will be presented is a trick some authors used when they haven't yet completed the study by the time of the abstract deadline, but this again is completely meaningless. In both examples, the abstract reviewer has nothing concrete with which to judge how good or bad the study was. It is impossible to give a good mark for Impact, design or conclusion if actual results are not given. Those empty statements achieved nothing except wasting the word count.

6.5　Make it easy to read

This sounds obvious, but it is a vital point. Remember that each abstract reviewer has a potential mountain of abstracts to read, and there is a deadline for him/her to meet for finishing all the reviews. After having read many other reviews that day, the abstract reviewer can be mentally exhausted. If an abstract is easy and 'pleasant' to read, it automatically leaves a good impression. If the abstract reviewer then finds the next abstract is clumsily worded and difficult to understand, then he/she will have a headache, moan, and then probably reject. Good writing does not mean using flowery, fanciful English. On the contrary, it means using simple language and short sentences. After a long day reviewing, it is these 'easy-to-digest' sentences that are most welcome by reviewers.

6.6　Write the Paper first!

Usually, many less experienced authors would choose to write the abstract first, present it at a conference, and then prepare the paper for a journal afterwards. This has the advantage of allowing the author to gather feedback from delegates at the conference regarding the study-and their comments can be used to improve the final paper. However, one tip offered by some experienced presenters is to write a draft of the paper for a journal before writing the abstract for a conference. This is because the process of writing a paper helps the author think clearly about the strengths and weaknesses of the study, and which are the most important results and conclusions. Once the paper is written, the authors can more plainly see the most relevant features to include in the abstract, and what details are more superfluous and can be left out. It is always possible to then submit and present the abstract at the conference, still get the feedback from the delegates, and then return to improve the draft of the paper before submitting it to the journal.

7　Tips for Submitting the Abstract

7.1　The Right Conference

Once the abstract is written, the choice of which conference to submit to will depend on a number of considerations. These may include: the 'prestige' of the conference; the nature of the conference; the location; the audience; and the supposed 'ease' of acceptance of submitted abstracts.

The 'prestige' of a conference is very subjective and can depend on its size, faculty, history, and word-of-mouth reputation. We personally do not think that this should be a key consideration when submitting an abstract. However, we recognize that for some clinicians, it is necessary to justify to their own institutions why they are going to a particular meeting, and in this case, going to a 'world famous' meeting can be a factor. More important is the nature of the meeting itself. Is this a large, comprehensive mega-conference; or is it a specialist symposium focused on a very specific subject? For the world of respirology, an example of the former might be an annual congress of an international society for respiratory medicine, whereas the latter may be a regional workshop on sleep medicine. For the trainee clinician, the former is attractive because while presenting one's own research to a large audience of peers, the trainee has the opportunity to learn about a huge range of topics presented within that specialty at that conference. If an abstract is likely to have broad impact for a large number of patients, it is also preferable to share it at a larger meeting so that the message can be more effectively spread. For the more experienced author who is beyond the stage of attending conferences to only learn from others, such general conferences may lack focus, and he/ she may prefer the latter specialist meetings that more specifically appeal to his/her personal clinical interests. Sharing an abstract on a very specialist topic among expert peers who better appreciate it may appeal more to more experienced clinicians.

Location is important for some clinicians, not because they want to choose a nice holiday destination, but because of travel expenses. Visa requirements for overseas conferences must also be checked. In most cases, conferences can provide attendees with invitation letters to the conference that some countries require for issuing visas. Submitters should be reminded that while it may sound pleasant to travel to a faraway conference to present, the impact of presenting abroad may not be great. A study from country A will not necessarily influence management in country B, and that may lessen the abstract's impact. Back home, the presenter's peers in his/her own country will also most likely be uninterested in the fact that the abstract was presented at a fancy conference in another country. If a clinician is still trying to build his/her own reputation in the specialty, it may sometimes be more useful to present in his/her own town, country or region.

The anticipated audience at a conference is another factor that must be considered. This has to do mostly with the professional society organizing that meeting. For example, a cardiac surgeon may wish to submit to a conference organized by a cardiology society if he/she wants to publicize a surgical procedure to cardiologists that may consequently refer patients to receive that procedure. On the other hand, the cardiac surgeon may choose to submit to a smaller meeting hosted by a cardiac surgery society if the abstract's content is more specialized, so that only peers from the author's own specialty will appreciate the nuances. Obviously, if a clinician wants to network within a given professional society, then it is also essential to present at conferences run by that society. It may take repeated good presentations at consecutive meetings before the presenter is noticed by the higher echelons of a society, so this may take perseverance.

Many people believe that the chances of their abstracts being accepted by bigger, more 'prestigious' conferences are lower. This is not necessarily true. The big conferences do attract many more submissions, so a lot will get rejected; but on the other hand, such big conferences have more sessions to fill with presentations, so the opportunities for acceptance do exist. As already mentioned earlier, bigger conferences also appreciate diversity, so in some instances submissions from overseas or less 'famous' institutions may even get slightly preferential consideration.

7.2　The Right Category

It has already been mentioned earlier that most conferences sort submitted abstracts into different subject categories, with specific sessions reserved during the meeting for presentations in each category. Those wishing to improve their chances of acceptance should pay attention to what categories are available and submit to the one they think is most likely to be under-subscribed. For example, in thoracic surgery, categories such as 'lung cancer' or 'minimally invasive surgery' are often very popular and receive a large number of submissions. Despite more sessions being allocated to these categories, the acceptance rate may be relatively low. On the other hand, categories such as 'mediastinum' or 'experimental/innovative' may receive fewer submissions.

However, submitters should be aware that getting an abstract accepted by choosing the category can occasionally backfire. Even if accepted, an abstract presented in a less popular category may end up being presented at a less well attended session.

7.3　The Right Timing

A final consideration regarding submission is the abstract submission deadlines. There are certain times during the year when the larger conferences tend to be held: often a peak in early summer, and another peak in late autumn/early winter. These tend to correspond to times of less extreme weather and off-peak holiday travel. These in turn mean that the deadlines for abstract submission for a number of meetings (around 6-9 months before a meeting as mentioned earlier) often come very close together at around two 'seasons' during the year. It is theoretically possible to submit an abstract to a conference with an earlier deadline, so that if it is rejected one can submit to another conference with a later deadline in the same deadline 'season'. However, in practice, the abstract review process takes too long. By the time an abstract is rejected, it is usually too late to submit to any major meeting in the same 'season'. One can either wait for the next 'season' or submit to a smaller meeting whose deadline is in-between the usual deadline 'seasons'. Our advice is simply to ignore playing games with time, and simply submit to the one conference one wants to attend.

8　Warning: Two Unforgiveable Sins

There are two things which anyone submitting to a conference must never do.

8.1　Duplicate Submission

It is very tempting to send abstracts to more than one conference, and then wait to see which conference accepts. Do not do this. The major societies organizing meetings are often in contact with each other, and sometimes abstract reviewers for different conferences can overlap. It is not too difficult to spot duplicate submissions. Anyone found guilty of duplicate submission will not only get rejected, but will likely get blacklisted and be banned from future submissions. The offence may also get reported to the submitter's institution, resulting in disciplinary action and irreparable damage to one's academic reputation.

An abstract presented at one meeting must not be presented at another one at a later date. This will also be regarded as a duplicate submission, and will also be punished strictly. Many clinicians believe that minor changes to an abstract (for example, adding a few more patients to the cohort) qualifies it to be a brand new abstract which is alright for submitting to another meeting. However, most major conferences do not view it this way, and will likely still regard it as a duplicate submission. The safest advice is to refrain from trying to 'milk' one abstract too hard, and try to get too many presentations from just one study. The consequences if caught are not worth the risk.

8.2　"No show" at the conference

Surprisingly, after managing to get an abstract accepted, some authors then do not turn up at the meeting. This is especially true for poster presentations more than oral presentations. These 'no show' authors often think that it is no big deal if they do not come. This thinking is deadly wrong. Conferences care very, very much about all 'no shows'. Anyone whose abstract is accepted but does not attend to present is liable to receive a ban from future submissions. In addition, many professional societies are now choosing not only to ban the presenter him/herself, but also *anyone else* from the same institute. This is very serious, as it means one's own 'no show' can hurt the entire hospital or university.

If a presenter is unable to present, it is his/her responsibility to seek one of the other co-authors to present instead. This is acceptable, but the conference must be notified in advance. If nobody can come to present, the author should also write to the conference to formally request withdrawal of the presentation. This must also be done well before the conference starts. The conference will not like withdrawals, but these are nonetheless much better than having a 'no show' on the day.

9　The Bottom Line

Even though they both come from the same research study, a conference abstract is different from a journal paper. They are prepared differently, and they are certainly judged differently by the abstract reviewer and the editor respectively. In some ways, the assessment of a conference abstract is more formulaic because of the scoring scheme used by many conferences nowadays. However, in other ways, there are more intangible considerations. When it comes to accepting or rejecting conference abstracts because the demands of the delegates and the organizing professional society are more variable than the predominantly scientific focus of journals and their readers. Clinicians wishing to present their abstracts at a given conference should study the nature and preferences of the organizing society, the likely composition of the delegates, and the responsibilities of the abstract reviewer serving them.

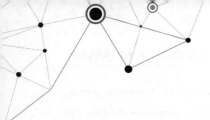

第 34 章
大会发言技巧

Chapter 34
How to Effectively Present a Scientific Paper

Jerzy B Gajewski, Janusz Springer

1 Introduction

Your scientific work may be excellent; however you have to know how to "sell" your research. Even if you want just to publish the paper you are often presenting the data at the scientific meeting. Participation at a scientific conference and delivering a presentation is one of the tangible rewards for your time and dedication in research work. It is a perfect opportunity for making potentially valuable research and job contacts in your field of work (so-called networking). Active participation at a conference is another line in your CV. Furthermore, you have a chance to visit a new city, taste different dishes and take a break from the daily routine. In sum: working in research is worth it.

How your paper will be received, depends on your presentation. Ludwig Mies, a German-American architect, designed buildings according to the principle "*less is more*". This approach accurately describes the process of designing slides and speech for a scientific conference. The more you follow this principle, the easier it will be for you to prepare and the better impression you will make at the conference.

2 Main principles:

- Your presentation=your business card
- Respect the judges and the audience: obey the time limit and slide limit
- One slide per minute
- Simple slide=easy to read=professional
- Short introduction=good introduction
- "*a picture is worth a thousand words*"
- Focus on your results and their relevance in practice
- More graphs and tables $\neq$ more professional presentation
- Practice with a stopwatch and in front of a camera
- You control the audience-not the other way around
- "*Less is more*"

3 Presentation=speech+slides

Both parts are equally important. Visually attractive slides will not rescue an incomprehensible speech. Similarly, a powerful speech will not take the audience's attention away from poorly-prepared slides.

4　Where to start?

Start by carefully reading the information and guidelines for conference participants.

Organizers send you this valuable information in the emails confirming your registration and/ or post it on the conference website. You **must** adjust the length of your presentation and number of slides to the limits determined by the organizers. If the organizers do not specify the slide limit, follow the principle of *"one slide per minute."*

5　Preparation

Paraphrasing the words of the legendary boxer Muhammad Ali; *"the fight is won or lost far away from witnesses"*-during training. This applies to any public speeches you make-your success will directly depend on how much time and effort you devote behind the scenes.

NO　reading of the text on the slide. This seems very obvious, yet often speakers do this at conferences and lectures.

NO　improvising

YES　plan and choose every word you will say

■ People who are not fluent in the language of the presentation instinctively write a "screenplay" of their speech and after many revisions they memorize it. Therefore, their presentations are thought out and planned.

■ Whereas it is the fluent speakers who are most likely to speak without preparation and to make the most common mistakes (speaking too fast, using slang words, using sentences that are too long, repeating what was already said, etc.)

■ Does your speech have words that are difficult to pronounce? → replace them with simpler and stronger, more direct words

■ Scientific terminology that is long and difficult to pronounce? → say those terms only once, show their abbreviation on the slide and from then on say only the abbreviation

YES　practice your speech with a stopwatch and video camera

- You do not need to buy any additional equipment. All mobile phones have a stopwatch application and all digital cameras (including the cameras in smartphones) have a video camera capability

- Even if you have a large mirror available, still practice in front of a video camera (because you will not be looking at the mirror during your entire practice presentation and therefore you will not notice what the camera will notice)

YES　analyze in detail all the recordings of your practice presentations

- Pay attention to what you say, how you say it, how you move and what are you looking at

- Identify all the weak points of your presentations

- In each practice presentation systematically correct and eliminate the weak points

YES　practice as many times as it takes for you to speak loudly and clearly

YES　look in the direction of the audience

- Your task is to present information to the people in the audience, therefore make eye contact with them

- When looking at the people in your audience, you can be sure that they can hear you well (because your head is lifted up and points in the same direction as the listeners)

YES shorten, shorten, shorten

- If you are speaking quickly in order to exceed the time limit=you are trying to say too much=you are more likely to make mistakes=you must shorten your speech

- Say short and strong sentences (remember that all people, including expert researchers or clinicians, have a limited attention span)

- Practice as long as it takes for you to finish your speech without hurry and have >1 minute of the time limit left (the less you say, the more the audience and the judges will understand and remember)

NO hiding behind the stand

- Usually you will present in rooms that are small enough so that you will not need to use a microphone

YES when discussing results, emphasize key words such (e.g. "is/is not, " "increases/decreases, " "causes/does not cause" etc.)

- Change the tone of your voice or make a short pause

- This will work well with the visual emphasis on your slide (e.g. an arrow, frame, red font pointing out the result/s)

6 Slides

How to start designing your slides? The easiest way is to paste each part of your abstract onto a separate slide. But that is not the end, it is just a start. You must show more than just the sentences from your abstract because the judges (and part of the audience) have already read them in the conference abstract book.

Therefore, your tasks are:

- to select from your abstract the **absolutely most important** information about your project

- to devote the most attention (speech time and on the slides) to your results

- to summarize the **significance** of your results to other researchers, clinicians or patients.

7 Slide design (Fig 34-1 & 34-2)

NO full sentences on the slides

- slides with full sentences and a lot of text are useful when there is no presenter available (e.g. lectures slides posted on a website as a study tool), however this not the situation at scientific conferences

- do not force your audience to choose between listening to what you are saying and reading what you wrote on the slides (majority of people are so-called"visual learners", therefore you can be sure that majority of the audience will stop listening to you and read instead)

YES sentence fragments (just like in newspaper headlines)

YES keywords

YES arrows instead of words such as "increase, " "decrease" or "causes/leads to"

NO writing many references on the slide (it shows that you are directly copying the text of your published paper and that your introduction is too long)

NO separate slide with a list of references (you will not show it long enough for the audience to read it)

YES select information on the slide so that only 1-2 most important references are needed. Write the references in the bottom part of the slides and use a smaller font. (e.g. the international guidelines on which your experiment is based on)

NO using images to fill the empty spaces on each slide (instead, each element of the slide must be meaningful)

YES images instead of words (use the slide as a tool for visual communication)

- old saying *"a picture is worth a thousand words,"*

e.g. do not list/describe the changes in a tissue sample, but show one high-quality image of a tissue with those changes)

NO low-quality/low-resolution images

-simple principle: if the image is not clear/sharp on your computer screen, then you can be sure that it will look even worse on the projector screen)

Too much text and references

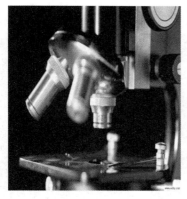

•Do not write full and long sentences on the slides, because the audience will stop listening to you and instead will focus on reading your sentences.

•This is another long sentence that distracts the audience, causes it to lose track of your speech and is not able to read everything your wrote anyway...

•Kowalski et al. Early IJK survival single-center study. Journal of X and Y 2010
•Smith, Adams, Johnson. Clinical trial number 2. Journal of Clinical Y 2009
•Gonzalez, Morales, Rodrigez. The influence of X in the analysis of Y. European Journal of Z. 2012

Random image that does not describe what you are discussing

Fig 34-1　Not a good design

A more reasonable amount of text

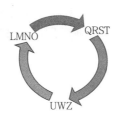

· Large, clear font
· Sentence fragment
· Keywords
· Most important facts only
· Image that describes what you are discussing

Kowalski et al. Early IJK survival single−center study. Journal of X and Y 2010

Fig 34-2　good design

8　Logo of the Department, University, Clinic or Hospital

If the background of the logo image is identical to the background of your slide AND if the logo image is optimal in size (small enough not to be distracting attention away from the slide content BUT large enough to be readable), then the logo will convey your professionalism. If the logo image does not fulfill all of the above three criteria, then it is better to skip it and instead write your institution's full name underneath your last name on the title slide

9　Background and font (Fig 34-3 & 34-4)

The PowerPoint and Impress programs offer you dozens of slide templates. Via google you can find 100s of even more creative-looking templates. Unfortunately, most of these templates use multi-color backgrounds which make it very difficult to match a clearly readable font color and type.

YES　Use the simplest possible slide background. A good compromise between simplicity and creativity is a 90% white background with a colorful stripe across one of the edges.

YES　Match the font color and type to background color.

YES　You must make the font color, size and type consistent on every slide (e.g. all the slide titles, text, table text, figure legend, references) in the entire presentation. Thanks to this, when on one of the slides a word or number is written in red font, it means you are purposefully pointing the audience's attention to this.

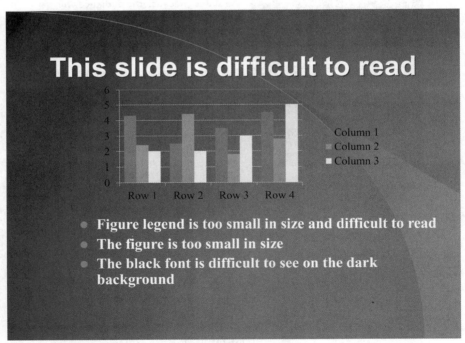

Fig 34-3　Not a good design

10　Tables and graphs (Fig 34-4)

Tables and graphs play an important role in research papers and presentations. The greater the scope of the project, the more results can be described using tables and graphs. However, follow the principle: more tables and graphs ≠ more professional slides

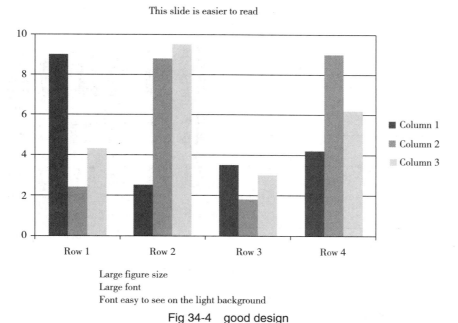

This slide is easier to read

Large figure size
Large font
Font easy to see on the light background

Fig 34-4　good design

YES　show only those tables and graphs which illustrate the **absolutely most important** results and correlations (in other words, those which "answer" the research questions)

YES　make sure that the text inside the table and the graph legend are written with a font large enough to be read from the last row of the room

YES　if the table has many columns and data, consider creating a smaller table that will contain only the data that is most important or most surprising

YES　use animated arrows, circles or frames to emphasize and point attention to the most important data in the table or graphs

- an animated frame will allow you to focus on speaking without the need to use a laser pointer (Fig 34-5)

- the more clearly you show and tell what is the most important, the more understandable your presentation will be.

11　Introduction

It is very easy to make mistakes in the introduction, both during the speech and while designing slides.

NO　reading of your presentation title out loud

of all your slides, the title slide is shown for the longest time; therefore you can be sure that everyone in the audience has read it

YES　limit the basic information about your subject to the absolute minimum

- the conference organizers pay attention to include your presentation in a subject-related session, therefore you can be sure that the majority of the audience already understands the basics

- in case your subject is very different from the others included in the session (e.g. an anesthesiology subject in a surgery session), you only need to say 2-3 sentences to get the audience's

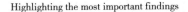

Highlighting the most important findings

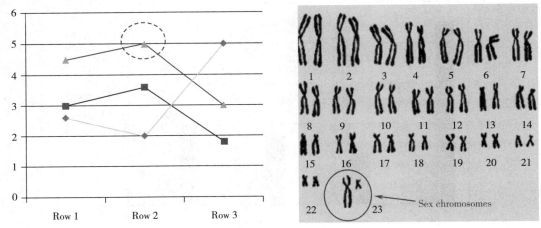

Fig 34-5 good graphics

attention and explain "what is what" in your subject

12 The last slide

NO it is not enough to just write the conclusions (e.g. "marker X is useful for testing the expression of gene efgh")

YES clearly write the **significance** of your findings in research and/or medical practice (e.g. "marker X is more sensitive than markers M and N, ""marker X is cheaper than the currently used markers, therefore it could make it affordable to screen for the IJK disease")

13 Saving the presentation

YES save your presentation in several formats

- always save a back-up copy in. pdf format

- always save your presentation in the **old** PowerPoint format "ppt (97/2000/XP)"-(this way you will avoid technical problems with opening your presentation file)

- if you created your presentation in software other than MS PowerPoint, then you must save a copy in the ppt format

- if you prefer to use Prezi, email the conference organizers and make sure that they will allow you to present in Prezi (if yes, make sure to save a back-up copy in the. pdf format)

14 Speech

Remember: you control the audience, not the other way around.

You decide what the audience sees and hears.

Fully take advantage of this situation in your presentation, regardless of how fluent you are in the language you are presenting or how strong your accent is. The former UN Secretary General Kofi Annan speaks English with a very strong accent, however that has no influence on his confidence and effectiveness as a public speaker.

15 Questions from the judges and the audience

The "*question & answer session*" is the part of the presentation that causes conference participants to worry and lose confidence. Although you can control even the smallest element of your presentation, you have no influence on what the judges and the audience will ask you.

However do not let this affect your confidence during the presentation.

Here is what you can do:

- Listen your practice recordings and think about what questions "automatically" come to mind and prepare answers to these questions

- Control *how* you answer the questions

Here are some fundamental principles:

(1) Never begin your answer by saying *"that's a good question."*

(2) Never answer a question with a question.

(3) Answer the question directly and briefly-in other words do not change the subject the way politicians often do.

(4) You can redirect the question to another co-author, who worked on the aspect of the research which the question is asking about.

(5) If you do not know the answer, it is best to say *"I don't know"* instead of making up an answer.

Those are the main principles and tips. The rest depends on your attention to details and the amount of time you spend practicing your presentation.

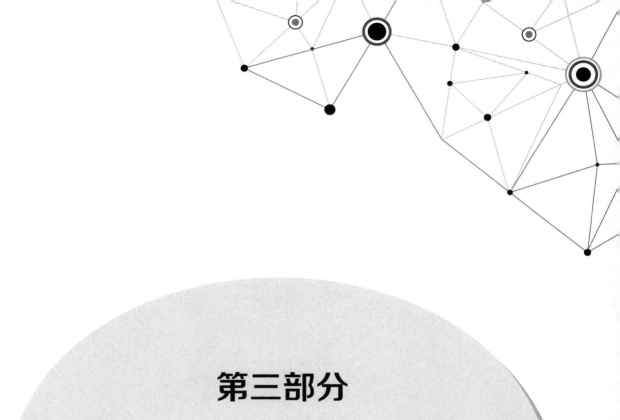

第三部分

附录

Part 3

Appendix

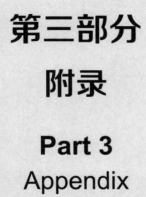

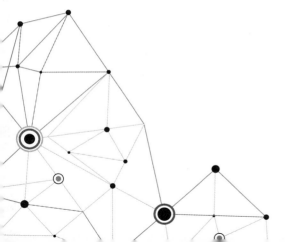

附录
中英文计量单位及论文写作应注意的问题

Appendix
Measurement Units in Chinese and English & Tips During the Writing

1. 常见法定计量单位（见表1、表2、表3）

表1 国际单位制的基本单位

量的名称	单位名称	单位符号
长度	米	m
质量	千克	kg
时间	秒	s
电流	安（培）	A
热力学温度	开（尔文）	K
物质的量	摩（尔）	mol

表2 国际单位制中具有专门名称的导出单位

量的名称	单位名称	单位符号	其他表示示例
频率	赫（兹）	Hz	s^{-1}
力	牛（顿）	N	$kg \cdot m/s^2$
压强	帕（斯卡）	Pa	N/m^2
能量;热量	焦（耳）	J	$N \cdot m$
功率	瓦（特）	W	J/s
电压	伏（特）	V	W/A
电荷量	库（仑）	C	$A \cdot s$
摄氏温度	摄氏度	℃	
吸收剂量	戈（瑞）	Gy	J/kg
放射性活度	贝克（勒尔）	Bq	s^{-1}
剂量当量	希（沃特）	Sv	J/kg

表 3　用于构成十进制倍数和分数单位的词头（SI 词头）

因数	词头名称		符号
	英文	中文	
10^{24}	yotta	尧［它］	Y
10^{21}	zetta	泽［它］	Z
10^{18}	exa	艾［可萨］	E
10^{15}	peta	拍［它］	P
10^{12}	tera	太［拉］	T
10^{9}	giga	吉［咖］	G
10^{6}	mega	兆	M
10^{3}	kilo	千	k
10^{2}	hecto	百	h
10^{1}	deca	十	da
10^{-1}	deci	分	d
10^{-2}	centi	厘	c
10^{-3}	milli	毫	m
10^{-6}	micro	微	μ
10^{-9}	nano	纳［诺］	n
10^{-12}	pico	皮［可］	p
10^{-15}	femto	飞［母托］	f
10^{-18}	atto	阿［托］	a
10^{-21}	zepto	仄［普托］	z
10^{-24}	yocto	幺［科托］	y

2. 法定计量单位在论文写作中应注意的问题

不同的杂志、期刊对计量单位的书写格式及其他要求都有详细说明，可在期刊杂志或相关网站上查看。以下列出一些常见要求，仅供参考。

（1）全稿使用法定计量单位符号，不用中文单位名称，中文单位名称只用于叙述性文字中。如：

时间用"d、h、min、s"

长度用"m、cm、mm、μm、nm……"

重量用"kg、g、mg、μg、ng……"

物质的量浓度用"mol/L……"

物质的量用"mol、mmol……"

旋转速度用"r/min"

温度用"℃"

热量用"kJ、J……"

（2）注意常见的不规范用法。如：

38±3℃　应为"38℃±3℃或（38±3）℃"

100±30Hz 应为"100Hz±30Hz或（100±30）Hz"

mg/kg/d 应为"mg/（kg·d）"

ml/ 小时应为"ml/h"

10~20% 应为"10%~20%"

2×4mm² 应为"2mm×4mm"

3×3×4mm 应为"3mm×3mm×4mm"

5~10 万应为"5 万 ~10 万"

5mg/ 湿（干）重 g 应为"5mg/g"

N（当量）应为"mol/L"

5Å 应为"0.5nm"

5μ 应为"5μm"

（3）SI 词头的使用：SI 词头共有 20 个（表 3）。词头不能单独使用,必须用于各种单位符号之前。如：

5μm 不能写成 5m

10kg 不能写成 10k

10kPa 不能写成 10k

20cm 不能写成 20c

（4）当量浓度（N）换算为摩尔每升（mol/L）。换算公式：

Mol/L=N÷ 离子价数

如：1N NaOH=1mol/L NaOH

血钾 1mEq/L=1mmol/L

血钙 4mEq/L=2mmol/L

2N H_2SO_4=1mol/L H_2SO_4

（5）不再使用英尺、英寸、码、品脱、夸脱、加仑、盎司、磅、里、丈、尺、寸、分这些计量单位,应换算成法定单位。

（6）统计学符号的使用：平均数用英文小写 $\bar{x}$,不用 $\bar{X}$;标准差用英文小写 s,不用 SD;标准误差用英文 sx,不用 SE;t 检验用英文小写 t;F 检验用大写 F;卡方检验用希文小写 χ^2;相关系数用英文小写 r;自由度用希文小写 v;样本数用英文小写 n;概率用英文大写 P。以上符号均用斜体。

（7）关于血压计量单位的使用：根据国家质量技术监督局和卫生部文件（质技监局量函［1998］126 号）规定,出版物中可使用毫米汞柱（mmHg）或千帕（kPa）,如果使用 mmHg 应注明 mmHg 与 kPa 的换算关系。

3. 常用医学相关法定计量单位之间的换算

各种单位		换算关系	举例	备注
压力之间的换算	从 mmHg 到 kPa	mmHg 数 ×0.133=kPa 数	5mmHg=（5×0.133）kPa=0.665kPa	适用于血压，O_2 分压，CO_2 分压等
	从 cmH₂O 到 Pa	cmH$_2$O 数 ×98.07=Pa 数	5cmH$_2$O=（5×98.07）Pa=490.35Pa	
	从 mmH₂O 到 Pa	mmH$_2$O 数 ×9.807=Pa 数	5mmH$_2$O=（5×9.807）Pa=49.035Pa	
温度之间的换算	从 ℉ 到 ℃	（℉数 -32）×0.555 6=℃数	100 ℉=[（100-32）×0.555 6]℃=37.780 8℃	
mg/dl 到 mmol/L	葡萄糖	mg/dl 数 ×0.055 5=mmol/L 数	50mg/dl=（50×0.055 5）mmol/L=2.775mmol/L	适用于全血，脑脊液等
	尿素氮	mg/dl 数 ×0.357=mmol/L 数	50mg/dl=（50×0.357）mmol/L=17.85mmol/L	适用于全血
	尿素	mg/dl 数 ×0.166 5=mmol/L 数	50mg/dl=（50×0.166 5）mmol/L=8.325mmol/L	
	非蛋白氮	mg/dl 数 ×0.713 9=mmol/L 数	50mg/dl=（50×0.713 9）mmol/L=35.695mmol/L	
	血钠	mg/dl 数 ×0.435=mmol/L 数	50mg/dl=（50×0.435）mmol/L=21.75mmol/L	适用于血清
	血钾	mg/dl 数 ×0.255 8=mmol/L 数	50mg/dl=（50×0.255 8）mmol/L=12.79mmol/L	
	血钙	mg/dl 数 ×0.249 5=mmol/L 数	50mg/dl=（50×0.249 5）mmol/L=12.475mmol/L	
	血磷	mg/dl 数 ×0.322 9=mmol/L 数	50mg/dl=（50×0.322 9）mmol/L=16.145mmol/L	
	胆固醇	mg/dl 数 ×0.025 9=mmol/L 数	50mg/dl=（50×0.025 9）mmol/L=1.295mmol/L	
	甘油三酯	mg/dl 数 ×0.011 3=mmol/L 数	50mg/dl=（50×0.011 3）mmol/L=0.565mmol/L	
	氯化物	mg/dl 数 ×0.282 1=mmol/L 数	50mg/dl=（50×0.282 1）mmol/L=14.105mmol/L	适用于血清、脑脊液

续表

	各种单位	换算关系	举例	备注
mg/dl 到 μmol/L	肌酐	mg/dl 数 × 88.402=μmol/L 数	5mg/dl=(5 × 88.402)μmol/L=442.01μmol/L	适用于全血
	胆红素	mg/dl 数 × 17.10=μmol/L 数	5mg/dl=(5 × 17.1)μmol/L=85.5μmol/L	适用于血清
g/24h 到 mmol/24h	尿素	g/24h 数 × 16.651=mmol/24h 数	50g/24h=(50 × 16.651)mmol/24h=832.55mmol/24h	适用于尿液
mg/24h 到 mmol/24h	肌酐	mg/24h 数 × 0.008 84=mmol/24h 数	500mg/24h=(500 × 0.008 84)mmol/24h=4.42mmol/24h	
μg/dl 到 μmol/L	氨	μg/dl 数 × 0.587 2=μmol/L 数	50μg/dl=(50 × 0.587 2)=29.36μmol/L	适用于全血
μg/dl 到 nmol/L	碘	μg/dl 数 × 78.8=nmol/L 数	5μg/dl=(5 × 78.8)=394nmol/L	适用于血清
μg/L 到 nmol/L	粪卟啉	μg/L 数 × 1.527=nmol/L 数	5μg/L=(5 × 1.527)nmol/L=7.635nmol/L	适用于尿液
mg/24h 到 μmol/24h	尿胆原	mg/24h 数 × 1.687=μmol/24h 数	5mg/24h=(5 × 1.687)μmol/24h=8.435μmol/24h	
mg/L 到 μmol/L	δ 氨基酮戊酸	mg/L 数 × 7.626=μmol/L 数	5mg/L=(5 × 7.626)μmol/L=38.13μmol/L	
酶活力	从 IU(国际单位)到 nmol/s	IU 数 × 16.67=nmol/s 数	5IU=(5 × 16.67)nmol/s=83.35nmol/s	
廓清率(清除率)	从 L/min 到 L/s	L/min 数 × 0.016 67=L/s 数	100L/min=(100 × 0.016 67)L/s=1.667L/s	
	从 ml/min 到 ml/s	ml/min 数 × 0.016 67=ml/s 数	100ml/min=(100 × 0.016 67)ml/s=1.667ml/s	
照射量	从 R(伦琴)到 mC/kg(毫库/千克)	R 数 × 0.258=mC/kg 数	5R=(5 × 0.258)mC/kg=1.29mC/kg	
吸收剂量	从 rad(拉德)到 Gy(戈瑞)	rad 数 × 0.01=Gy 数	50rad=(50 × 0.01)Gy=0.5Gy	
剂量当量	从 rem(雷姆)到 Sv(希沃特)	rem 数 × 0.01=Sv 数	50rem=(50 × 0.01)Sv=0.5Sv	
放射性活度	Ci(居里)到 GBq(吉贝可)	Ci 数 × 37=GBq 数	5Ci=(5 × 37)GBq=185GBq	
热量	从 kcal 到 kJ	kcal 数 × 4.184=kJ 数	5kcal=(5 × 4.184)kJ=20.92kJ	

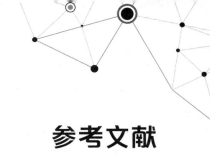

参考文献

References

1. Abantanga FA, Nimako B, Amoah M. The range of abdominal surgical emergencies in children older than 1 year at the Komfo Anokye Teaching Hospital, Kumasi, Ghana[J]. Ann Afr Med, 2009, 8(4):236-242.

2. Azad N, Molnar F, Byszewski A. Lesons leamed from a mulidisiplinary heart failure clinic for older women: a randomised controlled trial[J]. Age Ageing, 2008, 37(3):282-287.

3. Briscoe MH. Preparing scientific illustrations. New York: Springer, 1996.

4. Block SM. Do's and don't's of poster presentation[J]. Biophys J, 1996, 71(6):3527-3529.

5. Braun PM, Hoang-Böhm J, Alken P. Urolihiasis in Children—ESWL and Auxiliary Measures//Akimoto M, Higashihara E, Kumon H, Masaki Z, Orikasa S. Treatment of Urolithiasis. Recent Advances in Endourology. Tokyo: Springer, 2001:135-142.

6. Barbara G. 如何撰写和发表科技论文. 第6版. 北京: 北京大学出版社, 2007.

7. Calfee RC, Valencia RR. APA guide to preparing manuscript for joumal publication (revised). Washington D.C: American Psychological Association, 2007.

8. Chen Y, Wen JG, Li Y, et al. Twelve-hour daytime observation of voiding pattern in newborms <4 weeks of age [J]. Acta Paediatr, 2012, 101(6):583-586.

9. Council of Europe. Developing a methodology for drawing up guidelines on best medical practice (Recommendation Rec(2001)13 and explanatory memorandum). Strasbourg: Council of Europe Publishing, 2002.

10. Donev D. Principles and ethics in scientific communication in biomedicine[J]. Acta Inform Med, 2013, 21(4): 228-233.

11. Dai L, Ren P, Liu M, et al. Using immunomic approach to enhance tumor-associated autoantibody detection in diagnosis of hepatocellular carcinoma[J]. Clin Immunol, 2014, 152(1-2):127-139.

12. Gaw A. Reality and revisionism: new evidence for Andrew C Ivy's claim to authorship of the Nuremberg Code [J]. J R Soc Med, 2014, 107(4):138-143.

13. Grant MJ. What makes a good title?[J]. Health Info Libr, 2013, 30(4):259-260.

14. Gjersvik P, Gulbrandsen P, Aasheim ET, et al. Poor title—poor manuscript?[J]. Tidsskr Nor Laegeforen, 2013, 133(23-24):2475-2477.

15. George MH. How to Write a Paper.5th ed. Malaysia: Vivar Pinting Sdn Bhd, 2013.

16. Hoque MO, Soria JC, Woo J, et al. Aquaporin l is overexpressed in lung cancer and stiulates NIH-3T3 cell proliferation and anchorage-independent growth[J]. Am J Pathol, 2006, 168(4):1345-1353.

17. Hall GM. How to Present at Meetings. Hoboken: John Wiley & Sons, 2011.

18. Hall GM. How to Present at Meetings.3rd Edition. Hoboken: John Wiley & Sons, 2012.

19. Hall GM. How to Write a Paper. 5th Edition. Hoboken: John Wiley & Sons, 2013.

20. Hurst SA. Declaration of Helsinki and protection for vulnerable research participants[J]. JAMA, 2014, 311 (12): 1252.

21. International Committee of Medical Journal Editors. Uniform Requirements for Manuscriplts Submited to Biomedical Journals[J]. N Engl J Med, 1991, 324(6): 424-428.

22. Kjell ER, Rae RN. Surviving Your Dissertation: A Comprehensive Guide to Content and Process. Thousand Oaks: SAGE Publications, 2008.

23. Kotz D, Cals JW. Effective writing and publishing scientific papers, part X I: submitting a paper[J]. J Clin Epidemiol, 2014, 67(2): 123.

24. Lam HS, Ng PC, Chu WC, et al. Renal screening in children after exposure to low dose melamine in Hong Kong: cross sectional study[J]. BMJ, 2008, 337: a2991.

25. Li Y, Qi L, Wen JG, et al. Chronic prostatis during puherty[J]. BJU Int, 2006, 98(4): 818-821.

26. Li ZZ, Xing L, Zhao ZZ, et al. Decrease of renal aquapoins 1-4 is associated with renal function impairment in pediatric congenital hydronephrosis[J]. World J Pediatr, 2012, 8(4): 335-341.

27. Li ZZ, Zhao ZZ, Wen JG, et al. Early alteration of urinary exosomal aquaporin 1 and transforming growth factor β 1 after release of unilateral pelviureteral junction obstruction[J]. J Pediatr Surg, 2012, 47(8): 1581-1586.

28. Min KJ, Ouh YT, Hong HR, et al. Muscle weakness and myalgia as the initial presentation of serous ovarian carcinoma: a case report[J]. J Ovarian Res, 2014, 7: 43.

29. Northridge ME, Susser M. Amnotation: Seven Fatal Flaws in Submited Manuscripts[J]. Am J Public Health, 1994, 84(5): 718-719.

30. Patrias K, Wendling D. Citing Medicine: The NLM Style Guide for Authors, Editors, and Publishers[Intemet]. 2nd ed. Bethesda(MD): National Library of Medicine(US), 2007.

31. Pablo R. Medical English. Heidelberg: Springer, 2006.

32. Ramon Ribes, Pablo R. Medical English. Heidelberg, Germany: Verlag Berlin, 2006.

33. Robert AD, Barbara G. How to write and publish a scientific paper.6th ed. New York: Greenwood Press, 2006.

34. Robert AD, Barbara G. 科技论文写作与发表教程. 第6版. 曾剑芬, 译. 北京: 电子工业出版社, 2009.

35. Robert BT. Medical Writing. New York, America: Science+Business Media, 2011.

36. Robert AD, Barbara G. How to write and publish a scientifie paper. 7th ed. New York: Cambridge University Press, 2012.

37. Russey WE, Ebel HF, Bliefert C. How to Write a Successful Science Thesis: The concise guide for students. Weinheim, Berlin: Wiley-VCH, 2006.

38. Roben A. Day. How to Write & Publish a Scientific Paper. 5th ed. LonDon: ORYX PRESS, 1998.

39. Syam AF. Tips and tricks in writing review article[J]. Acta Med Indones, 2007, 39(3): 143-144.

40. Taylor R B. Medical writing. 2nd ed. New York: Springer, 2011.

41. Wallwork A. English for Writing Research Papers. New York: Springer, 2011.

42. Woolsey JD. Combating poster fatigue: How to use visual grammar and analysis to effect beter visual communications[J]. Trends Neurosci, 1989, 12(9): 325-332.

43. Wang G, Li C, Kim SW, et al. Ureter obstruetion alers expression of renal acid-base transport proteins in rat kidney[J]. Am J Physiol Renal Physiol, 2008, 295(2): 497-506.

44. Wang QW, Wen JG, Zhu QH, et al. The effect of familial aggregation on the children with primary noctumal enuresis[J]. Neurourol Urodyn, 2009, 28(5): 423-426.

45. Wen JG, Li Y, Wang QW. Urodynamic investigation of valve bladder syndrome in children［J］. J Pediatr Urol, 2007, 3(2): 118-121.

46. Wen JG, Wang QW, Chen Y, et al. An epidemiological study of primary noctumal enuresis in Chinese children and adolescents［J］. Eur Urol, 2006, 49(6): 1107-1113.

47. Wen JG, Yang L, Xing L, et al. A study on voiding pattern of newborns with hypoxic ischemic encephalopathy ［J］. Urology, 2012, 80(1): 196-199.

48. 白春学, 王向东, 韩江娜. 国际医学期刊论文撰写指南. 北京: 人民军医出版社, 2011.

49. 陈力丹. 硕士论文写作. 北京: 中国广播电视出版社, 2001.

50. 单良. 英文科研论文的撰写和发表技巧. 北京: 人民卫生出版社, 2012.

51. 何权瀛. 如何写好医学论文中的讨论部分［J］. 中国生育健康杂志, 2007, 18(5): 317-320.

52. 刘海. 医学科研方法与论文写作. 北京: 科学普及出版社, 2007.

53. 孟庆仁. 实用医学论文写作. 北京: 人民军医出版社, 2002.

54. 钱程. Fas 信号和 TLR 信号促进调节性树突状细胞负向调控 CD4$^+$T 细胞反应及相关机制研究. 第二军医大学, 2008.

55. 王海强, 刘志恒, 罗卓荆. 浅析医学博士培养的三个重要问题［J］. 医学研究杂志, 2011, 40(7): 167-168.

56. 王征爱, 宋建武. 摘要的类型及英文摘要写作中常见的问题［J］. 第一军医大学学报, 2002, 22(4): 383-385.

57. 徐天和, 石德文. 医学论文写作. 济南: 山东科学技术出版社, 2007.

58. 杨大春. 激活 TRPV1 改善血管功能和预防高血压的机制研究. 第三军医大学, 2009.

59. 殷国荣, 杨建一. 医学科研方法与论文写作. 北京: 科学出版社, 2009.

60. 于双成, 李玉玲, 张子骐. 医学综述性文献的特点及写作规范［J］. 医学与哲学, 2006, 27(2): 76-77.